Laparoscopic Ventral Hernia Repair

Springer-Verlag France S.A.R.L

Salvador Morales-Conde

Laparoscopic Ventral
Hernia Repair

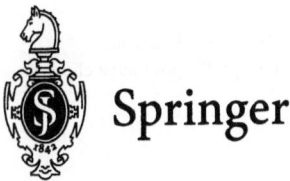 Springer

Salvador Morales-Conde (EDITOR)
Laparoscopic Surgery Division
University Hospital Virgen Macarena
Sevilla
Spain

Salvador Morales-Méndez (CO-EDITOR)
Chief of the General, Digestive and Laparoscopic Surgery Unit
University Hospital Virgen del Rocio
Sevilla
Spain

ISBN 978-2-287-59755-8   ISBN 978-2-8178-0752-2 (eBook)
DOI 10.1007/978-2-8178-0752-2

© Springer Verlag France 2003

Originally published by Springer-Verlag France in 2003.

SPIN : 10898550

Dedication

...inspiration...

...to Rosa

> *"...where are the limits of these categories wife, mother, friend, doctor, artist? Is more creative teaching than motherhood or love? Everything is complex and exigent and we see that art goes further than paint-brushes. This has been your legacy...a multifacetic personal realization... a globalization... Rrose Selavy (Rose, c'est la vie)... and the tunnel becomes a bridge..."*

...and her love

List of authors

A. Al Abdul Kareem
Division of General Surgery
King Khalid University Hospital
Riyadh
Saudi Arabia

F.R. Abiad
Specialized Medical Center Hospital
Riyadh
Saudi Arabia

A. Al Dohayan
Division of General Surgery
King Khalid University Hospital
Riyadh
Saudi Arabia

J.L. Aguayo
General Surgery Unit
Hospital JMª Morales Meseguer
Murcia
Spain

J.H. Alexandre
Hospital Broussais-Hôtel Dieu de Paris
University Paris IV
Paris
France

J.A. Almeida
Texas Endosurgery Institute
San Antonio, Texas
USA

A. Al Otiaby
Division of General Surgery
King Khalid University Hospital
Riyadh
Saudi Arabia

MªA. Argüelles
Department of Anesthesia
University Hospital Virgen del Rocío
Sevilla
Spain

M. Al Sebayel
Division of General Surgery
King Khalid University Hospital
Riyadh
Saudi Arabia

M.E. Arregui
St. Vincent Hospital and Health Center
Indianapolis, Indiana
USA

K. Aouad
Hospital Broussais-Hôtel Dieu de Paris
University Paris IV
Paris
France

M. Asensio
Laparoscopic Surgery Unit
Hospital Virgen de la Paloma
Madrid
Spain

C. Ballesta
Laparoscopic Center of Barcelona
Medical Center Tecnon
Barcelona
Spain

D. Berger
Department of Surgery
Stadtklinik
Baden-Baden
Germany

B. Bokobza
Hospital Le Havre
Le Havre
France

J.L. Bouillot
Hospital Broussais-Hôtel Dieu de Paris
University Paris IV
Paris
France

M. Bustos
Division of Laparoscopic Surgery
Digestive and General Surgery Unit
University Hospital Virgen del Rocío
Sevilla
Spain

H. Cadet
Division of Laparoscopic Surgery
Digestive and General Surgery Unit
University Hospital Virgen del Rocío
Sevilla
Spain

A. Cano
Division of Laparoscopic Surgery
Digestive and General Surgery Unit
University Hospital Virgen Macarena
Sevilla
Spain

J. Cantillana
Digestive and General Surgery Unit I
University Hospital Virgen Macarena
Sevilla
Spain

M.A. Carbajo
General Surgery Unit
Hospital Medina del Campo
Valladolid
Spain

L. Carrasco
One Day Surgery Unit
General Surgery Unit
Hospital JMª Morales Meseguer
Murcia
Spain

J.A. Castillo
One Day Surgery Unit
Anesthesia and Post-Anesthesia Recovery Department
Hospital J.Mª Morales Meseguer
Murcia
Spain

I. Charuzi
Department of Surgery B
The E. Wolfson Medical Center
Holon
Israel

J.-P. Chevrel
Digestive and General Surgery Unit
Hospital Avicenne
Bobigny
France

A. Cuzzocrea
Department of Plastic Reconstructive Surgery
Ospedale Cannizzaro
Catania
Italia

J. De Jaime
Laparoscopic Surgery Unit
Hospital Virgen de la Paloma
Madrid
Spain

E.J. DeMaria
Department of Surgery
Center of Minimally Invasive Surgery
Medical College Of Virginia at Virginia Commonwealth University
Richmond, Virginia
USA

C. Durán
Laparoscopic Surgery Unit
Hospital Virgen de la Paloma
Madrid
Spain

X. Feliu
General Surgery Unit
Hospital of Igulada
Barcelona
Spain

A.Z. Fernández
Department of Surgery
Center of Minimally Invasive Surgery
Medical College Of Virginia at Virginia Commonwealth University
Richmond, Virginia
USA

V. Fernández
Digestive and General Surgery Unit
University Hospital Virgen del Rocío
Sevilla
Spain

E. Fernández Sallent
General Surgery Unit
Hospital of Igulada
Barcelona
Spain

J.B. Flament
Service de Chirurgie Generale et Digestive
C.H.U. Reims.
Reims
France

M.E. Franklin
Texas Endosurgery Institute
San Antonio, Texas
USA

M.S. French
St. Vincent Hospital and Health Center
Indianapolis, Indiana
USA

H.R. Freund
Hadassah University Hospital Mount Scopus
Jerusalem
Israel

M. Gagner
Division of Laparoscopic Surgery
Mount Sinai School of Medicine
New York, New York
USA

P. Gentileschi
Division of Laparoscopic Surgery
Mount Sinai School of Medicine
New York, New York
USA

C. Gracia
Minimally Invasive Surgery & Technology Division
ValleyCare Health System
Pleasanton, California
USA

J.A. Guerrero
General and Digestive Surgery Unit A
Clinic University Hospital San Cecilio
Granada
Spain

A. Gutiérrez
Department of Anesthesia
University Hospital Virgen Macarena
Sevilla
Spain

K.L. Harold
Department of Surgery
Carolinas Medical Center
Charlotte, North Carolina
USA

B.T. Heniford
Carolinas Laparoscopic and Advanced Surgery Program
Carolinas Medical Center
Charlotte, North Carolina
USA

M. Hidalgo
Digestive Surgery Unit
Doce de Octubre University Hospital
Madrid
Spain

T. Hui
Department of Surgery
Cedars-Sinai Medical Center
Los Angeles, California
USA

A. Iuppa
Departament of Surgery and Minimally Invasive Surgery
Casa di Cure Distefano Velona
Catania
Italia

T. Jaber
Division of General Surgery
King Khalid University Hospital
Riyadh
Saudi Arabia

S. Kini
Division of Laparoscopic Surgery
Mount Sinai School of Medicine
New York, New York
USA

U. Klinge
Surgical Department
University of Aachen
Aachen
Germany

R.H. Koehler
Massachusetts General Hospital
Martha´s Vineyard Hospital
Oak Bluffs, Massachusetts
USA

S. Kyzer
Department of Surgery B
The E. Wolfson Medical Center
Holon
Israel

K.A. LeBlanc
Surgical Specialty Group
Baton Rouge, Louisiana
USA

F. López-Bernal
General and Digestive Surgery Unit
University Hospital Virgen del Rocío
Sevilla
Spain

F. Martín-Acebes
General Surgery Unit
Hospital Medina del Campo
Valladolid
Spain

J. Martín-Cartés
División of Laparoscopic Surgery
General and Digestive Surgery Unit
University Hospital Virgen del Rocío
Sevilla
Spain

M. Martín-Gómez
División of Laparoscopic Surgery
General and Digestive Surgery Unit I
University Hospital Virgen Macarena
Sevilla
Spain

W.C. Marujo
Liver Transplantation Unit
Hospital Albert Einstein
São Paulo
Brazil

B.D. Matthews
Department of Surgery
Carolinas Medical Center
Charlotte, North Carolina
USA

M. Miras
Laparoscopic Surgery Unit
Hospital Virgen de la Paloma
Madrid
Spain

M. Miserez
Department of Abdominal Surgery
University Hospital Leuven
Leuven
Belgium

S. Morales-Conde
División of Laparoscopic Surgery
Digestive and General Surgery Unit I
University Hospital Virgen Macarena
Sevilla
Spain

S. Morales-Méndez
Digestive, General and Laparoscopic Surgery Unit
University Hospital Virgen del Rocío
Sevilla
Spain

A. Moreno-Egea
Wall Defect and Hernia Unit
General Surgery Unit
Hospital JM^a Morales Meseguer
Murcia
Spain

F. Novell
Digestive and General Surgery Unit
Sant Pau Hospital
Barcelona
Spain

J. Novell
Digestive and General Surgery Unit
Sant Pau Hospital
Barcelona
Spain

J. Mª Ortega
Digestive and General Surgery Unit I
University Hospital Virgen Macarena
Sevilla
Spain

J.M. Pacheco
Digestive and General Surgery Unit
Hospital Puerta del Mar
Cádiz
Spain

E.H. Phillips
Division of Minimally Invasive Surgery
Department of Surgery
Cedars-Sinai Medical Center
Los Angeles, California
USA

H.S. Pollinger
Department of Surgery
Carolinas Medical Center
Charlotte, North Carolina
USA

J.F. Ponce
Digestive and General Surgery Unit
University Hospital Virgen del Rocío
Sevilla
Spain

I. Poves
Laparoscopic Center of Barcelona
Medical Center Tecnon
Barcelona
Spain

E. Prendes
Digestive and General Surgery Unit
General Hospital of Rio Tinto
Rio Tinto, Huelva
Spain

A. Prescher
Institute of Anatomy I
University of Aachen
Aachen
Germany

B. Ramshaw
Letton & Mason Surgical Group
Atlanta, Georgia
USA

S. Roll
Sao Paulo Institute of Minimally Invasive Surgery
Sao Paulo
Brazil

F. Sánchez-Ganfornina
Digestive and General Surgery Unit
University Hospital Virgen Macarena
Sevilla
Spain

J. Sanz
Anesthesia and Post-Anesthesia Recovery Department
Hospital JMª Morales Meseguer
Murcia
Spain

V. Schumpelick
Surgical Department
University of Aachen
Aachen
Germany

J.R. Schwab
Letton & Mason Surgical Group
Atlanta, Georgia
USA

E. Segovia
General and Digestive Surgery Unit A
Clinic University Hospital San Cecilio
Granada
Spain

N.J. Soper
Minimally Invasive Surgery
Washington University School of Medicine
St. Louis, Missouri
USA

R. Stoppa
Centre hospitalier universitaire (University Hospital)
Amiens
France

E.M. Targarona
Digestive and General Surgery Unit
Sant Pau Hospital
Barcelona
Spain

D.S. Thoman
Division of Minimally Invasive Surgery
Department of Surgery
Cedars-Sinai Medical Center
Los Angeles, California
USA

M. Toledano
General Surgery Unit
Hospital Medina del Campo
Valladolid
Spain

J.L. Tovar
General and Digestive Surgery Unit A
Clinic University Hospital San Cecilio
Granada
Spain

M. Trias
Digestive and General Surgery Unit
Sant Pau Hospital
Barcelona
Spain

J.D. Tutosaus
Division of Laparoscopic Surgery
General and Digestive Surgery Unit
University Hospital Virgen del Rocío
Sevilla
Spain

G. Voeller
University of Tennessee
Memphis, Tennessee
USA

Contents

Foreword

René Stoppa

Although never having personally performed laparoscopic hernia surgery, I can say that I have an important indirect experience of it: I dedicated much attention to it asearly as it has appeared and I have watched laparoscopic repairs many times, performed by expert friends. On another hand, I actively participated in the French contribution in solving the difficult problem of large ventral hernias surgical treatment by open procedures, together with GREPA, European and American Hernia Societies' fellow-friends. Then this is a latest novelty book and about it, Salvador Morales-Conde right away told me his curageous intentions: to edit the first compilation book exhaustively dealing with all aspects of the controversial topic of laparoscopic ventral hernias repair, written by more than seventy experts contributors. I received his project as a deed of belief!

Now under its final shape, the book is a remarkable accumulation of skilled surgeons testimonies which will allow an indispensable evaluation of the technical contributions in this particular surgical field. Editor and Co-authors must be congratulated for the result of their work. The Index encompasses all informations about history, anatomy, epidemiology, pathology, documentation on materials, biomaterials, procedures of repair, complications and results. And it is not surprising to note such honorable tutelages as those ones given by the Presidents of the European Hernia Society and the American Hernia Society.

Let me, now, take the difficult role of a "devil advocate" for helping the reader (and myself) to well understand the proposed changes, specially in large ventral hernias repair, for small and medium sized hernias treatment is a less complex problem. Be, here after, reminded of what I believe to be valuable, in open surgery, and is accepted in a large consensus by the European and American Hernia Societies fellows, for mending hernias with more than 10cm of collar diameter: Owing to frequent systemic, regional and local disorders, a careful preoperative management of the patient is mandatory, including, on demand, dermatologic care, respiratory physiotherapy, Goñi Moreno preoperative pneumoperitoneum, etc. With J. Rives & Associates, again I underline that patient preparation for surgery is as much important as the operation itself in obtaining satisfactory results. The main objectives of surgery are: closure of the wall defect without tension, reattachment of the muscles by the tendon-like action of a mesh prosthesis (if necessary, using relaxing incisions of the rectus sheath), restoration of a normal intraabdominal pressure at the time of closure of the defect. In practice, three methods are currently used, in France, in large ventral hernia cures: the large retromuscular prefascial prosthesis (Rives, 1973), the large preperitoneal and retrofascial prosthesis (Stoppa, 1973), and the large premuscular prosthesis (Chevrel, 1979); noticeably, intraperitoneal placement of any mesh is strongly disagreed. That is my vision of the starting point of all possible technical progresses.

Thus in this challenging surgery, I can see some interrogations to be answered and some apparent or real contradictions to be solved: In often multioperated patients, how to regularly create a fair working room through dense and complex adhesions? Laparoscopic adhesiolysis, when possible, is it not too much time consuming in patients at risk? Peritoneal cavity distension by insufflation and impossibility to use relaxing incisions impede any surgical reattachment of muscles on the midline, thus the abdominal wall gap is only bridged by the mesh: Many consider that a last resort solution in open repair. Placing any foreign body of any kind into the peritoneal cavity is not recommended as creating adhesions, potentially obstuctive or subject ed to migration into the bowel; research on antiadhesion barrier is not over.

As in every field of human activities, definitive certitudes or negations are rare in surgery, but the surgeon must only obey duly observed and confirmed facts. In addition, deontological correctness is mandatorily required in every medical decision.Thus the conditions for introducing laparoscopic repair in ventral hernias, in a large scale, seem to be the following: Be perfectly skillful in open surgical repair, and necessarily do not ignore anything in laparoscopic repair! Do what is to be done, applying evidence or, at least, consensus based principles! Refuse the dictature of technique, even one being of high tech nature...Conform the operation to the patient, not the patient to the operation ! Changing your technique: ask for which patient benefit and with which improved final results? I am confident and believe, with RP Sawyer, that: "...Surgeons are strong people, physically and mentally...decision makers, responsability takers..."

I hope those remarks will ditinguish the present wonderful volume as being a point of reference for full spectrum datas, as well as a guidance on prudently using mini-invasive surgery, in correct indications for mending ventral hernias. All general practicing surgeon and every training surgeon must have this book within reach of hand. We must thank Salvador Morales-Conde and his team of contributors for the nice gift they gratify our curiosity about knoledge and knowing how to do!

Finally, in homage to the time and the work the co-authors took for our satisfaction, this citation of Nicholas Stenon (Proem. Dem. Anatomic.Hafn. 1673), by Jacques Benigne Winslow (in *Expositions anatomiques du Corps Humain*, 1732), dear to Henri Fruchaud, my mentor: "Pulchra quae videntur", "Pulchroria quae sciuntur", "Longe pulcherima quae ignorantur"...or : What we ignore is far more beautiful than what we see or know.

Amiens, France July 27th, 2001.

Preface from the European Hernia Society

M. Hidalgo Pascual
President - European Hernia Society

In the last two decades abdominal wall surgery has gained a prominent position among the various surgical fields. From its former status as a procedure generating little or no interest it has now been taken up by major groups of renowned surgeons. This fact indicates the importance of ventral hernias, a common condition that can result from abdominal wall defects, from alterations or deficiencies acquired over the patient's lifetime or as a consequence of medical complications in general surgery, gynecology, urology, vascular surgery, etc.

This rapid and surprising shift in attitude has come about by the emergence of various factors during this period that have had created a favorable climate for change.

A) New surgical techniques based on the "tension-free" concept were described during the 1980s and 1990s, and numerous works evaluating these procedures in subsequent years have confirmed the initial findings and contributed new results, ideas and expectations.

B) The appearance of state-of-the-art biomaterials with properties that approach the ideal for this purpose have also played a part in the advancement of this surgery. Techniques for abdominal wall repair have extended rapidly and surgeons who were previously reluctant to handle this condition (probably due to the high recurrence rates) are now reconsidering their posture and accepting it without reserve.

C) The development of local and regional anesthesia and outpatient surgery has also contributed to the current increased importance of abdominal wall surgery.

D) The most recent advance along this line is laparoscopic surgery, an approach to the treatment of this condition that initially received significant criticism. Thanks to the effort and determination of groups of experts who have opened the way for this technique, laparoscopy is now considered a standard procedure for certain processes affecting the abdominal wall and not an isolated method within this surgery.

The publication of this monographic book, Laparoscopic Ventral Hernia Repair, which discusses all aspects related to laparoscopic surgery of the abdominal wall, can be considered a major achievement. A large number of experts have contributed their ideas, techniques and results to enhancing and enriching this comprehensive work.

Several sections of the book merit special mention. For example, one chapter centering on the various surgical methods discusses the technical considerations and modifications laparoscopy has gone through in recent years. It points out that European and American surgical teams appear to coincide in their study efforts to achieve improved results.

One of the most significant sources of criticism of the laparoscopic approach and surgical technique concerns postoperative complications. The high morbidity rate, almost always cited in the related publications, and the small but constant mortality rate have slowed the development of these techniques. For this reason the section dealing with these problems and providing valuable information of significant scientific interest, can be of great practical use for future groups dealing with this condition. In the hands of experts the morbidity associated with the laparoscopic approach to abdominal wall surgery has decreased to levels resembling those of conventional surgery.

The chapters on diaphragmatic, parastomal and lumbar hernias are also extremely interesting.

The presentation of the various problems, the organization of the chapters and the search for the ideal contribution for each subject has been handled by the book coordinator, Dr. Salvador Morales-Conde, who has admirably achieved the proposed objectives. His dedication to laparoscopic surgery and his contribution to this monograph with modern concepts and approaches that permit new techniques have made Dr. Morales the key figure in this work.

The book addresses all facets related to ventral hernias, making it an essential reference work for surgeons treating this condition.

The European Hernia Association is enormously pleased to witness the publication of this monograph, which is sure to have an enormous influence on this type of surgery in the future.

Preface from the American Hernia Society

K. A. LeBlanc
President – American Hernia Society

The laparoscopic repair of incisional and ventral hernias is becoming a popular procedure for the treatment of this difficult problem. There has been a need for a comprehensive text that can serve as a source of reference for the general surgeon interested in this technique. This work represents an exhaustive effort to fill this void in the surgical literature.

It is readily apparent from a review of the table of contents that even the smallest considerations that regard this procedure have been covered. Additionally, the list of authors that have contributed to this text are truly the leading proponents and experts of this operation. It is very difficult to achieve this level of a textbook without the input of the surgeons that are carefully studying and teaching this methodology. This has been accomplished.

The book will answer the questions from the laparoscopic novice while providing new insights to the experienced laparoscopist. The most current information has been provided in a practical easy-to-read format. It is obvious that great pains have been made to provide significant guidance to all levels of the surgical community. The history of this operation and the basic scientific underpinnings of it are revealed early in this text. There is a careful explanation of the indications and contraindications of this procedure also. All of the current variations in the instrumentation and technical surgical aspects are covered in every detail. The surgeon can apply this information to his or her method of choice.

Much credit is deserved to the contributors but most especially to the editor, Salvador Morales-Conde. This immense task to provide the world with this reference has resulted in the publication of this textbook. I hope that the reader will appreciate the contents as much as I. We continue to explore new frontiers in the field of surgery. Undoubtedly, this text will be available for us to continue our growth and satisfy our intellectual, scientific and practical needs.

SECTION I

Introduction

CHAPTER 1

Introduction

S. Morales-Conde, S. Morales-Méndez

Primary and incisional ventral hernias are common conditions often encountered in surgical practice. Because of the frequency of this problem it has come to be managed by surgeons in general, regardless of the type of hospital or the conditions dealt with in their daily practice. The incidence of incisional hernias is 2 to 11% according to some series (1, 2), and 3 to 13% according to other authors (3), increasing to over 40% if the surgical wound becomes infected during the postoperative period (3).

Although these types of hernias are very common, surgeons do not fully agree on the best method for repairing ventral hernias, and a number of procedures, both with and without the use of prosthetic materials, have been described by various authors for this purpose. Many factors are related to the recurrence of hernias, including hernia size, obesity, surgical wound infection, existence of concomitant disease (e.g., diabetes mellitus or chronic obstructive pulmonary disease), smoking, steroid and/or immunosuppressant therapy, and longitudinal incisions in the lower abdomen (1, 4).

Nevertheless, all authors appear to agree on the concept of "tension-free" procedures, involving the use of prosthetic materials in most cases, to prevent recurrence. Recurrence rates of up to 30-50% (1, 5-15) have been reported in patients who have undergone surgery without prosthetic materials; with a figure as high as 63.4% being cited (16). This recurrence rate decreases to about 12.5% (16, 17) when mesh is used, as the mesh reduces tension at the suture line. Some series, however, report that the rate holds steady at 19% (18).

But, the use of prosthetic materials is not problem-free since various related complications have been reported, including failure to tolerate the material, infections, intestinal fistulas, obstructive conditions, etc. (4, 7, 11, 16). This has led to the search for an ideal biomaterial that exactly meets the criteria of Lumberland and Scales (19). Although this material has not as yet been invented, some prosthetic materials closely match these criteria.

On the other hand, the implantation of prosthetic materials involves significant dissection. Tension-free placement of the prostheses is achieved by anchoring them to healthy tissue, with drains required in most cases. The maneuvers associated with prosthesis placement increase the possibility of complications at the surgical wound and at the level of the implanted materials. Some series report infection rates of up to 12% (3) in this respect. Also related to these complications is the considerable percentage of reoperations required to remove the prosthetic materials, due to the patients' lack of response to conservative medical treatment with antibiotics. Thus, the need for extensive dissection, the use of drains, and frequent wound complications mean that these procedures are associated with significant short-term and medium-term discomfort for the patient, longer postoperative recovery periods and a delay in the patient's resumption of daily activities.

Because of the necessity to implant prosthetic materials and the complications derived from their use, advances are being made in ventral hernia repair in two main areas:

a. - the search for prosthetic materials that possess ideal characteristics

b. - the development of surgical techniques associated with lower morbidity rates and lower recurrence rates.

a.- Improvements are being made in existing mesh materials to attain the ideal prosthetic material, namely, one that is biologically inert producing little or no foreign body reaction, that is strong yet pliable, that maintains its shape after implantation and that resists the formation of adhesions while supporting fibrous ingrowth of connective tissue (17). Polypropylene mesh has been the most widely used prosthetic material in hernia repair since it was introduced in 1963 (20, 21). However, clinical (22-24) and experimental (25) experience indicates a variety of complications that may be related to the physical properties of the mesh. There are numerous materials currently available, such as PTFE-e and its variants, with excellent properties closely resembling the ideal prosthesis, a biologically inert material, producing fewer adhesions (26, 27) and little or no inflammatory reaction; with its porous microstructure providing a lattice for the incorporation of connective tissue (19, 28, 29). Composites that combine various materials and attempt to obtain the best properties of each material for better results are also available.

b.- The laparoscopic approach has resulted from the search for surgical techniques that decrease the morbidity associated with conventional repair of ventral hernias. The advantages of laparoscopic surgery in numerous procedures such as cholecystectomy, colon resection, fundoplication, splenectomy and suprarrenalectomy were evident. These included enhanced patient recovery and reductions in complications related to the surgical wound, precisely the two main issues requiring improvement in conventional surgery for ventral hernias.

It was clear that there was a niche for the treatment of ventral hernias by laparoscopic approach. However a series of factors were in opposition. The traditional anatomic principles of ventral hernia repair, e.g. the need to approximate the anterior recti muscles in order to improve abdominal wall functionality, were not met. Moreover, prosthetic material had to be placed in contact with the bowel. These conditions meant that the technique was accepted only gradually after it was first described in the literature by LeBlanc, et al. (30).

There are, however, numerous advantages to laparoscopic repair of ventral hernias, many of which have been proven in laparoscopy for other pathologies. Apart from this, the functionality of the abdominal wall is not clearly diminished by this type of repair when intra-abdominal mesh is used to cover the hernia defect without approximating the muscles and preserving the sac. Moreover there are now optimal prosthetic materials for implantation within the abdomen. The treatment of ventral hernias by laparoscopy adheres to the principles of "tension-free" repair, i.e. without involving extensive dissection of tissues or the use of drains. The procedure uses three or four trocars at some distance from the hernia site, thereby significantly reducing (31-33) complications related to the wound and associated contamination, infection and rejection of the mesh, factors that promote early recovery, faster resumption of normal activities and decreased general costs resulting from this procedure (34) . In addition to these advantages, the recurrence rate is lower than with open surgery. As a result the indications for this surgical technique are currently being debated since the advantages are evident and progressive implementation is ensured. Now is the time to analyze the usefulness, results, technical variants and implications involved in implementation of laparoscopy as the technique of choice.

References

1. Hesselink VJ, Luijendik RW, De Wilt JHW, Heide R. An evaluation of risk factors in incisional hernia recurrence. Surg Gynecol Obstet 1993; 176:228-234.

2. Santora TA, Roslyn JJ. Incisional hernia. Surg Clin North Am 1993; 73:557-570.

3. Mudge M Hughes LE. Incisional hernia: a 10 year prospective study of incidences and attitudes. Br J Surg 1985; 72:70-71.

4. Leber GE, Garb JL, Alexander AI, Reed WP. Long-term complications associated with prosthetic repair of incisonal hernias. Arch Surg 1998; 133:378-382.

5. Langer S, Christiansen J. Long-term results after incisional hernia repair. Acta Chir Scand 1985; 151:217-219.

6. Van der Linden FT, Van Vroonhoven TJ. Long-term results after correction of incisional hernia. Neth J Surg 1988; 40:127129.

7. Berliner SD. Biomaterials in hernia repair. In: Nyhus LM, Condon RE, eds. Hernia (3rd ed). Philadelphia: JB Lippincott 1989: 541-554.

8. George CD, Ellis H. The results of incisional hernia repair: a twelve year review. Ann R Coll Surg Engl 1986; 68:185-187.

9. Houck JP, Rypins EB, Sarfeh IJ, Juler GL, Shimoda KJ. Repair of incisional hernia. Surg Gynecol Obstet 1989; 169: 397-400.

10. Lamont PM, Ellis H. Incisional hernia in re-opened abdominal incision: an overlooked risk factor. Br J Surg 1988; 75:374-376.

11. Read RC, Yoder G. Recent trends in the management of incisional herniation. Arch Surg 1989; 124:485-488.

12. Richards P, Balch C, Aldrette J. Abdominal wound closures. A randomized prospective study of 571 patients comparing continuous vs interrupted sutures techniques. Ann Surg 1983; 197:238-243.

13. Schildberg FW, Vatankhals M, Nissen R. Chirurgische Behandlung des Narbenbruchs. Langenb Arc Chir 1983; 361:319-323.

14. Stoppa RE. The treatment of complicated groin and incisional hernias. World J Surg 1989. 13:545-554.

15. Zimmermann G, Müller G, Haid A. Chirurgische Therapie der Narbenhernien. Chirurg 1991; 62:656-662.

16. Koller R, Miholic J, Jalk RJ. Repair of incisional hernias with expanded polytetrafluoroethylene. Eur J Surg 1997; 163:261-266.

17. Condon RE, DeBord JR. Expanded polytetrafluoroethylene prosthetic patches in repair of large ventral hernia. In: Nyhus LM, Condon RE, eds. Hernia (4th ed). Philadelphia: Lippincott Williams and Wilkins; 1995; 20:328-336.

18. Bauer JJ, Harris MT, Kreel I, Gelernt IM. Twelve-year experience with expanded polytetrafluoroethylene in the repair of abdominal wall defects. The Mount Sinai Journal of medicine 1999; 66(1):20-25.

19. Hamer-Hodges DW, Scott NB. Replacement of an abdominal wall defect using expanded PTFE sheet. J R Coll Surg Edinb 1985; 30:65-67.

20. Smith RS. The use of prosthetic materials in the repair of hernias. Surg Clin North Am 1971; 51:1387

21. Usher FC. Hernia repair with knitted polypropylene mesh. Surg Gynecol Obstet 1963; 117:239.

22. Kaufman Z, Engelberg M, Zager M. Fecal fístula: a late complication of Marlex mesh repair. Dis Colon Rectum 1981; 24:543.

23. Schneider R, Herrington JL Jr, Granada AM. Marlex mesh in repair of a diaphragmatic defect later eroding into the distal esophagus and stomach. Am Surg 1979; 45:337.

24. Voyles CR, Richardson JD, Bland KI. Emergency abdominal wall reconstruction with polypropylene mesh: short-term benefits versus long-term complications. Ann Surg 1981; 194:219.

25. Ponce González JF, Barriga Beltrán R, Martín Zurita I, Morales-Conde S, Morales Méndez S. Prosthetic materials in incisional hernia. Experimental study. Cir Esp 1998; 63(3):189.194.

26. Brown G. Comparison of prosthetic materials for abdominal wall reconstruction in the presence of contamination and infection. Ann Surg 1985; 201:705.

27. Murphy JL, Freeman JB, Dionne PG. Comparison of Marlex and Gore-tex to repair abdominal wall defects in the rat. Can J Surg 1989; 32:244.

28. Bauer JJ, Salky BA, Gelernt IM, Kreel I. Repair of large abdominal wall defects with expanded polytetrafluoroethylene (PTFE). Ann Surg 1987; 206:765.

29. Law NW, Ellis H. Adhesion formation and peritoneal healing on prosthetic materials. Clinical Materials 1988; 3:95.

30. LeBlanc KA, Booth WV. Laparoscopic repair of incisional abdominal hernias using expanded polytetrafluoroethylene: preliminary findings. Surg Laparosc Endosc 1993; 3 (1): 39-41.

31. LeBlanc KA, Booth WV, Spaw AT. Laparoscopic ventral herniorrhaphy using an intraperitoneal onlay patch of expanded polytetrafluoroethylene. In: Arregui ME, Nagan RF (eds). Inguinal hernia: advances or controversies?. Radcliffe Medical Press, Oxford 1994:515-517.

32. Park A, Gagner M, Pomp A. Laparoscopic repair of large incisional hernias. Surg Laparosc Endosc 1996; 6:123-128.

33. Saiz AA, Willis IH, Paul DK, Sivina M. Laparoscopic hernia repair: a community hospital experience. Am Surg 1996; 62:336-338.

34. Morales-Conde S, López F, Tutosaus JD, Cadet H, Ortega JM, Cantillana J, Martín, M, Morales S. Cost-effectiveness of "double crown" technique for laparoscopic ventral hernia vs open repair. 9th International Congress of the European Association for Endoscopic Surgery. Maastricht 2001.

CHAPTER 2

The Influence of the Laparoscopic Approach in Abdominal Surgery: The Third Surgical Revolution

N.J. Soper

In the mid-1980s, general (abdominal) surgery was relatively stagnant and at risk of being overshadowed by non-surgical specialties performing less invasive procedures for what had previously been major "open" surgical operations. These challenges to general surgery included flexible endoscopy (removal of mucosal tumours and endoscopic treatment of choledocholithiasis, management of gastrointestinal hemorrhage, endoscopic placement of feeding tubes, etc.) and interventional radiology (percutaneous drainage of abscesses, biopsy of tumor masses, etc.). Furthermore, great efforts were being made to develop non-invasive treatment of gallstones by using extracorporeal shock wave lithotripsy and gallstone dissolution agents. In the late 1980s, surgeons in Germany, France and the United States, working independently, began performing procedures that would revolutionize the practice of general surgery. Using traditional laparoscopic instruments and techniques (CO_2 pneumoperitoncum, trocar/sheath assemblies and long narrow instruments), but coupling the laparoscope to a CCD-video camera, the first laparoscopic cholecystectomies were performed. Although the academic community was slow to embrace the development, practicing surgeons and patients alike rapidly accepted and even demanded this new "minimally invasive" approach to the treatment of gallstones. As the 21st century unfolds, surgical experience has increased markedly, the initially crude instruments have been improved tremendously, and many additional general surgical procedures have been performed using laparoscopic techniques.

Virtually every intra-abdominal procedure previously reported using standard laparotomy (except major solid organ transplantation), has now been performed using laparoscopy. A growing experience with several of these operations, and carefully performed outcome studies have confirmed or refuted the potential advantages of laparoscopy for several of these procedures. The rationale for performing laparoscopy as opposed to standard laparotomy are multifactorial. Laparoscopy entails the use of small incisions with minimal blunt and penetrating injury to the abdominal wall and decreased exposure to the ambient atmosphere. The proposed advantages are that there is less postoperative pain, shorter hospitalization, reduced recuperation time and improved cosmetic results. Laparoscopy may also be beneficial by causing less perioperative suppression of the body's immune system. However, these purported advantages come at a price. The theoretical disadvantages of laparoscopy include increased costs, higher operative risk for certain procedures, and enhanced technical difficulty associated with learning curve complications. As with all surgical decision making, the risk versus benefit ratio must be assessed for each individual operation. Laparoscopy makes eminent sense when it replaces an operation previously done using a large incision to perform relatively simple intra-abdominal procedures. It is more difficult, however, to prove the superiority of laparoscopic procedures that replace operations requiring either complex intra-abdominal reconstructive techniques (such as pancreaticoduodenectomy) or those which were traditionally performed with small incisions or using local anesthesia (appendectomy or inguinal hernia repair).

Much time and effort has been spent in attempting to establish the veracity of these theoretical differences between laparoscopic and traditional open surgery. Several studies have shown that laparoscopic surgery does cause less pain and a shorter period of disability than open surgery (1,2). When performed by experienced surgeons, the overall rates of morbidity and mortality of laparoscopic surgery seems to be less than those for the same procedures performed by laparotomy (3). Calculations of the direct and indirect costs of operations are difficult at best and impossible at worst – the influence of the health care system, variations between different operations and an equitable estimate of indirect cost savings by accelerating the period before returning to gainful employment render making a definitive statement impossible. There are also emerging data strongly suggesting that laparoscopic surgery leads to less immunosuppression in the perioperative interval and thus might improve outcomes for the surgical management of cancer (4, 5).

A common theme in the practice of surgery is that while the real and perceived morbidity/mortality of an operation decreases, the frequency of performing the operation increases. In the mid-1970s, the mortality rate for the Whipple operation was very high and many surgeons were nihilistic about the treatment of pancreatic cancer. Improvements in surgical technique have resulted in the near-zero mortality rate of the Whipple operation (6) which has increased the number of these operations and has even allowed discussion of the Whipple procedure to be performed as a "prophylactic" procedure. Similarly, in multiple prospective randomized trials, laparoscopic cholecystectomy has been proven to be superior to open cholecystectomy (7, 8). As a result of the performance of laparoscopic cholecystectomy, the incidence of cholecystectomy in the United States has increased approximalety 30 % over the last 15 years (9). Likewise, establishment of laparoscopic anti-reflux surgery as a viable alternative to open surgical therapy has engendered an explosion in the number of surgical procedures performed for the treatment of gastroesophageal reflux disease (10, 11). However, comparisons of laparoscopic versus open appendectomy, laparoscopic versus open inguinal hernia repair, and laparoscopic versus open colectomy have so far not shown definitive advantages, and the laparoscopic alternative has not flourished as reality.

Laparoscopic ventral herniorrhaphy is a relatively new procedure. The traditional methods of repairing ventral hernias by primary closure or placement of prosthetic material by laparotomy are associated with a relatively high perioperative morbidity and rate of recurrence. Certainly, the concept of placing a large piece of prosthetic material which widely overlaps the fascial defect from its inner aspect makes eminent sense. However, the operation may be technically difficult and uncertainties remain regarding the intra-peritoneal of placement prosthetic material. Relatively few cases have been reported to date and long term outcomes are lacking. Thus, the editors of this textbook should be applauded for compiling the current state of knowledge regarding this procedure to be used as a foundation for further clinical and investigative research efforts.

The development of laparoscopic surgery has had a major positive impact on the practice of surgery today. Patient care has been improved and General Surgery as a discipline has been revitalized. Thus, laparoscopy may truly be considered the third surgical revolution. The appropriate place of laparoscopic ventral hernia repair in the surgeon's armamentarian will certainly be clarified by the authors' efforts contained herein.

References

1. Payne JH, Grininger LM, Izawa MT, et al. Laparoscopic or open inguinal herniorrhaphy? A randomized propective trial. Arch Surg 1994; 129; 973-979.

2. Trondseu E, Reiertsen O, Andersen OK, Kjaersgeard P . Laparoscopic and open cholecystectomy: A prospective randomized study. Eur J Surg 1993; 159: 217-221.

3. Shea JA, Healey MJ, Berlin JA, et al. Mortality and complications associated with laparoscopic cholecystectomy: A meta-analysis. Ann Surg 1996; 224: 609-620.

4. Sietses C, Havenith CEG, Eijsbouts QAJ, et al. Laparoscopic surgery preserves monocyte-mediated tumour cell killing in contrast to the conventional approach. Surg Endose 2000; 14: 456-460.

5. Allendorph JDF, Bessler M, Cayton ML, et al. Increased tumour establishment and growth after laparotomy versus laparoscopy in a murine model. Arch Surg 1995; 130:649-653.

6. Cameron JL, Pitt HA, Yeo CJ, et al. 145 consecutive pancreaticoduodenectomies without mortality. Ann Surg 1993; 217: 430-438.

7. Barkun JS, Barkun AN, Sampalis JS, et al. Randomized controled trial of laparoscopic versus minicholecystectomy. Lancet 1992; 340:1116-1119.

8. McMahon AJ, Russell IT, Baxter JN, et al. Laparoscopic versus mini-laparotomy cholecystectomy; A randomized trial. Lancet 1994; 343:135-38.

9. Steiner CA, Bass EB, Tallamini MA, Pitt HA, Steinberg EP. Surgical rates and operative mortality for open and laparoscopic cholecystectomy in Maryland. N Eng J Med 1994; 330: 403-8.

10. Nilsson G, Larsson S, Johnsson F, Randomized clinical trial of laparoscopic versus open fundoplication; Blind evaluation of recovery and discharge. Brit J Surg 2000; 87: 873-878.

11. Laine S, Rantala A, Gullichsen R, Ovaska J. Laparoscopic versus conventional Nissen fundoplication. A prospective, randomized study. Surg Endosc 1997; 11: 441-444.

Basic Considerations
of Ventral Hernias

CHAPTER 3

Anatomy and Physiology of the Abdominal Wall

U. Klinge, A. Prescher, V. Schumpelick

ANATOMY OF THE VENTRAL ABDOMINAL WALL

The ventral abdominal wall is bounded above by the xiphoid process and the costal arches and below, from lateral to medial, by the iliac crest, the anterior superior iliac spine, the inguinal ligament of Poupart, the pubic tubercle, and the symphysis. The integrity of the abdominal wall essentially influences the physical capability and thereby the life-quality of our patients (23). The extraordinary dynamics result from the complex interactions within this frame-work of bones, muscles and fascias, which are impossible to keep motionless even for a short period. The complicated anatomical architecture of the ventral abdominal wall presents some weak areas, which are predisposing factors for the origin of hernias. Thorough anatomical kowledge of these regions is essential for understanding these pathological appearances as well as for understanding the classical and laparoscopical surgical reparation techniques.

Muscles

The muscles of the ventral abdominal wall are integrated into an osseous frame composed of the lower ribs and the pelvis. Laterally, the muscular part consists of three flat muscles (from external to internal: the external oblique muscle, the internal oblique muscle and the transverse abdominal muscle. The medial part consists solely of the rectus abdominis muscle, which is enclosed into the rectus sheath. The rectus abdominis muscle originates with three dentations from the costal cartilages of Th5 to Th7 as well as from the xiphoid process. Then the muscle descends vertically beside the midline in order to insert at the pubic crest. The muscle is interrupted by three or four transverse tendinous bonds, the intersectiones tendineae. One lies at the level of the umbilicus, one at the level of the xiphoid process, and one between the two others. The facultative fourth one may be present somewhat below the umbilicus. These intersectiones tendineae are fused firmly with the anterior lamella of the rectus sheath but not with the posterior one. Thus, there is a large space between the dorsal surface of the muscle and the posterior lamella of the rectus sheath. The tendinous intersections are the relics of the former metameric trunc architecture and enable the bending of the trunk instead of simply shortening the distance between the xiphoid and the os pubis. Medially the intersections are fixed at the linea alba as well as the rectus muscle itself.

The arterial supply of the rectus muscles originates from the superior and inferior epigastric artery which are embedded in the dorsal surface of the rectus abdominis muscle. The nerve supply originates from the ventral rami of Th7 to Th12, frequently completed by additional branches of Th6 and L1. The nerves run on the dorsal surface of the internal oblique muscle, then cross the semilunar line and enter the muscle from lateral and dorsal.

The external oblique muscle originates at the 5th to 12th rib with an almost horizontal orientation of the fibres in the cranial part, whereas in the lower ones the fibres are orientated caudally. The muscle inserts at the external labium of the iliac crest, at the pubic tubercle and within the linea alba. The orientation of the fibres corresponds to the fiber-arrangement within the aponeurosis, which crosses the median line and penetrates the fibres of the contralateral side. The muscle is supplied by branches from Th5 – Th 12, often completed by L1. The vessels originate from the deep circumflex iliac artery, from the inferior and superior epigastric artery, from the musculophrenic artery, and from the lateral thoracic artery.

The internal oblique muscle starts at the linea intermedia of the iliac crest, at the superficial lamina of the lumbodorsal fascia, and at the lateral part of the inguinal ligament. The muscle inserts with a cranial margin from the tip of the 10th to the tip of the 12th costal cartilage and with a ventral margin in a line from the pubic tubercle to the tip of the 10th rib. The lower part of the muscle together with fibres of the transverse muscle constitute the cremasteric muscle of the spermatic cord. The fiber-arrangement of the aponeurosis generally corresponds to the orientation of the muscle fibres. At the back side of the muscle the segmental nerves (TH8-L1) ae well as the vascular structures (mainly of the vasa circumflexa ilium profunda) are embedded in a thick layer of connective tissue. Only at the distal part the nerves and vessels perforate the muscle and continue on the ventral surface in mediocaudal direction.

The transverse abdominal muscle is the most inner muscular structure with predominantly horizontal fiber orientation, covered dorsally by the fascia transversalis. The transition of the muscle into its aponeurosis forms the semilunar line of Spighel. There are two important but very variable accessory pelvic insertions of the transverse abdominal muscle: the falx ingui-nalis (also called conjoint tendon) and the interfoveolar ligament of Hesselbach. The conjoint tendon is a triangular sheet of connective tissue with a sickle-shaped lateral margin. Medially this structure is fused to the lateral border of the rectus muscle and caudally its base inserts at the medial part of the inguinal ligament as well as at the superior margin of the pubic bone. The interfoveolar ligament of Hesselbach is a fiber plate, which branches from the aponeurosis of the transversus muscle in the region of the arcuate line, runs caudally and inserts at the inguinal ligament as well as at the pecten osssis pubis. The interfoveolar ligament separates the laterally positioned deep inguinal ring from the medial inguinal fossa. The inferior epigastric vessels rest on the interfoveolar ligament. Both structures, the conjoint tendon as well as the interfoveolar ligament can contain muscular fibers. If the muscular fibers become obvious within the interfoveolar ligament, the interfoveolar muscle of Hesselbach will be described.

The transverse abdominal muscle is supplied by branches of Th5 (6) running on the ventral surface, occasionally supported by branches from the iliohypogastric and ilioinguinal nerves.

Fascial structures

The rectus sheath encloses the rectus muscle and consists of dense connective tissue, forming an anterior and posterior lamella. The architecture of these lamellas is different below and above the arcuate line of Douglas, which lies 4 to 5cm below the umbilicus. Above the line of Douglas the anterior lamella consists of the aponeurosis of the external oblique muscle and of the anterior part of the aponeurosis of the internal oblique muscle, whereas the posterior lamella is formed by the posterior part of the aponeurosis of the internal oblique muscle, the aponeurosis of the transverse abdominal muscle, covered by the transversalis fascia. Below the arcuate line all aponeuroses are composing the anterior lamella, whereas the posterior part of the rectus sheath is only formed by the transversalis fascia (fig. 1).

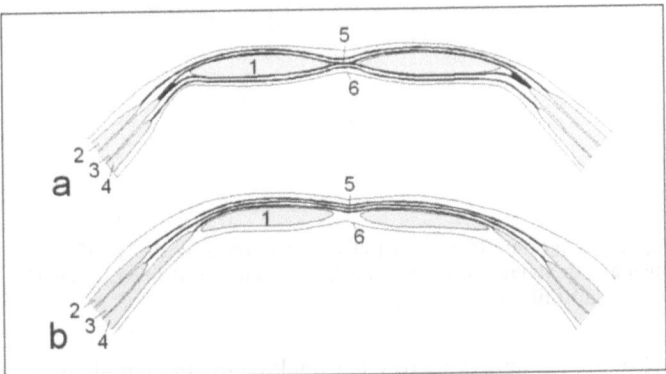

Fig. 1. Architecture of the ventral abdominal wall. a: Horizonal section through the ventral abdominal wall above the arcuate line of Douglas. b: Horizontal section through the ventral abdominal wall below the arcuate line of Douglas. 1. M. rectus abdominis, 2. M. obliquus externus abdominis, 3. M. obliquus internus abdominis, 4. M. transversus abdominis, 5. Linea alba, 6. Fascia transversalis.

Therefore the posterior lamella is very thin below the line of Douglas, whereas the anterior lamella shows an increased mechanical strength. Sometimes the arcuate line is doubled (20, 25) or a not distinctly delimited arcuate area or zone is present (14).

With a length of 35 to 40 cm the linea alba is a dense and strong stripe of fibrous tissue expanded between the xiphoid process and the symphysis (18). The linea alba results from the crossing and fusion of the bilateral aponeuroses of the lateral abdominal muscles, described above. Up to now the crossing was explained with the complicated criss-cross pattern described by Askar (1) (1984). Recent investigations (2, 3) present a different, more clear, architecture (fig. 2): the linea alba is composed of three zones characterised by different fiber orientations (from ventral to dorsal): the lamina fibrae obliquae consists of intermingling oblique fibers, the lamina fibrae transversae contains mainly transverse fibers while an inconstant, small lamina fibrae irregularium is composed of oblique fibers. In contrast to former investigations no separate lines of fiber-decussations are described.

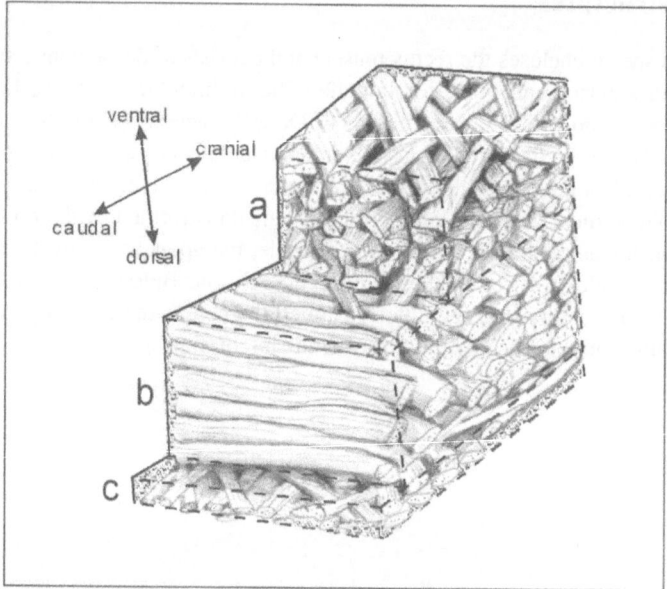

Fig. 2. Architecture of the linea alba according to Axer et al. (2, 3): a: lamella with oblique fibers, b: lamella with transversal fibers, c: lamella with irregular fibers.

Although the linea alba is narrow but thick below the umbilicus it may be as much as 2.5cm wide and flat above it. This anatomic feature may account for the rarity of midline hernias below the umbilicus. In the area of the former insertion of the umbilical cord a small defect remains in the linea alba and forms the umbilicus, surrounded by the umbilical anulus. Sometimes accessory minor openings are positioned above it. These little foramina are closed by adipose tissue.

Another essential fascial structure is the transversalis fascia, is a very complicated structure, which cannot be discussed at this place. For an overview see Prescher & Lierse (17).

Anatomy of the posterior surface of the ventral abdominal wall

Looking at the posterior surface (fig. 3) of the ventral abdominal wall, several peritoneal folds can be seen. In the midline the median umbilical fold runs from the vertex of the urinary bladder towards the umbilicus. This fold is established by an embryologic remnant, the obliterated urachus. Beside this structure the medial umbilical fold runs in an oblique way upwards to the umbilicus. The ligamentous, obliterated former umbilical artery lies within this fold. Further laterally the epigastric fold is formed by the inferior epigastric vessels, running up-wards and entering the rectus sheath. These peritoneal folds contain variable amounts of fat and present characteristic anatomical variations, classified by Hammond et al. (7). Fig. 4 illlustrates these entities.

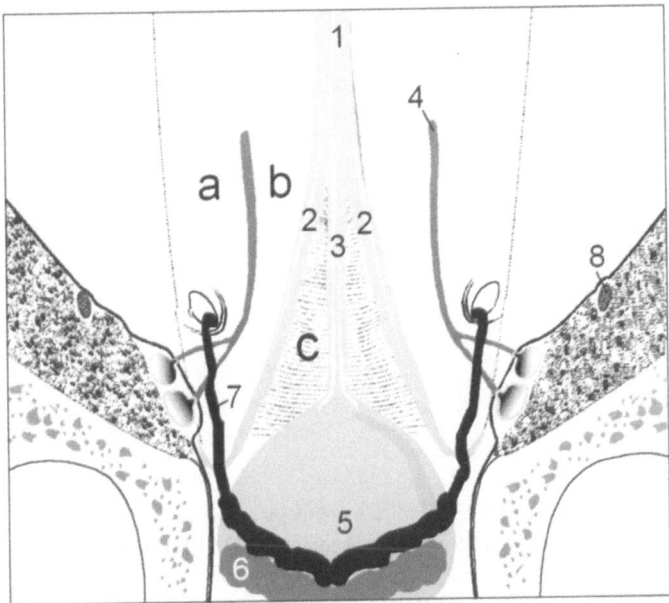

Fig. 3. Dorsal aspect of the ventral abdominal wall. 1. Lig. commune, 2. Plica umbilicalis medialis, 3. Lig. umbilicalis mediana, 4. Plica epigastrica, 5. Vesica urinaria, 6. Vesicula seminalis, 8. N. femoralis. a: Fossa inguinalis lateralis, b: Fossa inguinalis medialis, c: Fossa supravesicalis.

Between the peritoneal folds peritoneal fossae are formed (fig. 3). Between the median and the medial umbilical fold the supravesical fossa is described, between the medial and the epigastric fold lies the medial inguinal fossa, and laterally to the epigastric fold the important lateral inguinal fossa is situated. In the lateral inguinal fossa the internal (lateral, profund) inguinal ring can be seen. This structure is surrounded by characteristic structures (fig. 5): the medial margin is strengthened as plica semilunaris of Krause, which is a thickened part of the transversalis fascia. Furthermore the transversalis fascia forms a sling-like structure, called Henle's sling, which opens to the craniolateral side. It is discussed (12, 13), that this sling is able to close the internal inguinal ring by a sphincter mechanism and prevents therefore the development of an indirect inguinal hernia.

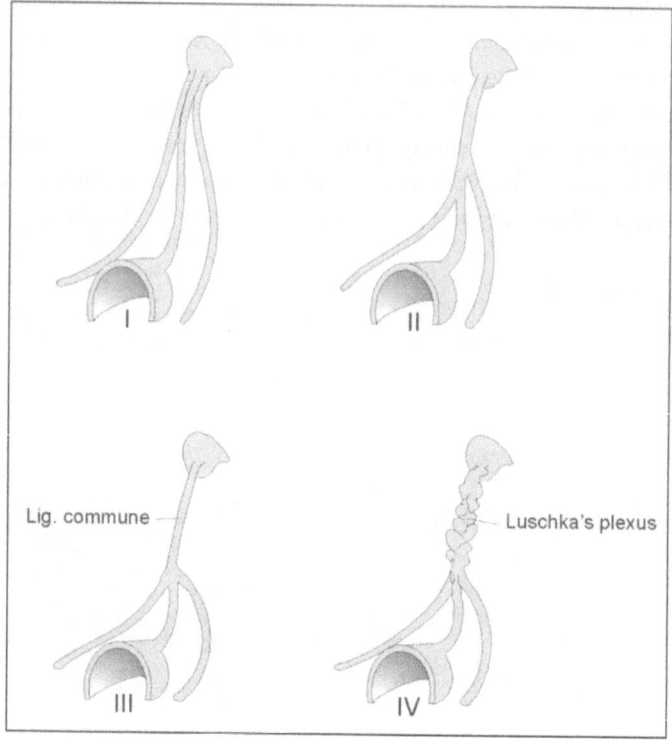

Fig. 4. The four main types of plica mophology on the posterior side of the
ventral abdominal wall according to Hammond et al. (1941) (7).

Another essential area of the ventral abdominal wall is the triangle of
Hesselbach, lying within the medial inguinal fossa (fig. 5). This triangle is an
especially weak area and establishes the anatomical basis for the direct (medial)
inguinal hernia. The boundaries of Hesselbach's triangle are: superomedial: the
arcade of the transverse abdominal muscle and the lateral margin of the rectus
abdominis muscle, lateral: the interfoveolar ligament with the inferior epigastric
vessels lying upon it, and laterocaudal: the inguinal ligament of Poupart. The
arcade of the transverse abdominis muscle is a tendinous thickened part of the
inferior border of the transversus muscle, which shines white through the
transversal fascia. Therefore this structure is often called "white line" by surgeons.
The triangular area of Hesselbach is the weakest part of the abdominal wall for
two reasons: first there are no muscles supporting the wall, and second the
aponeurosis of the external oblique muscle at the anterior side forms the medial
(superior) and lateral (inferior) crus in order to form the external (medial,
superficial) inguinal ring. The triangle of Hesselbach is completed by a further
weak area, the lacuna vasorum, lying beneath the inguinal ligament (fig. 5). Both
weak areas together are termed as myopectineal orifice of Fruchaud (6).

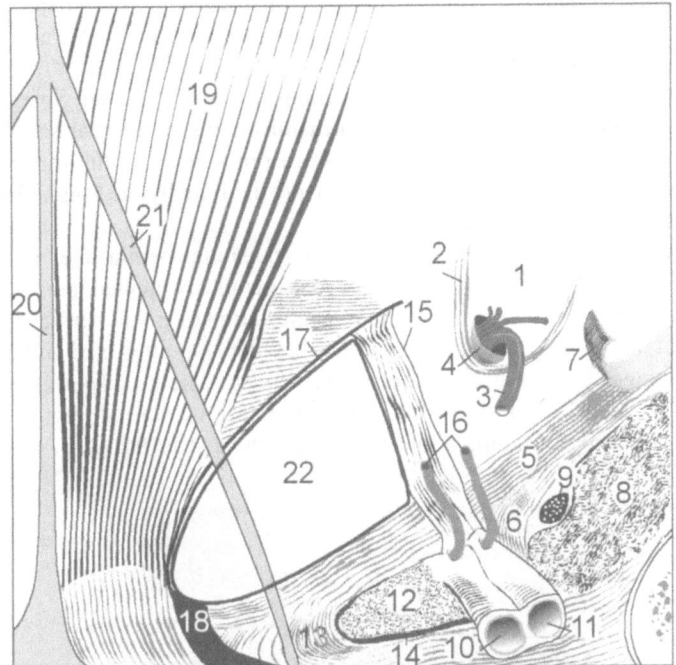

Fig. 5. Anatomical details of the dorsal aspect of the ventral abdominal wall. 1. Anulus ingui-nalis profundus, 2: Henle's loop, 3: Ductus deferens, 4: Plica semilunaris (Krause), 5: Lig. inguinale (Poupart), 6: Arcus iliopectineus, 7: Tractus iliopubicus (Thomsen), 8: M. iliopsoas, 9: N. femoralis, 10: V. femoralis, 11: A. femoralis, 12: Septum femorale (Cloquet), 13: Processus falciformis lacunaris, 14: Lig. pectineale (Cooper), 15: Lig. interfoveolare (Hesselbach), 16: A. / V. epigastrica inf., 17: Arcus m. transversi, 18: Falx inguinalis (conjoint tendon), 19: M. rectus abdominis, 20: Plica umbilicalis mediana, 21: Plica umbilicalis medialis, 22: Hes-selbach's triangel.

Anatomy of the hernia gap

Apart from the frequent incisional hernias following laparotomy or even laparoscopy there exist numerous primary hernias of the abdominal wall, e.g. umbilical, epigastric, Spieghelian and inguinal hernias. Defects may vary in diameter from several centimetres to only a few millimetres.

The umbilical hernias in adults, mostly in females, are herniations through the umbilical anulus within the linea alba. In contrast the epigastric hernias occur above the umbilical cicatrix, and perforate the linea alba too. They may occur in association with umbilical hernias and have to be differentiated from the rectus diastasis, that usually does not require any treatment. Epigastric hernias may form a true hernia with a peritoneal sac. If only preperitoneal fat bulges through a defect of the linea alba, this event should be termed as preperitoneal fat prolapse. Its origin is still obscure, either as a consequence of congenital defects of the linea alba or induced by local tissue damage or by perforating blood vessels.

With approximately a thousand cases published the hernia of the semilunar line of Spighel is another rare primary hernia of the abdominal wall (22). This entity was first described by Henry-Francois Lu Dran in 1742. Later it was termed as hernia of Spieghel after the Belgian anatomist, Adriaan van den Spieghel (1578 – 1625). A Spieghelian hernia is a protrusion of the peritoneal sac through a congenital or acquired defect within the linea semilunaris as the transition from the transverse abdominal muscle to its aponeurosis. Usually the Spighelian hernias manifest in the area below the umbilicus.

In contrast to these primary hernias the incisional hernia does not prefer a certain anatomic area but can develop at every previously applied incision. Even at the small incisions after laparoscopy the manifestation of trokar hernias is reported to be about 1 to 3%. However, most often they develop after median laparotomy with an incidence of up to 20% after major surgery. The usually oval defects are bordered by a dense fibrous ring and the laterally shifted rectus muscles. Frequently they appear multiple throughout the whole scar (fig. 6).

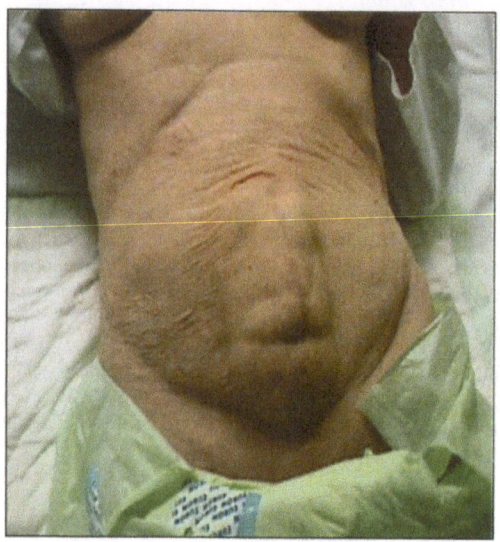

Fig. 6. Large incisional hernia following lower median laparotomy.

Particularly in respect to recent reports on a disturbed collagen metabolism in patients with incisional hernia, this hernia type has to be regarded mainly as a disease of the scarring process. Thus it must be supposed that the whole scar tissue is of insufficient strength, and that the hernial repair with a simple repetition of the primary applied surgical technique will fail again. Thus, it has to be recommended that the entire area of the insufficient scar tissue has to be reinforced by alloplastic material, a so-called mesh. Because even the anchorage of the mesh can suffer from the development of unstable scar tissue, the defect should be overlapped extendedly. The poor experiences with inlays underline the importance of large meshes, although this can be difficult in the neighbourhood of osseous structures, e.g. ribs and pelvis.

PHYSIOLOGY OF THE ABDOMINAL WALL

The restoration of the physiologic properties of the abdominal wall as the main task of any repair has to consider the complex interactions of the anatomic structures and therefore has to focus in particular on the resulting tensile strength and flexibility.

Functionality

The anatomic structures with the segmental innervation form complex functional loops of muscles and fascial structures (fig. 7), that not only have to protect the abdominal cavity but are essential for bending and rotating of the trunk as well as for the erect position.

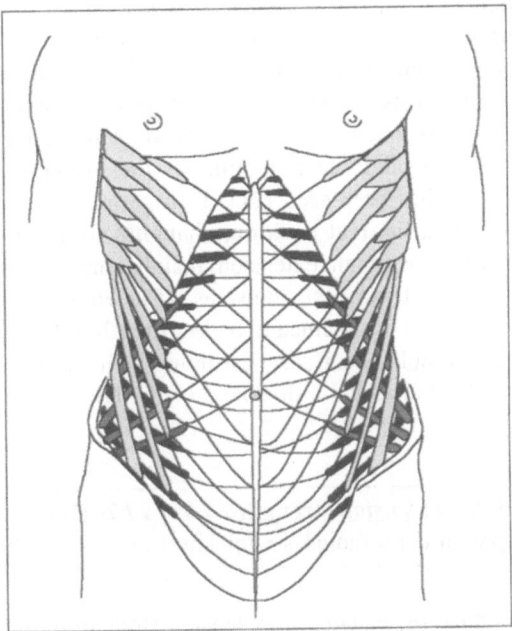

Fig. 7. Functional loops of the ventral abdominal wall.

As mentioned above the abdominal wall is stretched out between the osseous thorax and the pelvis. The origin of the muscles at the ribs and far away from the spine results in the development of considerable leverage. The intact abdominal wall function is essential for the stabilisation in erect position, for any kind of intentional movement, for the support of breathing, and for the regulation of the intraabdominal pressure for defecation. This is achieved either by simultaneous activation of contralateral muscles or by selective innervation of functionally corresponding and synergistically working pairs of muscles.

1. The horizontal loop of both transversal muscles girdles the waist and enables carrying the weight of the intraabdominal organs. The spontaneous activity of both muscles mostly defines the intraabdominal pressure.

2. The voluntary activation of the oblique loops, consisting of the contralateral external and internal oblique muscles tenses up the whole abdominal wall and allows specific rotational movements.

Mechanics

Tension and tensile strength

Whereas tension strength as a sort of pressure means force per cm^2, tensile strength is defined as force per cm and thus reflects the stability of the anatomic structures in a more suitable way. According to Tauber and Seidel (24) the tensile strength of the rectus sheath measured horizontally is about 70 to 80 N/cm, but is reduced to ¼ vertically. Because the force for tearing out the seam is only ⅓ to ¼ of the tensile strength of the tissue as measured by tearing out stripes, there results an effective load-bearing capacity of about 10 to 20 N/cm.

The mechanical requirements for any repair largely depend on the intraabdominal pressure. This ranges from 0,2 kPa in rest to a maximum pressure of almost 20 kPa (= 150 mm Hg) (8). Already at comparatively low pressure values of 1,3 kPa a considerable reduction of the blood supply within the abdominal wall to 42% has been seen (21). Transgastric measurements reveal a pressure of 11 to 15 kPa in erect position, changing from 10 - 12 kPa during flexion to 8.5 - 10 kPa at maximum extension, mainly corresponding to alterations in the activity of the transverse muscles (5). However, the maximum intraabdominal pressure can be assumed to be less than 20 kPa.

According to the formula of LaPlace, assuming a circumference of 100 cm, a maximum pressure of 20 kPa, and a thickness of the layer of 0,08 cm, a tension strength of about 200 N/cm^2 results.

La Place: *tension* strength $\tau = P * r / 2s$ (N/cm^2)
P = pressure, r = radius, s = thickness of muscle-layer

Though usually done (8) equating this tension strength to the tensile strength required for repair is not suitable. Instead, to estimate the necessary strength the human body can be regarded as a thin-walled hollow cylinder: by multiplying the supposed contact area of 8 cm^2 with the value of the tension strength at a circumference of 100 cm, a total force of 1600 N results. Division by the circumference allows to omit the vague size of the layer and results in a for-mula where the tensile strength depends only on the intraabdominal pressure and the diameter.

$F = P * d/4$ (N/cm)
d = diameter, P = pressure, F= force per cm circumference

Assuming a circumference of 100 cm and a maximum pressure of 20 kPa, theoretically a maximum tensile strength of about 16 N/cm results for humans (9) (fig. 8).

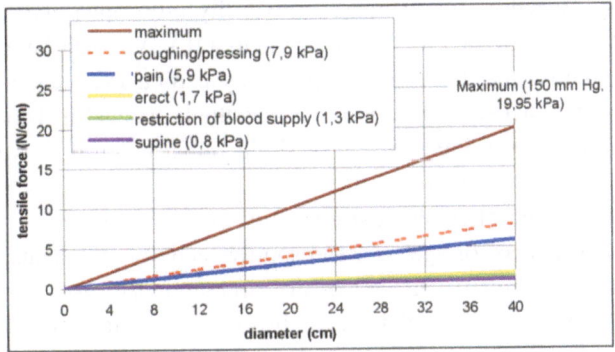

Fig. 8. Calculated tensile strength in relation to the diameter.

Apart from extreme strain, physiologically we have to deal with rather low tensile forces of 1-4 N/cm. These calculated data are in accordance with experimental studies where the tensile forces of applied sutures are recorded. All reports, Lipton et al. (11) for a Bassini repair as well as Read and McLeod (19) for a McVay, Calcagno and Wantz (4) for a Shouldice Repair, or Peiper et al.'s investigation of the groin's ability to withstand stress in humans (16), measured forces of far less than 10 N/cm. Thus we can conclude, that physiologically the required tensile strength even at maximum strain does not exceed the calculated value of 16 N/cm as an upper limit.

In regard to the widespread use of various mesh materials for the repair of incisional hernias it has to be mentioned that most of these materials exceed this range and thus appear to be considerably oversized (fig. 9).

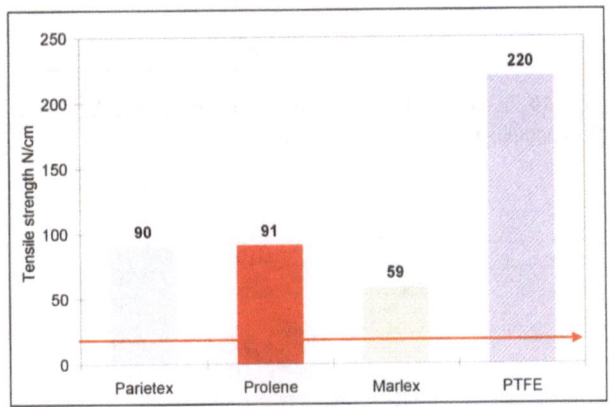

Fig. 9. Tensile strength of currently available mesh materials, Æ maximum tensile strength of 16 N/cm.

Elasticity

It is mainly the flexibility of the abdominal wall, whose impairment can cause severe complaints of the patients. It is well known that each laparotomy is followed by considerable pain together with a marked restriction of abdominal wall mobility. Recently, the decreased flexibility after open and laparoscopic surgery could be objectified by 3D-stereography (10). As could be expected, the data clearly confirm that the median laparotomy particularly leads to significant decrease of abdominal wall curvature, whereas the horizontal incision as well as the laparoscopic access induces only a slight impairment after two weeks as compared to preoperative data (fig. 10).

It is obvious that the physiological elasticity of the abdominal wall can vary distinctly in dependence of age, sex, and sportive activity of patients, and simple measurements of voluntary changes of the circumference reveal differences of about 30%. This is confirmed by own investigations at corpses, where the stretching of excised abdominal walls is determined. At a tensile strength of 16 N we frequently saw the high vertical elasticity of more than 30%, particularly in the area of the rectus muscles (mean: male 23%, female 32%), whereas the mean elasticity in horizontal direction with 15 to 20% is markedly lower (fig. 11, 12).

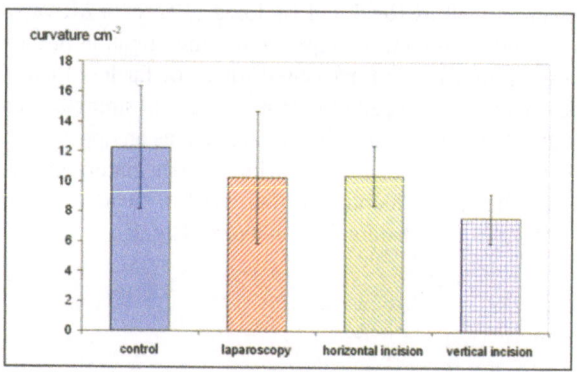

Fig. 10. Abdominal wall curvature as measured by 3D-Stereography two weeks after operation.

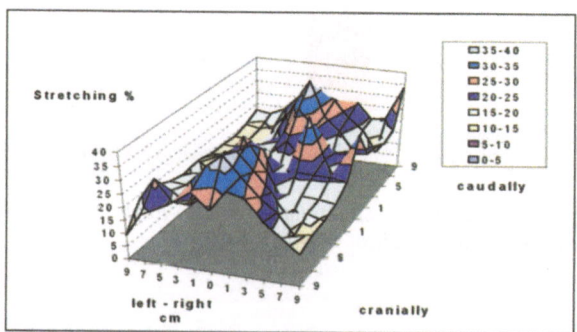

Fig. 11. Example of the high elasticity of the abdominal wall, measured at an excised abdominal wall.

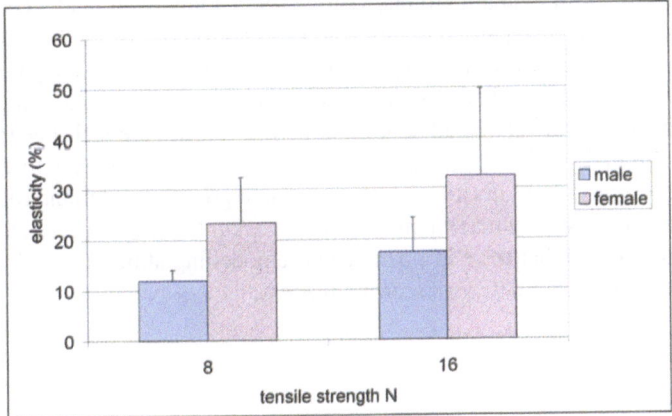

Fig. 12. Mean elasticity of the abdominal wall at 8 and 16 N (male and female n=7 each).

Particularly due to the reported restriction of the abdominal wall mobility after open implantation of polypropylene meshes (15), the physiological data has to be compared with the textile properties of meshes. Again, as for the tensile strength many materials do not show an appropriate elasticity, even in its textile form (fig. 13). It has to be supposed, that the tissue incorporation will lead to further stiffness.

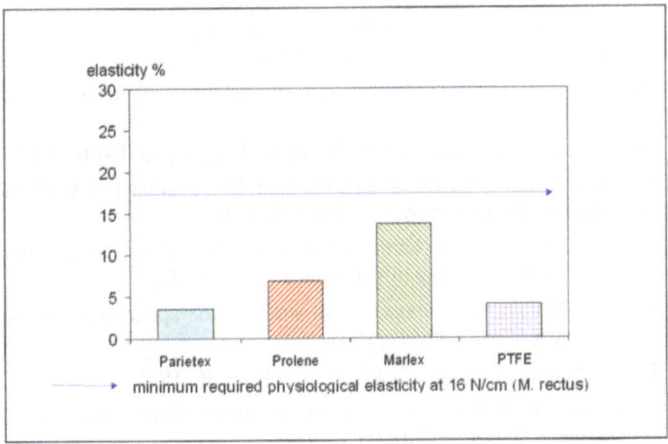

Fig. 13. Textile elasticity (%) of meshes at 16 N.

Fascial wound healing

The data about the ability of the repaired structure to withstand mechanical stress are contradictory. The duration till development of 90% of the original stability varies between 9 days, which might explain that absorbable sutures work successfully for abdominal wall closure, and up to one year. In 1975 Tauber and Seidel could show, that in rabbits a suture repair constantly can keep 50 to 60% of the fascial strength (24). However, in regard to the comparatively low physiologically required tensile strength, the currently available meshes and sutures should be able to withstand the strain. Animal experiments could show, that porous meshes are well integrated into the tissue within 2 weeks, so that at least for these materials a longer fixation does not seem necessary. Only in case of lacking tissue ingrowth the durable fixation has to withstand the described maximum strain of 16 N/cm for long periods. However, it has to be considered that there is a permanent remodelling at the scar and that these patients probably have a defective scarring process.

References

1. Askar OM. Aponeurotic hernias. Recent observations upon paraumbilical and epigastric hernias. Surg Clin North Am 64: 315-333, 1984.

2. Axer H, Graf v. Keyserlingk D, Prescher A. Collagen fibers in linea alba and rectus sheaths: P. 1: General scheme and morphological aspects. J Surg Res 96: 127-134, 2001.

3. Axer H, Graf v. Keyserlingk D, Prescher A. Collagen fibers in linea alba and rectus sheaths: P. 2: Variability and biomechanical aspects. J Surg Res 96: 239-245, 2001.

4. Calcagno D, Wantz G. Suture tension and the shouldice repair. Lancet 1(8443): 1446, 1985.

5. Cresswell A, Grundstrom H, Thorstensson A. Observations on intraabdominal pressure and patterns of abdominal intramuscular activity. Acta Physiol Scand 144: 409-18, 1992.

6. Fruchaud: cited after Skandalakis JE, Colborn GL, Skandalakis PN, Skandalakis LJ. Anatomy of the abdominal wall. In: Schumpelick V, Kingsnorth AN (Eds.). Incisional Hernia. Berlin, Heidelberg, New York: Springer 1999.

7. Hammond G, Yglesias L, Davis JE. The urachus, its anatomy and associated fasciae. Anat Rec 80: 271 – 287, 1941.

8. Kirsch U. Zu Naht und Knoten. Melsungen: Braun-Melsungen, pp. 104 ff, 1973.

9. Klinge U, Conze J, Limberg W, Brucker C, Ottinger AP, Schumpelick V. [Pathophysiology of the abdominal wall]. Chirurg 67 (3): 229-233, 1996.

10. Klinge U, Müller M, Brücker C, Schumpelick V. Application of three dimensional stereography to assess abdominal wall mobility. Hernia 2: 11-14, 1998.

11. Lipton S, Estrin J, Nathan I. A biomechanical study of the aponeurotic inguinal hernia repair. J Am Coll Surg 178 (6): 595-599, 1994.

12. Lytle WJ. The internal inguinal ring. Br J Surg 32: 441 – 446, 1945.

13. MacGregor WW. Demonstration of a true internal inguinal sphincter and its etiologic role in hernia. Surg Gynecol Obstet 49: 510 - 515, 1929.

14. Mempel, W. Zona, nicht Linea semicircularis! Untersuchungen über die sogenannte Linea semicircularis Douglasi. Morph Jahrb 109: 353-375, 1968.

15. Müller M, Klinge U, Conze J, Schumpelick V. Abdominal wall compliance after Marlex® Mesh implantation for incisional hernia repair. Hernia 2: 113-117, 1998.

16. Peiper C, Junge K, Füting A, Conze J, Bassaly P, Schumpelick V. Intraoperative Mes-sung der Nahtkräfte bei der Shouldice-Reparation primärer Leistenhernien. Chirurg 69: 1077-1081, 1998.

17. Prescher A, Lierse W. Anatomie der vorderen Leibeswand. In: Schumpelick V. Hernien. 4 ed. Stuttgart: Georg Thieme-Verlag, 2000. p. 3-27.

18. Rath AM, Attali P, Dumas JL, Goldlust D, Zhang J, Chevrel JP. The abdominal linea alba: an anatomo-radiologic and biomechanical study. Surg Radiol Anat 18: 281-288, 1996.

19. Read RC, McLeod PC. Influence of relaxing incisions on suture tension in Bassini's and McVay´s repairs. Arch Surg 116: 440-445, 1981.

20. Rizk NN. The arcuate line of the rectus sheath – does it exist? J Anat 175: 1-6, 1991.

21. Saxe JM, Ledgerwood AM, Lucas CE. Management of the difficult abdominal closure. Surg Clin North Am 73 (2): 243-251, 1993.

22. Schumpelick V, Klinge U. Epidemiologie In: Schumpelick V. Hernien. 4 ed. Stuttgart: Georg Thieme-Verlag, 2000. pp. 36-41.

23. Schumpelick V, Klinge, U. Reparationsprinzipien. In: Schumpelick V. Hernien. 4 ed. Stuttgart: Georg Thieme-Verlag, 2000. pp. 89-118.

24. Tauber R, Seidel W. Bedeutung mechanischer Faktoren bei der Entstehung der abdominellen Wunddehiszenz. Zentralbl Chir 100: 1178-82, 1975.

25. Yuan Lung-Chin. Constitution of the rectus sheath. Acta anatomica sinica 8: 234-238, 1965.

CHAPTER 4

Etiopathogenic and Physiopathologic Aspects of Ventral Hernias

M. Trias, E.M. Targarona, F. Novell, J. Novell

INTRODUCTION

A grasp of the etiopathogenesis and physiopathology of ventral and incisional hernias is the key to understanding their importance in terms of both prevention and treatment (1).

ETIOPATHOGENESIS

A number of factors may influence the development of an incisional hernia; such factors can be local, general or a combination of both (5).

Some of the factors listed below are clearly understood to be responsible for incisional hernias. Others are not universally accepted as single factors and are only regarded as contributors to the presence of an incisional hernia. We also mention some aspects that should be taken into considerations so that incisional hernias related to these factors can be prevented (3).

Local factors

Factors related to the local conditions of the surgical wound

Wound infection

Wound infection with proteolysis and necrosis of abdominal wall tissues, is probably the most important etiological factor for incisional hernias. Eviscerations can occur during the immediate postoperative period or sometime thereafter. Infection is basically related to contamination of the wound during the operation, hence a higher or lower infection rate can be expected, depending on the type of procedure. Prophylaxis protocols against surgical wound infection should be implemented to keep infection within acceptable limits. Preventive measures can also be taken.

As is discussed in the next section, in addition to operative contamination, other factors, such as the development of hematomas, seromas, etc. or the presence of foreign bodies, can promote wound infection.

In the case of incisions that may produce a residual empty space, lymphorrhea or bleeding, drain insertion should be considered to achieve negative pressure to close the residual space or to prevent retention of fluids in the abdominal wall.

Tension at the margins of the wound

Tension in abdominal wall sutures is the result of the specific characteristics of the abdominal wall or its contents: abdominal distention (intestinal occlusion, edema, etc.), missing portions of the abdominal wall (excision, recurrent hernias, trauma, etc.) or uncontrolled increase in pressure on the abdominal wall (due to coughing or constipation) (6, 7).

Some authors consider that the risk of incisional hernias will vary depending on the incision sites. Their rationale is the presence of various layers, the direction of the muscle fibers and the presence of the different layers of the aponevrosis of the muscles, since they produce different tension levels at the margins of the surgical wound (5,6,7,11). Several authors state that vertical incisions produce more hernias than transverse incisions; others contend that incisions following Lange's lines show a lower rate of hernias. Still others consider that suturing on the aponeurosis planes results in a lower risk of incisional hernias. There are contradictory clinical and experimental studies, hence no categorical conclusions should be drawn, as other technical or infection-related factors are at least as important, if not more (2, 5, 6).

In another section we discuss the advantages and disadvantages of placing tacks or anchors in cases involving some risk of evisceration or tension at the margins of the wound. In other cases, such as re-operations, generalized swelling, hypoproteinemia, etc., tension at the wound can be decreased or resistance increased by introducing prosthetic mesh that can reinforce or replace the abdominal wall. This may be indicated despite the risk of infection and rejection.

Factors related to the surgical technique

Although not all factors depend on the surgeon's skill (some incisional hernias occur, regardless of the steps taken), we feel that proper surgical technique can lower the risk of hernia (5, 8). In any case, the surgeon's skill is essential since he/she must close the laparotomy properly (minimum trauma, good hemostasis, etc.) and take additional measures (tacks, drains, etc.), depending on the characteristics of each patient.

Surgical contamination

During laparotomy contamination of the surgical wound can occur from extra-abdominal sources (instruments, surgical staff, patient's skin) as well as intra-abdominal sources (peritonitis, etc.), hence all necessary aseptic and antiseptic measures must be taken. Closure of the laparotomy should be considered a new operation and, depending on the degree of contamination produced during the surgical act, the surgical team's gloves and the operative fields, instruments, etc., should be changed to decrease the risk of infection.

Factors that increase infection rate

When hematomas occur at the surgical wound or there are residual empty spaces, foreign bodies, or dead or necrotic tissue, the risk of infection rises to levels above those normally expected with this kind of surgery. Good surgical technique should eliminate these factors entirely. If not possible, precautionary measures such as drains, antibiotic treatment, etc. must be taken.

Laparotomy closure techniques

During the development of the different surgical technique (and even nowadays), there has been some controversy around certain aspects of laparotomy closure. We do, however, feel there is sufficient evidence to support some of the techniques for this purpose (3, 15, 19).

The sutures used to close the laparotomy must be anchored to the aponeurosis or to tissues in good condition. Otherwise, an incisional hernia can develop over time, even though initial fibrosis may prevent it from appearing immediately.

Moreover, the space between sutures and over the border of the wound should be adequate to prevent excessive free space and ischemia of the wound margins that would favor evisceration or incisional hernias (11). Although this depends on various factors such as tissue type, wall thickness, existence of various layers, etc., the distance between each suture should not exceed 1.5 cm and should extend 1 cm beyond the margin of the wound.

Another controversial point has been the material used and the suturing technique. The current trend is to use sutures that are absorbed slowly (months). The same results have been reported with this type as with nonabsorbable sutures, with the added advantage that infected or non-tolerated sutures generally do not require removal (3, 10, 16, 19).

In terms of suturing technique for closure, there are various opinions regarding the use of continuous or interrupted sutures and of closure by planes or in a single plane. Slowly absorbing continuous sutures can be used in cases where no complications are expected and interrupted sutures (absorbable or nonabsorbable) in cases involving some risk. Several articles report that single-layer is superior to separate-layer suturing (3, 9-12, 16, 19).

Wound dehiscence

Eviscerations, as such, require emergency re-operations, whereas closed eviscerations can often be treated conservatively. However, almost all eviscerations progress to incisonal hernia in the immediate postoperative or early recovery period. They are usually quite large and characteristically have intestine adhered to the incision. If there are perioperative risk factors for serious wound infection such as abdominal distention or poor healing, or these could be expected to appear during the postoperative period, tack placement should be considered to prevent evisceration or incisional hernia (5, 6).

General factors

Obesity

All books and articles mention obesity as a factor related to the development of incisional hernia (17). Excess weight requires greater physical effort for breathing and movement, with the resulting transmission of greater tension to the margins of the suture. In addition, other factors that could be considered "local" should be kept in mind, such as the existence of a large, poorly vascularized subcutaneous tissue where contamination, "dead" spaces and foreign bodies can play an important role in surgical wound infection.

Elderly patients

Advanced age has always been considered a negative factor, due to a slower healing process, decreased collagen resistance, etc. Since the mean age of surgical patients is higher due to longer life expectancy and better overall condition of patients, some series have reported an increase in the risk of incisional hernia during the fifth and sixth decade of life; this increase as more noticeable in men than women (5).

Diabetes

Diabetes is widely recognized as another factor favoring wound infection, due to delayed wound healing and increased susceptibility to infection (17, 18).

Medical therapies

Some patients receive temporary or long-term drug therapies that can influence healing of the surgical wound or encourage the development of complications.

Corticoids

Patients with systemic diseases may be receiving high doses of corticoids, which increase protein catabolism, thereby altering collagen synthesis and other healing factors (5,18).

Anticoagulants or platelet antiaggregants

An increasing number of patients are treated with anticoagulants and platelet antiaggregants and, therefore, frequently present peri- and/or postoperative problems. Although the effect of these agents should be corrected before the operation, this is not always possible and/or therapy must be resumed immediately after surgery, increasing the risk of bleeding (5, 18).

Radiotherapy

Radiotherapy increases the risk of incisional hernia, both when performed preoperatively and in the immediate postoperative period, since it alters surgical wound healing due to lesion of the affected tissues. Generally speaking, depending on the type of irradiation, immunosuppression occurs, thereby increasing the risk of infection and leading to poor healing of the wound. Although the application of these drugs is increasingly more precise, their use should still be taken into account (5,18).

Chemotherapy

As a therapeutic agent, one of the functions of chemotherapy is to slow or block tumor proliferation. Hence, it can influence healing of the surgical wound, depending on which of the chemotherapy drugs is used. The effect is even greater when combinations of chemotherapy drugs are used (5,18).

PHYSIOPATHOLOGY

Small incisonal hernias generally produce only local changes such as pain, swelling, discomfort from clothing, etc. Large hernias, on the other hand, produce significant local and general alterations that affect both the patient's normal activities and the treatment. The anterior and lateral abdominal muscles form a cylinder of several muscle layers, in which the fibers lay at different angles, thereby allowing thorax and chest movements in all directions as well as mobility and co-ordination of chest and diaphragmatic muscles during breathing (2,5,7,18)

Local alterations

When laparotomy and subsequent closure are performed, inter-layer anchoring and retraction secondary to healing produce changes in mobility due to lack of elasticity, even when the clinical signs are minimal or tolerable. This is true even when there is no incisional hernia. In this hernias, the lack of muscle continuity involves missing portions of the abdominal wall and a change in the action of the muscle fibers. This favors a progressive increase in the area of the hernia and a progressive distortion of abdominal wall movement, a situation that is aggravated when muscle fibers have been sectioned perpendicularly. Muscle atrophy also occurs due to lack of activity, an effect that is enhanced when vascular-nervous pedicles are sectioned (1, 5, 18).

Intra-abdominal pressure favors an increase in the volume of the incisional hernia. When the hernia encounters an area of low resistance, such as the area of a previous incision, comprised of the peritoneum, subcutaneous cell tissue and skin, the hernia sac volume grows progressively and acts as an "escape valve" for pressure on the normal abdominal wall (Fig. 1 and 2).

Incisional hernias can contain free abdominal viscera or viscera with adhesions between each other and/or to the abdominal wall, causing clinical conditions such as incarceration, strangulation, occlusion or fistulas. Discomfort can be local and non-specific. However, if the hernia is large, it may cause significant discomfort, leading to limited movement that results in even further weakness and atrophy of the abdominal muscles whose main function resides in maintaining walking (1, 5, 18).

These local alterations are also significant for surgical treatment of incisional hernias. Whether the operation involves closing the hernia or introducing a prosthetic mesh, the subcutaneous tissue must be dissected down from the musculo-aponeurotic fasciae in good condition, since retraction and atrophy could mean that this layer is deeper than suggested by the physical examination. As much skin and peritoneum as possible should be preserved until the closure technique to be used has been decided. The intra-abdominal viscera may be adhered to the skin, particularly if the incisional hernia is secondary to an evisceration or has experienced an occlusion. In cases of large hernias, some authors recommend preoperative pneumoperitoneum to distend the retracted abdominal muscle and minimize tension in the subsequent closure (7, 18).

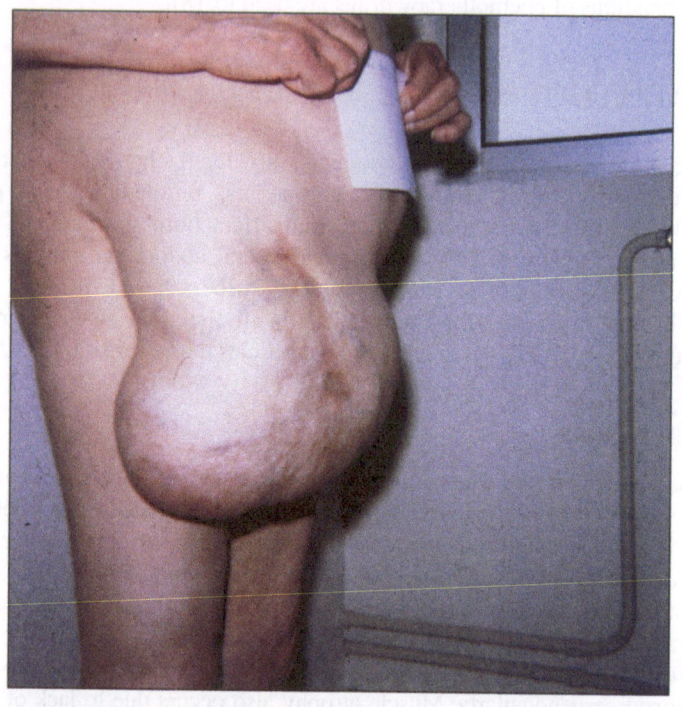

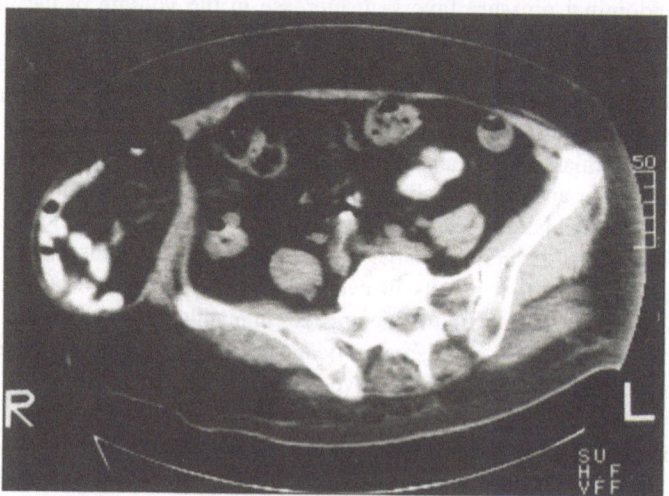

Figs. 1 and 2. Large incisional hernias, which involve pathophysiological changes and therapeutic difficulties.

General alterations

We have already discussed the importance of the abdominal wall muscles for thoracic and respiratory movement.

Even in patients with moderately large hernias, local discomfort for movement and breathing means that the patients' physical activity will be reduced, thereby promoting muscle atrophy and decreasing the cardiac and respiratory capacity in addition to improving the local factors described earlier. In large hernias, the abdominal muscles tend to offset static-dynamic alterations secondary to the increase of abdominal diameter and to the atrophy and localisation of the muscles, causing lordosis of the spinal column, which enhances growth of the hernia and produces secondary morbidity (5, 18).

Large hernias significantly influence the respiratory function, since abdominal muscles contract in coordination with the thoracic and diaphragmatic muscles to produce the intrathoracic and intra-abdominal pressure changes needed for inspiration and expiration. In fact, in large hernias with "loss of space", a "second abdominal cavity" is created and receives pressure from the abdominal cavity itself, behaving like a thoracic "volet" or paradoxical respiration. Abdominal pressure will always be low or at least below normal levels when lack of abdominal wall continuity and a second abdomen of elastic walls exist. This leads to inefficient muscle function, since abdominal movements are paradoxical, and result in respiratory insufficiency, a condition that is particularly obvious at the time of expiration when the combination of diaphragmatic relaxation and abdominal muscle contraction should increase the abdominal pressure and cause expiration, but pressure is actually lost due to filling of the incisional hernia (Fig. 3) (5, 7, 18).

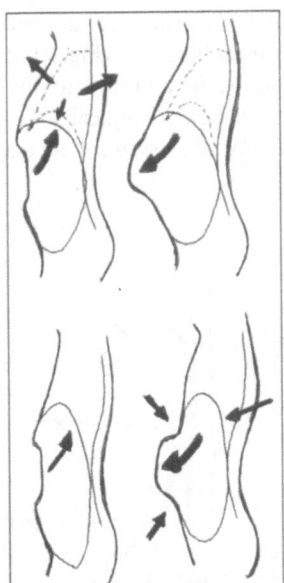

Fig. 3. The four basic diagrams of paradoxical respiration occurring in large incisional hernias, according to Rives (5).

These changes in abdominal pressure also have direct consequences on the splanchnic and systemic vascular systems. In terms of the splanchnic system, abdominal hypopressure produces venous stasis, with vascular dilation and mesenteric edema, which can result in decreased portal vein return and cardiac output. With regard to systemic circulation or inferior vena cava circulation, abdominal hypotension causes slower return, increasing the risk of venous thrombosis of the lower extremities and thromboembolism (5, 18).

Ventilatory and vascular alterations can be corrected when the hernia is repaired, although serious complications may arise if the patient's adaptation is limited. A large number of articles describe the how to calculate the diaphragmatic performance in each case, although overall patient response represents an individual risk. Preoperative study of cardiac and respiratory function is extremely important and the possibility of performing the hernia repair by using a prosthetic material without tension should be considered in serious cases(5, 18).

Special cases

Ostomies

Etiopathogenesis

Ostomies, colostomies, ileostomies and other urological ostomies are currently performed on a frequent basis. Many of these procedures are temporary in nature and intestinal continuity will be reestablished after several months; others will persist for some time or will be permanent. The presence of a hernia causes particular discomfort in the case of long-term ostomies, as well as greater complexity and higher risk in cases where they must be closed (Fig. 4) (2, 5, 7, 9).

In terms of etiopathogenesis, in addition to the factors mentioned for all laparotomies, the risk of contamination of surgical wound is greater in this case since the colostomy must be moved. Nevertheless, there are also some specific factors.

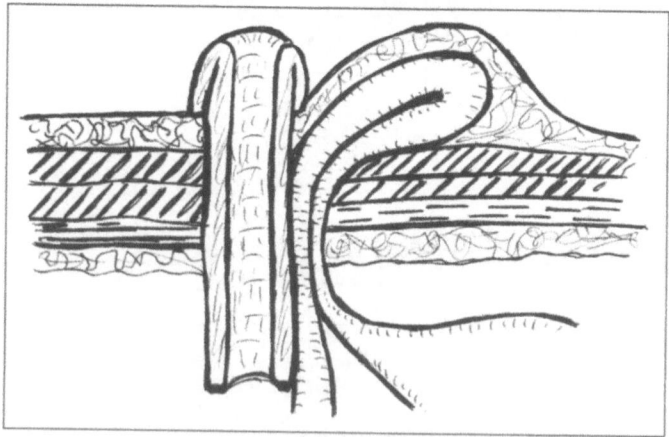

Fig. 4. Pericolostomy incisional hernia. Can occur in the various anatomic layers of the abdominal wall.

Ostomy site

The colostomy site is key and must be planned before the operation in the case of elective surgery (2, 5, 7, 9, 11).

The type of surgery will condition the colostomy site, particularly in emergency procedures. Whenever possible, however, it should be placed in a position that is easily accessible to the patient and does not cause problems regarding clothing.

According to some authors, colostomies created between the anterior rectus muscle fiber of the abdomen have a lower incidence of hernia than those performed between the oblique muscles of the abdomen (2, 5, 7).

Fixation of the intestine to the abdominal wall

Some authors feel that the number of anchoring layers is highly significant, particularly the peritonization, although there is no agreement on this issue (2, 5, 7). We feel that the intestinal wall should be attached to the peritoneum and to some of the muscle layers in order to prevent free space that would allow passage of the abdominal contents due to the intra-abdominal pressure.

Excessively large parietal incision

Adaptation of the intestine to the parietal incision is sometimes difficult to predict. On other occasions, however, it is inevitable such as when treating hernias due to a definitive colostomy. Although this closes to surround the ostomy, hernias tend to appear with some frequency (2, 5, 7).

Physiopathology

In periostomal hernias, functional alterations and risks of occlusion must be considered in addition to all the other characteristics mentioned for incisional hernias. Reconstruction is complex, since the surgery is contaminated both in terms of healing the hernia and the position of the new ostomy (2, 5, 7).

Laparoscopic surgery

The increased popularity of laparoscopic surgery in the final decade of the 20th century has led to reduced surgical aggression through small incisions and less intra-abdominal manipulation. Normally 5 and 10-mm trocars are used, although trocars with a smaller or larger diameter can be applied, depending on the surgical indications and the surgeon's skill (3).

Authors appear to agree that incisions under 5 mm do not require closure of the muscle wall. However, there are a variety of opinions about cases involving incisions of 10 mm or more. Some authors argue that a 10-mm incision does not require specific closure, since it is within the limit of an acceptable distance between suture stitches for a laparotomy. Others feel that the incision must be closed, hence specific instruments have been designed since suturing of the musculo-aponeurotic plane through a 10-mm orifice is not easy. When larger trocars or assisted minilaparotomy are used, the incisions should be closed according to the same criteria used for conventional laparotomy (10).

We have not observed hernias in incisions produced by 5-mm trocars but have seen it in 10-mm incisions, in some cases they had been in fact closed, leading us to believe that the technique had not been correctly performed.

References

1. Alvarez J, Hidalgo M. Hernia incisional. Una complicación demasiado frecuente. Cir Esp 2000;68:91-92.

2. Baker, RJ. Incisional Hernia. Capítulo 19. Hernia. Nyhus, LIM, Condon RE. JB Lippincott Company. Philadelphia. 1989

3. Bakkum EA, Dalmeijer RAJ, Verdel MJC, Hermans J, Van Blitterswijk CA, Trimbos JB. Quantitative analysis of the inflammatory reaction surrounding sutures commonly used in operative procedures and the relation to postsurgical adhesion formation. Biomaterials 1995;16:1283-1289.

4. Coda A, Bossoti M, Ferri, Mattio R, Ramellini G, Poma A, Quaglino F, Filippa C, Bona A. Incisional hernia and fascial defect following laparoscopic surgery. Surg Laparosc Endosc Percutan Tech 2000.

5. Chevrel JP, Flament JB. Les éventrations de la paroi abdominale. Masson, Paris, Milan, Barcelona, Mexico, 1990.

6. Chevrel JP, Flament JB. Traitement des éventrations de la paroi abdominale. Techniques chirurgicales-Appareil digestif. Editions Techniques. Encycl. Méd. Chir. Paris1995;40-165.

7. Devlin HB: Management of Abdominal Hernia. Butterworths. London, 1988.

8. Gislason H, Soreide O, Viste A. Wound complications after major gastrointestinal operations. The surgeon as a risk factor. Dig Surg 1999;16(6):512-4.

9. Hodgson N, Malthaner R, Ostybe T. The search for an ideal method of abdominal fascial closure. A meta-analysis. Ann Surg 2000;231:436-442.

10. Hsiao WC, Young KC, Wang ST, Lin PW. Incisional hernia after laparotomy: prospective randomized comparison between early-absorbable and late-absorbable suture materials. World J Surg 2000 Jun;24(6):747-51;discusion 752.

11. Israelson LA, Jonsson T, Knutsson A. Suture technique and wound healing in midline laparotomy incisions. Eur J Surg 1996 Aug;162(8):605-9.

12. Kasperk R, Klinge U, Schumpelick V. The repair of large parastomal hernias using a midline approach and a prosthetic mesh in the sublay position. Mesh. Am J Surg 1996;171 (1) suppl.:80-84.

13. Nezhat C, Nezhat F, Seidman DS, Nezhat C. Incisional hernias after operative laparoscopy. J Laparoendosc Adv Surg Tech A 1997 Apr;7(2):111-5.

14. Ortiz H, Sara MJ, Armendariz P, De Miguel M, Martí J, Chocarro C. Does the frequency of paracolostomy hernias depend on the position of the colostomy in the abdominal wall?. Int J Colorectal Dis 1994 May;9(2):65-7.

15. Ranaboldo C.J, Rowe-Jones DC. Closure of laparotomy wounds: skin staples versus sutures. Br J Surg 1992;79:1172-1173.

16. Sahlin S, Ahlberg J, Granstrom L, Ljungstrom KG. Monofilament versus multifilament sutures for abdominal closure. Br J Surg 1993 Mar;80(3):322-4.

17. Sugerman HJ, Kellum J, Reines D, DeMaria E, Newsome H, Lowry J, Greater risk of incisional hernia with morbidly obese than steroid-dependent patients and low recurrence with prefascial polypropylene mesh. Am J Surg 1996 jan;171(1):80-4.

18. Urquijo, H, Garcia-Sancho L. Etiopatigenia y fisiopatologia de las eventraciones. Indicaciones del neumoperitoneo progresivo preoperatorio. Capítulo 36. Cirugía de la pared abdominal. Porrero, JL Masson. Barcelona, 1997.

19. Weiland D, Curtis Bay R, Del Sordi S. Choosing the best abdominal closure by meta-analysis. Am J Surg 1998;176:666-670.

CHAPTER 5

Classification of Incisional Hernias of The Abdominal Wall

J.-P. Chevrel

As with inguinal hernias, incisional hernias (I.H.) of the abdominal wall assume many clinical forms in terms of functional symptomatology, the site and the size of the parietal defect, the number of orifices and the number of any previous recurrences.

Numerous factors are involved in the genesis of these I.H. and the quality of the results of their repair. To mention only the principal ones, these include age, anemia, which leads to tissue hypoxia (1, 2), malnutrition (3, 4, 5, 6, 7), obesity (8, 9, 10, 45% of primary I.H. and 61% of recurrent I.H. in our series), systemic diseases such as cancer, chronic cardiopulmonary failure, jaundice (2, 6, 8, 10, 11, 12), steroid therapy (8, 13, 14), radiotherapy (14), the closure technique of the previous procedure (6), arising of and complications, especially sepsis and wound infection after the last operation (9, 15, 16, 17, 18).

In so far as any serious prospective and possibly comparative scientific study dealing with the results of treatment, we must begin by defining the type of I.H., and therefore it seemed necessary to resort to a classification allowing the study or comparison of homogeneous groups. It is very clear that it is impossible to integrate into such a classification all the factors listed above.

So we have chosen a restricted number of factors having the greatest predictive value, in order to propose a simple classification of I.H. This classification makes it possible to carry out prospective or retrospective studies on homogeneous groups and facilitate the choice of the most appropriate techniques for the different types of I.H.

MATERIAL AND METHODS

For this purpose, a retrospective study of a series of 435 abdominal I.H. operated between 1980 and 1998 was started in 1999. This series of 435 patients included 177 men (40.68%) and 258 women (59.31%). The mean age was 56 years (ages ranging from 21 to 95 years). 267 patients (61.3%) presented a primary I.H., while 168 (38.6%) patients had had one recurrence or more.

Initially, to simplify matters, we recorded only three parameters, to determine if there was a statistically significant relationship with recurrence rate: the site of the I.H.(S), its width (W), and the presence or absence of one or more previous recurrences (R).

About the site

Every surgeon knows that the repair of a lateral I.H. is different from that of a medial I.H., and that the repair of a medial subumbilical hernia is easier than the repair of a subxiphoid hernia.

Thus, the site of I.H. was classified as follows:

- medial incisional hernias are coded as M, with 4 subgroups:
M1: supraumbilical I.H.,
M2: juxtaumbilical I.H.,
M3: subumbilical I.H.,
M4: xipho-pubic I.H.

- lateral incisional hernias are coded as L, with 5 subgroups:
L1: subcostal I.H.,
L2: transverse I.H.,
L3: iliac I.H.,
L4: lumbar I.H.,
L5: parastomial hernias.

About the width

For many years some authors have sought to classify incisional hernias in terms of their dimension (19, 20). Some use the two main measurements of length and width, some use the surface area calculated by a sometimes rather complicated formula, and others use grids placed over the orifice of the incisional hernia perioperatively (21). We have preferred to take the width of the incisional hernia as the only criterion of its severity, since, for equal surface areas, as shown in Fig. 1, it is easier to repair an I.H. of small width and greater length than one that is more wide than long. The two I.H. shown in Fig. 1 have exactly the same surface area, but all surgeons familiar with the treatment of I.H. are aware that it is easier to repair I.H. measuring 4 cm in width by 20 cm in length than one measuring 10cm in width and 8cm in length.

So, the width of the incisional hernias, measured perioperatively with a metric band, are classified by 5cm increments as follows:
W1: < 5cm,
W2: 5 to 10cm,
W3: 10 to 15cm,
W4: > 15cm.

For multiorificial I.H., we take the final width of the defect obtained once the fibrous bridges separating the openings have been sectioned.

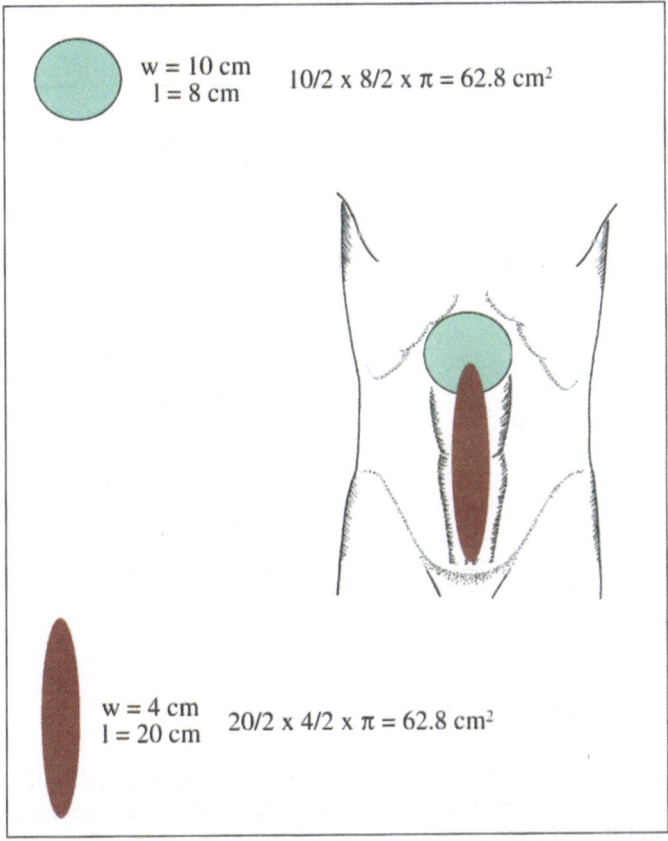

w = 10 cm
l = 8 cm   10/2 x 8/2 x π = 62.8 cm²

w = 4 cm
l = 20 cm   20/2 x 4/2 x π = 62.8 cm²

Fig. 1. Measurement of an incisional hernia orifice surface using the calculation formula for the surface of an ellipse.

About the recurrences

It is generally acknowledged that, as for inguinal hernias, recurrent I.H. are more difficult to repair than primary hernias. In our series, we find that, in fact, the number of previous recurrences has no significant influence on the post-operative results.

This can be explained by the fact that the procedures used are more efficient (unabsorbable sutures, aponeuroplasties, meshes, biologic or synthetic glue...) for recurrent I.H. than for primary.

The recurrences are classified by their number:

no recurrence: R0- or R-,

first recurrence: R1,

second recurrence: R2,

etc.

Table I. Proposed classification for midline and lateral incisional hernias of the abdominal wall

Site	Type	
M (1 to 4)	W1 <	R0
		Rx
or	W2 <	R0
		Rx
L (1 to 5)	W3 <	R0
		Rx
	W4 <	R0
		Rx

w = width ; W1: < 5 cm; W2: 5-10 cm; W3: 10-15 cm; W4 > 15 cm
R = recurrences; 0 = number of recurrences

The statistical relationship

The statistical relationship between these three parameters (site of incisional hernia, width of orifice, and number of recurrences) and the recurrence rate, on the one hand, and the type of repair of the incisional hernia performed (prosthetic or non-prosthetic) on the other, was studied by means of the chi square test. Values of p less than 0.05 were considered statistically significant.

Patients were examined three times during the first postoperative year, then annually. Minimum follow-up was then 1 year, maximum up to more than 10 years.

Each time that the follow-up was less than 90% we have corrected the percentage of recurrences by the coefficient of the maximal bias developed some years ago for the study of inguinal hernias treatment (22, 23); we recall that when the follow-up is less than 90%, it is conceded that 18% of all the patients without follow-up are considered as having recurrences.

RESULTS

Study of the relationship between the site of the incisional hernia and the development of recurrences

-Midline incisional hernias: There is no significant difference between the 3 groups M1 (supraumbilical), M2 (juxtaumbilical) and M3 (subumbilical) and the noted recurrence rate. Paradoxically, the M4 group (xipho-pubic), which included

15 primary and 18 recurrent I.H., yielded the best results with no recurrences. This can be explained by the fact that, for this group, we always reconstruct a linea alba with a plasty using overlapping flaps of anterior rectus sheath reinforced by a mesh in onlay situation (24).

-Lateral incisional hernias: The results of treatment of I.H. for type L1 (subcostal) was less satisfactory than those of treatment for type L3 (iliac). However, the difference was not statistically significant.

Study of the relationship between the width of parietal defect and recurrence rate

As might be expected, there is a significant difference between I.H. of subgroup W4 R+ (recurrent I.H. wider than 15cm), for which the recurrence rate was 16%, and I.H. of type W3 R- or R+ or W4 R-, where the recurrence rate varied from 0 to 6.25%.

On the other hand, we were surprised to find that incisional hernias of types W1 and W2 had higher recurrence rates than incisional hernias of type W3 or W4 R-. This can be explained by the fact that, for small I.H., the repair is often performed by a simple absorbable running suture, which is a bad technique.

Study of the relationship between the existence of previous recurrences and the development of new recurrences

In groups W1 and W2 the results were better in the subgroups R+ than in the subgroups R-, although the difference was not statistically significant.

There was no significant difference between the group W3 R+, with 6.25% recurrence rate, and group W3 R-, with 5.71% recurrence rate.

There was a significant difference between the subgroups W1 R-, W1 R+, W2 R- and W2 R+ taken together and subgroups W3 R-, W3 R+ and W4 R- taken together: the latter three subgroups had the better results.

These results seem to prove that the number of previous recurrences had no statistically significant impact on the results.

DISCUSSION

About the results concerning the relationship between the site of the I.H. and the recurrence rate

-For midline I.H., the better results obtained in the M4 group are explained, not by the extent in height of the incisional hernia, which logically should lead to a higher risk of recurrence, but by the fact that more selective and reliable techniques were used in this group of large incisional hernias, notably with a greater percentage use of prostheses (84.84%). Thus it seems that the site of the incisional hernia is not correlated with the quality of the results.

-*For lateral I.H.*, the better results were obtained with the treatment of iliac I.H. compared to that of subcostal incisional hernias. However, even if the difference is not statistically significant, it seems as if this difference may not be linked to the site of the I.H. but rather to the technique employed: in the iliac incisional hernias we inserted more prostheses than for subcostal I.H. (66.6% as against 54.28%) and sometimes even double prostheses, one between two muscle layers and the other in an onlay position.

About the results concerning the relationship between the width of the I.H. and the recurrence rate

We found that there was a significant difference between the group W4 R+ and the previous groups. This can be readily explained since it refers to I.H. which are more difficult to treat, especially if the number of previous recurrences is high, so that the result of their repair depended on the quality of the tissues and the techniques previously used.

We also saw that there was a significant difference between the two groups W1 and W2 taken together and the subgroups W3 R- and R+ and W4 R- taken together. Prosthetic repairs were more often performed in groups W3 and W4 than in groups W1 and W2, which were often treated some what rashly, sometimes by a simple continuous suture of absorbable material without even a relaxing incision in the context of group W1. Conversely, the wider the I.H., the more reinforcing prostheses were used and the better the results.

Therapeutic proposals

The analysis of our results leads us to the following therapeutic proposals. We feel that there is no single specific treatment for I.H., whether primary or secondary.

-For I.H. of type W1-R0 or W2-R0, we believe that these can be treated by a simple herniorrhaphy, provided this is done with nonabsorbable material, tension free, thanks to relaxing incisions as used by Gibson or Clotteau-Prémont.

-For the groups W1-R+ and W2-R+,we prefer an autoplasty of the Welti-Eudel type, reinforced by a pre-musculofascial prosthesis.

-For the groups W3 and W4, in cases of medial I.H. (M), we perform a reconstruction of the linea alba by means of an overlapping flap of the anterior rectus sheath reinforced by a prosthesis in onlay situation, fixed by a spray of fibrin or synthetic glue (24).

-For lateral I.H. (L) we prefer a prosthesis inserted sandwich-like between two muscle layers, a deep layer formed by the transversus abdominis and internal oblique mm. and a superficial plane formed by the external oblique m. A second prosthesis in the pre-musculo-fascial position may reinforce this arrangement.

Lastly, when it is not possible to begin the parietal repair by an anatomic reconstitution of the wall, and when there is a substantial loss of substance of the abdominal wall, we habitually fill this loss of substance with an absorbable prosthesis fixed to the margins of the orifice of the incisional hernia and lined superficially by a nonabsorbable prosthesis which widely overlaps the first one on the aponeurosis of the external oblique muscle.

CONCLUSION

The multiplicity of anatomic forms of abdominal I.H., the several factors interfering with normal wound healing, the diverse possibilities of parietal repair, and the difficulty of choosing the ideal treatment lead us to present this classification, in which we emphasize two characteristics: its simplicity and its predictive value (25).

From well-defined anatomo-clinical groups, it becomes easier to perform prospective studies in order to assess the influence of different factors on the quality of parietal repair.

References

1. Jonsson K, Jensen JA, Goodson WH, Scheuenstuhl H, West J, Hopf HW, Hunt TK. (1991) Tissue oxygenation, anemia, and perfusion in relation to wound healing in surgical patients. Ann Surg 214: 605-613.

2. Makela JT, Kiviniemi H, Juvonen T, Laitinen S (1995) Factors influencing wound dehiscence after midline laparotomy. Am J Surg 170: 387-390.

3. Belcher HJ, Ellis H (1991) An investigation of the role of diet and burn injury on wound healing. Burns 17: 14-16.

4. Greenhalgh DG (1987) Is impaired wound healing caused by infection or nutritional depletion? Surgery 102: 306-312.

5. Law NW, Ellis H (1990) The effect of parenteral nutrition on the healing of abdominal wall wounds and colonic anastomoses in proteinmalnourished rats. Surgery 107: 449-454.

6. Niggebrugge AH, Hansen BE, Trimbos JB, van de Velde CJH, Zwaveling A. (1995) Mechanical factors influencing the incidence of burst abdomen. Eur J Surg 161: 655-661.

7. Soisson AP, Olt G, Soper JT, Berchuck A, Rodriguez G, Clarke-Pearson DL (1993) Prevention of superficial wound separation with subcutaneous retention sutures. Gynecol Oncol 51: 330-334.

8. Baggish MS, Lee WK (1975) Abdominal wall disruption. Obstet Gynecol 46: 530-534

9. Bucknall TE (1983) Factors influencing wound complications: a clinical and experimental study. Ann Roy Coll Surg Engl 65: 71-78.

10. Regnard JF, Hay JM, Rea S, Fingerhut A, Flamant Y, Maillard JN (1988) Ventral incisional hernias: incidence, date of recurrence, localization and risk factors. Ital J Surg Sci 18(3): 259-265.

11. Makishima T (1989) Experimental study of the wound healing in liver cirrhosis. Nippon Geka Gakkai Zasshi 90: 1706-1712.

12. Sanders RJ, DiClementi D (1977) Principles of abdominal wall closure. Arch Surg 112: 1188-1191.

13. Dostal GH, Gamelli RL (1990) The differential effect of corticosteroids on wound disruption strength in mice. Arch Surg 125: 636-640.

14. Ellis H (1976) Wound healing. Ann Roy Coll Surg Engl 59: 382-387.

15. Smith M, Enquist IF (1967) A quantitative study of impaired healing resulting from infection. Surg Gynecol Obstet 125: 965-973.

16. Cameron AE, Parker ES, Gray RC, Wyatt AP (1987) A randomised comparison of polydioxanone (PDS) and polypropylene (Prolene) for abdominal wound closure. Ann R Coll Surg Engl 69: 113-115.

17. Gys T, Hubens A (1989) A prospective comparative clinical study between monofilament absorbable and non-absorbable sutures for abdominal wall closure. Acta Chir Belg 89: 265-270.

18. Israelsson LA, Jonsson T (1993) Suture length to wound length ratio and healing of midline laparotomy incisions. Br J Surg 80: 1284-1286.

19. Herzsage L. (1999) Indication and limitations of suture closure - Significance of relaxing incisions. In: V. Schumpelick, A.N. Kingsnorth Eds., Incisional Hernia, Springer-Verlag Berlin Heidelberg, 279-283.

20. Schumpelick V, A.N. Kingsnorth et al (1999) Panel discussion: classification. In: V. Schumpelick, A.N. Kingsnorth Eds., Incisional Hernia, Springer-Verlag Berlin Heidelberg, p 491.

21. Champault G. Personal communication.

22. Schwartz D, Flamant R, Lellouch J. (1980) The problem of missing subjects. In: Clinical trials. London, Academic Press, p 223-224.

23. Hay JM, Boudet MJ, Fingerhut A, Pourcher J, Hennet H, Habib E, Veyrières M, Flamant Y, and the French Association for Surgical Research. (1995) Shouldice inguinal hernia repair in the male adult: the gold standard? A multicenter controlled trial in 1578 patients. Ann Surg 222: 719-727.

24. Chevrel JP, Rath AM (1997) The use of fibrin glues in the surgical treatment of incisional hernias. Hernia 1: 9-14.

25. Chevrel JP, Rath AM (2000) Classification of incisional hernias of the abdominal wall. Hernia 4: 7-11.

CHAPTER 6

Surgical Alternatives for the Repair of Ventral Hernias

J.Mª Ortega, F. Sánchez Ganfornina, J. Cantillana

INTRODUCTION

Incisional hernias are protrusions of the abdominal viscera through areas of the abdominal wall where musculoaponeurotic continuity is lacking due to a trauma, specially postoperative (1). Some synonymous terms of incisional hernias are postoperative hernia or post-laparotomy hernia. It should not be confused with the terms like "laparocele" or diastasis, which define other types of abdominal wall defects.

Incisional hernias are frequent complications of abdominal surgery involving laparotomies. Depending on the series, they occur in 2 to 10% of all laparotomies (2-3), with a higher incidence in the first three years after surgery (4).

Incisional hernia surgery is a common procedure because of this high rate. A number of surgical techniques have been developed to treat this problem, since results have not been particularly good, with the recurrence rate being relatively high.

The main objective of this chapter is to present the alternative surgical techniques considered to be "traditional". We will first review several concepts that we believe are basic in terms of physiopathogenesis and preoperative preparation of the patient with an incisional hernia. We will avoid the use of eponyms as much as possible, although a number of equivalent terms exist, as in other hernia surgeries.

TYPES AND PATHOPHYSIOLOGICAL CONSEQUENCES OF INCISIONAL HERNIAS

Incisional hernias have been classified on the basis of size and location. The size is considered to be the largest transverse diameter, hence the hernias are classified as: small, medium-size and large. The figures reported by the various authors vary considerably(5-8).

	Small	Medium-size	Large
Jessen-Soerensen	< 2	2 - 5	> 5
Ponka	< 6	6 - 10	> 10
Barroetaveña	< 4	4 - 7	> 7
Rives	< 5	5 - 10	> 10

Based on their topographic region (9-10), they can be divided into two groups, namely, midline and lateral. Xiphoumbilical (epigastric and periumbilical, supraumbilical), umbilicopubic (subumbilical or infraumbilical) or xiphopubic (suprainfraumbilical); within the medial or midline sites.

The pathophysiological consequences of incisional hernias depend on the size, site and time of evolution of the lesion. They can be classified as follows:

a- Local or musculocutaneous level:
• Atrophy, sclerosis or scleroadipose degeneration of the wide muscle of the abdominal wall.
• Sagittal shape of the rectus muscles.
• Trophic skin ulcers of ischemic origin.
• Infected lesions.

b- General level:
• Latent chronic respiratory insufficiency.
• Dilation and distention of viscera.
• Dilation of large veins, with slowed return circulation.

If these consequences are not anticipated and prevented in the immediate postoperative period, the patient could present major general complications such as progressive respiratory distress or deep venous thrombosis - pulmonary thromboembolism (11-13).

PATIENT PREPARATION

Prior to surgery, the incisional hernia must be assessed for the presence of ulcers or intertrigo lesions; if there are any, they must be treated until cured, before surgical repair can be undertaken. In some cases, trophic ulcers require initial surgery, including excision and suture, for proper healing.

On the day of the operation, the skin must be washed with soap, shaved and carefully disinfected with povidone iodine.

Obese patients must go on a weight-loss diet before the surgical treatment.

The most important preparatory step is unquestionably the respiratory preparation. Respiratory function studies (spirometry, chest x-ray and arterial gasometry) should be performed in all patients. In addition, rehabilitation treatment for several weeks in respiratory physiotherapy units is imperative before admission, in order to achieve diaphragm reeducation, stimulation of coughing and expectoration. The use of incentive inspirometers is very important. The respiratory function tests are then repeated to assess the efficacy of this preparatory step.

After respiratory preparation, any patient with a maximum forced expiratory volume per second (FEV1) of less than 1 liter, and a Tiffeneau index below 50% should be excluded for surgical treatment (14).

Lastly, in patients undergoing incisional hernia repair, antibiotic and thromboembolic prophylaxis should be considered. On the first point, although a single dose of a wide spectrum antibiotic (e.g., 1st- or 2nd-generation cephalosporin) given intravenously during anesthesia induction is sufficient from a theoretical point of view, we recommend that the antibiotic be continued until the drains are removed. Regarding the prevention of thromboembolic disease, we believe the prophylactic agent should not be given in the abdomen near the incision.

Preoperative progressive pneumoperitoneum

This procedure was conceived by Iván Goñi Moreno (15), who presented it at an Argentinean Surgery Congress in 1940. At that time the technique was a genuine revolution for surgery of large incisional hernias, and it spread around the world in the years that followed.

The procedure involves the gradual insufflation of air into the peritoneal cavity in several sessions. The objective is to increase the capacity of the abdomen by distending the muscles and adapting the diaphragm to the intraabdominal hyperpressure, in order to prevent complications during reintegration.

Basic indications include incisional hernias where the reintegration of viscera in the abdominal cavity is physically impossible, juxtastomal hernias and hernias with infected prostheses that must be removed.

SURGICAL TREATMENT

Needless to say, an essential requirement for satisfactory repair of a hernia is appropriate knowledge of the anatomy of the anterolateral abdominal wall. The objectives of the treatment are to release and reintegrate the content of the hernia sac in the abdominal cavity and to reconstruct the abdominal wall, restoring its biomechanics.

The surgery consists of two basic phases: exposure and reconstruction. The first stage involves more or less the same steps regardless of the reconstruction technique, and consists mainly in dissection and treatment of the hernia sac. In the second stage, the surgical procedure depends on the transverse diameter of the hernia margins, and the condition and trophism of the rectus muscles and their sheaths (16).

On many occasions, the surgeon uses a hybrid procedure that solves problems as they arise during the surgery.

Exposure

The incision should excise the old scar in the form of ellipse. The incision should be 2 or 3cm longer than the length of the scar. Surgery is sometimes performed in association with a dermolipectomy. Any suture material from previous surgery must be removed.

The next step consists in dissecting the hernia sac; sometimes there is more than one (multisaccular incisional hernia). Initially the sac should not be opened. The dissection of subcutaneous cell tissue should go down as far as the area of fibrous scar tissue at the sac, continuing in the direction of the defect margins, and following the superficial aponeurosis (supra-aponeurotic dissection). The extent of the separation between the subcutaneous tissue and the aponeurosis may vary, and depends on the repair procedure being carried out. Care must be taken with hemostasis during this phase of the surgery, the margins must be protected and the skin isolated.

The sac is then opened; if it has been opened accidentally, this area is used. Before removing the sac, the surgeon should assess whether or not it will be needed for the closure. All intestinal or omental intrasaccular adhesions are then released. We recommend performing complete enterolysis in cases where the patient presented clinical symptoms of abdominal pain or subocclusive symptoms. Finally, the inner side of the wall must be examined for secondary orifices, and, if there are any, the bridges between them must be sectioned to create a single defect.

Reconstruction

In this section we address the various surgical procedures used to repair midline incisional hernias, which account for almost 80% of cases (2). Lateral, juxtastomal and strangulated incisional hernias will be covered in separate chapters.

The surgical procedures we will discuss are considered to be "traditional". We feel there is no sense in mentioning any obsolete techniques such as the use of grafts or suturing and prosthesis materials that are no longer used. There are three main groups of procedures: direct sutures (on one or more layers), aponeurotic plasties (overlapping the margins or making incisions to reduce the tension) and prostheses (depending on the anatomic space where they are placed).

The second group includes a number of techniques known by the name of author, although they are often small variations of other techniques. In these cases we will describe the most well-known procedure and limit ourselves to mentioning procedures that have derived therefrom.

Direct sutures

A distinction can be made between the following types of direct sutures: the simple, in two layers and with lateral incisions to reduce tension.

The *simple suture* is only indicated in defects with a maximum transverse diameter under 3 cm. This procedure has the poorest results, with recurrence rates estimated at 20-30%.

The *two layers of sutures* must also be reserved for small incisional hernias with no atrophied muscles. There should be no tension on the suture lines, otherwise recurrence is certain.

When classifying the various techniques, some authors include procedures that involve incisions to release tension within the group of aponeurotic plasties or autoplasties. The first author to describe lateral incisions to reduce tension away from the suture midline was *Gibson* in 1920 (17).

The *Gibson procedure* consisted of three steps:

1- Peritoneal suture (running suture).

2- Lateral incisions to reduce the tension on the suture line about 3 cm from the inner margin of the sheaths, in the vertical direction and exceeding the medial suture length at the top and the bottom.

3- Aponeurotic suture (interrupted sutures).

Gibson's concept inspired several authors to describe other procedures, such as *Cames and Acebal* who included a third suture line joining the lateral portions of the rectus sheaths after detaching them from the muscles (18); *Koontz*, who performed aponeurotic suture by far-and-near or Smead-Jones sutures (19); and *Rothschild*, who stated that his proposal developed from an erroneous interpretation of Gibson's technique (20).

The *Clotteau-Prémont operation* (21) is another classic suture technique with tension-reducing contraincisions. This consists of dissecting the anterior layer of the rectus sheath (which Barroetaveña calls the supra-aponeurotic dissection) after doing the simple or two-layer suture, and making small, 1.5-cm vertical incisions, separated by 1.5 cm and arranged in 3 or 4 parallel lines on each side of the midline.

Plasties

These procedures are known as autoplasties since they use endogenous material to cover the hernia defect. As mentioned earlier, various techniques have been described, but we will refer to the most well-known.

The *Welti and Eudel procedure* (22) described in 1941, was initially recommended for small xiphoumbilical midline incisional hernias. It was inspired by other older procedures such as those described by *Chrobak* (1887) (23) and *Quénu* (1896) . The principle is similar: a part of the anterior layer of the rectus sheaths is utilized as a hinge. Once the sac is treated, a longitudinal incision is made 1.5 cm from the internal diehedral of the sheath, only 1-2 mm is separated, turned over like a hinge, then sutured in one layer, taking the medial flap of the sheath, the hernia margins and the peritoneum. Some authors first perform one suture line including the sac and peritoneum. The lateral lips of the sheath openings are not sutured since this would create tension; Quénu used this suturing technique, although it had initially been designed for umbilical hernias (24).

The *Del Valle procedure* (25) is more complicated; it traces quadrangular 3x2 cm flaps, alternating them from one side to the other, with the anterior layer of the rectus sheath. Then these flaps are inverted toward the opposite side and sutured.

Other similar technique described by *Babcok* (26), consists of creating flaps in the form of strips that are subsequently interwoven and sutured.

Another type of autoplasty that uses the posterior layer of the sheath was devised by *Berman* (27). The procedure consists of opening one of the sheaths on its deep face, working with the posterior layer. The other sheath is opened on its anterior face, forming two flaps that are sutured in two planes.

In 1965 *Zavaleta* et al. introduced lateral incisions to reduce tension in the obliquus externus muscle over the costal wall (28).

Lastly we mention *Lázaro da Silva's procedure* (29). In 1979 this author introduced the use of the sac together with flaps of the rectus sheaths to cover the wall defect. The sac is first opened longitudinally at the middle, then the rectus sheaths are sectioned, one at the anterior layer and another at the posterior, both about 1 cm from the margin. Closure is then performed as follows (assuming that the right sheath was opened through its posterior layer):

1- interrupted suture of the left layer of the sac with the lateral margin of the posterior layer of the right sheath.

2- interrupted suture of the medial margin of the posterior layer of the right sheath with the medial margin of the left rectus sheath (the greatest resistance corresponds to this suture).

3- Suture (also discontinuous) of the right layer of the sac with the lateral margin of the anterior layer of the left sheath.

Prosthesis

In an attempt to repair medium-size and large incisional hernias, in which repair by direct suture or musculoaponeurotic plasty is accompanied by an unacceptable recurrence rate, exogenous materials were used to replace the wall defect or reinforce a parietal plasty technique (30).

Although the use of synthetic materials is first attributed to *Acquaviva* and *Bourret* in 1948, most authors consider that prosthetic material was first used extensively in incisional hernia surgery after *Usher* published his results with polypropylene mesh in 1963.

The use of prostheses (regardless of whether they are associated with some kind of plasty or not) has become widespread.

Before discussing technical details, we should mention that there are two types of synthetic prostheses: absorbable (polyglactin 910, polyglycolic acid) and nonabsorbable (dacron, polypropylene, PTFE-e). We have published several experimental works on the organic assimilation mechanisms of some of these materials, defining the advantages and disadvantages of each one (31,32). Other experimental studies (33) have concluded that absorbable materials are not effective for incisional hernia repair. These materials disappear after a short period of time and wall resistance depends only on the fibrous tissue that grew on the mesh, tissue that is insufficient to support tension.

We can divide the techniques involving prosthetic mesh into two groups, depending on the objective: replacement, in which the prosthesis is placed to bridge or overlap the parietal defect, thereby acting as a single retention layer; and reinforcement, in which the prosthesis is positioned as simply another layer above or below a musculoaponeurotic plastic reconstruction. The reinforcement techniques are generally speaking more widely used.

Another way to classify repair techniques with prostheses is based on the anatomical site (34). (from outside in):

1- supra-aponeurotic, premusculoaponeurotic or subcutaneous

2- subaponeurotic or prefascial retromuscular

3- preperitoneal

4- intraperitoneal.

Classic reinforcement techniques

Chevrel's operation (35): This consists of adding a premusculoaponeurotic polypropylene mesh to a plasty in superimposed layers. A large supra-aponeurotic dissection is required for this plasty, then the anterior layers of the rectus sheaths are placed vertically. An initial running suture line of the peritoneum is created.

The inner flaps of the anterior layers of the sheaths are folded toward the midline in a hinge-like fashion, then sutured in two layers with a double line of sutures. Lastly the mesh is placed above the aponeurosis, extending beyond the lateral margins of the sheaths and fixed with running suture.

Some authors have placed the mesh at this level, but based on other types of procedures such as that of *Welti and Eudel* or *Clotteau-Prémont*, with very good results.

In these reinforcement procedures with subcutaneous positioning of the prosthesis, some authors have introduced the application of fibrin glue on the mesh to prevent dead space and seromas (36, 37).

Rives technique (8, 38): The basic aspects of this technique consist in an opening in the posterior layer of the rectus sheaths, with dissection of the prefascial retromuscular layer. Running suture of the peritoneum and the posterior layer of the rectus sheath is performed. A mesh is then placed below the rectus muscles and anchored with loose sutures tied using a Reverdin needle. In the original technique these sutures are brought up to the skin, with the tie remaining in the subcutaneous cell tissue, but some surgeons prefer tying at the level of the anterior sheet of the rectus sheath.

Stoppa technique (39): This repair, originally designed for bilateral inguinal hernias, consists in placing a large mesh in the preperitoneal space at the height of the abdominal wall area below the arch of Douglas. This technique is indicated in low infraumbilical midline incisional hernias.

Usher technique (40): In this method, a reinforcing prosthesis is implanted at the intraperitoneal level on an omentoparietal bed to prevent complications due to adhesions or fistulas. A normal aponeurotic closure is subsequently performed.

Replacement techniques

Matapurkar or peritoneal "sandwich" technique (41): This technique requires a large ventral sac, that is opened longitudinally. The prosthesis is sandwiched by the two halves of the sac. This procedure prevents the mesh from coming into contact with the intestinal loops or subcutaneous tissue.

The other replacement repair technique is known as *direct intraperitoneal*, i.e. the mesh is secured with running suturing at the margins of the defect. A PTFE-e or Composite materials are used to prevent adhesions or fistulas.

References:

1. Jaboulay M et Patel M. Hernies. En: Le Dentu A et Delbet P. Nouveau Traité de Chirurgie. JB Baillière et fils, Paris, 1908.
2. Chevrel JP, Flament JB. Les éventrations de la paroi abdominale. 92ᵉ Congrès français de Chirurgie. Paris, 1990.
3. Larson GM, Vandertoll DJ. Approaches to repair of ventral hernia and full-thickness losses of the abdominal wall. Surg Clin North Am, 1984; 64: 335-349.

4. Mudge M, Hugues LE. Incisional hernia: a 10 year prospective study of incidence and attitudes. Br J Surg 1985; 72: 70-71.

5. Jessen C et Soresen BM. Incisional hernia. Acta Chir Scandinav; 1967; 133: 487.

6. Ponka JL. Hernias of the abdominal wall. WB Saunders Co., Philadelphia, 1980.

7. Barroetaveña J, Herzage L, Tibaudin H, Barroetaveña JL, Ahualli CE. Cirugía de las eventraciones. Buenos Aires: Ed. El Ateneo, 1988.

8. Rives J, Pire JC, Flamment JB, Palot JP, Body C. Le traitement des grandes eventrations. Nouvelles indications therapeutiques a propos de 322 cas. Chirurgie 1985; 111: 215-225.

9. Sibilla CE. Eventración postoperatoria. El Día Méd., 1940; 12: 15.

10. Garriz RA, González JM. Temas de Terapéutica Quirúrgica. Librería Acadia Editorial, Buenos Aires, 1984.

11. Flamment JB, Olivier F, Palot JP, Delattre JF. Histoire du traitement des éventrations. Bruneau. Monographie GREPA 1986; 8: 1-6.

12. Rives J, Lardennois B, Pire JC, Hibon J. Les grandes éventrations. Importance du volet abdominal et des troubles respiratoires qui lui sont secondaires. Chirurgie 1973; 99: 547-563.

13. Rives J, Pire JC, Flamment JB, Palot JP. Les grandes éventrations. In: Chevrel JP. Chirurgie des parois de l'abdomen. Springer Verlag. Paris. 1985; pp 118-145.

14. Chevrel JP et Flament JB. Traitement des éventrations de la paroi abdominale. Encycl. Méd. Chir. (Elsevier, Paris-France), Techniques chirurgicales – Appareil digestif, 40-165, 1995, 14p.

15. Goñi Moreno I. Eventraciones crónicas y hernias voluminosas. Preparación con el neumoperitoneo progresivo. Procedimiento original. Bol. Y Trab. Acad. Argent. Cir., 1946; 30: 1041.

16. Martínez Gómez DA, García Marcilla JA, Morcillo Ródenas MA et al. Resultados de las prótesis en las eventraciones moderadas y grandes. Cir Esp 1997; 62: 24-29.

17. Gibson Ch L. Operation for cure of large ventral hernia. Ann Surg 1920; 72: 214.

18. Cames OG, Acebal JA. Técnica operatoria en el tratamiento de las eventraciones medianas. An Cir Rosario, 1940; 7: 255.

19. Koontz AR. An operation for large incisional epigastric hernia. Surg Gynec Obstet, 1962; 114: 117.

20. Rothschild NJ. Treatement of recurrent incisional hernia by flaps of anterior sheath of rectus. Ann Surg, 1935; 101: 754.

21. Clotteau JE, Prémont M. Cure des grandes éventrations cicatricielles médianes par un procédé de plastie aponévrotique. Chirurgie 1979; 105: 344-346.

22. Welti H, Eudel F. Un procédé de cure radicale des éventrations postopératoires par auto-étalement des muscles grands droits, après incision du feuillet antérieur de leurs gaines. Mem Acad Chir 1941; 28: 791-798.

23. Chroback FR: In Zimmerman LM, Anson BJ: Anatomy and Surgery of Hernia. 2nd. Ed. The Williams and Wilkins Co., Baltimore, 1967.

24. Quénu E. Traité de Technique Chirurgicale, IV Masson, Paris, 1955.

25. Del Valle D. Una técnica para el tratamiento de las eventraciones de la línea alba. Sem Méd, 1934; 1: 1586.

26. Babcock WW. Interdigitation in the repair of large ventral hernias with observations on lipectomy. Surg Gynec Obstet, 1924; 40: 853.

27. Berman EF. Epigastric hernia. An improved method of repair. Am. J. Surg.1945; 68: 84.

28. Zavaleta DE, Bun RF, Solian JA y Bresan E. Las incisiones costales de relajación en el tratamiento de las grandes eventraciones supraumbilicales. Prensa Méd Argent 1965; 52: 1349.

29. Lázaro Da Silva A. Surgical correction of longitudinal median or paramedian incisional hernia. Surg Gynec Obstet 1979; 148: 579.

30. Vaquero Pérez MM. Integración orgánica de materiales protésicos en hernias postlaparotómicas. Estudio experimental. Tesis Doctoral. Sevilla: Universidad Hispalense, 1993.

31. Vaquero M.M., Ortega Beviá J.M., Capitán L., Cantillana J, Asimilación de materiales homólogos en el tratamiento de hernias postlaparotómicas. Estudio experimental. Inflamación. 1.998; 9, 2, 53-57.

32. Vaquero M.M., Capitán L., Cantillana J, Ortega Beviá J.M. Asimilación orgánica de prótesis sintéticas en el tratamiento de hernias post-laparotómicas. Estudio experimental. Cir. And. 2.000; 11: 341- 345.

33. Ponce González JF, Barriga Beltrán R, Martín Zurita I, Morales Conde S y Morales Méndez S. Materiales protésicos en la hernia incisional. Estudio experimental. Cir Esp 1998; 63: 189-194.

34. Porrero JL. Cirugía de la pared abdominal. Masson, S.A. Barcelona, 1997.

35. Chevrel JP, Dilin C, Morquette H. Traitement des éventrations abdominales médianes par autoplastie musculaire et prothèse prémusculo-aponévrotique. A propos de 50 observations. Chirurgie 1986; 112: 612-622.

36. Chevrel JP, Rath AM. The use of fibrin glues in the surgical treatment of incisional hernias. Hernia 1997; 1: 9-14.

37. Fernández Lobato R, Fernández Luengas D, Serantes A, Cerquella C, et al. Aplicación de Histoacryl ® en dermolipectomías y eventraciones. Cir Esp 2000; 67: 119-120.

38. Porrero Carro JL, Sánchez-Cabezudo Díaz-Guerra C, Salomón Giordani P, Ramos García I, et al. Técnica de Rives con prótesis de politetrafluoroetileno expandido (PTFE-E) en el tratamiento de las hernias laparotómicas. Cir Esp 1997; 62: 278-281.

39. Stoppa RE. The treatment of complicated groin and incisional hernias. W J Surg 1989; 13: 545-554.

40. Usher FC. New technique for reparing incisional hernias with marlex mesh. Am J Surg 1979; 138: 740-744.

41. Matapurkar BG, Gupta AK, Agarwal AK. A new technique of "Marlex-Peritoneal Sandwich" in the repair of large incisional hernias. World J Surg 1991; 15: 768-770.

SECTION III

Basic Considerations of Laparoscopic Ventral Hernia Repair

CHAPTER 7

Anatomical Basis of Ventral Hernia Repair: Is There a Place for Laparoscopic Surgery?

K.A. LeBlanc, J.B. Flament

INTRODUCTION

The abdominal wall is a complex structure that has a multitude of components that include skin, muscles, aponeuroses, fat, and mesothelium This musculoaponeurotic structure is attached to the vertebral column posteriorly, the pelvic bones inferiorly and the ribs superiorly. The integrity of the abdominal wall is essential to protect the underlying organs, allow for movement of the truck of the body, provision of assistance in respiration and to prevent the herniation of the intra-abdominal contents.

Unfortunately, little attention has been paid to the importance of this portion of the human body by surgeons. All physicians know of the need for its structural disruption during the course of every laparotomy. The factors that influence the prevention and development of hernias and adhesions are frequently overlooked during the closure of the celiotomy wound. The result can be the predisposition of the occurrence of the fascial defect that will allow the extra-abdominal migration of the contents of the abdomen. This hernia, in turn, can eventuate in complications such as incarceration, strangulation, loss of domain, and significant cosmetic deformities. Therefore, the approximation of the abdominal wall as the final act of the laparotomy should be considered as important as the intra-abdominal procedure that necessitated the incision. This represents the optimum opportunity to avert the development of herniation in the future.

Once the hernia has developed and the surgeon is to repair the fascial defect, many considerations shall influence the herniorraphy chosen. The laparoscopic repair of incisional and ventral hernias may require the surgeon to adopt new concepts and methods. Additionally, an understanding of the anatomical basis of the repair of the incisional and ventral hernias of the abdomen is necessary to assure an optimal structural, functional and cosmetic result.

FUNCTIONAL ANATOMY OF THE ABDOMINAL WALL

The functional anatomy of the abdominal wall centers on the flat muscles that provide protection of the abdominal viscera, retention of the contents of the abdomen, assistance in respiration and provision of movement of the mid-portion of the body. These components include the rectus abdominus, external oblique, internal oblique, and transversus abdominus.

Rectus Abdominus Muscle

This muscle extends from the xiphoid process and the lower rib margins to the pubis. The entire length of this muscle contains the linea alba in the mid-portion. Because the linea alba is the site of the most frequent point of entry into the abdomen for surgical procedures, this is the site most commonly becomes the site of herniation. This muscle, when contracted, will bring the xiphoid and ribs closer to the pubis. It also acts to contain the viscera in concert with the flat muscles. The function of the rectus will be compromised after the development of a hernia at the site of the linea alba. The laparoscopic repair of midline hernias does not re-approximate the linea alba. Consequently, the normal function of the rectus is not restored to its native state. The placement of the prosthetic biomaterial will reconstruct the containment function of the muscle but only minimally, if at all, improve its motor functions.

Some laparoscopic surgeons use the posterior rectus sheath of the rectus within which to perform the operative procedure and to place the prosthetic material. This posterior rectus sheath is entered, the hernia is reduced and the repair is performed within that space. This provides for an extraperitoneal operation similar to that of the laparoscopic inguinal herniorraphy. The space limitations of that operative field make this approach impractical for very large hernias, incarcerated hernias or hernias that do not reside within the rectus sheath. It has also not been proven that this method of repair improves the functionality of the muscles to an extent greater than that of the intraperitoneal placement of the prosthetic biomaterial.

External Oblique Muscle

The outermost layer of the flat muscles of the wall of the abdomen arises from the lowest seven or eight ribs, courses obliquely downward and towards the midline. There, it interdigitates with the fibers of the contralateral external oblique. The fleshy muscle fibers insert on the anterior iliac spine and the iliac crest. This muscle, along with the internal oblique and the transversus abdominus, functions to retain the viscera of the abdomen. Contraction of the external oblique lowers the ribs, thereby bringing the thorax closer to the pelvic brim. In this manner, it functions as an accessory muscle of expiration. Unilateral contraction of this muscle causes the opposite hemithorax to depress and rotate toward the side of muscle contraction.

This muscle function can be compromised with the hernias that develop outside of the midline. Such hernias include subcostal incisional hernias, postappendectomy hernias and post-colostomy hernias. Because of the lack of re-approximation of the edges of the hernia defect during the laparoscopic repair, the expiratory function will not resume its function consistent to the efficiency that was present prior to the herniation.

Internal Oblique Muscle

These fibers course beneath that of the external oblique and in an opposite direction. The muscle runs from the pelvic brim upward and medially to the thoracic cage and the linea alba. The function of this muscle is similar to that of the external oblique, however, its unilateral contraction results in rotation and lowering of the thorax on the ipsilateral side of the contraction. Consequently, laparoscopic herniorraphy has a comparable effect on this muscle as that of the external oblique.

Transversus Abdominus Muscle

The innermost muscle layer of the abdominal wall inserts posteriorly on the lower six ribs, the lumbo-dorsal fascia, iliac crest and the iliopsoas fascia. It also inserts on the medial surface of the costal portion of the lower seven or eight ribs and interdigitates with the insertions of the diaphragm. It is a very important component of respiration as it is the main antagonist of the diaphragm. As such, it could be considered a key muscle of expiratory function. It acts in this role by displacing the visceral contents under the diaphragm at the end of the initial stage of diaphragmatic inspiration.

Because of its position within the layers of the abdominal wall, it is also the major component of the containment functions of these muscles. It has a powerful function that provides traction on the abdominal wall. This action results in the tendency of the margins of the laparotomy incision to separate. This act of rapid retraction explains the frequency of dehiscence that occurs with the vertical midline laparotomy incision. It also accounts for the difficulty that is encountered during attempts to provide closure of the midline following dehiscence or the development of midline incisional hernias. The advantage of the laparoscopic herniorraphy and the placement of a prosthetic biomaterial is the elimination of the forces of that muscle that would weaken or destroy a tissue re-approximating type of repair. Conversely, the use of the prosthetic material to bridge the gap within this muscle that is created by the development of a large hernia does little to correct the respiratory function that is lost after such an occurrence. Much is known about the function of the muscles of the abdominal wall prior to the occurrence of a hernia. Few studies have examined the effects of the muscle function after incisions through them or after the development and subsequent repair of the hernias. These are needed to assess the ability of these operations to restore the function of these muscles other than that of the retention of the viscera within the abdomen.

ANATOMY OF A HERNIA

Approximately 90% of non-inguinal hernias of the abdominal wall result from an incision through the aponeurotic layer. The loss of integrity of the transversalis fascia predates its development. Additionally, poor nutritional status, infection, pulmonary disease, steroid usage, or morbid obesity can potentiate the weakening effects of such an incision. Initially, one may not recognize that a hernia has developed as it could take several months for this to become apparent. Sometimes, however, a postoperative incisional infection will be of such severity so as to delineate the fascial defect prior to discharge of the patient from the hospital.

The fascial defect that becomes apparent may be difficult to demarcate by the surgeon. Obesity and incarceration can make this particularly difficult. The muscle layers will be forced aside from the herniation of the preperitoneal tissues or intra-abdominal contents of the hernia. The herniated structures can be preperitoneal fat, omental fat, and/or small or large intestine in most cases. Frequently these organs will be fixed to one another due to adhesions that will have developed after the initial operation. Generally, the more numerous the intra-abdominal operations, the more likely will be the probability of encountering more numerous and denser adhesions. Each additional operative procedure increases these odds.

Most incisional and ventral hernias will be single defects within the fascia. The layers of muscle and fascia will be displaced from the normal position into all directions from the hernia. This results from the traction effects of the flat muscles of the abdomen. In 18-25% of the patients, there will be two or more defects along the incision. In these instances, the muscle will be displaced laterally from the defect but the fascia will be intact between the hernias. This will create one or many "fascial bridges" separating the various hernias. In either situation, the peritoneal surface of the hernia will then be covered with preperitoneal fat (if any exists), subcutaneous fat and the skin of the abdominal wall. In some patients, there may be a lack of any tissue between the hernia sac and the skin. If this is encountered, good judgment will dictate that no energy source, such as electrocautery be utilized in that area during the dissection of adhesions. This will avoid causing necrosis of the compromised skin surface.

There are numerous types of incisions that are used to enter the abdomen, obviously influenced by the intra-abdominal procedure to be performed. Because of this, some patients may have hernia in more than one location. This is not infrequent in the patients that have temporary colostomies placed after perforation of the colon. These are particularly well suited for the laparoscopic approach as both can be repaired simultaneously. A similar situation is seen in the patient that presents with both an incisional and an inguinal hernia(s).

Hernias are also seen following the flank incisions for anterior lumbar interbody fusions and nephrectomies. These are usually not a true defect in the fascia but are the result of denervation of the musculature caused by the incision itself. The flat layer of muscle becomes paralytic. The loss of support gives the patient a broad area of weakness that is unsightly and frequently symptomatic. There is no true fascial defect in the usual case. The "hernia" is due instead to the loss of structural support by the paralyzed musculature.

Finally, the hernias that occur without a premorbid event are known as primary hernias. These include epigastric and umbilical hernias. These can represent 10-20% of abdominal wall hernias in most series (excluding inguinal hernias). These patients, however, will incur a weakness in the transversalis fascia that results in herniation of the intra-abdominal contents. Predisposing factors include low birth weight, steroid usage, pulmonary disease, urological disorders, trauma or obesity. Despite the origin, the concepts in the laparoscopic repair of these hernias are not changed.

Little is known of the function of the abdominal wall once a herniation develops. Of course, the development of a hernia mandates a loss of the retention function of these muscles. It is felt that there is also some compromise of the respiratory function of the flat muscles.

ANATOMIC CONSIDERATIONS IN THE REPAIR OF ABDOMINAL WALL DEFECTS

The goal of any repair of a defect of the abdominal wall is to restore the integrity of the covering of the abdominal contents. The oldest method in which to do so is the sutured technique. This method will approximate the linea alba and attempt to restore the normal architecture of the abdominal wall. It is felt that this will provide the best long-term functional and cosmetic result for the patient. Unfortunately, this method of repair is fraught with a recurrence rate from 25-51% in most centers (1, 2). There are reports, however, that show recurrence rates as low as 5% (3).

The use of a prosthetic biomaterial in the open repair of incisional hernias has reduced the rate of recurrence to 10-25%.(2,4) The manner of placement of this biomaterial can vary widely, however (5). The biomaterial can be placed intraperitoneally, extraperitoneally, below the rectus muscle, above the rectus muscle or above the fascia. Additionally, there are several methods in which to handle the fascial defect itself during the insertion of the prosthesis. Some surgeons will place the mesh at the edge of the fascial defect, others will close the fascial defect before or after the insertion of the mesh (6).

Additionally, the method of fixation of the biomaterial will also vary greatly with the area of the world that this biomaterial is inserted. Indeed, it is very common for the method of fixation to vary within the hospital staff within a single institution. Thus, a comparison of the method of a prosthetic repair of the open incisional hernias can be difficult and inaccurate.

The proponents of the laparoscopic repair of incisional and ventral hernias (LIVH) share the common belief that an effective repair of the defect requires the insertion of a prosthetic biomaterial. Only the very smallest of hernias (less than one cm) are closed with sutures alone; although most series have not mentioned this fact (7). The method of fixation and location of the prosthetic can vary as it does with the open repair. The biomaterial can be placed intraperitoneally, extraperitoneally, or in the retro-rectal position. Most commonly, however, it is placed in the intraperitoneal position. The method of fixation is usually tacks alone or tacks and transfascial sutures. In only one series the literature has an effort been made to close the fascial defect (8). It has not been the practice of the other published reports to close the fascial defect. In fact, little attention has been paid to the necessity of the closure of the linea alba in the laparoscopic herniorraphy of incisional and ventral hernias. It is believed that the repair of the fascial defect will place tension on the repair and offer no improvement in outcome.

The anatomical considerations of the closure of the fascial defect and, in most cases, the linea alba will be the reconstitution of the normal anatomy and function of the anterior abdominal wall. It has not been definitely proven that any long-term benefits will be seen if this is done. Many proponents of the open repair will insist on the approximation of the linea alba. It is felt that this will restore the "respiratory" function of the abdominal wall. This can be done in many but certainly not all cases of a hernia that involves portions of the abdominal wall other than the inguinal and femoral areas. The patients that have hernia defects that are larger than 5 cm^2 will make the fascial closure difficult. In fact, closure of most of these hernias will result in a considerable amount of tension of the repair. The success of both open and laparoscopic herniorraphy depends on the elimination of tension on the tissues. This can only be accomplished, in the majority of patients, with the use of a prosthetic biomaterial. The question of the anatomical modification of the laparoscopic approach becomes moot if acknowledgement of the concept of tension free herniorraphy is applied to every hernia repair.

Is it necessary to re-approximate the edges of the hernia defect? This is the question that has not been answered adequately in the literature. The restitution of the function of the abdominal wall musculature is said to depend on the reconstitution of the flat surfaces of these muscles. Only the open method can do this but even in these patients it is not possible in many cases.

BIOMATERIAL PLACEMENT IN LAPAROSCOPIC HERNIORRAPHY

During the repair of incisional and ventral hernias the prosthesis will usually be placed in the intraperitoneal position. In some areas and in some patients, this may not be the case, but in the majority of published series; the location is within the abdomen. While there is a theoretical risk of patch migration such as has been seen in the open repair, to date, none have been reported with the laparoscopic repair. In only the series mentioned above has the defect within the fascia been closed. The usual operation will simply place the prosthesis under the defect with an overlap of the patch of three cm or more. The biomaterial is then fixed into position and the operation terminates without regard to the re-approximation of the linea alba. Certainly, in hernias that are located in sites not in the midline, the linea alba is not involved in the repair of the hernia. These typically are not of large size and not considered significant in the overall function of the wall of the abdomen. The open repair does provide for the resection of the peritoneal sac. When the sac is not resected, seromas occur very frequently. In some instances, these seromas may require additional procedures to treat them. Fortunately, this is infrequent.

The prosthesis acts as a barrier to the protrusion of the intra-abdominal contents. It does not assume any functional role in the abdominal wall. The muscles of the abdomen will not have any significant change in their own function after the operation. The repair of the hernia, especially the larger ones, will probably improve the function of the flat muscles of the abdomen. There is no supportive data to prove this but one would assume that the elimination of the hernia will paradoxical motion of the hernia and its contents in relation to the normal movements of the abdominal wall.

The method of fixation could potentially impact their function, although this has never been studied. The use of tacks alone in the fixation of the biomaterial will probably not allow the prosthesis to act in tandem with the muscles as would the use of transfascial sutures. The tacks will only penetrate 4-5mm thereby attaching the biomaterial to the posterior layers of the transversus abdominus and possibly the internal oblique muscles. It could be postulated that only the movement of the transversus abdominus muscle will affect the patch attached in this manner.

The fixation of the biomaterial with transfascial sutures will more likely assure that the movement of each of the three layers of muscle of the abdominal wall will impact the prosthesis in some manner. The prosthesis becomes a significant portion of the abdominal wall function once it has been fixed in this manner. I believe that the patch will respond to movement of these muscles and have a greater impact in the function of the wall of the abdomen. However, the sutures will also fix all of the layers of the flat muscles together. This will diminish the independence of each of their function. If the biomaterial is placed in the retro-rectal position, the effects of this fixation will be felt as well. Usually, however, the hernias are smaller and only in the midline if this method is utilized. The same functional result should be seen. More experimental data is needed to evaluate the impact of these issues.

During dissection and at the time of the fixation of the biomaterial there is a risk of injury to the vessels of the abdominal wall. The significant vessels of the abdominal wall are that of the inferior epigastric arteries and veins. These are usually out of harms way with the more traditional repairs of the hernias of the abdomen. Generally, this would be recognized on the operating table and controlled. The most common method of control would be the transfascial placement of sutures similar to that of the fixation of the patch. This will easily and effectively control the hemorrhage. Late hematomas have been described in several series in the literature. One could assume that these represented late development of hemorrhage from these vessels either die to partial tamponade or delayed necrosis of the vessel wall secondary to electrocautery.

The sutures may also impinge the small nerves of the subcutaneous space. This is unavoidable but is has not proven to be a significant complaint following the operation. Most of the pain is probably related to neuroma formation but there are patients that seem to have prolonged pain (1-2%) that may be due to suture constriction. One of the authors (KAL) has had two patients that were relieved of symptoms after laparoscopic incision of the offending sutures. The other (JBF) had to remove several of these laparoscopically placed tacks in patients with chronic pain. These maneuvers resulted in relief of the symptoms, as well.

The type of biomaterial that is used in the LIVH will also impact the functionality of the abdomen. The polypropylene meshes are usually quite stiff and result in a significant amount of cicatrization during the healing process. The contraction of the scar that occurs will result in a firm area of the abdomen at the site of the previous hernia sac and defect. This site will not be pliable in the manner of the normal anatomy. It is not an area that acts in unison with the muscles of the abdomen but instead is an independent site in which the muscles of the abdomen act "around" rather than "with" the biomaterial. The thicker, two-layered Composix® mesh has an even greater effect of solidifying the site of implantation than does the single layer of PPM. In the few patients that I have seen that have had this implanted, the abdominal wall was more "board-like" than flexible.

The ePTFE products result in an organized healing process that more closely resembles that of the normal progression. As a result, the abdominal wall is more likely to act "with" rather than against the patch in the function of the muscles. While this prosthesis is not "stretchable" and does not contract to any significant degree, the softness of the product and the characteristics of the collagen infiltration into the biomaterial allow this to conform more naturally to the abdominal wall. Although it is certainly not as soft as the native tissues and does not function as do they, it is apparent that there is a marked improvement over the comparison of the PPM or polyester biomaterials. Follow-up computerized tomography of the abdomen after this procedure will verify the conformability of the prosthetic biomaterial (Figure 1).

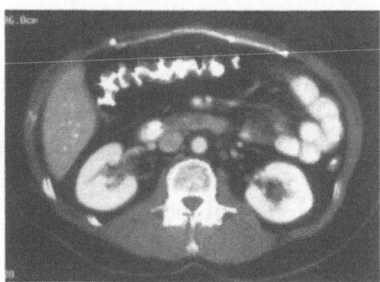

Fig. 1. Follow-up computerized tomography of the abdomen after laparoscopic ventral hernia repair observing the conformability of the prosthetic biomaterial.

MATURATION OF THE HERNIA REPAIR

Once the LIVH is completed, the healing processes will begin. Scar contraction will generally be completed within 90 days. Following this time period, the effects of the biomaterial choice will become apparent. The PPM products can contract as much as 20%, although this process may take place over the ensuing one or two years. In so doing, the original defect will correspondingly contract, which results in a closer re-approximation of the abdominal wall muscles. This could improve the function of these muscles but again the dense scar may actually be more of a detriment to this fact but no studies are available to verify this statement.

The ePTFE biomaterials do not contract to any significant degree if the product has been fixed firmly and circumferentially at the initial operation. It would not be anticipated that the fascial defect should change in size to any significant degree subsequent to the maturation process. In effect, the function of the abdominal wall will be more "matured" at the completion of the LIVH if the ePTFE rather than the other materials is used in the repair. The level of tissue penetration and collagen invasion with other biomaterials such as polypropylene or polyester will be more intense than that seen with the older ePTFE products.

During the healing phase of the patient following the operation, many clinical changes will be seen that are frequently new to the surgeon that has just begun to use this technique. Initially, many patients will not have any noticeable protrusion at the site of the original hernia, particularly if a pressure dressing or abdominal binder is used following the procedure. Many, if not all, patients, however, will develop a seroma at the site of the hernia sac. The size and significance of this varies greatly. It can be worrisome and unsightly, but will usually resolve without intervention.

Following its resolution, the patient will generally have an abdominal wall that is very similar in appearance to the pre-morbid condition prior to the development of the hernia. The cosmetic result in the vast majority of patients will be acceptable to both the surgeon and the patient because of the resumption of a normal contour as perceived by the patient. Most patients will have a lax abdomen due to lack of tone in the muscles of the abdominal wall, particularly in obese individuals. In these individuals, the larger patches will actually result in a "flattened" appearance as compared to the other areas of the abdomen. This is probably related to the support of the abdominal wall that is improved with the prosthetic. In some, the lateral aspects of the abdomen will seem to protrude disproportionately as compared to the midline where the repair was done. These effects are more pronounced with the PPM biomaterials rather than the ePTFE products.

This can be noted more frequently, however, in the thinner individuals because the site of the prior fascial defect could be more easily apparent due to the lack of significant subcutaneous tissue. This is not unsightly but will be noted by the patient. I have not had any patient complain of this result cosmetically or functionally. In some of these patients, if followed for a longer period of time, the abdomen will seem to protrude on either side of the biomaterial. This is due to the relative weakness of the muscles in relation to the strength and lack of distensibility of the prosthesis itself (as noted above). A few patients will need reassurance of this phenomenon. In those individuals, that have a particularly lax abdomen, I prefer to make a note of this to the patient preoperatively so that this can be anticipated.

COSMETIC RESULT

Many surgeons are concerned with the skin that overlies the hernia protrusion. In many cases, this represents a fairly large amount of tissue that is much larger than the defect of the fascia itself. Those patients that have a large amount of redundant skin after the hernia repair may need to wear the binder for a longer period of time. This will help to eliminate the dead space that is created by the repair of the hernia. Despite this effort, however, many will have changes that will take a few months to resolve. Initially, this area will be soft owing to the presence of a seroma in many cases. After a few weeks or months, this will become firmer as a result of the healing processes. The seroma fluid will be absorbed and the scar tissue will replace this fluid. The scar will then contract within several weeks or months. The time frame of these events will be dictated by the size of the hernia at the original operation. The larger eventrations will, of course, take a longer period of time to complete the processes that occur will healing. Generally, however, this will be completed within 90-120 days.

The redundant skin will contract as these events are taking place. Once this is complete, the skin will almost always resume the appearance that it had prior to the development of the hernia. The preperitoneal fat that was scarce preoperatively overlying the hernia sac will sometimes be replaced by new fat. The patch will not be felt underneath the skin and a more normal curve of the abdomen will be seen regardless of the size of the hernia that was repaired. In essence, the cosmetic result will be excellent. In no patient, either in my personal series (KAL) or in those that have been published, has any mention been made as to the need for reconstruction or revision of the skin and subcutaneous tissues overlying the hernia defect after this period of time has transpired.

However, some surgeons believe that the cosmetic result is unacceptable to themselves and their patients. For this reason, the open repair is preferred so that a paniculectomy can be performed at the same time. This is particularly apparent with the very large hernias. In these instances, this may lead the choice toward the open rather than the laparoscopic repair.

FUNCTIONAL RESULT

There is a paucity of information regarding the functional result following the LIVH. The compliance of the abdominal has been noted to change after the repair of incisional and ventral hernias. This seems to be dependent on the type of biomaterial that has been used in the repair of the fascial defect. Because of this fact, there has been a move to decrease the amount of PPM material that is used in the open repair of incisional hernias when repaired with PPM. The effect of this can be shown in the laboratory but the actual clinical significance of this improvement has not been shown conclusively. There is even less data related to the ePTFE products.

It can certainly be said that there is no re-approximation of the fascia or the muscles of the abdominal wall with the LIVH. The long-term effects of this remaining defect in the fascia of these muscles have not been studied. The follow-up of our patients over a long period of time has not revealed a single problem related to this remaining functional defect. I believe that these patients have long before lost the benefit of a normal anatomical functioning abdominal wall. The repair of the single defect does not impact the innate laxity of the "normal" muscles. The development of a hernia in and of itself, alerts the physician to the fact that this patient's fascia has been weakened.

The physiology of the abdominal wall has been studied by many techniques. Because of the expiratory function of these muscles, the importance of the re-approximation of the linea alba has bee demonstrated by several authors. The efforts of relaxing incisions and the lateral placement of prosthetics rather than in the midline during the open repair of incisional hernias are to restore that function. No data is available with this newer procedure.

CONCLUSION

The laparoscopic repair of incisional and ventral hernias requires the use of a prosthetic biomaterial. In all but the smallest of hernias, no tension is placed on the repair. This may explain the decrease in the length of hospitalization of the patients because of diminished levels of pain and ileus. This does not provide for the reconstitution of the normal anatomy of the abdominal wall. In so doing, the expiratory function may be compromised. In no instances, however, has these proven to be a clinical problem. More experimental and clinical studies are needed to accurately assess the actual functionality of the wall of the abdomen following the laparoscopic ventral and incisional herniorraphy.

References

1. Hesselink VJ, Luijendijk RW, deWilt JHW, et al. An evaluation of risk factors in incisional hernia recurrence. Surg Gynecol Obstet 176:228-234, 1993.

2. Luijendijk RW, Hop WCJ, Tol van den P, et al. A Comparison of Suture Repair With Mesh Repair for Incisional Hernia. N Engl J Med 343:392-398, 2000.

3. Herszage, Leon. Personal communication, 2000.

4. Leber GE, Garb JL, Alexander AI, Reed WP. Long-term Complications Associated With Prosthetic Repair of Incisional Hernias. Arch Surg 133:378-382, 1998.

5. Flament JB, Avisse C, Palot JP, Delattre JF. Biomaterials. Principles of implanation. In Incisional Hernia, Ed. Schumpelick V, Kingsnorth, Springer-Verlag, Berlin, 1999.

6. Flament JP, Palot JP, et al. Treatment of major incisional hernias, in Abdominal Wall Hernias, Ed. R. Bendavid. Springer-Verlag, Berlin 2000.

7. LeBlanc KA, Booth WV, Whitaker JM, Bellanger DE. Laparoscopic Incisional and Ventral Herniorraphy in 100 Patients. American Journal of Surgery 180(3):193-197, 2000.

8. Franklin ME, Dorman JP, Glass JL, Balli JE, Gonzales JJ. Laparoscopic Ventral and Incisional Hernia Repair. Surgical Laparoscopy & Endoscopy 8(4):294-299, 1998.

CHAPTER 8

From Open to Laparoscopic Ventral Hernia Repair Placing a Mesh intraperitonally

J.H. Alexandre, K. Aouad, J.L. Bouillot

In order to repair a large ventral hernia, a surgeon must opt for an adapted technique for each individual patient.

A laparoscopic approach is only decided upon after careful analysis of the advantages, the risks and the benefits of the wall repair.

THE AIM OF WALL REPAIR

For a long time it has been our policy (since we decided as members of the GREPA Group to add meshes as reinforcement in large ventral hernia repair) to reconstruct a solid muscular abdominal wall, with excision of the sac, and bring together the anterior and posterior fascias towards the midline (1).

We believe two concepts of wall repair have to be opposed: the anatomical repair, and the "viscera reservoir" repair.

Primarily, the surgeon reconstructs a solid, tonic, anatomical wall, like the original wall. This implies the restitution of pulmonary and diaphragmatic function, and the normal dynamic, the physiological aptitudes of the wall to make the usual efforts, including those of all sports.

To obtain such a result, the muscles need to be replaced in their initial position, principally the rectal muscles. Due to the defect, these muscles laterally and sagitally retracted. They have to be replaced, as RIVES said, together and frontally (2).

In so far as the goal is a functionalist repair, as in the case of large ventral hernias, we consider the concept of a "tension-free operation" as inapplicable and undesirable. We feel it is necessary to remake a wall under tension.

On the other hand, another goal is to cover the defect, without any muscular reconstruction, by the procedure of a meshsutured intraperitonally.

This is always possible, by open or laparoscopic route. Sometimes if there is no alternatative, the procedure is acceptable. For limited defects (i.e. a defect of no more than 10cm), the laparoscopic method is very effective. However, for very large defects it is maladjusted, and the surgeon practises only the "viscera reservoir" repair.

Thus, the surgeon's choice depends on the "quality" of the wall he plans to reconstruct and sometimes on the state of the patient's abdomen, as well as what the surgeon feels is preferable.

As the reader can understand we have also, in the majority of cases, preferred an anatomic repair, because of its functional implications. It has been done in every case by the open route, with the use of a large mesh placed intra or extra-peritonally intra or extra-peritonally .

PAST AND PRESENT REPAIRS: OUR EXPERIENCE 1986-1998

Technique

Before the laparoscopic approach, we preferred using a large, multifixed polyester mesh, placed in the prefascial retromuscular site in order to reconstruct an anatomical wall of each patient. This was not because of the simplicity of the technique, nor because it meant a shorter stay in hospital but due to the physiological quality of the wall.

In the majority of cases of median large hernias, we inserted a very large prothesis fixed from the xyphoid appendix to the Cooper ligaments. The mean size was 15 to 18 cm.

To bring together the rectal muscles and the fascia, we used a median incisional route and excised all the scars, granulomas, and the sac and freed all the viscera.

The posterior transverse sheath was closed from the xyphoïd appendix to the peritoneum, above the umbilical area, freeing the preperitoneal space, exposing the Cooper ligaments.

We always polyfixed by Vicryl sutures using a Polyester Mersuture or Parietex supple mesh behind the rectal muscles.

The closure of the anterior rectal fascia was carried out with a running absorbable suture of N°1 PDS. We frequently used three little vertical incision lines of 15mm, made on the aponeurosis of the anterior sheath.

For parastomal hernias, we always changed the location of the stoma. For the new stoma placement, we reinforced the wall with a polyester mesh (with a hole for the colon), placed between 2 muscular layers (3).

In 42 cases, we selected the intraperitoneal procedure, because of the impossibility to free the rectal sheath, or because an extra peritoneal dissection was too difficult after 1, 2 or more previous operations, or after an infection.

Until 1998, we placed a large ePTFe Goretex Dual mesh intraperitonally: it was fixed laterally on the deep part of the lateral muscles, using multiple non absorbable sutures.

Suction drains were inserted at the anterior surface of the patch.

The anterior flap of the rectal sheath was sutured in front of the patch. Relaxation incisions were made so that midline closure could be achieved. In these cases, an omento-parietal bed was always created with the omentum in order to isolate it from the loops.

During two years, for intraperitoneal procedures, we tested the Parietex-Composite mesh. This polyester material is doubled with a hydrophilic resorbable film placed against the visceras to avoid adhesions.

We did not use blood transfusions.

Patients

Between January 1986 and January 1998, 578 patients were operated on in our Department of Surgery (University Hospital: Paris VI) and 435 received a prosthetic mesh. In this study all the patients had a hernia orifice **larger than 10 cm** (10 – 30 cm or more).

There were 194 men and 241 women with an average age of 61 years (age range 43 – 85).

The location of the incisional hernia was midline in 278 cases, lateral and transversal in 157 cases (39 iliac, 29 subcostal, 22 transversal, 6 lumbar, 18 parastomal, 43 complex hernias: paramedian and other).

In 64 cases, the hernia was operated on for the second time, 11 for the third time, 8 for a fourth time.

For lateral and transversal repairs, mostly large meshes were placed between 2 muscular layers.

Intraperitonal procedures were performed in only 42 cases.

Results

Mortality

Six patients died (1,3%) post operatively during the first twenty days, (2 obese patients by pulmonary embolism, 1 by septic shock, 1 by post-op haemorrhage, 1 by cerebral haemorrhage, 1 by aspiration pneumonia).

We informed the patients, in particular the obese patients, that each surgical procedure for large giant incisional hernias represents an important surgical risk, needs to be studied in regard of the advantages and benefits.

We have been impressed by the absence of death using the laparoscopic procedure.

We believe, therefore,that today laparoscopic repairs are beneficial for certain types of patient, especially the old or obese.

The mortality rate published by the French Association of Surgery was 1.2% (1825 operations). The flament mortality rate was 0.6% (517 operations) (4).

Morbidity

Sixty out of four hundred and thirty-five patients (13%) had various complications.
- 12 infectious complications (8 superficial, 4 deep infections which necessitated the removal of the prosthesis)
- 17 hematomas (14 required evacuation of a superficial hematoma, without infection) Hematomas were found twice in the prosthetic bed, but there was no need to remove the prosthesis.

- 9 seromas (this complication appears more frequently in intra-peritonal procedures).
- 12 pulmonary complications,
- 9 deep vein thrombosis.

We did not observe postoperative enteric fistula, but we never used polyester Mersilène intra-peritonally so as to avoid this. At this site some surgeons described such complications using polypropilene or polyester meshes (Flament, Chevrel) (4).

We did not notice digestive migrations of prosthetic material, as reported in the litterature: they occur more often after intra-abdominal prosthetic placement than after prefascial retromuscular placement (Kaufman 1981, Seelig 1995). The diagnostic can be made by fistulography (Seelig 1995) (5-6).

We did not notice late infections: Amid insisted on the need to differenciate between macroporous and microporous prosthesis, and even between multifilament macroporous prosthesis (7).

For these reasons we always preferred polyester prosthesis.

In our study, no chronic pain was reported postoperatively. We always used supple meshes, never rigid material (such as Marlex). We never used metallic clips, and sutured all our prosthesis by Vicryl sutures.

We did not find any induced cancer.

We did not report any rupture of a polyester prosthesis as experienced by others.

Recurrences

In our study, the follow up was undertaken by a physician for 85% of our patients, during 2 to 9 years and with a mean follow up of 4.3 years.

Seven recurrences (1.6%) were discovered.

The quality of the follow up is very important in hernia repairs, for a statistical evaluation of a technique the patient should be therefore examined by a surgeon.

If the percentage of deaths of patients is above 10%,which was observed in our study, the statistical method of Maximal Bias should be applied.

In our study the definitive result is 4,3% recurrence.

For the French Association of Surgery, the recurrence rate after using a prosthetic repairs was 8.6% (53/326 operations) (4).

Chevrel 's recurrence rate is 5.5% (13/326 operations) by using the prefascial mesh technique.

At the GREPA Meeting in 1986, the same results were published (1% – 5.8%) (4).

Flament (1999) published about 5.6% recurrence rate (27/474 operations) (9).

Authors	Year	N° oper.	Material	Mortality	Morbidity	Recur. %
Adloff	1987	130	Mersilene	1.5		4.5 %
GREPA	1986	326	Mersilene	0	14 %	8.6%
Amid	1998	75	Marlex	0		1.3%
Schumplick	1996	82	Marlex	0	6.8%	6.8%
Flament	1999	474	Mersuture	0	3%	5.6%
Stoppa	1996	554	Mersuture	0	14%	12.7%
Alexandre	1998	393	Mersuture	1.3	13%	4.36%

Morbidity, mortality and recurrence rates by prefascial mesh procedures (10, 11, 12).

Personal considerations

Quality of a repair

What is a "good result" in terms of wall quality ?

It is a difficult question to answer. For us, apart from the usual quality index, the pain score and the quality of life index, two criteria can help evaluation: the clinical examination of the patient (after preoperative classification of the ventral hernia, as practised by Chevrel), and a CT scan.

• *Clinical evaluation*

A clinical evaluation has to be done by the surgeon during the first month, the first year (50% of recurrence appears during the first year); and each year following. In the erect position, the wall has to be flat, without any protrusion, and without any palpable new defect, even when coughing or straining. A pulmonary examination with inspection of the diaphragmatic contraction is also necessary. Lying down, with both legs streched straight in elevation, has to demonstrate a strong wall, without defect or bulging.

• *CT scan*

The CT scan, in our opinion, is the only impartial test. In the "up" position to demonstrate to verify there is no more defect, or a small space between the rectus muscles, and the position of the prosthesis up, down and against the wall. It is easy to analyse with a ePTFe prosthesis which is X ray opaque.

In our experience, the best C.T. quality repair is obtained by the prefascial technique. In the case of the intraperitoneal mesh procedure, even after laparotomy, the prosthesis appears as festooned sticking out of the muscle. Never theless we have seen some excellent prosthetic position after laparoscopic procedures.

We believe that the major reasons for recurrence of ventral hernias is the use of a too small prosthesis or its displacement (after inadequate fixation).

Every default can be observed post-operatively by a C.T. scan, and we ask for one to be done, in each case.

Recent results after laparoscopic intra-abdominal prosthetic repair

To compare the results, we must also compare similar patients (same defect size, same risk factors) according to the same criteria. Between the risk factors the most frequent parameters have been:
- the ASA status,
- the body mass index,
- the BMI, the age (> 70 years),
- a chronic pulmonary disease,
- a coronary artery disease,
- a diabetes mellitus,
- hypertension.

The most frequently evaluated criteria are :
- mortality rate
- morbidity rate
- recurrence rate
- hospital stay
- post op pain index
- quality of repair.

Most of the publications (Heniford, Leblanc, Koehler and Voeler, Chari, Park, Franklin, Nassam) demonstrated that the laparoscopic technique is beneficial with regards to decreased pain, a shorter hospital stay, few bad complications, a low initial recurrence rate, and no mortality (13, 14, 15, 16, 17, 18).
Most of the publications describe limited or umbilical defects, and others all the type and size of defect. The follow up is often insufficient.
Recent publications prove these findings.

Lap-Authors	Year	N° patients	Morbidity %	Recurrence%	H. stay: days
Heniford	2000	100	14%	3%	1.6%
Ramshaw	1999	79	19%	2.5%	1.7%
Carbajo	2000	100	15%	2%	1%
Toy	1998	144	32/144	3.5%	2.3%
Charuzi	1999	53	6%	1%	3.3%
Chowbey	2000	202	32%	1%	1.8%

Morbidity

When comparing open intraperitonal and lap intraperitonal mesh procedure we find that the mortality rate is about the same, 15%. There are more seroma in the lap procedure, and some perforations of the intestine, requiring a conversion.
It seems there is less post-op hematomas by the laparoscopic route.

Hospital stay

The hospital stay appears very short after laparoscopic procedures (1-3 days); Berger (personal communication).
According to our experience, the mean hospital stay is longer after open procedures, but for us, it is 10 days.
In other publications, we see that after open procedure the hospital stay is shorter, 6-8 days, but always superior than by the laparoscopic procedure.
It is an economic advantage.

Recurrence rate

Low recurrence rates represent the first goal in hernia surgery.
All publications on the laparoscopic approach are impressive with their low recurrence rate: 3 - 4%.
However, the follow up is often very short and the details on the hernia defects and the patients are sometimes imprecise and non comparable.

Rawshaw compared two groups operated on using the open or laparoscopic route. In the first group, the size of the defect was larger than in the second. Nevertheless there was a 20.7% recurrence rate in the open group and 2.5% in the laparoscopic group. It is impossible to conclude (14).

In other publications, the patients operated on by laparoscopic surgery presented only limited defects, inferior to 10cm in diameter.

In conclusion, comparing the open technique with that of the laparoscopic; it seems that the recurrence rate is similar, but in the majority of described cases, the defects were limited (less than 15cm).

The global morbidity was a little higher for open the open technique, but induced by a lot of benign seromas and hematomas. We have noticed some perforations of the intestine with a conversion. The significant progress is a short hospital stay of less than 3 days.

THE CHOICE OF THE PROSTHESIS IN INTRAPERITONAL MESH PROCEDURES (19)

With the majority of the authors, we think that ePTFe Dual Mesh, placed intraperitonally, gives a good security rate. Many publications defend this practice using this particular prosthesis by laparoscopic or open procedure (Gillion)(20). In this book, K.A. LeBlanc explains the distinctive qualities of the various materials that are possible to choose for laparoscopic surgery.

After having used ePTFe Goretex Dual-meshes, we can say that we appreciate the solidity, the suppleness and the tolerance of this material, especially against the intestine. Nevertheless, we have noticed its regrettable default; which is the failure of adhesion to the wall and the difficulty to stretch it during the fixation to the wall.

This explains the frequency of the seromas between the wall and the prosthesis and also the possibility of sepsis. In case of sepsis, it is necessary to remove the prosthesis, which, of course is usually very easy.

For this reason; we have experimented with, whether in open and laparoscopic surgery; the placement of a new material: a polyester composite mesh (Parietex – Sofradim).

This prosthesis is able to make strong adhesions with the wall, (which we need), and avoid intestinal adhesions.

We published a multicentric prospective clinical trial (21) using this innovative composite mesh. About 80 patients were operated on; 64% by the open approach and 30% laparoscopally. We have evaluated the anti-adhesive capability of the mesh as regards the viscera ultrasonically.

80% of the patients were ultra-sonically "adhesion free" after 2 months (88% in the laparoscopic group, 77% in the incisional group). Seroma were present in 16%. We did observe post-operative complications relative to adhesions after 1 year.

The advantage of the adhesion to the wall by a porous polyester mesh, and without adhesions with the visceras, has to be evaluated for many years.

CONCLUSION

We have exposed our surgical steps for ventral hernia repair.

Until 1998 we used the intraperitonal approach only in the cases where the pre-fascial procedure was impossible, for anatomical reasons, and when the dissection seemed to be too aggressive for a patient.

Some authors such as Arnauld (10), and others such as Beaulieux, used this open approach with an intra peritonal mesh as a routine.

With our personal new experience in laparoscopic surgery, (in 24 cases), and with the results that we have shown in many publications because of its advantages, we think that there are specific indications for this enthousiastic laparoscopic hernia repair.

For us the laparoscopic approach is indicated in the case of patients with risk factors, (obesity and oldage), and those who don't need a sportive wall, with a defect under 6cm.

We think there are multiple indications in case of an umbilical hernia or a defect not more than 6cm, in the iliac site or in the midline, for patients who do not need an anatomical reconstruction.

We still indicate an open approach for large or giant ventral hernias, in the younger population, and for the patients who hope to recover their initial wall with aesthetic and anatomic implications. We prefer in these conditions, with the risks, a prefascia-mesh technique, because we have major experience with this operation, excellent results and a very low recurrence rate after a good follow up.

We think that the presence of a intraperitonal mesh is not desirable for the young population if it is possible to do differently.

The open procedure placing a mesh intraperitonally is reserved for giant or recurrent ventral hernias.

Laparoscopic repairs for ventral hernias depend, of course, on the experience of the surgeon in laparoscopic surgery.

References

1. Alexandre J-H, Bouillot JL, 1994. Traitement des hernies de la ligne blanche. Med. Chir. Techniques chirurgicales -App. digestif 40-150, 1-6.

2. Rives J, Pire JC, Flament JB, 1885. Le traitement des grandes éventrations. Nouvelles indications thérapeutiques à propos de 322 cas. Chirurgie 111;215-225.

3. Alexandre J-H, Bouillot JL, 1993. Parastomal hernias repair with use of Dacron prosthesis.World J. Surg 17, 680 -682.

4. Chevrel JP, Flament JB,1990. Les éventrations de la paroi abdominale. Rapport présenté au 92ᵉ Congrès Français de Chirurgie. Monographie de l'AFC Paris, Masson.

5. Kaufman Z, Engelgerg M, Zager M. 1981.Fecal fistula a late complication of marlex mesh repair. Dis Colon Rectum 24; 243-244.

6. Scelig M H, Kaprek R, Tietze L, Schumpelick V.1995. Enterocutaneous fistula after Marlex net implantation. A rare complication after incisional Hernia repair. Chirurg 66;739-741.

7. Amid PK. 1997.Classification of biomaterials and their related complications in abdominal wall hernia surgery Hernia 1;15-21.

8. Chevrel JP, Rath AM. 1997. The use of fibrin glues in the surgical treatment of incisional hernias. Hernia 1;19-24.

9. Flament JB, Avisse C, Palot JP, Delattre JF. 2000. Complications in incisional hernia repairs by the placement of a retromuscular prosthesis. Hernia :4 (suppl);S25-S29

10. Adloff M, Arnaud JP.1987. Surgical management of large incisional hernias by an intraperitoneal mersilene mesh and an aponeurotic graft. Surg Gyn Obst 165;204-206

11. Stoppa R, Henry X, Canarelli S. 1979. Les indications des méthodes opératoires sélectionnées dans le traitement des éventrations post-opératoires de la paroi abdominale antérolatérale. Chirurgie ;105;276-286.

12. Stoppa R.1989. The treatment of complicated groin and incisional hernias World J. Surg 13;545-549.

13. Heniford BT, Ramshaw BJ .2000 Laparoscopic ventral hernia repair; a report of 100 consecutive cases. Surg Endosc. May ; 14(5):419-423.

14. Ramshaw BJ, Esartia P, Scwab J, Mason EM, Wilson RA, Duncan TD, Miller J, Lucas GW 1999. Comparison of laparoscopic and open ventral herniorrhaphy. Ann Surg Sept : 65 (9) 827-831.

15. Carbajo MA, Martin del Olmo JC, Blanco JL, De la Cuesta C, Toledano M. 1999 Surg Endosc Mars ; 13(3) ;250-2.

16. Toy FK, Bailey RW, Carey S, Chapuis CW, Gagner M, Joseph LG, Mangiante E C, Park AE, Pomp A, Smoot RT, Uddo JF, Voeller GR. 1998. Prospective multicenter study of laparoscopic ventral hernioplasty. Preliminary results Surg Endosc 1998 Jul ; 12 (7) :955 -9.

17. Kyzer S, Alis M, Alonbi y, Charuzi 1 1999 Laparoscopic repair of post operative ventral hernia. Early post operation results. Surg Endosc Sept ;13(9) ;928-31.

18. Chowbey PK, Sharma A, Khullar R, Mann V, Baijal M, Vashistha A. 2000, Laparoendosc Adv Surg Tech Apr 10;(2)79-84.

19. Alexandre J-H, Aouad, K, Bethoux JP, Bouillot JL. 2000. Recent advances in incisional hernia treatment. Hernia 4. Suppl S1-S2.

20. Gillion JF, Begin GF, Maresco C, Fourtanier G, 1997 Expanded polytetrafluoroethylene patches used in the intra or extra peritoneal position for repair of incisional hernias of the antero lateral abdominal wall. The American J. of Surgery ;Vol 174 ;16-19.

21. Balique JC, Alexandre JH, Arnaud JP, Benchetrit S, Bouillot JL, Fagniez PL, Flament JB, Gouillat C, Jarsaillon P, Lepère M, Magne E, Mantion G. 2000. Intra peritoneal treatment of incisional and umbilical hernias: intermediate results of a multicenter prospective clinical trial using an innovative composite mesh; Hernia, 4 Supl, S10-S16.

CHAPTER 9

Evolution of Laparoscopic Ventral Hernia Repair

K.A. LeBlanc

The concept of the posterior repair of abdominal wall hernias had its earliest beginnings in 1871 when Marcy (1) noted that the closure of the internal inguinal ring could accomplish the repair of an indirect inguinal hernia. He later reported the intra-abdominal approach of this repair during a laparotomy for another purpose (2). One year earlier, Tait described the use of a laparotomy to repair inguinal hernias (3). These repairs all approached the inguinal floor from inside the abdominal cavity. Because of the morbidity of this approach to this problem, the interest in this method of repair was never very great.

In 1920, Cheatle described a newer type of approach that utilized the preperitoneal space to perform the operation (4). This repair was rediscovered in the latter part of this century as an effective method of herniorraphy (5). Rignault (6), Nyhus (7), Stoppa (8), and Wantz (9) showed the benefits of this repair using a prosthetic biomaterial. These surgeons did not have the availability of the laparoscopic methodology at that time to investigate this method of access to the abdominal or preperitoneal spaces. The results that they achieved with the use of a giant prosthetic to repair the visceral sac was impressive.

The first report of the use of the laparoscope in the repair of an abdominal hernia was made by Ger in 1982 (10). He reported a series of thirteen patients in which he closed the peritoneal opening of the sac using Michel clips. All but the last patient in this series was repaired through an open incision. The thirteenth patient was repaired in 1979 under laparoscopic guidance with a special stapling device. The three-year follow-up of that patient revealed him to be free of an identifiable recurrence. Ger continued his efforts to repair these hernias laparoscopically. He reported the closure of the neck of the hernia sac using a prototypical instrument called the "Herniostat" in beagle dogs (11). The results in these models appeared to be promising. In that same article, he reported the potential benefits of the laparoscopic approach to groin hernia repair as: 1) creation of puncture wounds rather than formal incisions, 2) need for minimal dissection, 3) less danger of spermatic cord injury and less risk of ischemic orchitis, 4) minimal risk of bladder injury, 5) decreased incidence of neuralgias, 6) possibility of an outpatient procedure, 7) ability to achieve the highest possible ligation of the hernial sac, 8) minimal postoperative discomfort and a faster recovery time, 9) ability to perform simultaneous diagnostic laparoscopy, and 10) ability to diagnose and treat bilateral inguinal hernias. These potential advantages and advances in the laparoscopic repair of hernias continue to be the recognized goals that each method is attempting to achieve. Subsequent to the publication of his article, the majority of inguinal hernia repairs are being repaired on an outpatient basis.

Bogojavalensky, a gynecologist, presented the first known use of a prosthetic biomaterial in the laparoscopic repair of inguinal and femoral hernias in 1989 (12). He placed a roll of polypropylene mesh into indirect hernias of female patients. The neck of the internal inguinal ring was then closed with sutures. Popp repaired a coincidental direct hernia that was found at the time of a uterine myomectomy. He recognized the need to provide coverage of a wider area than that of the defect itself. To accomplish this, he placed a 4 x 5-cm oval dehydrated dura mater patch over the defect. This was secured to the peritoneum with catgut sutures that were tied extracorporeally. Popp expressed concerns that the intra-abdominal repair of inguinal hernia could lead to adhesive complications and suggested that a preperitoneal approach might be preferable (13).

Schultz published the first patient series of laparoscopic herniorraphy (14) in 1990. Rolls of polypropylene were stuffed into the hernial orifice, which was then covered by two or three flat sheets of polypropylene mesh (2.5 x 5 cm) over the defect. These rolls of mesh were not secured to either the fascia or peritoneum. The peritoneum, however, was closed using clips. This probably represents the earliest attempt at a type of transabdominal preperitoneal (TAPP) repair that is commonly used today. Corbitt (15) modified this technique by inverting the hernia sac and performing a high ligation with sutures or with an endoscopic stapling device. The initial reports above were promising but longer follow-up revealed recurrence rates that were 15-20% (16). This unacceptably high rate of recurrence forced the quick abandonment of these techniques.

The lack of extensive dissection with the above methods, however, remained appealing. A similar concept was applied in the intraperitoneal onlay patch (IPOM) technique. This repair, investigated by Salerno, Fitzgibbons and Filipi (17), used a polypropylene patch material in a porcine model. They placed rectangular pieces of the prosthesis against the abdominal wall covering the internal inguinal ring and secured it with a stapling device. The success of these repairs led them to apply this method in clinical trials.

At about the same time, Toy and Smoot (18) reported upon their first ten patients that were repaired with the IPOM technique. They secured an expanded polytetrafluoroethylene patch (ePTFE) to the inguinal floor with staples that were introduced by a prototypical-stapling device of their own design. Their stapler was called the "Nanticoke Hernia Stapler" (Fig. 1, chapter 15). They successfully used this fixation device in 20-30 patients without adverse results. A subsequent report of their first 75 patients was published in 1992 (19). In this later series, the same prosthetic biomaterial (7.5cm x 10cm) was attached with the Endopath EMS® stapler. After a follow-up of up to 20 months, the recurrence rate was 2.4%. They noted a significant decrease in postoperative pain and an earlier return to normal activity as compared to the open repair of the hernia defect. Others reported similar results (20, 21, 22).

Fitzgibbons (23) later abandoned the IPOM repair except for simple indirect inguinal hernias. One patient developed a postoperative scrotal abscess that may or may not have been related to the placement of the mesh in that position. This patient was noted to have firm attachment of the appendix to the site of the polypropylene mesh. He also noted that, in follow-up of these patients, the patch material could be pulled into the hernial defect because it was affixed to the peritoneum alone rather than fascia. He felt that the transabdominal preperitoneal (TAPP) approach, which had also been reported by Arregui (24) for the other types of groin hernias, was more appropriate. In this repair, the peritoneum is incised and dissected away from the transversalis fascia to expose the inguinal floor. The mesh material is then secured to that fascia which was believed to ensure superior fixation and tissue ingrowth. This, as did the IPOM method, required the entry into the abdominal cavity.

Popp (25) described a method to dissect the peritoneum away from the abdominal wall prior to the incision of the peritoneum in the TAPP repair. Saline was inserted into the preperitoneal space via a transcutaneous syringe. This "aquadissection" was found to be helpful in the dissection of this area to allow for "working room". This early concept probably led to the idea that the entire dissection could be accomplished from within the preperitoneal space, thereby eliminating the need to enter the abdominal cavity.

Other operations that were attempted at that time included the "ring-plasty" and a preperitoneal iliopubic tract repair. The former method was a sutured repair that approximated the deep structures of the lateral iliopubic tract to the proximal arching musculotendinous fibers of the transversus abdominis muscle. (20,26) The latter technique was also a "tissue" repair but secured the iliopubic tract to the transversus abdominis muscle (27, 28). This repair incorporated the use of an inlay of a prosthetic material but still had the disadvantage of being a repair under tension.

As the technique of laparoscopic inguinal herniorraphy matured, the predominant method that was used to accomplish this task was the TAPP repair using either a polypropylene mesh (16, 29) or an expanded polytetrafluoroethylene material (30). Arregui (31) and Phillips (32) introduced a technique that did not utilize a peritoneal incision in the repair of the inguinal floor. The dissection of the preperitoneal space was accomplished under direct visualization of the area via a laparoscope placed into the abdominal cavity. The laparoscope was then moved into the newly dissected preperitoneal space to complete the repair. Dulucq (33, 34) was the first surgeon to perform the laparoscopic repair of the inguinal hernia without any direct entry into the abdominal cavity. Ferzli (35) and McKernan (36) later popularized this technique. Using the "open" entry into the preperitoneal space, the dissection of the space was carried out under direct visualization. The completed totally extraperitoneal (TEP) repair was identical to that of the TAPP but decreased the risk of injury to the intra-abdominal organs.

Currently, the majority of laparoscopic inguinal hernia repairs are approached by either the TAPP or TEP method and utilize a polypropylene mesh biomaterial. The majority of the surgeons that perform the TEP repair utilize the commercially available dissection balloons to create the space within the preperitoneal area to perform the repair.

In a recent report (37), the recurrence rate of these repairs was 0.4% in 10,053 repairs with a median follow up of 36 months. The surgeons that continue to perform the laparoscopic herniorraphy believe that the goals that were anticipated by Ger (11) have been realized.

The improvement in recovery in the laparoscopic cholecystectomy and herniorraphy patients led us to attempt the repair of the ventral and incisional hernias in 1991 (38). This initial report involved only five patients using an ePTFE patch biomaterial. The quick recovery and the safety of the procedure were encouraging. At that time we believed that an overlap of the hernia defect by the prosthesis of 1.5-2cm was adequate. Despite these shortcomings, these patients were free of recurrence after seven years of follow-up. The fixation used was that of the "box-type" of hernia stapler without the use of sutures. Interestingly, we used sutures to aid in the positioning of the patch but then cut these out at the end of the procedure. With further patients and follow-up, no recurrences were noted (39, 40). The use of the ePTFE prosthetic is believed by this author to be the preferential biomaterial because of its in-growth characteristics and its ability to diminish the development of intra-abdominal adhesions (41). Barie (42) proposed the use of a polyester material covered on the visceral side with a mesh of absorbable polyglactin.

Park (43) modified our technique for the repair of large ventral hernias by utilizing the transfascial fixation of the ePTFE or Prolene® mesh with transabdominally placed Prolene® sutures passed through a Keith needle. In their series of thirty cases, only one recurrence was noted. This repair used a fascial overlap of 2cm. Holzman (44) placed a Marlex® prostheses with a 4cm. overlap onto normal fascial edges and secured them with an endoscopic stapler. He found this technique to be safe and effective. In separate investigations, Holzman (47) and Park (45) found that the laparoscopic repair took longer to accomplish but was associated with fewer postoperative complications and a shorter hospital stay. The largest study published to date confirms that the laparoscopic repair of incisional and ventral hernias can be accomplished with reproducibility and with excellent results (46). Additionally, the long-term follow up of patients has proven that this is a durable procedure when the tenets that are noted below are followed (47).

Currently, it is felt that a minimum of a 3cm. overlap is required for an adequate repair. The biomaterial is preferably fixed to the abdominal wall with both transfascial sutures and the helical tacks. The size of the biomaterial and the method of fixation are the paramount concerns to a successful hernia repair. The recurrence rate declines with better fixation methods as shown by the use of staples alone (13%), helical tacks alone (13%), or tacks with transabdominal sutures (0%) (47). Based on our ongoing experience, I believe that this procedure requires three essential ingredients for success. These are: 1) a minimum prosthetic overlap of 3cm; 2) helical tacks placed 1-1.5cm intervals; and 3) transfascial sutures placed at 5cm intervals.

Others, however, do not share this view. Some surgeons, notably in Spain, prefer the use of the "double crown" technique (48, 49). In this technique no sutures are used. Instead, two rows of helical tacks are placed. One at the periphery of the biomaterial as in the sutured technique and the second, inside of this one, near the hernia defect itself. The initial reports seem to have similar results as that of the authors using the transfascial sutures but only a longer interval of follow-up will prove or disprove of either one or both of these approaches is best.

In a careful review of the literature, the biomaterial that is selected for this procedure in 75% of the patients is that of the ePTFE. The latest form is that of the dual sided material that had a very rough "corduroy-like" surface. This has superior in-growth characteristics to that of the original product. Other authors have generally used a polypropylene biomaterial (50) or have used polypropylene and then covered this with ePTFE (51). The majority of surgeons continue to hold the belief that the bowel should not come into contact with either a polypropylene or polyester biomaterial for fear of the complications such as fistula formation, etc. (52). Other prosthetic biomaterials are undergoing development for the use with this procedure.

CONCLUSION

The history of open inguinal hernia repair spans many centuries. The use of the laparoscope in the repair of inguinal hernias has been proven to be effective and represents another method to approach this entity. The laparoscopic repair of incisional and ventral hernias can only be considered in its infancy, if the past is revisited. In experienced hands, the recurrence rate is significantly better than that of the open repair with or without a prosthetic biomaterial. The complication is low and, in many cases, lowers rate than the open technique. The operative times may or may not be faster but the cost of the procedure is lower when performed laparoscopically because of the diminution in the length of hospitalization of these patients. Longer follow up of the variations of this repair as well as the development of innovative technology, newer biomaterials and the adoption of this procedure by the of the world will provide us with the chance to be a part of the history of this operation.

References

1. Marcy HO. A new use of carbolized catgut ligatures. Boston Med Surg J 85:315-316, 1871.
2. Marcy HO. The Anatomy and Surgical Treatment of Hernia. New York: D. Appleton & Co., 1892.
3. Tait L. A discussion of treatment of hernia by medial abdominal section. Br Med J (Clin Res) 1891;2:685.
4. Cheatle GL. An operation for the radical cure of inguinal and femoral hernia. Br Med J 1920;2:68-69.

5. Nyhus LM Preperitoneal herniorraphy. Western J Surg, Obstret and Gynec 1959;7:48-54.

6. Rignault DP. Preperitoneal prosthetic inguinal herniorraphy through a Pfannennestiel approach. Surg Gynecol Obstet 1986;162:465.

7. Nyhus LM, Pollak R, Bombeck TC, Donahue PE. The preperitoneal approach and prosthetic buttress repair of recurrent hernia. Ann Surg 1988;208:722-727.

8. Stoppa RE, Warlaumont CR. The preperitoneal approach and prosthetic repair of groin hernia. In: Nyhus LM, Condon RE, Eds. Hernia. Philadelphia, PA: JP Lipponcott, 1989;199-225.

9. Wantz GE. Prosthetic repair groin hernioplasties. In: Atlas of Hernia Surgery. New York, Raven Press, 1991;101-151.

10. Ger R. The management of certain abdominal herniae by intra-abdominal closure of the neck of the sac. Ann R Coll Surg Engl 1982; 64:342.-344.

11. Ger R, Monro K, Duvivier R, et al. Management of Inguinal Hernias by Laparoscopic Closure of the Neck of the Sac. Am J Surg 1990;159:370-373.

12. Bogojavalensky S. Laparoscopic treatment of inguinal and femoral hernia (video presentation). 18th Annual Meeting of the American Association of Gynecological Laparoscopists. Washington, DC, 1989.

13. Popp LW. Endoscopic patch repair of inguinal hernia in a female patient. Surg Endosc 1990;5:10-12.

14. Schultz L, Graber J, Pietrafitta J, et al. Laser laparoscopic herniorraphy: a clinical trial, preliminary results. J Laparoendosc Surg 1990;1:41-45.

15. Corbitt J. Laparoscopic herniorraphy. Surg Laparosc Endosc 1991;1:23-25.

16. Corbitt J. Laparoscopic herniorraphy: A preperitoneal tension-free approach. Surg Endosc 1993;7:550-555.

17. Salerno GM, Fitzgibbons RJ, Filipi C. Laparoscopic inguinal hernia repair. In Zucker KA, Ed. Surgical Laparoscopy. St. Louis: Quality Medical Publishing, 1991;281-293.

18. Toy FK, Smoot RT. Toy-Smoot laparoscopic hernioplasty. Surg Laparosc Endosc 1991;1:151-155.

19. Toy FK, Smoot RT. Laparoscopic Hernioplasty Update. 1992;2(5):197-205.

20. Spaw AT, Ennis BW, Spaw LP. Laparoscopic hernia repair: The anatomical basis. J Laparonedosc Surg 1991;1:269-277.

21. LeBlanc KA, Booth WV. Avoiding Complications with Laparoscopic Herniorraphy. Surg Laparosc Endosc 1993;3(5):420-424.

22. LeBlanc KA, Spaw AT, Booth WV. Inguinal herniorraphy using intraperitoneal placement of an expanded polytetrafluoroethylene patch. In Arregui ME, Nagan RF,Eds. Inguinal hernia:advances of controversies? Oxford: Radcliffe Medical Press 1994:437-439.

23. Fitzgibbons RP. Laparoscopic Inguinal Hernia Repair. In Zucker KA, Ed., Surgical Laparoscopy Update, St. Louis, Quality Medical Publishing. 1993;373-934.

24. Arregui ME. Preperitoneal repair of direct inguinal hernia with mesh. Presented at Advanced Laparoscopic Surgery: The International Experience. Indianapolis, Ind.: May 20-22, 1991.

25. Popp LW. Improvement in Endoscopic Hernioplasty: Transcutaneous Aquadissection of the Musculofascial Defect and Preperitoneal Endoscopic Patch Repair. J Laparoendosc Surg 1991;1(2):83-90.

26. Dion YM, Morin J. Laparoscopic inguinal herniorraphy. Can J Surg 1992;35:209-212.

27. Gazayerli MM. Anatomic laparoscopic repair of direct or indirect hernias using the transversalis fascia and iliopubic tract. Surg Laparosc Endosc 1992;2:49-52.

28. Gazayerli MM, Arregui ME, Helmy HS. Alternative technique: Laparoscopic iliopubic tract (IPTR) inguinal hernia repair with inlay buttress of polypropylene mesh. In Ballabtyne GH, Leahy PF, Modlin IR, EDS. Laparoscopic Surgery. Philadelphia, WB Saunders 1993.

29. Kavic MS. Laparoscopic hernia repair. Surg Endosc 1993;7:163-167.

30. Campos L, Sipes E. Laparoscopic Hernia Repair: Use of a fenestrated PTFE Graft with Endo-Clips. Surg Laparosc Endosc 1993;3(1):35-38.

31. Arregui ME, Navarrette J, Davis CJ, et al. Laparoscopic Inguinal Herniorraphy: Techniques and Controversies. Surg Clin N Am 1993;73(3):513-527.

32. Phillips EH, Carroll BJ, Fallas MJ. Laparoscopic preperitoneal inguinal hernia repair without peritoneal incision: technique and early clinical results.
Surg Endosc 1993;7:159-162.

33. Dulucq JL. Treatment of inguinal hernia by insertion of a subperitoneal patch under preperitoneoscopy. Chirurgie 1992;118(1-2):83-85.

34. Dulucq JL. Treatment of Inguinal Hernias by Insertion of Mesh through Retroperitoneoscopy. Post Grad Surg 1992;4(2):173-174.

35. Ferzli GS, Massad A, Albert P. Extraperitoneal Endoscopic Inguinal Hernia Repair. J Laparoendosc Surg 1992;2(6):281-286.

36. McKernan JB, Laws HL. Laparoscopic repair of inguinal hernias using a totally extraperitoneal prosthetic approach. Surg Endosc 1993;7:26-28.

37. Felix E, Scott S, Crafton B, et al. Causes of recurrence after laparoscopic hernioplasty. Surg Endosc 1998;12:226-231.

38. LeBlanc KA, Booth WV. Laparoscopic repair of incisional abdominal hernias using expanded polytetrafluoroethylene: preliminary findings. Surg Laparosc Endo 1993;3(1):39-41.

39. LeBlanc KA, Booth WV, Spaw AT. Laparoscopic ventral herniorraphy using and intraperitoneal onlay patch of expanded polytetrafluoroethylene. In Arregui ME, Nagan RF. Eds. Inguinal hernia: advances or controversies? Oxford: Radcliffe Medical Press;1994;501-510.

40. LeBlanc KA, Booth WV, Whitaker JM. Laparoscopic Repair of Ventral Hernias Using an Intraperitoneal Onlay Patch: Report of Current Results.
Contemp Surg 1994;45(4):211-214.

41. LeBlanc KA. Two-phase in vivo comparison studies of the tissue response to polypropylene, polyester, and expanded polytetrafluoroethylene grafts used in the repair of abdominal wall defects. In Treuter KH, Schumpelick, Eds. Peritoneal Adhesions, Berlin Springer-Verlag;1997:352-362.

42. Barie PS, Mack CA, Thompson WA. A Technique for Laparoscopic Repair of Herniation of the Anterior Abdominal Wall Using a Composite Mesh Prosthesis. Am J Surg 1995;170:62-63.

43. Park A, Gagner M, Pomp A. Laparoscopic Repair of Large Incisional Hernias. Surg Laparosc Endosc 1996;6(2):123-128.

44. Holzman MD, Parut CM, Reintgen K, et al. Laparoscopic ventral and incisional hernioplasty. 1997;11:32-35.

45. Park A, Birch DW, Lovrics P et al. Laparoscopic and open incisional hernia repair: A comparison study. Surgery 1998;124:816-822.

46. Heniford BT, Park A, Ramshaw BJ, Voeller G. Laparoscopic Ventral and Incisional Hernia Repair in 407 Patients. Journal of the American College of Surgeons 2000;190(6): 645-650.

47. LeBlanc KA, Booth WV, Whitaker JA, Bellanger DE. Laparoscopic Incisional and Ventral Herniorraphy: Our Initial 100 Patients. Am J Surg 180(3): 193-197, 2000.

48. Carbajo MA, Martin del Olmo JC, Blanco JI, de la Cuesta C, Martin F, Toledano M, Perna C, Vaquero C. Laparoscopic Treatment of Ventral Abdominal Wall Hernias: Preliminary Results in 100 Patients. Journal of the Society of Laparoendoscopic Surgeons 2000;4:141-145.

49. Morales-Conde S, Martin-Gomez M, Cadet H, Morales-Méndez S. Laparoscopic ventral hernia without sutures: Double Crown technique. Surg Endosc (in press).

50. Franklin ME, Dorman JP, Glass JL, Balli JE, Gonzales JJ. Laparoscopic Ventral and Incisional Hernia Repair. Surgical Laparoscopy & Endoscopy 1998;8(4):294-299, 1998.

51.Farrakha M. Laparoscopic treatment of ventral hernia. Surgical Endoscopy 2000;14:1156-1158.

52.Leber GE, Garb JL, Alexander AI, Reed WP. Long-term Complications Associated With Prosthetic Repair of Incisional Hernias. Arch Surg 1998;133:378-382.

CHAPTER 10

Controversies of Laparoscopic Ventral Hernia Repair: A Review of the Literature

H.S. Pollinger, K.L. Harold, B.D. Matthews, B.T. Heniford

Ventral hernia repair has been the topic of great debate over the past two decades. The use of prosthetic material in the repair of incisional hernias has clearly been shown to be superior to primary repair (1). The issue of recurrence was definitively addressed by Luijendijk, et al., and shown to be 4-24% when mesh was utilized vs. 24-50% with primary repair (1).

During the evolution of ventral hernia repair, Rives and Stoppa eloquently demonstrated the importance of utilizing the potential space posterior to the rectus muscle and anterior to the peritoneum for the placement of prosthetic material (2, 3). This anatomic location was more physiologic. It allowed for adequate dissipation of abdominal wall forces, as well as protection of the prosthetic material from the peritoneal cavity. Despite the decreased recurrence rates associated with this technique, it has a significant risk of morbidity. The extensive dissection required for the creation of the tissue flaps has a 20% wound complication rate and often requires re-operation (2). This type of surgical repair often requires drain placement and involves a lengthy hospital stay (3).

Laparoscopic incisional hernia repair has evolved to be feasible and safe. It has been shown to be as effective as the time-tested open repair (4). There is a lower recurrence rate when incisional hernias are repaired laparoscopically (21, 25). One possible explanation for this is that the laparoscopic vantage point allows the operator to assess the entire abdominal wall. Small defects, which can be missed with the open approach, can be easily visualized with the laparoscope (10). The laparoscopic approach has been shown to be cost effective. This is due in part to the lower recurrence rates, and reduced incidence of complications (21). Health care costs are potentially reduced due to shorter length of stay. Average length of stay has been reported to be 1.4 to 1.8 days (14).

Despite the excellent preliminary results of laparoscopic ventral hernia repair, there are numerous controversies which are associated with this operation. The primary aim of this chapter is to address many of these issues, and provide data surrounding the debated topics.

PATIENT SELECTION: SEVERAL FACTORS

A debate often arises when it comes to the size of the ventral hernia defect which should be repaired with mesh. The consensus in the literature states that any defect greater that 4 cm. should be repaired with mesh (6, 7). It has also been suggested that hernias smaller than 4 cm. should be considered for repair with prosthetic material as well (1, 3). Two specific clinical situations when this holds true are for recurrent hernias and hernias in the obese patient (5, 6, 8). Large hernias can also be approached laparoscopically with no specific size as being too big (6, 14, 21). As the operator becomes more familiar with the technique, even the most complicated hernias such as incarcerated or multiply recurrent hernias can be repaired successfully with the laparoscopic approach.

Any patient who can tolerate general endotracheal anesthesia and pneumo-peritoneum is a candidate for the laparoscopic technique. Contraindications to laparoscopic ventral hernia repair would include pregnant patients, children, and patients with intra-abdominal sepsis (6, 9, 14). The youngest patient in whom a laparoscopic ventral hernia repair has been preformed was 13 years of age (6). No data is available concerning the use of this technique in children. For patients with a limited life expectancy, or who are extremely debilitated, ventral hernia repair could be associated with more morbidity than the hernia defect itself (10). Portal hypertension is a relative contraindication to laparoscopic ventral hernia repair, although it has been reported (10). The prolonged pneumoperitoneum has the potential to decrease liver function in the face limited hepatic reserve. Overall, laparoscopic ventral hernia repair is safe, with few contraindications. It can be recommended with confidence in most patients (7, 11, 12).

Preoperative imaging studies

It is controversial whether pre-operative radiographs are needed for any hernia repair. There has been a suggestion that imaging studies might be helpful in patients with recurrent hernias and hernias in unusual anatomic locations (10). Having a "road-map" preoperatively can aid with decision making, such as the best way to access the reoperative abdomen, or to determine the location of the bladder, iliac crest, or other important structures relative to a hernia defect. Likewise, it is essential to know the anatomic relationship between the kidney and ureter when planning a lumbar hernia repair (13).

Patient preparation

The rate of prosthetic infection in laparoscopic ventral hernia repair is extremely low, however the morbidity associated with this complication can be devastating.

Due to the extremely low rate of infection (approximately 1%), it is controversial as to whether measures to avoid skin contamination should be implemented beyond a betadyne skin prep (10). An additional step that be taken is to cover the entire ventral skin surface with a bio-drape material. Using an iodophor impregnated plastic adhesive drape has been shown to reduce wound contamination from 15% to 1.6% in open surgery (15). There is no evidence that prevents or reduces mesh infection in laparoscopy, but it will protect the mesh from the skin. Pre-operative antibiotics also help decrease wound or mesh infection. A first generation cephalosporin is typically administered intravenously prior to the skin incision. For obese patients, 2 grams of the cephalosporin is chosen to attain adequate blood levels. Patients often receive antibiotics every 2 hours throughout the duration of the operation when a prosthetic is being inserted. Again, little or no scientific data is available concerning the need for peri-operative antibiotics in laparoscopic operations.

Establishing pneumoperitoneum

Accessing the reoperative abdomen can be challenging for even the most experienced laparoscopic surgeon. The two most common techniques are the open, "Hasson" technique and the Veress needle approach. Neither technique has been proven to be better or safer than the other. The operator's experience with the particular access technique is the most important factor associated with its safety.

A controlled muscle-splitting technique using "S"-shaped Hasson retractors was utilized in one report more than three-hundred times with no reported visceral injury to date (6). The entry site chosen was high and lateral in the abdomen at the right or left costal margin. This open approach utilizes a 1.0-1.5cm muscle splitting incision using the retractors to separate each muscle and fascial layer. Once the peritoneum is incised, a balloon-tipped Hasson trocar can easily be inserted into the peritoneal cavity. A benefit of the balloon-tipped trocar is that it helps to maintain pneumoperitoneum through the larger incision.

The alternative technique is to use the Veress needle to establish pneumoperitoenum. Again, the left or right upper quadrants are the most common entry site. After establishing pneumoperitoneum, a "see-through" or optical trocar, where a laparoscope can be placed into the trocar, is used to allow direct visualization of its placement (10). A advantage of the Veress approach is that it allows the operator to easily change the site of the initial port placement if the abdominal contour is drastically modified by pneumoperitoneum (19, 10). This technique requires good judgement and experience.

Adhesiolysis

Lysis of adhesions is considered to be the most dangerous and rate limiting aspect of laparoscopic ventral hernia repair (12). The incidence of enterotomy during laparoscopic ventral hernia repair has been reported to be 1% to 6%.(14,16,17) Minimal use of energy sources during adhesiolysis has been advocated to avoid bowel injury (6, 10, 17, 19, 21). If the surgeon is familiar with, and recognizes the correct tissue planes when taking down adhesions, energy sources are often not needed. If bleeding is encountered in an area around the intestine or a questionable area, hemoclips can be employed which will control most bleeding sources. In the instance when the intestine is out of the field, electrocautery at low wattage or an ultrasonic shears can be used to stop oozing tissue.

Ultrasonic energy has been proposed as an effective modality for adhesiolysis in laparosopic ventral hernia repair. Some believe that if this alternative energy source, if used carefully, can be a true asset during adhesiolysis. A benefit of the ultrasonic scalpel is its ability to take down adhesions as well as seal small vessels simultaneously, limiting thermal spread to about 3mm (22). Also, many believe that tissue planes separate ahead of the blade of the ultrasonic energy source due to the gas released from the transected tissues, allowing for visualization of the tissue plane before it is dissected (23). However, when injury does occur with this device, the edges of the viscera can be sealed without bleeding, due to the lack of bleeding or the extravasation of intestinal contents. These injuries can go unrecognized, only to result in disaster postoperatively. By incorporating angled scopes and countertraction with the non-dominant hand on the anterior abdominal wall, even the most difficult adhesions can be taken down with minimal use of alternative energy sources (6).

Reapproxiamtion of mid-line fascia

Laparoscopic surgeons are often criticized by their colleagues who perform open ventral hernia repair exclusively because the posterior sheath can not be reapproximated laparoscopically. Wantz has stated that when closing a parietal defect, the hernia repair should restore normal function of the abdominal wall and normal intraabdominal pressure by reattaching in the midline the tendons of the retracted lateral abdominal muscles (24). It should be addressed that in the open Rives-Stoppa-Wantz repair, it is commonplace for the midline not to be reapproximated due to the large size of the defect. Second, in the largest published series of laparoscopic ventral hernia repairs (407 patients) it was shown that the average size of the defect exceeded 100 cm^2, with the largest fascial defect measuring 480 cm^2 (6). With anatomic defects this size, it is physically impossible to reapproximate the mid-line.

Laparoscopic repair has been definitively shown to have a low recurrence rate, despite the fact that the mid-line is not reapproxiamated (18). In fact, Heniford et al. reported a recurrence rate of 3.4% in a series of 407 patients, with a mean follow-up of 23 months and a range of up to 5 years (6). Conversely, the recurrence rate has been reported to be higher in most open series even when the mid-line is reapproximated (2, 3).

Mesh fixation

The technique used to fix the mesh to the abdominal wall in laparoscopic ventral hernia repair has engendered much controversy. Debate has centered around the need for trans-abdominal sutures, in addition to staple or tack fixation. Given that most mesh materials are 1mm thick and tacking devices only purchase 4mm, the maximum penetration into the peritoneum and posterior abdominal wall is only 3mm. Many surgeons have stressed the need for suture fixation to prevent the migration of the mesh into the defect with a subsequent recurrence.

As evidence for full thickness, trans-abdominal sutures surrounding the mesh prosthesis, several reports have demonstrated a substantially increased recurrence rate when they were not employed (6, 8, 11, 14, 19, 21). In a series by LeBlanc et al., it was reported that the recurrence rate was 13% when the tacking device was used as the sole fixation technique, compared to no recurrences when sutures were added (14). Heniford et al, confirmed these results in their series, reporting 14 recurrences out of 407 patients, with 6 of the 14 occurring in patients when no sutures were used in the repair (6). It has been suggested that placement of non-absorbable sutures should be spaced 4 to 5 cm. apart (6, 10). Placement at more frequent intervals is sometimes necessary with large defects to prevent the mesh from pulling loose when the tissue at the defect edge is poor.

Alternatively, some surgeons believe that the use of a tacking device alone is sufficient to secure the mesh to the abdominal wall (16). Carbajo and colleagues randomized 60 patients into two groups over a 3-year period. Thirty patients underwent open repair of their ventral hernia, and the remaining 30 were operated on laparoscopically. Within the laparoscopic cohort, the first 18 patients had the mesh secured with trans-abdominal suture and 5 mm helicoidal tacks. Mesh fixation in the last 12 patients was done exclusively with the helicoidal tacking device (16). The authors were able to obtain equivalent results with respect to coverage and fixation with both techniques. Despite the lack of long-term follow up in this series, there were no episodes of recurrence reported in either laparoscopic group (16). However, it was noted that the time required to use both the suture and tacks was significantly longer than the tacking device alone.

BIOMATERIALS

Laparoscopic ventral hernia repair and novel biomaterials have evolved together over the past decade, with each entity lending some facet to the other to propel its development. Essentially, there are 3 biomaterials available for use today that have undergone extensive testing. These consist of polypropylene mesh, polyester mesh, and expanded polytetrafluoroethylene (ePTFE) mesh.

In 1997, Holzman et al. reported a series of 21 ventral hernias repaired laparoscopically using Marlex mesh (25). They concluded that the utilization of intraperitoneal Marlex mesh is not a forbidden practice, reporting 1 wound infection, 1 bowel obstruction, and no incidence of fistula formation (25). However, it is has been well established that when polypropylene or polyester are placed intraperitoneally, an intense inflammatory response is induced (9, 20, 26). Leber et al. showed that when compared to ePTFE, both polypropylene and polyester meshes had a statistically significant increased rate of infection, adhesion formation, small bowel obstruction, fistula formation, and recurrence rate.[9] It has been shown that the incidence of fistula formation associated with the use of polypropylene approaches 2%-5% when the polypropylene is placed in contact with the intestine (9, 21). These meshes are often extremely difficult to remove if reoperation is necessary.

For these reasons, a dual sided ePTFE (Dual Mesh,- W. L. Gore, Flagstaff, Arizona, USA) is the mesh of choice for many surgeons who perform laparoscopic ventral hernia repair (6, 8, 10-12, 14, 17-18, 19, 21). The visceral surface of the mesh has a pore size of 3 μm. which prohibits or, at least, limits adhesion formation. In fact there are no reported cases of PTFE erosion into the intestine or small bowel obstruction due to mesh adhesions. The peritoneal surface has an extensive microstructure which enhances tissue ingrowth and may help with mesh fixation. Newer composite biomaterials have recently been introduced into the clinical arena, but research is limited, and no clinical trials have shown them to be as efficacious as ePTFE in adhesion prevention or to improve recurrence rates. Until clinical data is available, these meshes cannot be recommended for use in laparoscopic ventral hernia repair.

Seroma formation

Seroma formation is not unique to the laparoscopic approach. Because the hernia sac is not removed during laparoscopic ventral hernia repair, many patients develop a seroma at the hernia site. In the vast majority of patients, these seromas are palpable, but asymptomatic. Most will resolve spontaneously by 8 to 10 weeks following surgery.

The treatment of these seromas is controversial. Most surgeons will offer treatment only if the seroma becomes symptomatic, or has not resolved after a course of conservative management. Voeller reports liberal needle aspiration of a hernia site seroma. He advocates only that the skin be sterilely prepped prior to inserting the needle.[10] However, infection of the prosthesis must be considered as a possible complication associated with seroma aspiration, but as yet, it has not been reported.

Prolonged pain at suture sites

After laparoscopic ventral hernia repair, patients will occasionally complain of point pain and tenderness at a site on the abdominal wall where a suture has been placed. The incidence of this complication has been reported to be approximately 2% (6). Treatment of this problem has not been well delineated and remains controversial. The first line of treatment for this type of post-operative pain could be a course of oral non-steroidal anti-inflammatory therapy. If the pain persists, it can often be permanently alleviated with a one time injection of bupivacaine and lidocaine into the muscular fascia at the suture site (6). For many patients prolonged relief is obtained, but the procedure can be repeated if the pain persists. The mechanism of action of this technique is not well delineated. If the techniques described do not provide the patient with relief, then the suture which is felt to be responsible for the symptoms can be removed.

Enterotomy during laparoscopic repair

The incidence of small bowel enterotomy during laparoscopic ventral hernia repair has been reported to be from 1% to 6% (6, 14, 16, 17). When enterotomies are not identified intra-operatively, the outcome is often ominous. When an injury is identified, if it cannot be repaired laparoscopically, the patient must be converted to an open repair.

There are two main options when it comes to the management of a bowel injury and the placement of mesh. The safest measure may be to make the repair a two stage operation. This entails repairing or resecting the injured bowel laparoscopically or in an open fashion, and bringing the patient back for a second operation to repair the hernia defect from a few days to a few weeks later. The second option must be considered with caution. If there is minimal spillage associated with the enterotomy, and the enterotomy was in the small intestine, the injury can be repaired and the mesh placed at the same operation. This scenario has been reported in 5 patients, all of whom have done well, without mesh infection or other sequela (6)

CONCLUSION

Over the past 8 years, laparoscopic incisional hernia repair has been shown to be safe and effective. Increasing numbers of reports have documented this point. As with most other areas of surgery in which new procedures have been developed, various areas of controversy remain. In this regard, we all remain in our "learning curve" for laparoscopic ventral hernia repair. As experience grows and randomized, prospective trials become available, these and other questions will be answered.

References

1. Luijendijk RW, Hop WC, van den Tol MP, et al. A comparison of suture repair with mesh repair for incisional hernia. N Engl J Med 2000:343(6):392-8.

2. Rives J, Pire JC, Flament JB, Convers G. Traitement des eventration. *Minerva Chir.* 1977;32(11):749-756.

3. Stoppa RE. The treatment of complicationed groin and incisional hernias. World J Surg. 1989;13:545-554.

4. Sampsel J. Delayed and recurring infection in postoperative abdominal wounds. Am J Surg. 1976;132:316.

5. Ellis H, Gajraj H, George CD. Incisional Hernias: when do they occur? Br J Surg 1983;70:290-1.

6. Heniford BT, Park A, Ramshaw BJ, Voeller G. Laparoscopic ventral and incisional hernia repair in 407 patients. J Am Coll of Surg. 2000; 190 (6):645-50.

7. Hesselink VJ, Luijendijk RW, de Wilt JHW, et al. An evaluation of risk factors in incisional hernia recurrence. Surg Gynecol Obstet. 1993;176:228-234.

8. Voeller GR. Repair of Incisional Hernias and Midline Defects. Abdominal Wall Hernia. Springer. 2000:519-524.

9. Leber GE, Garb JL, Alexander AI, et al. Long-term complications associated with prosthetic repair of incisional hernias. Arch Surg. 1998;133:374-82.

10. Heniford BT, Park A, LeBlanc KA, et al. Laparoscopic repair of Incisional Hernias: Patient selection and pre-op evaluation. Cont Surg.2001;57:171-182.

11. LeBlanc KA, Current Considerations in Laparoscopic Incisional and Ventral Herniorrhaphy. JSLS.2000;4:131-139.

12. Heniford BT, Ramshaw BJ. Laparoscopic Ventral Hernia Repair. A Report of 100 Consecutive Cases. Surg Endo. 2000;14: 419-423.

13. Arca MJ, Heniford BT, et al. Laparoscopic Repair of Lumbar Hernias. J Am Coll of Surg. 1998;187:147-152.

14. LeBlanc KA, Booth WV, Whitaker JM, et al. Laparoscopic Incisional and Ventral Herniorraphy in 100 patients. Am J Surg. 2000;180:193-197.

15. Fairclough JA, Johnson D. The prevention of wound contamination by skin organisms by the pre-operative application of an idophor impregnated plastic adhesive drape. J Int Med Res. 1986;14: 105-109.

16. Carbajo MA, Martin del Olmo JC, Blanco JI. Laparoscopic treatment vs. open surgery in the solution of major incisional and abdominal wall hernias with mesh. Surg Endosc. 1999;13: 250-252.

17. Koehler RH, Voeller G. Recurrences in laparoscopic incisional hernia repairs: a personal series and review of the literature. J Soc Laparoendosc Surg. 1999;3:293-304.

18. Toy FK, Bailey RW, Carey S, et al. Multicenter prospective study of laparoscopic ventral hernioplasty: preliminary results. Surg Endosc. 1998;12:955-959.

19. Roth JS, Park AE, Witzke D, et al. Laparocopic incisional/ventral herniorraphy: a five year experience. Hernia. 1999;4:209-214.

20. Ellis H. The causes and prevention of intestinal adhesions. Br J Surg. 1982;69:241-243.

21. Park A, Birch DW, Lovrics P. Laparoscopic and open incisional/ventral herniorraphy: a five year experience. Hernia. 1999;4: 209-214.

22. Hambley R, Hebda PA, et al. Wound healing of skin incisions produced by ultrasonically vibrating knife, scapel, electrosurgery, and carbon dioxide laser. J Dermatol Surg Oncol 14:1213,1988.

23. Amaral JF. The Experimental Development of an Ultrasonically Activated Scalpel for Laparoscopic Use. Surg Laparosc Endoscopy.1994; 4:92-99.

24. Wantz GE. Letters to the Editor. J Am Coll Surg. 1999;189:635-637.

25. Holzman MD, Purut CM, Reintgen K, et al. Laparoscopic ventral and incisional hernioplasty. Surg Endosc. 1997;11:32-35.

26. Matthews BD, Pratt BL, Backus CL, et al. Assessment of Adhesion Formation to Intra-Abdominal Polypropylene Mesh and Polytetrafluoroethylene Mesh. Accepted for presentation at Surgical Forum- American College of Surgeons October, 2001.

CHAPTER 11

Advantages and Disadvantages of Laparoscopic Ventral Hernia Repair

M. Miras, C. Durán, M Asensio, J. De Jaime

INTRODUCTION

Ventral hernias are defects of the abdominal wall and are the second most frequent type of hernia after those occurring in the inguinal region. Ventral hernias may be primary or secondary to a previous laparotomy, in which case they are known as incisional hernia, a condition with an incidence of 3 to 13% (1). Surgical repair of this type of defect is a significant challenge for the surgeon, since 18 to 41% of ventral hernias recur after the initial surgical procedure. In addition, the incidence of recurrence can be as high as 50% when a second operation is performed to repair these defects (2).

An effective technique for the treatment of ventral hernias must be accompanied by low morbidity in the immediate postoperative period and a low rate of recurrences. A variety of techniques aimed at achieving these results have been described, including lateral incisions to reduce tension on the suture line, rotation of muscles, large parietal dissections, etc. Nevertheless the only techniques offering a lower recurrence rate are those incorporating a prosthetic material to repair the defect (3).

The use of prosthetic material in ventral hernia repair requires considerable dissection of tissues, which can result in increased rates of infection, leading to a longer hospital stay, the need for abdominal wall drainage and a longer recovery time.

The laparoscopic approach to this type of hernia can prevent the complications associated with the conventional approach. There are significant advantages to using tension-free techniques in which only three or four small incisions no larger than one centimeter are made during the procedure. As compared to the results of conventional surgery, patients undergoing laparoscopic ventral hernia repair require shorter hospitalization, have a reduced need for analgesics, and can resume normal activities faster (4, 5, 6).

A laparoscopic technique for ventral hernia repair was first described by LeBlanc (7). Since then numerous publications have analyzed the results, and the advantages and disadvantages of this new approach.

Our experience covers the period from January 1993 to December 2000 and includes a total of 90 patients (Table I); 82 presented incisional hernia and 20 were recurrences (25%).

Table I. Ventral hernias patient characteristics

FEMALES/MALES	56/34
TYPE OF HERNIA	
Incisional	81
Umbilical	7
Epigastric	2
HERNIA RECURRENCES	20 (25%)
MULTILOCULAR	79
UNILOCULAR	11

SURGICAL TECHNIQUE

The technique is based on the surgical principles outlined by Stoppa and Rives (8), consisting in the placement of a large mesh below the anterior rectus muscle of the abdomen, anterior to the aponeurotic and preperitoneal fasciae. Fixation and securing with the tissues is assisted by intra-abdominal pressure (Laplace's law). The laparoscopic approach benefits from these principles, but applies the prosthesis at a deeper position (abdominal cavity), thereby eliminating the need for extensive dissection of the tissues.

The technique we use in our series does not differ from the standard technique, and, although it is not the subject of this chapter, we would like to mention several key details: We create the pneumoperitoneum by using a Veress needle at some distance from the previous surgical incisional until obtaining an intra-abdominal pressure of 14 mmHg. We work with a 5-11 mm trocar, into which a 30° lens is introduced. After examining the abdominal cavity to assess the characteristics of the hernia defect and the presence of adhesions we place two other 5 mm trocars.

After releasing all adhesions from the abdominal wall and confirmation of the defect, we introduce PTFE Dual Mesh Plus (WL Gore & Assoc.), which should extend beyond the border of the defect by at least 4 to 5 cm. The mesh is fixed with tacks (Protack, USSC, Norwalk, CT, U.S.A.), followed by second crown tacks at the edge of the hernia defect. In our earlier cases, we added four full-thickness sutures of nonabsorbable material in the subcutaneous layer to secure the mesh, but no longer include this step, as it leads to pain in the suture area. No drains are inserted.

RESULTS

Laparoscopic surgery was performed in all patients except three, in which conversion was required due to multiple adhesions. Nine patients (10%) presented complications in the immediate postoperative period (Table II). In one an intestinal pseudo-occlusion occurred due to slippage of the bowel between the anterior abdominal wall and the prosthesis; surgery was required. In this patient the mesh was not secured with tacks of nonabsorbable material as recommended by Heniford (17) and, in general, by all North American authors. Despite the above complication, we tend not to secure the mesh as it can produce pain at the suture sites even though positioned subcutaneously. In any case, this factor does not seem to influence the rate of recurrence. In fact the only recurrence in our series was in a patient in whom the mesh had been anchored with four suture stitches. Eight patients presented seroma, which resolved spontaneously in five patients and required puncture in three, with no further complications. As mentioned earlier, we had one immediate recurrence (1.1%) in a patient with subcostal incisional hernia, due to shifting of the mesh at its upper margin. Long-term follow-up showed no recurrences.

ADVANTAGES AND DISADVANTAGES

Definitive assessment of the advantages and disadvantages of the laparoscopic approach to ventral hernia repair requires analysis of several other aspects in addition to those already considered and proven: shorter hospitalization, less postoperative pain, faster resumption of normal activities.

In this regard there are few studies comparing the conventional and laparoscopic approaches. The two most complete works, published in 1999 by Ramshaw (9) and De Maria (6), analyzed several variations of these procedures, and reported considerably shorter hospital stays, with 2.8-4.5 days in the open surgery group versus 0.8-1.7 days in the laparoscopic surgery group. A significant difference was also observed in the rates of both major and minor complications, at 4.6% and 21.8% respectively versus 2.5% and 16.5% in patients undergoing laparoscopic repair. Open surgery had 20.7% of recurrences, a much higher rate than the 2.5% for laparoscopy.

As mentioned earlier, the two main objectives of good ventral hernia surgery are the minimization of both complications and recurrences. Hence, the potential contribution of laparoscopic surgery to these two important factors should be analyzed separately.

Table II. Laparoscopic ventral hernias. Results

CONVERSION	3 (3.3%)
COMPLICATIONS	9 (10%)
Seroma	8 (9%)
Intestinal oclusion	1 (1.1%)
HOSPITAL STAY	2 days (2-7)
RECURRENCES	1 (1.1%)

Advantages

Recurrence

The incidence of recurrence following open surgery of ventral hernias is 40-60% (10). These rates can be lowered to 10-15% with the use of tension-free techniques and prosthetic material (11). An analysis of the largest laparoscopic repair series (Table III) shows recurrence rates no higher than 6%, with the exception of results from Park (5) and Koehler (12), who report 11 and 9%, respectively. In a multicenter study performed with 144 patients, Toy (13) reported an incidence of 4%.

What is the reason for this significant reduction in recurrence rate?

Since the main drawback of open surgery is the high number of recurrences, we have analyzed the factors that can influence this complication, including age, weight, incision type and site, surgical technique, size of hernia defect, etc. The conclusions derived show that the factors of actual importance in recurrence are surgical wound infection and tension-free surgery, which involves the use of prosthetic material.

Wound infection

This type of complication is naturally more frequent in open surgery due to the inherent characteristics of the technique, since the incision is made on the previous scar and on tissues with some degree of deterioration, hence the potential for infection is considerably higher. Moreover, prosthesis placement also requires considerable tissue dissection, since the material must extend beyond the margins of the abdominal wall defect by at least 4 cm.

The laparoscopic approach solves these problems, as is evident in our discussion of the technique. No tissue dissection of any kind is required since an approach other than the site of the hernia defect is used. In addition, by introducing the prosthesis through the trocar, it does not come into contact with the skin and the risk of infection is lower.

Tension-free technique

The use of a prosthesis has contributed significantly to reducing the number of recurrences. The characteristics of the mesh used to cover the defect are directly related to the development of complications, such as infection or enteric fistulas, which may be important to the subsequent progress of the patient. Two types of mesh are used, polypropylene (PP) and expanded polytetrafluoroethylene (ePTFE). In a comparative study of the two surgical approaches, Ramshaw (9) reported a high rate of infection in open surgery patients in which the PP prosthesis was used, whereas the infection rate in patients with the PTFE was 0.

As mentioned earlier, prosthesis placement via laparoscopy implies contact between the prosthesis and the contents of the abdominal cavity. Therefore, a type of prosthesis that does not adhere to the bowel must be used to prevent the development of abdominal fistulas. Moreover, the risk of infection of the prosthesis must be minimized, as this is an additional determinant in the etiopathogenesis of recurrences (14), which will require a second operation to remove the mesh.

In terms of which mesh type should be used, studies performed by Gagner (5), Salky (15) and LeBlanc (16) have shown that ePTFE is the most suitable material, as it leads to fewer infections, causes no foreign body reaction, and ensures good adhesion to the tissues but not to the bowel (due to its characteristics), thereby preventing the appearance of enteric fistulas.

Adhesiolysis

Another advantages of laparoscopic repair are the benefits of pneumoperitoneum in the adhesiolysis process (adhesions due to previous surgery are always seen in incisional hernias.

Cost-benefit

Data on cost-benefit are limited, although a comparative study of the two techniques carried out by De Maria (6) analyzing a series of parameters such as the need for analgesics during the postoperative period, hospitalization in days, etc., showed that costs were significantly lower in the case of the laparoscopic procedure, being $8,273 versus $12,461 for open surgery.

Tabla III. Laparoscopic ventral hernias. Recurrences

AUTHOR	CASES	RECURRENCES (%)
Park (5) 1996	30	3
Toy (13) 1998	144	4
Koehler (12) 1998	34	9
Ramshaw (9) 1998	49	2
Franklin (19) 1998	176	1
Constanza (17) 1998	16	6
De María (6) 1998	21	0
Var Gish (20) 1998	45	6
Park (18) 1998	56	11
Kyzer (22) 1998	53	1.8
Bickel (23) 1998	23	0
Reitter (24) 2000	49	7.1
Carbajo (21) 2000	100	2

DISADVANTAGES

Although this type of laparoscopic technique is conceptually simpler to perform than other techniques, it also has a learning curve, as it requires extensive removal of adhesions between the abdominal wall and the bowel and, therefore, requires some skill to prevent major complications, such as inadvertent lesions to the contents of the abdominal cavity.

Enterotomy during maneuvers carried out to free the adhesions is the most important complication of laparoscopy repair. These lesions may go unnoticed in some cases, due to poor visualization or inexperience on the part of the surgeon. The incidence of enterotomy ranges from 1.5% in the multicenter study performed by Toy (13) to 6% in Koehler's series (12). The use of monopolar electrocautery is another determining factor in these lesions. Although the use of bipolar coagulation or harmonic scalpel theoretically avoids this complication, lesions have also been reported with these techniques.

There is some controversy concerning the placement of mesh in these cases. If the intestinal lesion is detected immediately and can be successfully repaired during the surgical procedure, use of a prosthesis is acceptable. However, depending on the surgeon's experience, it may be advisable not to use a mesh because it can favor the development of infection, an extremely important factor associated with recurrence and subsequent surgeries. Toy's multicenter study found that two of eight recurrences (25%) were due to mesh infection, and Heniford (17) reported a single recurrence also due to infection of the mesh and requiring subsequent removal. Roth and Park's study (18) with 75 patients showed seven recurrences, two of them (28%) related to infection of the prosthesis.

CONCLUSION

Based on our experience and on the results from other series, we conclude that laparoscopic surgery for ventral hernia repair is feasible and effective in comparison with open surgery, although these findings should be confirmed by long-term follow-up.

From the purely surgical standpoint, use of this technique improves the examination and diagnosis of both the hernia defect and the entire abdominal cavity. It does not affect previously operated areas of the abdominal wall that are in poor condition and basically prevents tension in the tissues.

Therefore, laparoscopic repair offers important advantages over conventional surgery that include significant reductions in local and general complications, practically no mesh contamination, extremely low recurrence rate and considerable reductions in the duration of surgery and hospitalization.

References
1. Mudge M, Hughes LE. Incisional hernia: A 10-year prospective study of incidence and attitudes. Br. J. Surg 1985;72:70-1.
2. Hesselink VJ, Luijendijk RW, de Wilt JHW, et el. An evaluation of risk factors in incisional hernia recurrence. Surg Gynecol Obstet 1993;176:228-34.
3. Temudom T, Siadati M, Sarr MG. Repair of complex giant or recurrent ventral hernias by using tension-free intraparietal prosthetic mesh: Lessons learned from our initial experience (50 patients). Surgery 1996;120:738-43.

4. Holzman MD, Purut CM, Reintgen K, et al. Laparoscopic ventral and incisional hernioplasty. Sur Endosc 1997;11:32-5.

5. Park A, Gagner M, Pomp A. Laparoscopic repair of large incisional hernias. Surg Laparoscopy Endoscopy 1996;6:123-8.

6. DeMaria EJ, Moss JM, Sugerman HJ. Laparoscopic intraperitoneal polytetrafluoroethylene (PTFE) prosthetic patch repair of ventral hernia. Surg Endosc 2000; 14.326-9.

7. Leblanc KA, Booth WV. Laparoscopic repair of incisional hernias using expanded polytetrafluoroethylene: Preliminary findings. Surg Laparosc Endosc. 1993;3:39-41.

8. Stoppa RE. The treatment of complicated groin and incisional hernias. World J Surg 1989; 13:545-54.

9. Ramshaw BJ, Esartia P, Schwab J, Mason EM, Wilson RA, Duncan TD, et el. Comparison of laparoscopic and open ventral herniorrhaphy. American Surgeon 1999;65:827-32.

10. Gecim IIE, Kocak S, Ersoz S, et el. Recurrence after incisional hernia repair: results and risk factors. Surg Today. 1996; 26:607-9.

11. Condon RE. Incisional hernia. In Nyhus LM and Condon RE, ed. Hernia (4th ed.) Philadelphia: Lippincott CO; 1995:319-39.

12. Koehler RH, Voeller G. Recurrences in laparoscopic incisional hernia repairs: A personal series and review of the literature. Journal Of Society of Lapar Surgeons 1999;3:293-304.

13. Toy FK, Bailey RW, Carey S, et al. Prospective multicenter study of laparoscopic ventral hernioplasty. Surg Endo 1998;12:955-59.

14. Leber GE, Garb JL, Alexander Al, Reed WP. Long-term complications associated with prosthetic repair of incisional hernias. Arch Surg 1998;133:378-82.

15. Bauer JJ, Salky BA, Gelernt IM, Kreel I. Repair of large abdominal wall defects with ePTFE. Ann Surg 1987;206:765-9.

16. LeBlanc KA, Booth WV, Whitaker JM, Baker D. In vivo study of meshes implanted over the inguinal ring and external iliac vessels in uncastrated pigs. Surg Endo 1998;12:247-51.

17. Constanza MJ, Henniford BT, Arca MJ, et al. Laparoscopic repair of recurrent ventral hernias. Am Surg. 1998;64:1-7.

18. Park A, Roth S. Data presented at the American Hernia Society, 3rd Annual Meeting, Las Vegas, NV, February 1999; 23-25.

19. Franklin ME, Dorman JP, Glass JL, et al. Laparoscopic ventral incisional hernia repair. Surg Laparosc Endosc 1998;8:294-99.

20. Vargish T. Laparoscopic repair of ventral hernia. In American College of Surgeons, Postgraduate Course 7, 1998:36-37.

21. Carbajo MA, Martin del Olmo JC, Blanco JI, et al. Laparoscopic treatment of ventral abdominal wall hernias: Preliminary results in 100 patients. Jr Society of Laparoendoscopic Surgeons 2000;4:141-45.

22. Kyzer S, Alis M, Aloni Y,Charuzi I. Laparoscopic repair of postoperation ventral hernia. Surg Endosc 199;13:928-31.

23. Bickel A, Eitan A. A simplified laparoscopic technique for mesh placement in ventral hernia repair. Surg Endosc 1999; 13:532-34.

24. Reitter DR, Paulsen JK, Debord JR, Estes NC. Five-year experience with the "four-before" laparoscopic ventral hernia repair. The American Surgeon 2000; 66(5):465-69.

CHAPTER 12

Indications and Contraindications for a Laparoscopic Approach to Incisional Hernia Repair

R.H. Koehler

INDICATIONS

General considerations

In discussing the indications for a laparoscopic approach to incisional hernia repair, the easiest way to begin is with the simple and accurate statement that these are the same indications for the repair of any incisional hernia. As Condon, Stoppa and Wantz (3,13-17) have all said, the presence of a true incisional hernia is an indication to at least consider a repair.

More specifically with respect to the laparoscopic approach, the surgeon should be considering the placement of synthetic material reinforcement, and this then becomes the basis for a laparoscopic attempt. As a recent review pointed out, mesh placement offers significantly superior results to primary fascial closure in the repair of incisional hernias (9). Stoppa's simple statement, "Recurrent hernias must not be repaired by the same technique used to treat the initial hernias" (12) is an elegant cautionary note to the surgeon involved in incisional hernia repairs.

Multiple previous surgeries and adhesions are not a contraindication to an initial attempt at repair via laparoscopy. However, these situations should heighten the surgeon's, and the patient's, awareness about the likelihood of conversion to open or laparoscopically-assisted case. This is particularly true if previous mesh has been placed in the intraabdominal position.

It seems therefor useful to reason that all incisional hernias, with the exception perhaps of small initial port-site hernias, should be repaired with mesh reinforcement. This would also apply to even recurrent umbilical hernias, where secondary primary repair seems highly likely to fail (10).

Defect Size

The size of a defect is sometimes alluded to as a determining factor by several authors (1-4,8-14), using either "large", or more specifically greater than 10cm², as indicators of mesh requirement. Others have defined "large" as 3cm². Carbajo defines "small" as <5cm², "medium" as 5-10cm², and "large" as > 10cm², and suggest that all of these ranges are approachable via laparoscopy.(1,2) Leblanc, one of the first to report a laparoscopic repair of an incisional hernia, characterizes "large" as >25cm² (8). However, as many authors on the topic of laparoscopic incisional hernia repair will testify, the actual hernia defect is frequently surrounded by either satellite defects of varying sizes, or highly suspect-appearing weakened fascia-the so-called "swiss cheese" phenomenon (Fig. 1). The Netherlands group reported that comparative analysis of hernia sizes was difficult, and that tissue integrity surrounding the defect may a more important determinant to record as part of the overall defect "size" (9). The US multicenter trial results, using 4cm² as a baseline minimum size for laparoscopic repair, found that the actual fascial defect at the time of laparoscopy often involved more extensive tissue weakening than the physical exam findings would have predicted (6). They noted, as well, that multiple smaller defects often surrounded the principle hernia defect. As more accurate reporting of overall defective fascial dimensions is adopted, the hernia sizes being reported will appear to be larger, accounting for the inclusion-as should be the case-of all areas of fascia requiring repair.

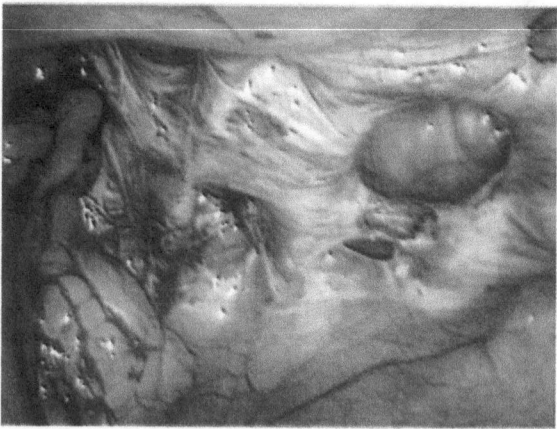

Fig. 1. Primary defect at right, with multiple small secondary defects which were nonpalpable by preoperative exam.

Patient size

The size of the patient is, alone, not a contraindication to a laparoscopic approach. Most every study has demonstrated that obesity is frequently a comorbid condition to the incisional hernia itself. Truly morbidly obese patients should be approached by the surgeon familiar with the unique logistical requirements of such cases, such as longer ports and specialized reinforced tables.

In large and/or particularly tall patients, and those patients with combined defects such as a previous ostomy site hernia in close proximity to a midline defect, patches may require customized tailoring (Fig. 2). However, success rates have never been shown to vary based upon patch size or patient size alone as independent variables. If anything, the avoidance of a particularly large open repair would seem of even more specific benefit to such patients (Fig. 3).

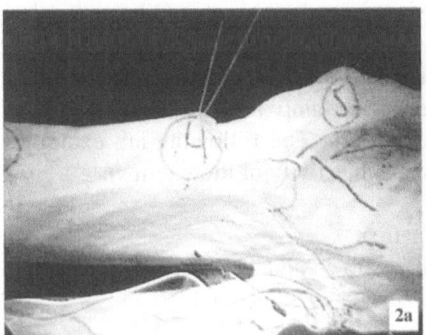 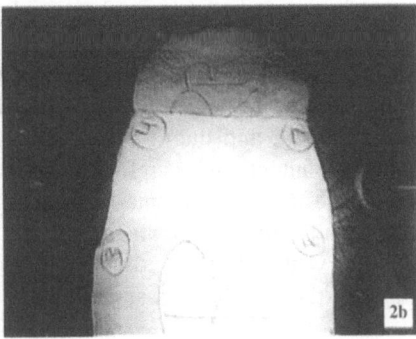

Figs. 2a and b. Large hernias may require customized tailoring of two patches sewn together, as shown here in the patient seen in figure three.

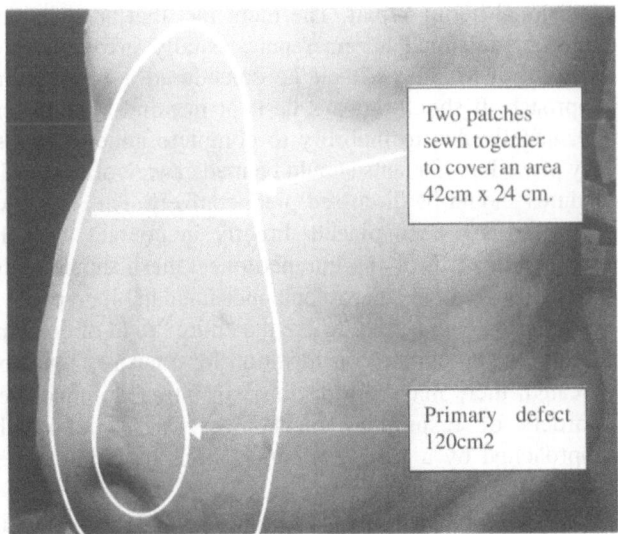

Two patches sewn together to cover an area 42cm x 24 cm.

Primary defect 120cm2

Fig. 3. This 39 year old male, six feet three inches tall and 315lb, suffered a ruptured abdominal aortic aneurysm, after which he developed a large (120cm^2) incisional hernia in the periumbilical region. However, multiple associated small fascial defects found at the time of laparoscopic repair led to this large composite patch covering the entire midline incision. He was discharged post-operative day 1, and is recurrence free at two years.

Incarcerated and emergent cases

With respect to the incarcerated incisional hernias, this should not be considered as an absolute contraindication to a laparoscopic approach. Many of the large series reported have included successful management of emergency procedures (5, 6, 8, 12, 15). Under these circumstances, it can in fact be quite helpful to make an initial evaluation laparoscopically. Often there is only omental strangulation rather than true intestinal strangulation. Although not an absolute contraindication to a laparoscopic approach, the emergent visceral strangulated incisional hernia should be undertaken after a reasonable experience is achieved with complex elective cases, and patients should be forewarned of a high likelihood of conversion to an open approach.

With regard to primary ventral hernias, there is certainly a role for synthetic mesh reinforcement, and thus for laparoscopic surgery. The following are examples (quotes are intentional, to reflect the inherent subjectivity of these terms):
- the "large" umbilical hernia
- the "small" umbilical hernia in a "large" patient
- multiple ventral defects, i.e. umbilical hernias with combined with epigastric hernias
- the recurrent trochar port-site hernia.

CONTRAINDICATIONS

There are relatively few absolute contraindications to an initial laparoscopic approach for incisional hernia repair. The mere fact that an individual has had multiple attempts at incisional hernia repair, usually involving several mesh placements, should not in and of itself be considered a contraindication to a laparoscopic approach. It should always be kept in mind that conversion to an open procedure, usually due to inability to complete adhesiolysis safely, is a possibility in any procedure. Patients should be made aware of this, and alternative "backup" procedures should be discussed preoperatively. This is particularly true where previous mesh has been placed directly in contact with the viscera. Recurrent hernias and those involving intraperitoneal mesh should be reserved for the more experienced surgeon in laparoscopic incisional hernia repair.

The true "giant" incisional hernia, where the entire "right of domain" has been lost, is probably not an appropriate consideration for a laparoscopic approach. As Stoppa has indicated, there may be a decrease in intraabdominal pressure with associated disorders of respiratory mechanics. These hernias have been successfully approached by a variety of open methods, as best described by Chevrel, Flament, Kingsworth and others.

Henniford and Ramshaw have suggested that there are few contraindications, noting possibly those hernias being strangulated, and the as yet unproven efficacy of mesh repair in children (< 13 years old) (5).

The following therefor is a list of contraindications for a laparoscopic approach to incisional hernia repair
1. Patient's inability to tolerate pneumoperitoneum and/or general anesthesia
2. A requirement for complete reconstruction of the anterior abdominal wall, where it is necessary to reaproximate the midline achieve musculoskeletal and respiratory function

3. Fistulas and/or gross contamination of infection within the confines of where the mesh is to be placed. (Note: This does NOT include the stable parastomal hernia)

4. Pediatric patients.

References

1. Carbajo MA, Martin del Olmo JC and Blanco JI et al. Laparoscopic treatment versus open surgery in the solution of major incisional and abdominal wall hernias with mesh. Surg Endosc 1999, 13:250-252.

2. Carbajo MA, Martin del Olmo JC and Blanco JI, de la Cuesta C, Martion F, Toledano M, Perna C, Vaquero C. Laparoscopic treatment of ventral abdominal wall hernias: preliminary results in 100 patients. JSLS 2000;4:141-145.

3. Condon RE. Incisional Hernia. In Nyhus LM and Condon RE, ed. Hernia (4th ed). Lippincott Co;1995:319-339.

4. Franklin ME, Dorman JP, Glass JL, Balli JE, et al. Laparoscopic ventral incisional hernia repair. Surg Laparosc Endosc 1998;8:294-299.

5. Henniford BT, Ramshaw BJ. Laparoscopic ventral hernia repair:a report of 100 consecutive cases. Surg Endo 2000;14:419-423.

6. Heniford BT, Park A, Ramshaw BJ,Voeller G. Laparoscopic ventral and incisional hernia repair in 407 patients. JACS 199;190:645-650.

7. Hesselink VJ, Luijendijk RW, deWilt J, Heide R et al. An evaluation of risk factors in incisional hernia recurrence. Surg Gyn Obst 1993;176:228-234.

8. LeBlanc KA, Booth WV, Whitaker JM, Baker D, Bellanger DE. Laparoscopic incisional and ventral herniorraphy in 100 patients. Am J Surg 2000;180:193-197.

9. Luijendijk RW, Hop W, van den Tol MP, de Lange DCD, Braaksma, MJ, IJzermans, JNM, Boelhouwer RU, de Vries BC, Salu MKM, Wereldsma JCJ, Bruijninckx CMA, Jeekel J. A Comparison of Suture Repair with Mesh Repair for Incisional Hernia. NEJM 2000;343:392-398.

10. Luijendijk RW, Lemmen MHM, Hop W, Wereldsma JCJ. Incisional hernia recurrence following "vest-over-pants" or vertical Mayo repair of primary hernias of the midline. World J Surg 1997;21:62-66.

11. Park A, Gagner M, Pomp A. Laproscopic repair of large incisional hernias. Surg Lapar Endo 1996;6:123-128.

12. Park A, Birch DW, Lovrics P. Laparoscopic and open incisional hernia repair: A comparison study. Surgery 1998;124:816-22.

13. Stoppa RE. The treatment of complicated groin and incisional hernias. World J Surg. 1989;13:545-554.

14. Temudom T, Siadati M, Sarr MG. Repair of complex giant or recurrent ventral hernias by using tension-free intraparietal prosthetic mesh (Stoppa technique): lessons learned from our initial experience (fifty patients). Surgery 1996; 120:73843; (disc 7434).

15. Toy FK, Bailey RW, Carey S, Chappuis CW, et al: Prospective, multicenter study of laparoscopic ventral hernioplasty. Surg Endo 1998;12:955-959.

16. Wantz G. Incisional hernioplasty with Mersilene. Surg Gyn Obst 1991;172:129.

17. Wantz GE. Incisional Hernia: the problem and the cure. JACS 1999;188:429-447.

Instruments and Materials for Laparoscopic Ventral Hernia Repair

CHAPTER 13

Prosthetic Biomaterials in the Laparoscopic Repair of Incisional and Ventral Hernias

K.A. LeBlanc

INTRODUCTION

Incisional hernias will develop in approximately 11-13% of laparotomy incisions. The risk of herniation is increased by fivefold if a postoperative wound infection occurs. Other factors that predispose to the development of a fascial defect include obesity, poor nutritional status, steroid usage, etc. While some of these may be avoided, those patients that are found to have such a hernia can present difficult management problems due to the high potential for recurrence. Without the use of a prosthetic biomaterial, the recurrence rate is as high as 51% (1, 2). The use of a synthetic prosthetic material will reduce this rate to 10-24% (3, 4).

The laparoscopic repair of incisional and ventral hernias was introduced in 1993 using the Soft Tissue Patch made by W.L. Gore and Associates (Flagstaff, AZ) (5). The recurrence rate that has been reported varies from 0-11% (6-10). The collective recurrence rate in all of the series that have been published to date averages 3.1%. This is a remarkable improvement. This is especially significant since this technique has been reported early in most of the experiences of the surgeons. Because of the apparent success of this operation and the fact that hospital length of stays and costs are decreased with this procedure, it is gaining popularity (11-13). The increasing adoption of this technique has encouraged many of the manufacturers of these biomaterials to seek the goals of the "ideal" product. Consequently other biomaterials have been and are being developed to meet the requirements of this procedure. This chapter will identify these goals and the properties of the various biomaterials that are on the market today. The rational for the choice of a material in the laparoscopic incisional herniorraphy will be developed.

INDICATIONS FOR USE OF PROSTHETIC BIOMATERIALS

The chief purpose of these materials will be the repair of a fascial defect in the abdominal wall. The main indications of use of the materials are listed in Table I.

Table I. Indications for Prosthetic Biomaterials

❖ Replacement of lost musculofascial tissue caused by:

♦ Trauma
  • External
  • Internal
♦ Infection
❖ Reinforcement of native tissue weakness
♦ Aging (laxity of tissues)
♦ Neurological deficit (denervation)

Musculofascial tissue strength can be lost in a variety of ways. The most common, of course, would be due to the external etiology following a laparotomy or any other abdominal incision that is larger than that of the 5mm laparoscopic trocar. Another example would be the loss of tissue subsequent to gunshot wounds or motor vehicle accidents. Life threatening infections such as fascitis and gangrene will produce large areas of necrosis with resultant tissue loss and represent areas of potential hernia formation.

The increase in intra-abdominal pressure that results from significant weight gain will result in an internal source of weakening of the abdominal wall musculature and/or the widening of the sites of potential weaknesses. Other problems such as emphysema or the chronic bronchitis of smokers that produces a constant increase in intra-abdominal pressure are significant factors. Poor nutritional and/or protein balances are also examples of an internal etiology that predisposes to hernia formation. The development of a postoperative wound infection will increase the risk of herniation by as much a five times. In fact, about 30% of patients that develop a postoperative incisional wound infection will ultimately develop an incisional hernia (14).

The effects of aging and the declining ability of the elderly patient to repair the native tissues will lead to the loss of fascial strength. This is commonly seen with the direct inguinal hernia. It also occurs with the enlargement of the linea alba that is referred to as a diastasis recti (although this is also seen in the younger age groups as well). These defects can enlarge to the size that they become symptomatic and require repair.

The most common defect that results from a denervation phenomenon follows the flank incision that is utilized in a nephrectomy. Similarly, a defect can also eventuate from the incision that is used for a lumbar sympathectomy or an anterior approach to the lumbar spine for lumbar inter-body fusion for degenerative disk disease. In these entities, there is not the usual well-defined fascial edge that is seen with the more common anterior abdominal wall defects. This is due to the broad surface of the denervated musculature that has intact fascia but lacks the reinforcement of the muscle tissue.

PROSTHETIC BIOMATERIALS

History

The use of materials for the repairs of hernias can be found in antiquity. It is believed that Heliodorus used the cellulose from a cotton or flax plant to effect scarification in the inguinal area to treat herniation in A.D. 25. The use of silver as a synthetic prosthesis was reported in 1900 (15). Metallic biomaterials have also included the use of tantalum gauze mesh and stainless steel mesh. None of these materials gained wide acceptance because of the complications that were associated with their usage. These included lack of pliability, seromas, wound infection, fatigue fractures (and herniation through the fracture sites), abnormal scarification, adhesions, loss of structural integrity and allergic reactions.

Natural prostheses were considered as myofascial replacement shortly after the use of silver filigree (16). Other materials that have been used are listed in Table II.

Table II. Natural Prosthetic Biomaterials

Autogenous dermal grafts	Whole skin grafts
Dermal collagen homografts	Porcine dermal collagen
Autogenous fascial heterografts	Lyophilized aortic homografts
Preserved dural homografts	Bovine pericardium

These materials were used with good results, in some cases, but scarcity and cost limited their widespread adoption. Additionally, there were concerns of viral transmission as one case of Creutzfeld-Jacobs disease developed in a patient that had the use of a dural homograft. The development of synthetic biomaterials that were easier to use and did not appear to have these adverse side effected the demise of these unsatisfactory products.

A series on nonmetallic synthetic prosthetic biomaterials were used as well. Some of these are listed in Table III. As with the metal biomaterials, there were significant disadvantages with these products. These included infections, sinus tract formation, alteration of the product *in vivo*, and lack of incorporation into the native tissues. Carbon fiber has never been used in humans because of concerns of potential carcinogenicity (although it functioned fairly well in the experimental model). Currently, only the silastic product is used clinically in the pediatric surgical correction of omphalocele and gastroschisis.

Table III. Nonmetallic Synthetic Prosthetic Biomaterials

Fortisan fabric (cellulose)	Polytetrafluoroethylene
Polyvinyl sponge	Polypropylene mesh/gelatin film
Polyvinyl cloth	Polyester-reinforced silicon sheeting
Nylon mesh	Silastic
Carbon fiber	Polyester
Silicon-velvet composite	Carbon fiber

All of these biomaterials were attempting to address the "ideal characteristics" that were promulgated by Cumberland (17) and Scales (18). While it is widely felt that the ideal material has yet to be found, these criteria (Table IV) are the goals that are sought by the manufacturers.

Table IV. The Ideal Characteristics of Synthetic Biomaterials

No physical modification by tissue fluids	Chemically inert
Does not incite inflammatory or foreign body reaction	Does not produce allergy or hypersensitivity
Noncarcinogenic	Resistant to mechanical strains
Can be fabricated to the form required	Sterilizable

While the clinical use of prosthetic biomaterials shares these considerations, the operating surgeon does, in fact, experience slightly different priorities in the use of the prosthesis within the patient. The clinical characteristics of the "ideal surgical" biomaterial are listed in Table V.

Table V. Ideal Surgical Clinical Characteristics of Synthetic Biomaterials

Permanent repair of the abdominal wall (i.e. no recurrences)
In-growth characteristics that result in a normal pattern of tissue repair and healing
No alteration of the compliance of the abdominal wall musculature
Lack of adhesion predisposition
Cuts easily and without fraying
Inexpensive

The synthetic prosthetic biomaterials can be divided into the absorbable and non-absorbable products. The absorbable biomaterials (polyglycolic or polyglactic acid) have been used to cover polypropylene prosthetics used to repair a fascial defect in an effort to protect the viscera from that product. While these materials may appear to have a role in the prevention of adhesions, they may, in fact, enhance their development. This can be explained because of the fact that there must be an inflammatory response as a natural consequence of the resorption of these materials. There is no clinical data to support this type of usage of the absorbable biomaterials. Recent laboratory studies have shown that this technique does not achieve its intended result (20).

The non-synthetic biomaterials are of many types, sizes and shapes. The use of these products is commonplace in the repair of inguinal hernias. The current use of the prosthesis in the tension-free concept of a repair of the incisional hernias has gained widespread acceptance within the last several years. Approximately 90% of incisional and ventral hernias in the United States are repaired with the use of some type of prosthetic biomaterial. Outside of the United States, however, the repair of these hernias is frequently performed without their use; the cost of these materials representing the major obstacle in their use. With the exception of the very smallest of hernias, every laparoscopic approach to the incisional or ventral hernia employs a prosthetic product.

Synthetic Prosthetic Biomaterials

The currently available products in use today are either polypropylene (PPM), polyester, expanded polytetrafluoroethylene (ePTFE) or a composite of these materials. The many PPM biomaterials that are available for the surgical repair of the incisional hernia are listed in Table VI.

Table VI. Polypropylene Biomaterials and Manufacturer

Atrium, Atrium Medical Corporation, Hudson, NH
Marlex, C. R. Bard, Murray Hill, NJ
Prolene, Ethicon, Somerville, NJ
Parietene, Sofradim International, Villfranche-sur-Saône, France
Surgipro, United States Surgical Corporation, Norwalk, CT
Trelex, Meadox Medical Corporation, Oakland, NJ
Hertra 1 mesh, HerniaMesh S.R.L., Torino, Italy

The scanning electron microscopic views of these products are shown in Figures 1-6. The differences in the appearance of the prosthetics are easily seen in these photos. The size of the pores of these materials as well as the thickness of the product will have a significant impact on its stiffness. These factors affect the degree of scarring within the tissues. There are other PPM products that are not included but please note that there are many other types. Polyester products that are currently available include Mersilene® (Ethicon, Inc., Somerville, NJ) and Parietex® (Sofradim International, Villefranche-sur-Saône, France).

All of the above biomaterials are associated with an aversion to their placement into the abdominal cavity without the protection of some structure. The most common, of course, is the omentum. Another method of placement is in the extraperitoneal space so that the peritoneum and/or fascia protect the intestines from contact with those products. This will prevent the complication of fistulization due to the contact of the bowel to these rough biomaterials. In my opinion, the best method of protection from the product is the use of a biomaterial that is not associated with such a complication. This would be limited to the expanded polytetrafluoroethylene (ePTFE) prostheses. The currently available ePTFE prostheses are listed in Table VII.

Table VII. ePTFE Biomaterials and Manufacturer

Soft Tissue Patch, W. L. Gore and Associates, Flagstaff, AZ
Reconix, C. R. Bard, Murray Hill, NJ
Mycromesh, W. L. Gore and Associates, Flagstaff, AZ
DualMesh, W. L. Gore and Associates, Flagstaff, AZ
DualMesh with Holes, W. L. Gore and Associates, Flagstaff, AZ
DualMesh Plus, W. L. Gore and Associates, Flagstaff, AZ

The two factors that have been found to increase the propensity of the development of adhesions are the pore sizes the thickness of the material. The larger the pore sizes and the thicker the biomaterial, the greater will be the incidence of adhesions. Additionally, these same factors will result in more tenacious adhesions. Laboratory studies involving both rabbit and porcine models have demonstrated the differences in the adhesive potential in these different products (19, 21). In these experiments the amount of adhesions and the difficulty that was encountered in the dissection of them off of the biomaterial at 30 and 90 days after implantation were evaluated. The percentage of the prosthetic that was covered by adhesions was noted and is shown in Graph 1 The data from these graphs were analyzed to produce an "adhesion score." The scores ranged from 1-7 (seven being the worst possible score). The extent of the prosthesis covered by adhesions was given a number from 1-4 based on 25% increments of coverage. A score of one indicated that 25% or less of the biomaterial was covered by adhesions. The tenacity was graded from 1-3 based upon whether the adhesions were easily pulled off, bluntly dissected off or cut off with scissor dissection. A score of three reflected the need for scissor dissection to release the adhesions. It was apparent that the stiffer the biomaterial and the larger the pore sizes of the product produced a corresponding increase in the amount of adhesions. Additionally these same factors were seen increase the difficulty of the removal of them from the prosthesis. The greatest extremes are noted between Marlex® and the original DualMesh® (Graph 2). The results of these studies are borne out in the clinical situation. The adhesions that are encountered with reoperation of the patients that have had a PPM implant are quite tenacious and frequently difficult to remove. The result is the well-known risk of fistualization. This complication has also been seen in polyester products as well (3). To overcome the problems with adhesions to the omentum and bowel as well as the risk of fistulization, manufacturers have responded with new materials. The need for this type of material is particularly acute with the laparoscopic repair of incisional hernias.

INCIDENCE OF ADHESIONS

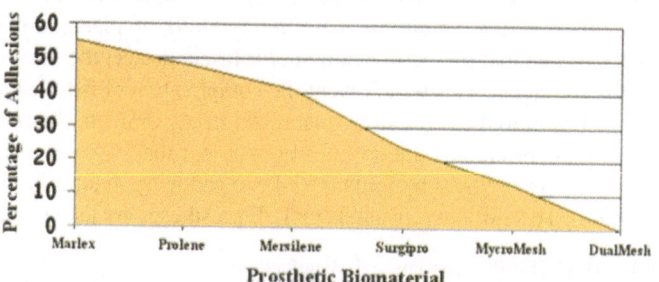

Graph 1. Incidence of Adhesions to Various Biomaterials in the Experimental Animal

ADHESION SCORES

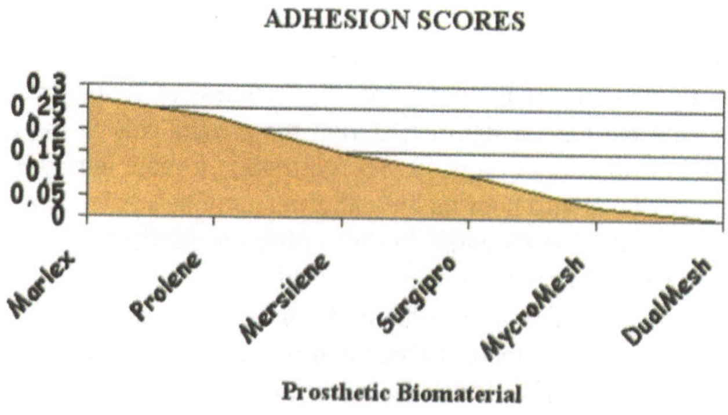

Graph 2. Adhesion scores to the Various Biomaterials in the Experimental Animal

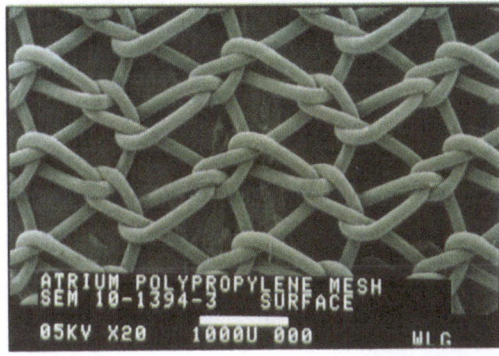

Fig. 1. Scanning Electron Microscopic View of Atrium® mesh.

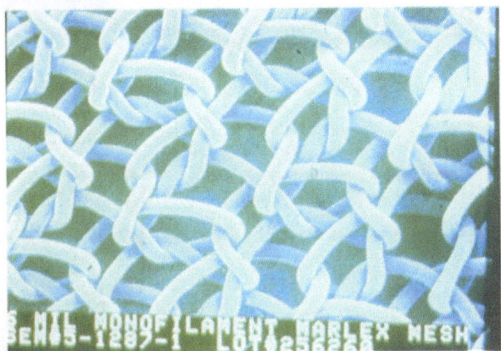

Fig. 2. Scanning Electron Microscopic View of Marlex® mesh.

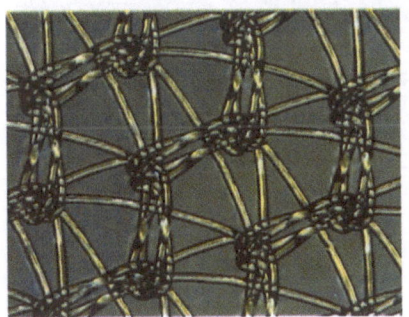

Fig. 3. Scanning Electron Microscopic View of Prolene® mesh.

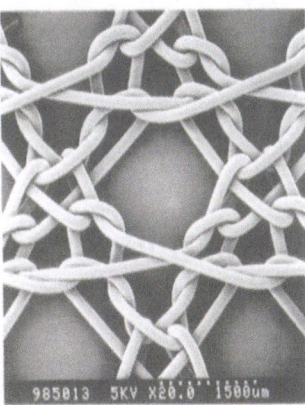

Fig. 4. Scanning Electron Microscopic View of Paritene® mesh.

Fig. 5. Scanning Electron Microscopic View of Surgipro® mesh.

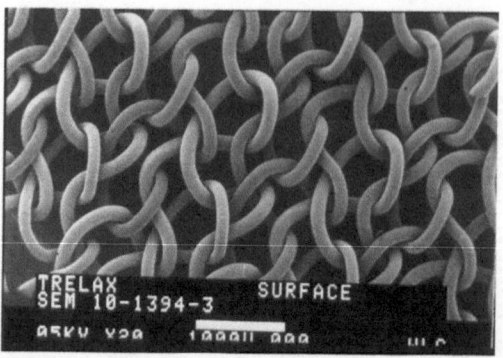

Fig. 6. Scanning Electron Microscopic View of Trelex® mesh.

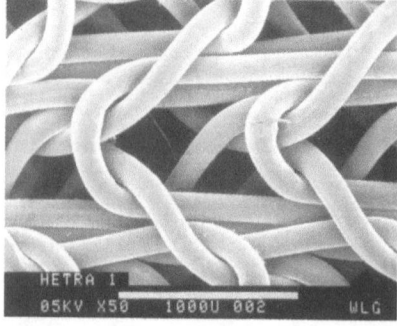

Fig. 7. Scanning Electron Microscopic View of Hertra 1 mesh®

BIOMATERIALS FOR LAPAROSCOPIC INCISIONAL HERNIORRAPHY

The currently available products for this operation are modifications of older materials or a composite type material of the older materials (Table VIII). In general, all of these prosthetic devices can or have been used in both open and laparoscopic incisional herniorraphies. Only a few of these products have long-term follow-up data to support the idea that there is a lack of problems related to adhesion formation (9-12).

Table VIII. Prosthetic Biomaterials for LIVH and Manufacturer

Composix®, C. R. Bard, Murray Hill, NJ, USA
Sepramesh‰, Genzyme Corporation, Cambridge, MA, USA
Parietex® Composite, Sofradim International, Villfranche-sur-Saône, France
DualMesh®, W. L. Gore and Associates, Flagstaff, AZ, USA
DualMesh® Plus, W. L. Gore and Associates, Flagstaff, AZ, USA
DualMesh® with holes, W. L. Gore and Associates, Flagstaff, AZ, USA
DualMesh® Plus with holes, W. L. Gore and Associates, Flagstaff, AZ, USA

Two composite materials incorporate polypropylene with an "anti-adhesive" barrier. The first of these to be introduced was Composix® mesh (C.R. Bard, Murray Hill, NJ). This material is shown in Figures 8-10. The "parietal" surface of this material is the PPM Marlex®, while the "visceral" surface of the product is a very thin layer of ePTFE. This product is stiff because it is made with two layers of Marlex® rather than one flat mesh. The ePTFE layer is easily punctured and can separate from the PPM during the surgical manipulation necessary for its implantation if sufficient care is not exercised in its placement. Additionally, it is impossible to roll this product into a sufficiently small size so as to permit its introduction into the abdominal cavity via a 5mm trocar site. It is usually necessary to remove a 12mm trocar and insert the product through this site. There are currently no reported clinical data regarding the long-term use and benefits of this biomaterial. One study has demonstrated that 30% of the rabbits that had an implant of Composix® developed adhesions (22). Figure 11 illustrates the microscopic appearance of the product in a patient that I removed the material because of chronic debilitating pain.

SepraMesh™ is the newest of these composite prosthetic synthetic materials (Figure 12). A single layer of polypropylene is covered by the previously released Seprafilm® which is marketed as an anti-adhesive biomaterial. The "visceral surface" of the product is a combination of carboxymethylcellulose and hyaluronic acid that is a foam. The foam is dry and must be rehydrated with saline prior to its implantation. This portion of the product is stated to last 7-14 days, at which point, it has been resorbed. The manufacturer recommends that the omentum should be used to cover the mesh material after its fixation. There are only reports regarding the Seprafilm® product in the use in the experimental animal (23). One report has shown that no adhesions were seen in 80% of the rabbits that were studied using an open laparotomy to repair a full thickness defect in the abdominal wall with Seprafilm™ (24). Clinical trials and long-term studies with this biomaterial are needed.

It has been said that one must be careful with its use because of the removal of the foam during manipulation. I have, in fact, found this to be true in the laboratory. Once this dry foam was rehydrated, it was very easily removed. My thumbprints are seen in Figure 13. After insertion into the abdomen of a porcine model, large areas of the anti-adhesive material were notably absent. This is noted as the bare areas in the laparoscopic views (Figure 14). Until this problem is overcome, one should consider the use of this prosthesis as subject to the same risks as bare PPM. The recommendation of the manufacturer to cover the biomaterial with omentum must be strictly followed when this product is used. It will be very difficult to use this material in the laparoscopic repair of incisional hernias because of this problem.

Parietex® Composite, mentioned above, is a three-dimensional weave of polyester. Its manufacturer has incorporated an absorbable hydrophilic film into the product (Figure 15). The film is made of a mixture of oxidized atelocollagen type I, polyethylene glycol and glycerol. This must also be rehydrated prior to implantation. Unlike the Sepramesh™, the absorbable material does not appear to separate from the mesh as easily with manipulation. This prosthetic has been used clinically with both the open and laparoscopic method of incisional hernia repairs. Early reports have shown that this material does not appear to have the risk of postoperative adhesive problems that are known with the PPM products (25, 26). In only the series of Balique et al. (25) was this composite material used in the intraperitoneal position in 29 patients. The relative inexperience with this biomaterial makes its long-term affects unknown. Because of the concerns that were shown with the use of polyester materials with the open repair, such as fistulization, one should be cautious of the long term outcomes subsequent its implantation (3).

The ePTFE biomaterials have been used since this operation was first described in 1993 (1). The Mycromesh® biomaterial is generally used in the tension free repair of inguinal hernias and is not recommended for the incisional and ventral hernia repair. The other materials come in both one and two millimeter thickness. The smaller size, however, is more than adequate to repair hernia defects of the abdominal wall. To my knowledge, there have been no reports with the use of the Reconix® prosthesis with the laparoscopic method. Once the DualMesh® product became available, I have used this material exclusively in the one millimeter thickness.

The original DualMesh® (Figure 16) was smooth on one surface and textured on the other surface. The smooth (visceral) surface, had interstices of approximately three microns. This was found to significantly diminish or even eliminate the risk of adhesions of the bowel and omentum (21). The opposite "parietal" surface had interstices of 17-22 microns, which allowed the infiltration of fibroblasts and collagen into the biomaterial (Figure 17). I have used this material for over seven years and have not seen any problems related to adhesions. On occasion, I have had an opportunity to re-laparoscope some of these patients and have noted filmy adhesions in several individuals (Figure 18). These were generally seen to develop to the neovascularization that is noted to occur on the visceral surface of the biomaterial. In the few instances that more tenacious adhesions were noted, none involved intestinal organs. In these patients, there was encapsulation of the visceral side of the patch. This could be easily separated from the biomaterial with minimal dissection and without the need for sharp dissection that is required with other prosthetic materials.

The DualMesh® biomaterial is also available in another form in which there are holes in the patch (Figure 19). These are spaced 7.0 millimeters apart and measure 0.9 millimeters in diameter. This material could be considered to diminish the occurrence of seromas that are common after the LIVH. However, the neomesothelium that develops over the visceral surface does so very rapidly. As such, it could not be stated with certainty that it would have the desired effect. In fact, in the only series that has been published using this product, the incidence of seroma was still 10% (27). This falls within the rate that is predicted with this operation. It is 1.5mm rather than 1.0mm thick making it somewhat more difficult to insert in to the abdomen when compared to the thinner product.

In an effort to increase the in-growth potential of the prosthetic, W. L. Gore and Associates have re-engineered the parietal side of the DualMesh®. This new surface is notably "rougher" than the original product and has the appearance of a corduroy type of material. The surface changes results from the increase in the interstitial pore sizes to approximately 150 microns. The visceral surface, however, has not been changed. The result is an even greater incorporation into the native tissues. The collagen infiltration that is seen in the original product is shown in Figure 20. The increase in this deposition is notable when compared to Figure 21.

Because of concerns as to the extent of the actual amount of clinically significant in-growth into this newer biomaterial, I performed an experiment using the rabbit model. Each animal was implanted with two biomaterials in a random fashion. The materials chosen were Marlex®, the original DualMesh®, the new DualMesh® with the "corduroy" surface. These materials were retrieved three days after surgical implantation. Each material was connected to a tensiometer and then forcibly pulled away from the abdominal wall. The force necessary to separate the biomaterial from the animal was recorded. The results (Graph 3) demonstrate that the newer DualMesh® achieves a level of in-growth, at just three days, that makes it more difficult to pull off of the tissues than that of either the older product or Marlex®. The difference is statistically significant.

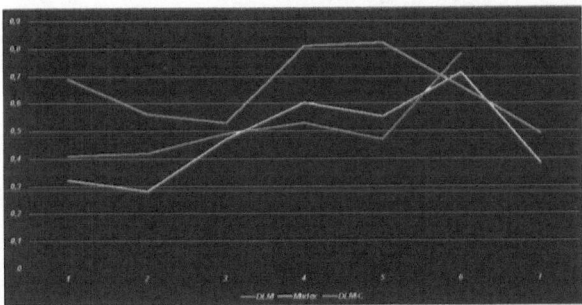

Graph 3. Tensiometer measurements of the force necessary to extract the biomaterials from the fascial surface (x axis-number of the animal; y axis-lbs/in2 of force to extract

The DualMesh® Plus bio,material (with and without holes) has the added benefit of the addition of antimicrobial agents. Silver and chlorhexidine have been incorporated into the material to provide for this activity. These agents are absorbed generally within seven days. A multicenter trial evaluated the possibility of adverse reactions by the patients into whom this material was implanted. No adverse events were noted in either the open or laparoscopic placement of the patches (28).

A beneficial result of the addition of the silver to the biomaterial is the impartation of a characteristic brown color to the prosthesis (Figures 17 and 21). This greatly diminishes the glare of the product during the laparoscopic procedures when compared to the traditional ePTFE biomaterials. The resulting enhancement of the ease of patch positioning because of this color is a further benefit of the use of this product. Additionally, because the brown color is greatest on the visceral surface of the patch, the surgeon should never have any uncertainty as to the correct orientation of the prosthetic against the abdominal wall.

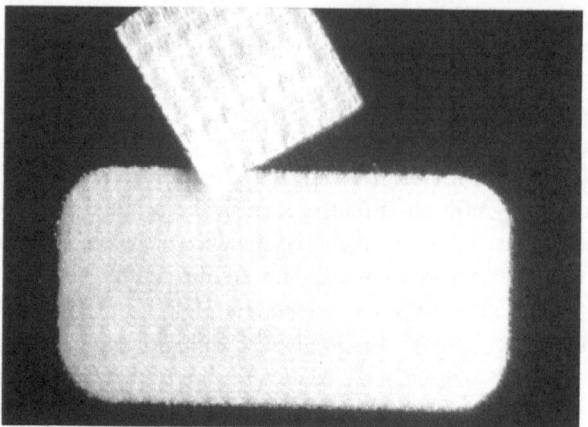

Fig. 8. Gross Photograph of Composix® mesh. Note the differences in appearance of the ePTFE and the PPM surfaces.

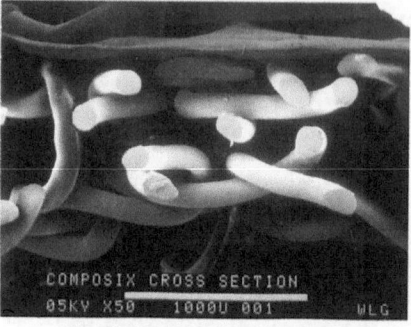

Fig. 9. Cross-sectional SEM view of Composix® mesh.

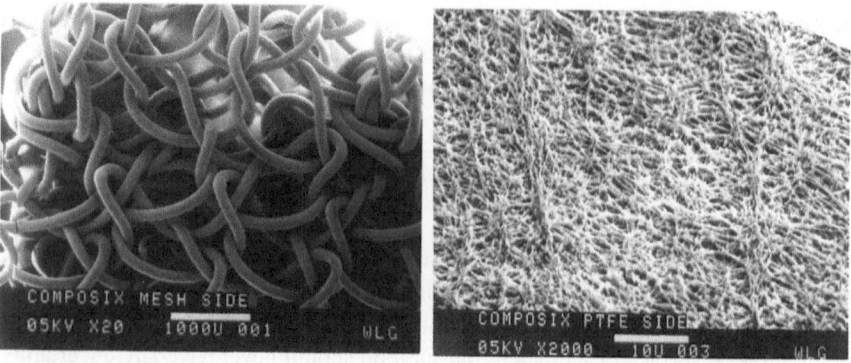

Fig. 10. SEM views of the PPM (left) and the ePTFE (right) surfaces of Composix® mesh.

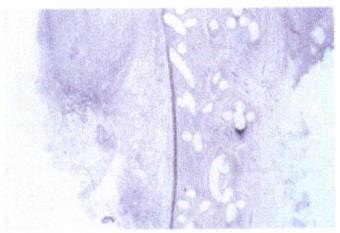

Fig. 11. Microscopic appearance of an explanted Composix® mesh.

Fig. 12. Gross View of Sepramesh™ Prior to Hydration.

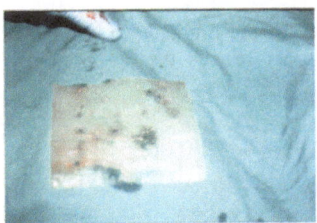

Fig. 13. Sepramesh™ after Rehydration. Note the separation of the anti-adhesive foam caused by the manipulation by my fingers and thumbs.

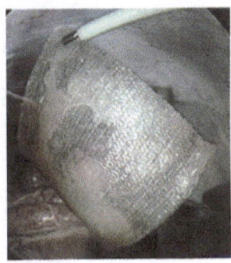

Fig. 14. Laparoscopic view of Sepramesh™ after insertion into the abdomen during laparoscopy.

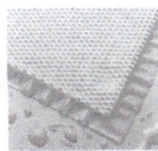

Fig. 15. Gross View of Parie-tex® Composite Prosthetic Bio-material.

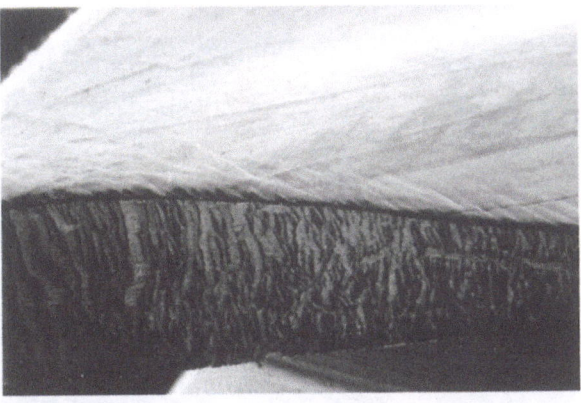

Fig.16. SEM View of the Visceral Surface of the original DualMesh®.

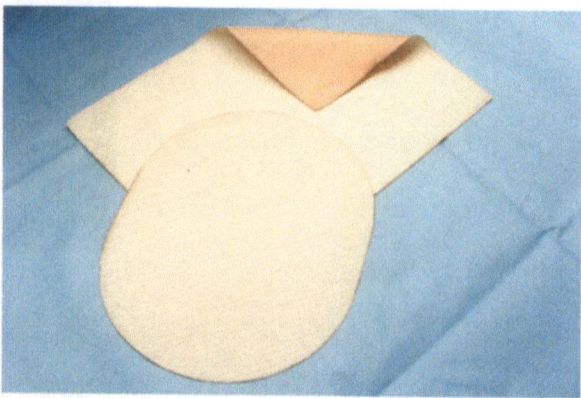

Fig. 17. SEM view of the "parietal surface" of the original DualMesh® Plus. The lower right hand corner reveals the visceral surface of the biomaterial.

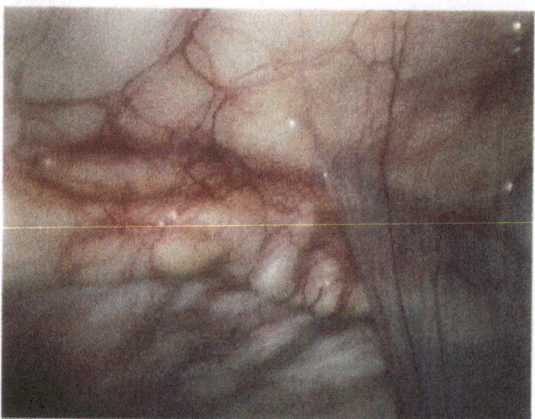

Fig. 18. Typical filmy adhesions that are occasionally seen with the DualMesh® biomaterial upon re-operation.

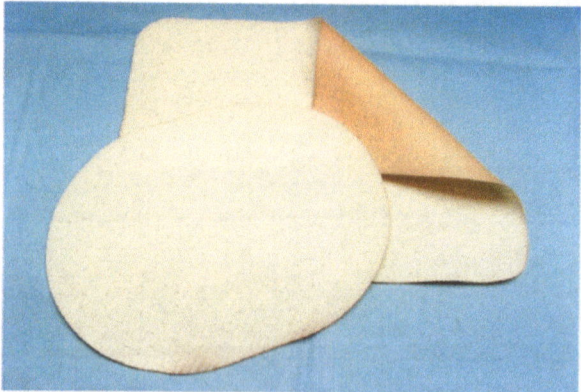

Fig. 19. DualMesh® with holes.

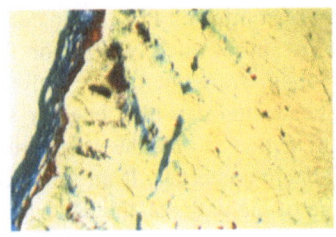 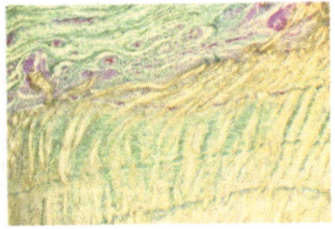

Fig. 20. Trichrome stain of the original implanted DualMesh®. Note the depth of penetration of the collagen in this SEM.

Fig. 21. Trichrome Stain of the new DualMesh® biomaterial. There is a significant increase in the amount of collagen deposition compared to the original DualMesh®.

CHOOSING THE BIOMATERIAL

Based on the information that has been provided above, the surgeon should have a better understanding of the various prosthetic biomaterials that are available. More importantly, a rational choice could be made when performing the laparoscopic repair of incisional and ventral hernias.

A thorough review of the currently available literature reveals that 75% of the series reported have used some type of an ePTFE biomaterial. Generally this will be the DualMesh® in its original form as the newer product has been in existence for a shorter time. The remaining 25% of the series have used a PPM product. There have been no reports of fistulization in any of these series but this has been reported with the inguinal herniorraphy using PPM (29). Two papers, referenced above, have reported the use of Parietex® Composite in a total of 30 patients. No long-term reports are known on the implantation of the Composix® mesh.

Other concerns should be the ability of the chosen prosthesis to be fixed to the abdominal wall by whatever method is used. In most, this will include both the use of the helical tacks and transfascial sutures. All of these prosthetics will provide enough structural support for both of these fixation methods. Some surgeons do not feel that sutures are necessary with this procedure irrespective of the biomaterial chosen. Longer follow-up will validate or negate this concept.

Effects of the Biomaterials

The implantation of a foreign material into the body can have either helpful or harmful results. The currently used biomaterials do not cause most of the myriad of problems that were seen in the earlier part of the last century with the early synthetic biomaterials. There are a few comments that are warranted, however.

One early concern with the implantation of any product that is foreign to the body is that of infection. The use of these products has a good history in this regard. None appear to incite infection. Once an infection develops, however, these materials behave differently. In general, an infected PPM biomaterial can be treated without removal of the product in approximately 80% of the cases. Additionally, there is a possibility of open drainage of the infection and subsequent granulation over the mesh. The wound can then heal by secondary intention or a split thickness skin graft could be placed onto the granulating bed.

The same cannot be said with the ePTFE biomaterials. If an infection occurs with these products, in at least 80% or more of the patients, the patch will require removal. In that instance, the patient will be left with a very high likelihood of recurrence of the hernia. To lessen this risk, the use of one of the absorbable biomaterials at the time of explantation may help in closure of the resulting fascial defect. When the hernia recurs, I would not hesitate to place the ePTFE again, unless there was some predisposition of the patient to infections. I would also recommend using the biomaterial with the impregnated antimicrobial agents. Fortunately, however, this problem is infrequent (7-13).

On rare occasion, one may attempt to temporize in the patient with severe infection who is critically ill and has a large fascial defect. In this instance, the surgeon could sequentially remove the midportion of the patch material and sew it together. In this manner, the fascial edges of the large hernia will come together slowly. Hopefully, this could occur rapidly enough to allow complete removal of the prosthesis and primary closure of the hernia. One would have to accept the likelihood of recurrence, however. If the patient survived, it could be repaired at a later date.

Seroma formation has been said to occur in the majority of patients after the LIVH. The difficulty in the review of the literature lies in the fact of the definition of the term "seroma" in each of the reported series.

The majority of the published papers have demonstrated a rate of some type of seroma formation varying from 2-13% (2, 6, 7, 9, 29, 30). These papers utilized the DualMesh® biomaterial. The majority used the product that lacked the antimicrobial agents although this does not seem to have had an impact on the occurrence of a seroma. In the only paper that has been published with a significant patient population in which PPM was used as the prosthetic biomaterial, the incidence of seroma was 1.1% (7). Generally these are defined as clinically significant if they lasted more than four weeks or were symptomatic to the patient. Until a standardized method to quantify and delineate the significance of any collection of fluid above the prosthesis, it shall be difficult to recognize the actual occurrence of the complication. Suffice it to say that at this time, many patients will develop some type of seroma and that in the majority, it will not result in clinical difficulties because these generally will resolve without intervention.

These seromas can, however, predispose to the development of an infection and a resulting abscess. In this instance, the prosthesis will usually require removal, which results in a recurrence of the fascial defect. This problem appears to be more related to those patients in whom an attempt is made to aspirate the seroma. With this in mind, I would refrain from attempting to aspirate these fluid collections. The vast majority will, in fact, remain benign and resolve spontaneously.

One of the factors that should be given consideration when choosing a prosthesis for either open or laparoscopic incisional hernia repair is the results of the healing and scarring processes that will normally occur. The in-growth characteristics of the PPM products involve a significant amount of cicatrization. The dense scar that forms is a desirable event to many surgeons who feel that this is necessary for a strong and permanent repair of the fascial defect. This will result in contraction of the scar as part of normal healing. The PPM products are well known to shrink as much as 20% once they in place for 90 or more days (31). This fact may predispose the patient to chronic pain (see below) or may increase the risk of recurrence of the hernia because of this fact. The ePTFE biomaterials, on the other hand, have not been shown to undergo contraction to any significant degree. This can be explained by the lack of large interstices of the material itself. Additionally, the healing process that occurs with this biomaterial more approximates the normal processes of the healing tissues. Both of these factors significantly diminish the scar contraction that is seen with the PPM products (20, 21, 32).

Chronic pain associated with the use of prosthetic is a poorly understood phenomenon. With the laparoscopic repair, it has been reported to vary from approximately 1-2% (7, 8). The cause of the pain has not been satisfactorily determined. The two series noted above used PPM and ePTFE respectively. Therefore, it is somewhat difficult to attribute the pain to the biomaterial itself. I have personally removed a Composix® mesh from one patient because of debilitating pain that persisted following an open repair of an incisional hernia 14 months after the implant. The fascial defect was repaired with a DualMesh® patch with an open technique that mimicked the laparoscope method. The patient remains pain free eight months after excision of the PPM.

To further confuse this picture, I have had two patients that had severe pain after an open and a laparoscopic repair of incisional hernias respectively using ePTFE. Both patients had permanent resolution of their pain subsequent to the laparoscopic release of the transfascial suture at the site of the pain. Consequently, one must not definitely attribute the occurrence of chronic postoperative pain to the biomaterial in every case. Generally, this type of pain will resolve with time with conservative measures. If it does not, consideration of either cutting the offending suture or complete excision of the prosthetic must be given. I would predict that with the ePTFE, the complete excision will be rarely needed.

As mentioned above, the choice of prosthesis that is placed intraperitoneally should be made with careful forethought, as this biomaterial will be in direct contact with the intestine. It is important to remember that there is a known occurrence of adhesion formation and fistulization with the PPM products. This has been seen in the past with the open repair of incisional hernias. It is anticipated that this will also been experienced with the laparoscopic placement of the PPM biomaterials. Certainly the occurrence of adhesions after this operation using PPM has been reported. Franklin (7) noted that only one third of the nineteen patients that were re-laparoscoped after the use of PPM had no adhesions. In one third of these patients, however, "severe" adhesions were seen. The passage of time will be necessary to evaluate the development of fistulas secondary to these adhesions.

There has not been a report of fistulization with the use of a ePTFE biomaterial. The only incidence of any fistula associated with a LIVH repair that used an ePTFE biomaterial was not related to the biomaterial but instead was due to the helical tack that was used to fixate the patch (13). During several re-operations on patients that we have placed an intraperitoneal ePTFE, we have seen filmy adhesions in some of these cases. Occasionally, as mentioned above, we have seen encapsulation of the visceral surface but this was easily removed to expose the DualMesh® underneath (Figure 22). I have personally used ePTFE in the open and laparoscopic repair of both inguinal and incisional hernias since 1985 and have never seen any problem related to adhesions nor have I seen a postoperative fistula.

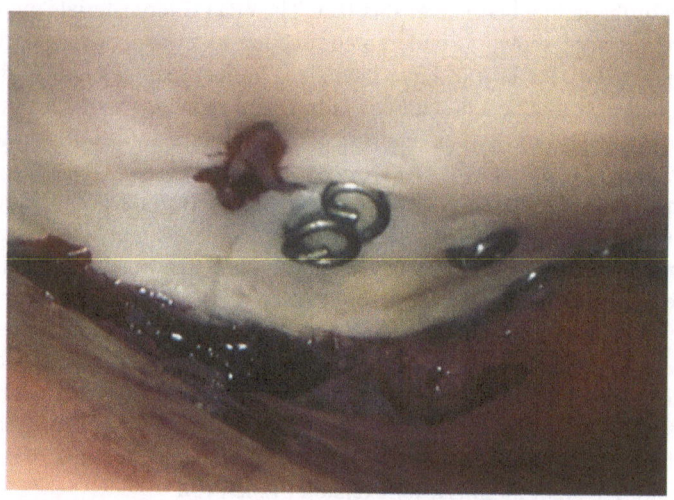

Fig. 22. Laparoscopic appearance of DualMesh® after dissection of the "visceral" surface capsule.

Results

Regardless of the biomaterial that has been utilized with the LIVH, the results of the procedure are favorable. In fact, in most early series, the results are superior to the open repair with the use of a prosthesis and particularly with sutured repairs. The long-term follow-up of these patients will be necessary to evaluate its effectiveness. Based on our findings, these patients must be followed for a minimum of three years to positively ascertain the exact rate of recurrence with the individual surgeon (9). The overall rate of recurrence in the literature averages 3.1%. I would consider that even this excellent number will be improved with the experience that is gained over the next several years.

FUTURE PROSTHETIC BIOMATERIALS

The discussion within this chapter delineates the currently available biomaterials. Without a doubt, others will be developed in the future. The goal of any new product will continue to be achievement of the "ideal" goals of the surgeon and the patient. The most important considerations will be the ease of use, normal tissue penetration and the elimination of adhesions. With the current materials, it may difficult to actually improve on the clinical results. Many future "improvements" may actually be marketing efforts rather than clinical benefits.

The true future of biomaterials may be in a completely new arena rather than that of new synthetic biomaterials. The technological advancements that have been noted on the biotechnical aspects of medicine will probably advance the science of biomaterials in the not so distant future. Genetically altered or bio-engineered biomaterials may address many of the disadvantages of the current materials. It is quite probable that such products will very nearly approximate the natural tissues that could be replaced with these biocompatible "reproductions" of human tissue. Such an advance would truly change the face of surgical correction of hernia defects.

CONCLUSION

The current enthusiasm for the LIVH is based on its success with minimal morbidity, cost effectiveness, and the low rate of recurrence. It may become the new "standard of care" for the treatment of incisional and ventral hernias.

The surgeon that adopts the LIVH for the treatment of these hernias must be familiar with the prosthetic biomaterial options that are currently available. In this manner, he or she will perform the most effective operation with the least amount of risk to the patient. Most importantly, the permanence of the repair will be assured. Many manufacturers will claim the benefits of the products but only a few have been proven. Until the "ideal" biomaterial is found, one must rely on the history of those currently in use. The future will hopefully provide for the development of the most perfect prosthetic, probably one that is based on human tissues.

References

1. Hesselink VJ, Luijendijk RW, deWilt JHW, et al. An evaluation of risk factors in incisional hernia recurrence. Surg Gynecol Obstet 176:228-234, 1993.

2. Linden van der FT, Vroonhoven van TJ. Long-term results after surgical correction of incisional hernia. Neth J Surg 40:127-129,1998.

3. Leber GE, Garb JL, Alexander AI, Reed WP. Long-term Complications Associated With Prosthetic Repair of Incisional Hernias. Arch Surg 133:378-382, 1998.

4. Luijendijk RW, Hop WCJ, Tol van den P, et al. A Comparison of Suture Repair With Mesh Repair for Incisional Hernia. N Engl J Med 343:392-398, 2000.

5. LeBlanc KA, Booth WV. Laparoscopic repair of incisional abdominal hernias using expanded polytetrafluoroethylene: preliminary findings. Surg Laparosc Endosc. 1993;3:39-41.

6. Kyzer S, Alis M, Aloni Y, Charuzi I. Laparoscopic repair of postoperation ventral hernia. Surgical Endoscopy 13:928-931, 1999.

7. Franklin ME, Dorman JP, Glass JL, Balli JE, Gonzales JJ. Laparoscopic Ventral and Incisional Hernia Repair. Surgical Laparoscopy & Endoscopy 8(4):294-299, 1998.

8. Heniford BT, Park A, Ramshaw BJ, Voeller G. Laparoscopic Ventral and Incisional Hernia Repair in 407 Patients. Journal of the American College of Surgeons 190(6):645-650, 2000.

9. LeBlanc KA, Booth WV, Whitaker JM, Bellanger DE. Laparoscopic Incisional and Ventral Herniorraphy in 100 Patients. American Journal of Surgery 180(3):193-197, 2000.

10. Park A, Birch DW, Lovrics, P. Laparoscopic and open incisional hernia repair: A comparison study. Surgery 124(4):816-822, 1998.

11. Carbajo MA, Martin del Olmo JC, Blanco JI, de la Cuesta C, Toledano M, Martin F, Vaquero C, Inglada L. Laparoscopic treatment vs. open surgery in the solution of major incisional and abdominal wall hernias with mesh. Surgical Endoscopy 13: 250-252, 1999.

12. Ramshaw BJ, Escartia P, Schwab J, Mason EM, Wilson RA, Duncan TD, Miller J, Lucas GW, Promes J. Comparison of Laparoscopic and Ventral Herniorraphy. American Surgeon 65:827-832, 1999.

13. DeMarie EJ, Moss JM, Sugerman HJ. Laparoscopic intraperitoneal polytetrafluoroethylene (PTFE) prosthetic patch repair of ventral hernia. Surgical Endoscopy 14:326-329, 2000.

14. Bucknall TE, Cox PJ, Ellis H. Burst Abdomen and Incisional Hernia: a Prospective Study of 1129 Major Laparotomies. Br Med J 284:931-933, 1982.

15. Goepel R. Uber die verschliersung von bruchpforten durch einleilung gerflochtener fertiger silberdrahtnetze. Verh Deutsch Ges Pathol. 1900;29:4.

16. Kirschner M. Die praktischen Ergebnisse der freien Fascien-Tranaplantation. Arch Klin Chir 1910;92:888-912.

17. Cumberland O. Ueber die Verschliessung von Bauchwunden und Brustpforten durch Bersenkte Siberdragrnetze. Zentralbl Chir 1900;27:257.

18. Scales JT. Discussion on metals and synthetic materials in relation to soft tissues: tissue reactions to synthetic materials. Proc R Soc Med 1953;46:647.

19. Vrijland WW, Bonthuis F, Steyerberg EW, Marquet RL, Jeckel J, Bonjer HJ. Peritoneal adhesions to prosthetic materials. Surg Endosc 14:960-963, 2000.

20. LeBlanc KA. Two phase *In Vivo* Comparison Study of Adhesion Formation of the Goretex Soft Tissue Patch, Marlex Mesh, and Surgipro using a Rabbit Model, in Inguinal Hernia: Advances or Controversies, eds. Arregui, ME and Nagan, RF, Radcliffe Medical Press Ltd. pp. 515-517.

21. LeBlanc KA. Two phase *In Vivo* Comparison Studies of the Tissue Response to Polypropylene, Polyester, and Expanded Polytetrafluoroethylene Grafts Used in the Repair of Abdominal Wall Defects, in Peritoneal Adhesions. Eds. Truetner KH, and Schumpelick V., Springer-Verlag. pp. 352-362, 1997.

22. LeBlanc KA, Booth WV, Whitaker JM, Baker D. *In vivo* Study of Meshes Implanted over the Inguinal Ring and External Iliac Vessels in Uncastrated Pigs. Surg Endosc 12:247-251,1998.

23. Greenwalt KE, Butler TJ, Rowe EA, et al. Preclinical Evaluation of Sepramesh‰ Surgical Composite Prosthesis in a Rabbit Incisional Hernia Repair Model. Presented at the American Hernia Society meeting, Toronto, Canada, June 15-18, 2000.

24. Greenawalt KE, Butler TJ, Rowe EA, Finneral AC, Garlick DS, Burns JW. Evaluation of a sepramesh biosurgical composite in a rabbit repair model. J Surg Res 2000;94:92-98.

25. Balique JG, Alexandre JH, Arnaud JP, Benchetrit S, et al. Intraperitoneal treatment of incisional and umbilical hernias: intermediate results of a multicenter prospective clinical trial using an innovative composite mesh. Hernia 4[suppl]:S10-S16,2000.

26. Benchetrit S, Debaert M, Detruit B, Dufilho A, Gaujoux D, et al. Laparoscopic and open abdominal wall reconstruction using Parietex® meshes: clinical results in 2700 hernias. Hernia 2:57-62.

27. Carbajo MA, Martin del Olmo JC, Blanco JI, de la Cuesta C, Martin F, Toledano M, Perna C, Vaquero C. Laparoscopic Treatment of Ventral Abdominal Wall Hernias: Preliminary Results in 100 Patients. Journal of the Society of Laparoendoscopic Surgeons 4:141-145, 2000.

28. DeBorg J, Bauer JJ, Grischkan DM, LeBlanc KA, Smoot RT, Voeller GR, Weiland LH. Short-Term Study on the Safety of Antimicrobial-Agent-Impregnated ePTFE Patches for Hernia Repair. Hernia 4(3):189-193, 1999.

29. Klein AM, Banever TC. Enteroctaneous Fistula as a Postoperative Complication of Laparoscopic Inguinal Hernia Repair. Surg Laparosc & Endo 9(1):60-62, 1999.

30. Toy FK, Bailey RW, Carey S, Chappuis CW, Gagner M, Josephs LG, Mangiante EC, Park A, Pomp A, Smoot RT, Uddo JF, Voeller G. Prospective, multicenter study of laparoscopic ventral hernioplasty. Surgical Endoscopy 12:955-959, 1998.

31. Amid P. Classification of biomaterials and their related complications in abdominal wall hernia surgery. Hernia 1:15-21,1997.

32. LeBlanc KA. Two-phase *in vivo* comparison studies of the tissue response to polypropylene, polyester, and expanded polytetrafluoroethylene grafts used in the repair of abdominal wall defects. In: Treutner KH, Schumpelick V, eds. *Peritoneal Adhesions*. Berlin: Springer-Verlag; 352-362, 1997.

CHAPTER 14

Adhesion Formation to Intraperitoneally-Placed Mesh: reoperative clinical experience after laparoscopic ventral incisional hernia repair

R.H. Koehler

INTRODUCTION

In the repair of abdominal incisional hernias, the need for synthetic reinforcement of the abdominal wall has been well established in the literature (1-7), and a recent multicenter study has confirmed the findings of these past reports (8).

The use of biomaterials in abdominal wall repair has been the topic of voluminous experimental research, and it is not the intent of this chapter to review the numerous studies to date. The extensive, 300-referenced work of Morris and Stiff is suggested to the reader (9), along with other chapters such as those in Schumpelink's recent text, "Incisional Hernia"(10), Bendavid's text (11), and that of Condon (12).

Comparatively little has been reported about reoperative experiences in the clinical setting with respect to adhesion formation to biomaterials used during abdominal incisional hernia repair. Most reports are largely anecdotal, and often can only be gleaned from reviewing the discussions. Much of it is found in the trauma literature, where biomaterials of many sorts have been popularly-and successfully-utilized for temporary closure of major abdominal wall defects.

The central clinical questions around the various biomaterials available remain two-fold: Does the material provide adequate strength to the repair (including the need for aponeurotic tissue incorporation), and is there a significant danger of severe visceral adhesion formation with the possibility of bowel obstruction and/or fistula development?

The latter question is the subject of this chapter, starting with a brief review of clinical reports on experiences with reoperations on the abdominal wall, comparing the various biomaterials available (principally involving polypropylene

(PP), polyesters (POL) and expanded polytetraflouroethylene (ePTFE). The significance of intraperitoneal patch location with respect to the advent of the laparoscopic approach to incisional hernia repair is discussed, and following that will be a preliminary report from this author, along with six colleagues, on their collective reoperative experience in 53 cases where a new, dual-layer ePTFE mesh (DualMesh: W.L. Gore & Asso. Flagstaff, AZ) was used for ventral incisional hernia repair.

REPORTS OF REOPERATIVE CLINICAL EXPERIENCES WITH BIOMATERIALS

As the use of biomaterial reinforcement in ventral and incisional hernia repair began, so too did early anecdotal reports of complications. A early as 1981, Kaufman (13) reported on a large bowel fistula with the use of polypropylene (PP), echoing concerns in 1979 raised by Schneider, who presented a case of diaphragmatically placed PP eroding into the esophagus and stomach (14).

The trauma literature became a frequent repository of reports on complications from meshes placed often in contact with the viscera. In 1981, Stone et al reported on their experiences with visceral adhesions to nonabsorbable materials used for temporary closure (15). In the same year, Voyles, et al found extensive PP mesh erosion, extrusion and fistula formation in 31 patients undergoing 23 reoperations after emergency abdominal wall closure with PP (16).

Fabian, et al reported in 1994 on reoperative experiences in trauma patients using a four-stage procedure involving removal of initially placed meshes (PP, ePTFE, polyglactin and plastic) (17). They found greater adhesions to polypropylene than to ePTFE, and the least adhesions to the polyglactin.

Brandt, et al in 1995 found fistula formation between PP and viscera in 7% of 70 trauma patient reconstructions (18). They also reported that an omental interposition appeared to eliminate fistula formation, a technique to be discussed later with respect to its advocacy by laparoscopic surgeons.

Nagy, et al in 1996 reported a retrospective experience with three materials(19)-PP, polyglycolate (Dexon) and ePTFE-in temporary abdominal wall closures in trauma patients. Their experience changed from using Marlex 7, then to Dexon in 8, then to soft-tissue ePTFE in 10: 8/25 patients died, leaving 4,6, and 7 patients respectively. Three out of four patients in the PP(Marlex) group developed fistulas. They removed the prosthesis at 19 days (all but one Marlex meshes were successfully removed), but adhesions were more severe to the Marlex. They found no wound sepsis in the ePTFE group. Based on this experience, the authors recommended ePTFE as temporary replacement material, and have "…abandoned the use of Marlex for temporary closure." They have also recently reported on ePTFE in experimental trauma protocols, and found it less adhesiogenic than polyglycolate (20).

In considering these reports of erosion and fistula formation to PP placed in the abdominal wall, it must be kept in mind that these cases involved extensive contamination due to the traumatic nature of the original injuries. Infection and multiple organ injury scenarios were part of the clinical spectrum. The PP meshes used were in contact with the viscera by necessity, and often there was no tissue covering over the patch externally. Caution, therefor, should be used in extrapolating these findings to the use of PP and POL meshes in elective incisional hernia cases.

There are several recent reports in non-trauma cases involving reoperative experiences with abdominal wall biomaterial implants. Karakousis, et al reported on cancer patients with abdominal wall defects (21). Of 56 patients undergoing reoperation with PP previously placed, 30 had an omental interposition at the time of the original surgery in an attempt to limit adhesion formation. In the 26 patients who did not have an omental interposition, fistula formation occurred in 26%.

Leber, et al recently reported a retrospective study of 200 patients, involving PP (Marlex), ePTFE (Gore-Tex soft tissue patch, W. L. Gore and Asso., Flagstaff, AZ), and POL(Mersilene) for closure of incisional hernias, that were apparently not trauma-related emergency cases (22). They further analyzed closure techniques as being with or without omental coverage and/or hernia sac coverage, and whether the mesh was onlay, subfascial, or a combination. In the series, 41% had the mesh placed subfascially all or in part, full fascial closure was done in 44%, and the omentum was used as coverage in 24%. Therefor at least 50% of the cases involved the mesh being potentially in contact with the viscera. The authors concluded that Mersilene had a significantly higher number of complications, including obstructions and fistulas. Unfortunately, the authors did not sub-categorize the type of closures and placement with respect to each material individually. Given the wide variations of closure techniques, and the independent significant difference if the mesh was in direct contact with the viscera, one could conclude (as the study implies) that closure technique had more to do with complications than the individual biomaterial used.

The advent of the laparoscopic approach to incisional hernia repair: the dilemna of covering the intraperitoneal patch

Even prior to the laparoscopic approach to incisional ventral hernia repair, it was clear from many authorities that avoiding mesh contact with the viscera was a critical part of the patch placement. Stoppa, and Wantz can both be quoted as saying "...the intraperitoneal prosthesis (Mersilene) must be prevented from touching the viscera either by the omentum or by an absorbable synthetic prosthesis" (7, 23). This warning is repeated by Shumpelink, stating (with respect to polypropylene and polyesters) that "...nonabsorbable meshes should never, if possible, be implanted adjacent to the hollow viscera..." (6). If the omentum is not present, both of these authors suggest using absorbable meshes as a barrier. Condon and Walker make the same pronouncement regarding PP: "...the bowel must be protected from the mesh,...because of the intense inflammatory reaction caused." (12). Recent reports on the open Stoppa approach echo these concerns as well (24).

With the laparoscopic approach to incisional hernia repair, first described by Leblanc and Booth (25), the choice of patch location was of necessity in the intraabdominal position. Many authors (not the above) in choosing PP or POL, were solving the viscera-contact problem by the use of an omental covering. Attempts at peritoneal dissection and covering over the mesh were found to be virtually prohibitive in most true incisional hernias. Holzman and Eubanks found this to be true in their early experience: "...a preperitoneal approach to incisional hernias is virtually impossible. Attempts to separate the peritoneum of the hernia sac are met with serious obstacles,...results in a large peritoneal defect,...and leaves exposed mesh." (26). Quoting from Abrahamson's chapter (27), they suggested omental interposition. Franklin suggested the same (28), while both Brandt (18) and Karakousis (21) felt this technique reduced or even eliminated adhesion of viscera to the PP. However, in Franklin's own reoperative experience in 19 cases, presumably using this technique, one third of patients had "severe" adhesions to the PP mesh.

Compounding the problem of mesh coverage are the larger mesh placements taking place laparoscopically. Park reported their early experience with large defects (29), noting patch sizes as large as 530cm². In the experience of this author, 38% of cases involved meshes of 18cm x 24 cm or larger, and 9% required two patches sewn together (30). This has also been the experience revealed in many other laparoscopic reports (28, 31-35). Avoiding the use of an omental cover by using ePTFE (DualMesh; W.L Gore and Asso., Flagstaff, AZ), Carbajo noted the difficulty one would face with covering a 18cm x 24cm patch in it's entirety by available omentum (36). It would seem concerning therefor, that larger PP and POL patches may be left exposed by attempts at omental coverage alone. Despite this, reports still exist with the use of direct intrabdominally placed POL (37).

If omentum is not available, Shumpelink suggests using absorbable mesh to protect the viscera from the nonabsorbable material, allowing that this will not eliminate severe adhesions but "...reduces the incidence by half" (6). This technique is also advised by Wantz (7, 23). One experimental study has suggested some efficacy to this technique (38).

However, with respect to nonabsorbable mesh placements during incisional hernia repair, there are no reoperative clinical experiences to suggest the effectiveness of such an absorbable barrier. The placement of an absorbable barrier to a large mesh, subsequently fixed to the extremely dynamic moving environment of the anterior abdominal wall, seems an improbable successful solution, even temporarily. This point is underscored in Luijendijk's multicenter study: "Contact between the polypropylene mesh and the viscera must be avoided because of the risk of adhesions, intestinal obstruction, and fistulas. When the peritoneum cannot be closed or when omentum cannot be interposed, polyglactin 910 (Vicryl) mesh may be interposed to protect the viscera, but experimental and clinical studies are not conclusive with respect to the efficacy of the interposition of the polyglactin mesh in preventing these complications"(8).

Baptista's study of adhesion formation in a rat model suggests that most adhesions fully developed within 7 days (39). They also found that adhesions started at the edges of the mesh, and worked toward the center, and that omentum adhered first, followed by bowel. This led to a suggestion that a temporary barrier would be required for perhaps as little as 7 days.

These observations have led to a significant research, and proprietarial, interest in coating and/or combining materials to achieve protection of the viscera from the nonabsorbable mesh. Much of this was promulgated by the report by Diamond that a hyaluronate-carboxymethylcellulose composite sheet prevented adhesions to pelvic organs in a multicenter trial (40). This much-quoted study led to the term "Diamond Scale" for adhesion descriptions, and as well to an arguably premature FDA approval of the substance, Seprafilm (Genzyme Corp., Cambridge, MA), extrapolating it's effectiveness not only in the gynecologic applications in which it had been tested, but in preventing adhesions additionally in a wide variety of general surgical applications. One study has shown decreased adhesion formation by using layers of Seprafilm as a barrier in a rat model with traumatized bowel and polypropylene abdominal wall closure (41). Their scoring system, however, was simply "dense" versus "filmy".

Amid however cautioned about the results of Baptista's suggestions, and sited their own experience in developing composite materials to achieve the combination of nonabsorbable mesh with visceral protection (42, 43). This area of interest has led to a bewildering array of materials with exotic properties combining nonabsorbable and absorbable properties: Composix (Davol, Cranston,RI), Vypro (see studies by Shumpelink, et al. (10, 44), and Flourosoft (polyglactin and POL-see Vrijland, et al. (45) are but a few examples. Unfortunately as well, many authors suggest different materials as being the most appropriate for use in incisional hernia repair: Polypropylene-Devlin (46), Chevrel (47), POL-Stoppa, Wantz, Arnaud (23, 37, 48), and ePTFE-DualMesh-Henniford, et al (30, 32-33, 49-50). Some have even reported covering POL with ePTFE (51).

The scope of research on these materials is beyond the intent of this chapter. Rather, what follows is a review of recent experiences in reoperative surgery, to be compared with those discussed above, with both ePTFE Gore-Tex Soft Tissue patches and with the newer dual-layer ePTFE, DualMesh (W.L.Gore and Asso., Flagstaff, AZ.)

REOPERATIVE EXPERIENCES WITH ePTFE IN INCISIONAL HERNIA REPAIRS

In light of the concerns raised as discussed above with respect to protecting the viscera from either PP or POL, the choice of ePTFE Soft Tissue Patch became popular in an attempt to limit adhesion formation. Reoperative experiences began demonstrating an apparent effectiveness.

Bellon reported on reoperative experiences in patients who had undergone incisional hernia repairs with ePTFE "soft tissue patches"(52). They performed electron microscopy as well as light microscopy on biopsies from these patients, and observed a "neoperitoneum" developing sometime after 40 days, and in all cases by 12 months. The same researchers followed up in an animal model, comparing ePTFE to PP, and found a similar neoperitoneum developing by 90 days in the ePTFE group, but not at all in the PP group (53).

Gillion reported 6 "second look cases" in 158 open repairs with ePTFE soft tissue patch (not DualMesh) (54): no adhesions were seen, and the authors commented that the "...tolerance to ePTFE prosthesis was excellent,...no obstructive complications."

Koller reported 2 reoperative cases out of 26 repairs with ePTFE, and noted the dissection was accomplished "without difficulty" (55).

Leber's review was discussed above (22) reporting fewer adhesions to ePTFE than POL, allowing again for the multiple closure techniques and clinical circumstances involved in their cohort.

REOPERATIVE EXPERIENCES WITH ePTFE-DUALMESH IN INCISIONAL HERNIA REPAIRS

After Leblanc and Booth's report (25), the use of ePTFE DualMesh for laparoscopic incisional and ventral hernia repair increased to the point where well over 1000 cases have been reported (29, 30-35, 49, 56). This material incorporates a standard ePTFE "smooth" surface to face the visceral side of the repair, while the opposite side has been engineered to open the surface to at least 22um sized pores ("rough" side), and later variations have included microperforations as well as the most recent engineering involving a corrugated surface to the "rough"side ("Corduroy" DualMesh). The technique for placement is detailed elsewhere in this textbook.

Reports with the new DualMesh are amongst the most recent to be seen. In this author's initial series (30), reoperative experiences with the DualMesh revealed either no adhesions, or filmy avascular adhesions that came down with gentle blunt dissection. Most impressive was the observation of a well vascularized "neoperitoneum" across the entire patch, similar to what had been described by Bellon et al. Carbajo reported the same finding in their series, where the two reoperative cases they described revealed a complete reperitonealization of the DualMesh patch (31).

This author has compiled preliminary results from personal experiences as well as those of six other surgeons, all with extensive experience with laparoscopic incisional hernia repair. These preliminary findings represent the first such review of its kind.

Fifty three patients underwent reoperations, who had all had DualMesh previously placed in the abdominal wall for ventral and incisional hernias. Adhesions were scored, retrospectively from operative reports, using the scale reported by Diamond (40).

The average time between initial implant placement and reoperation was 420 days (2-1739): 92% of the cases showed either no adhesions, or filmy avascular adhesions. Of the 8% with dense adhesions, these were to omentum only. No enterotomies occurred during adhesiolysis. Early reoperations, those less than 14 days, showed no adhesions and no neoperitoneum (Fig. 1). By later intervals, the previously described neoperitoneum across the entire patch was seen in all cases

(Fig. 2). (The plane of dissection therefor can be chosen either between omentum/viscera and neoperitoneum, or between neoperitoneum and patch surface; both were easily developed.) It is of note that one can in fact "harvest" this membrane, intact, off the underlying patch surface(Fig. 3) Whether this finding has application to endothelial membrane research is an intriguing question to be answered.

With respect to individual patient differences in adhesion formation to different biomaterials, several interesting observations in this author's experience along with those of Henniford and Ramshaw (32) are of note. Several patients had previous PP mesh placed as well as the subsequent DualMesh. Many of these patients had been noted to have dense adhesions to the PP at the time of original surgery At reoperation, dense adhesions were seen to the PP (Fig. 4), whereas adhesions were minimal to the DualMesh, implying that the adhesions seen were not patient specific, but due rather to the biomaterials themselves.

Interestingly as well, adhesions occur on the antimesenteric border of the bowel wall. Given the relative ischemia of the bowel wall in this region, coupled with the extensive adhesiolysis being performed, this may account for reports of "delayed" enterotomy as seen in this author's initial experience, where two enterotomies were not evident until 36 hours and 5 days postoperatively. This phenomenon has been reported by others as well (32, 33). Ramshaw reported that one of two enterotomies in their 100 cases was occult and not immediately recognized, and one of six enterotomies in the multicenter trial series did not manifest at the time of surgery. Many o f these investigators, including this author, believe that these cases represent delayed breakdown of the antimesenteric border rendered ischemic by the adhesiolysis. This underscores the need for careful post-operative evaluation of patients who have required extensive adhesiolysis.

Adhesions were also seen to exposed titanium tacks (Fig. 5). It should be noted that staples as well as tacks are equally adhesiogenic, and the 5mm tack, we believe, offers a superior holding ability with respect to the ePTFE mesh in the ventral abdominal wall.

Although we choice the "Diamond Scale" to describe adhesions, we all found significant limitations. We choice not to use the quantitative portion, since our concern was far greater with how difficult the separation of omentum/viscera was during adhesiolysis, rather than with the surface area involved. Easily sweeping aside several hundred square centimeters of filmy adhesions may take less than a minute, without incident. Conversely, even a few square centimeters of sever dense adhesions to PP can lead to an enterotomy (Fig. 6). Likewise, comparisons of studies such as those discussed above are very difficult, due to many different descriptions of what are "mild" versus "severe" adhesions.

This author favors an adhesion scale that reflects the ease, or difficulty, with which adhesiolysis is carried out. The one described by Zuhle, et al is close to this goal (57): 1: filmy , easy to separate; 2: blunt dissection possible, partly sharp dissection; 3: sharp only; strongly attached; 4: injury to organ likely.

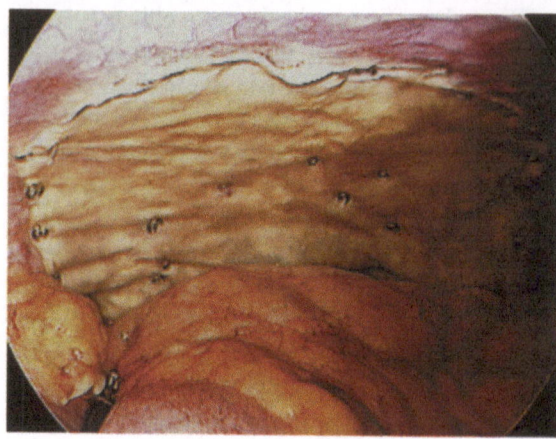

Fig. 1. DualMesh at 5 days. Patient had developed an incarcerated inguinal hernia five days after repair of this previously incarcerated flank nephrectomy hernia.

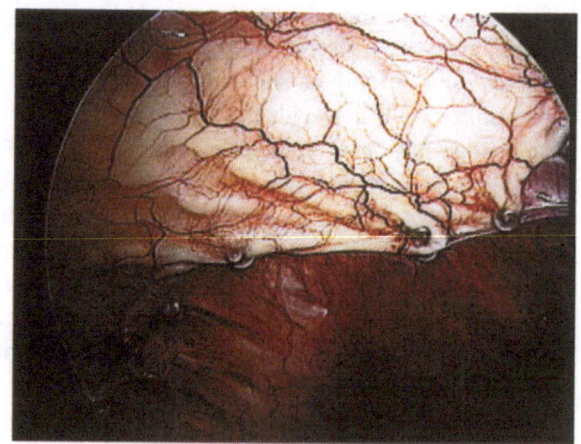

Fig. 2. DualMesh at 20 months. Note neoperitoneum and extensive vascularization across large patch surface (18cm x 24 cm).

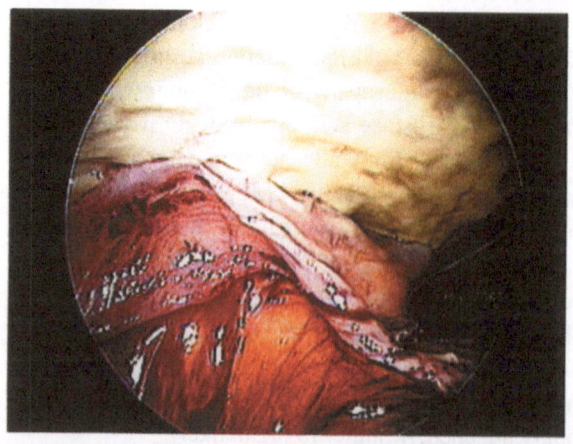

Fig. 3. Harvesting of neoperitoneum away from DualMesh surface in same case as Figure 2.

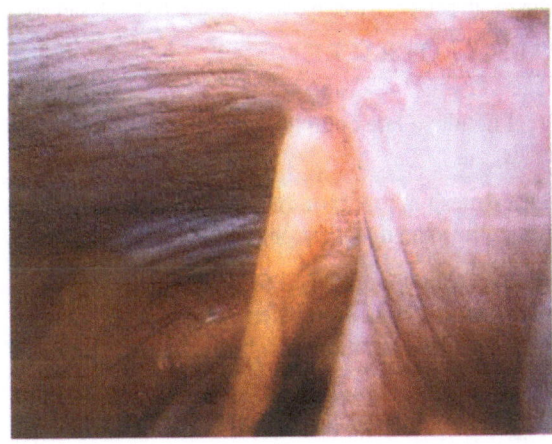

Fig. 4. Adhesion to polypropylene seen in patient where subsequent DualMesh placement resulted in no adhesion formation.

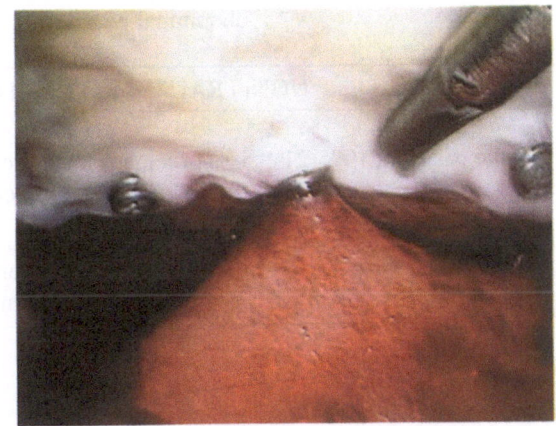

Fig. 5. Adhesion to titanium tack 12 days post-operatively; note lack of adhesions to DualMesh. (Patient had developed a small bowel obstruction due to enteroenteric adhesions unrelated to the repair).

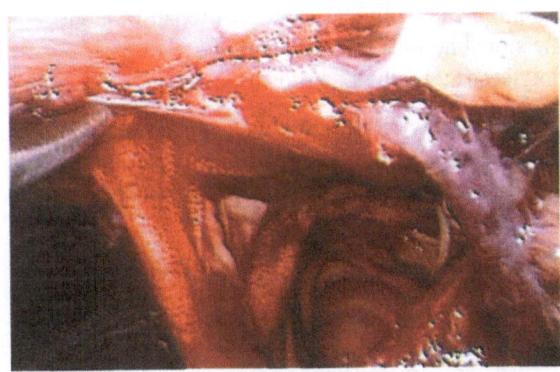

Fig. 6. Enterotomy in small bowel densely adhered to polypropylene: note polypropylene in right upper corner essentially completely incorporated into the bowel wall. (Patient had presented with small bowel obstruction after intraabdominally-placed polypropylene "protected" with a layer of polyglactan.

Table I. Clinical reports of complications with polypropylene meshes in abdominal wall surgery

TRAUMA LITERAURE	
Kaufman et al, 1981(13)	Fecal fistula: a late complication of Marlex mesh repair
Schneider et al, 1979 (14)	Marlex mesh in repair of diaphragmatic defect later eroding into the distal esophagus and stomach
Voyles et al, 1981(16)	Emergency abdominal wall reconstruction with polypropylene mesh: short-term benefits versus long-term complications
Fabian et al, 1994(17)	Planned ventral hernia: staged management for acute a abdominal wall defects.
Brandt et al, 1995(18)	Polypropylene mesh closure after emergency laparotomy: morbidity and outcome
Nagy KK et al, 1999 (20)	Optimal prosthetic for acute replacement of the abdominal wall
NON-TRAUMA LITERATURE	
Karakousis et al, 1995(21)	Use of a mesh for musculoaponeurotic defects of the abdominal wall in cancer surgery and the risk of bowel fistulas
Leber et al, 1998(22)	Long-term complications associated with prosthetic repair of incisional hernias

Table II. Clinical reports of reoperative experience with ePTFE: Soft tissue Patch (W.L. Gore, and Asso., Flagstaff, AZ)

Bellon et al, 1997(52)	Pathologic and clinical aspects of repair of large incisional hernias after implant of a polytetrafluoroethylene prosthesis
Gillion et al, 1997(54)	Expanded polytetrafluoroethylene patches used in the intraperitoneal or extraperitoneal position for repair of incisional hernias of the anterolateral abdominal wall
Koller et al, 1997(55)	Repair of incisional hernias with ePTFE
Leber et al, 1998(22)	Long-term complications associated with prosthetic repair of incisional hernias

Table III. Reoperative cases involving ePTFE DualMesh (W.L.Gore & Asso., Flagstaff, AZ)

Average age		55 (27-86)
Average time from original repair		420days(2-1739)
Reason for reoperation:		
Recurrence		11
Complication		9
New diagnosis		16
	Total	53
Adhesion Score*		
0		10 ⎫ 92%
1		39 ⎭
2		4

*Based on severity rate, Diamond et al. (40)

CONCLUSION

Laparoscopic ventral incisional hernia repairs involve, out of necessity, the placement of nonabsorbable mesh in an intraabdominal location. Extensive experimental research has been carried out to evaluate the adhesiogenic properties of synthetic mesh materials in an effort to determine the risk of visceral adhesion formation in clinical scenarios. Despite this, comparatively little has been written about clinical reoperative experiences with these materials, other than that reported in the trauma literature-where multiple extenuating circumstances make application of that data to elective hernia surgery very difficult.

The collective reoperative experiences discussed here, with respect to biomaterials used in abdominal ventral and incisional hernia repairs, suggest that ePTFE DualMesh is unique in effectively limiting, and at times eliminating, visceral adhesion formation under clinical conditions.

Extensive ongoing research is being carried out on newer materials involving the combination of both absorbable and nonabsorbable materials for use in abdominal wall hernia repairs. Clinical reoperative experiences, evaluated with meaningful adhesion-scaling systems, will be important determinants as to the comparative effectiveness of these newer materials.

Acknowledgment.
The author thanks the following colleagues for the use of their data on reoperative experience with DualMesh:
Dennis Begos MD (Lawrence, MA), Prof. Deiter Berger MD (Baden-Baden, Germany), Steve Carey MD and Roy Smoot MD (Seaford, DE), Karl LeBlanc MD (Baton Rouge, LA), and Bruce Ramshaw MD (Atlanta, GA).

References

1. Bendavid R (1994) The need for mesh. In: Bendavid R (Eds.) Prostheses and abdominal wall hernias. (pp. 116-122) Austin, TX: RG Landes Company.

2. George CD, Ellis H. The results of incisional hernia repair: a twelve year review. Ann Roll Coll Surg Eng. 1986;68:185-7.

3. Hesselink VJ, Luijendijk RW, deWilt J, Heide R et al. An evaluation of risk factors in incisional hernia recurrence. Surg Gyn Obst 1993;176:228-234.

4. Mudge M and Hughes LE Incisional hernia: A 10-year prospective study of incidence and attitudes. Br J Surg 1985, 72:70-71.

5. Stoppa RE The treatment of complicated groin and incisional hernias. World J Surg. 1989;13:545-554.

6. Wantz GE. Incisional Hernia: the problem and the cure. JACS 1999;188:429-447.

7. Wantz G. Incisional hernioplasty with Mersilene. Surg Gyn Obst 1991;172:129.

8. Luijendijk RW, Hop W, van den Tol MP, de Lange DCD, Braaksma, MJ, IJzermans, JNM, Boelhouwer RU, de Vries BC, Salu MKM, Wereldsma JCJ, Bruijninckx CMA, Jeekel J. A Comparison of Suture Repair with Mesh Repair for Incisional Hernia. NEJM 2000;343:392-398.

9. Morris-Stiff GJ, Hughes LE The Outcomes of Nonabsorbable Mesh Placed Within the Abdominal Cavity: Literature Review and Clinical Experience. J Am Coll Surg 1998;186:352-67.

10. Schumpelink V and Kingsnorth AN, eds. Incisional Hernia. Berlin, Heidelberg, New York: Springer-Verlag; 1999:294-302.

11. DeBord J.R. (1994) Prostheses and hernia surgery: the evolution of the ideal material. In: Bendavid R. (Eds.) Prostheses and abdominal wall hernias. (pp. 7-32) Austin, TX: RG Landes Company.

12. Condon RE.Incisional Hernia. In Nyhus LM and Condon RE, ed. Hernia (4th ed). Lippincott Co;1995:319-339.

13. Kaufman Z, Engelberg M and Zager M Fecal fistula: a late complication of Marlex mesh repair. Dis Colon Rectum 1981, 24:543-544.

14. Schneider R, Herrington JL Jr, Granda AM. Marlex mesh in repair of diaphragmatic defect later eroding into the distal esophagus and stomach. Am Surg. 1979;45:337-339.

15. Stone HH, Fabian TC, Turkleson ML and Jurkiewicz MJ Management of acute full-thickness losses of the abdominal wall. Ann Surg 1981, 193:612-618.

16. Voyles CR, Richardson JD, Bland KI, Tobin GR, Flint LM, Polk HC. Emergency abdominal wall reconstruction with polypropylene mesh: short-term benefits versus long-term complications. Ann Surg 1981;194:219-223.

17. Fabian TC, Croce MA, Pritchard FE, et al. Planned ventral hernia: staged management for acute abdominal wall defects. Ann Surg 1994;219:643-653.

18. Brandt CP, McHenry CR, Jacobs DG, et al. Polypropylene mesh closure after emergency laparotomy: morbidity and outcome. Surgery 1995;118:736-741.

19. Nagy KK, Perez F, Fildes JJ, Barrett J.J. Optimal prosthetic for acute replacement of the abdominal wall. J Trauma 1999 Sep;47(3):529-32.

20. Nagy KK, Fildes JJ, Mahr C, Roberts RR et al. Experience with three prosthetic materials in temporary abdominal wall closure. Am Surg 1996;62:331-5.

21. Karakousis C, Volpe C and Tanski J. Colby ED, Winston J, Driscoll DL. Use of a mesh for musculoaponeurotic defects of the abdominal wall in cancer surgery and the risk of bowel fistulas. J Am Coll Surg 1995, 181:11-16.

22. Leber GE, Garb JL, Alexander AI, Reed WP. Long-term complications associated with prosthetic repair of incisional hernias. Arch Surg 198;133:378-382.

23. Wantz GE. Open repairs of hernias of the abdominal wan. In: Scientific American Surgery 1995; Surg Tech:6:17-19.

24. Temudom T, Siadati M, Sarr MG. Repair of complex giant or recurrent ventral hernias by using tension-free intraparietal prosthetic mesh (Stoppa technique): lessons learned from our initial experience (fifty patients). Surgery 1996;120:73843; (disc 7434).

25. LeBlanc KA, Booth WV. laparoscopic repair of incisional hernias using expanded polytetrafluorethylene: preliminary findings. Surg Laparosc Endo. 1993;3:39-41.

26. Holzman MD, Purat CM and Reintgen K et al. Laparoscopic ventral and incisional hernioplasty. Surg Endosc 1997, 11:32-35.

27. Abrahamson J. Hernias. In Schwartz SI and Ellis h, ed. Maingot's Abdominal Operations (9th ed.). Appleton and Lang; 1989:273-296.

28. Franklin ME, Dorman JP, Glass JL, Balli JE, et al. Laparoscopic ventral incisional hernia repair. Surg Laparosc Endosc 1998;8:294-299.

29. Park A, Gagner M, Pomp A. Laproscopic repair of large incisional hernias. Surg Lapar Endo 1996;6:123-128.

30. Koehler RH, Voeller G. Recurrences in laparoscopic incisional hernia repairs: a personal series and review of the literature. J Laparoendosc Surg 1999;3:293-304.

31. Carbajo MA, Martin del Olmo JC and Blanco JI, de la Cuesta C, Martion F, Toledano M, Perna C, Vaquero C. Laparoscopic treatment of ventral abdominal wall hernias: preliminary results in 100 patients. J Laparoendosc Surg 2000;4:141-145.

32. Henniford BT, Ramshaw BJ. Laparoscopic ventral hernia repair:a report of 100 consecutive cases. Surg Endo 2000;14:419-423.

33. Heniford BT, Park A, Ramshaw BJ,Voeller G. Laparoscopic ventral and incisional hernia repair in 407 patients. J Am Coll Surg 2000;190:645-650.

34. LeBlanc KA, Booth WV, Whitaker JM, Baker D, Bellanger DE. Laparoscopic incisional and ventral herniorraphy in 100 patients. Am J Surg 2000;180:193-197.

35. Ramshaw BJ, Schwab J, Mason EM, et al. Comparison of laparoscopic and open ventral herniorrhaphy. Am Surg 1999;65:827–831.

36. Carbajo MA, Martin del Olmo JC and Blanco JI et al. Laparoscopic treatment versus open surgery in the solution of major incisional and abdominal wall hernias with mesh. Surg Endo 1999, 13:250-252.

37. Arnaud JP, Tuech JJ, Pessaux P, Hadchity Y. Surgical treatment of postoperative incisional hernias by intraperitoneal insertion of dacron mesh and an aponeurotic graft: a report on 250 cases. Arch Surg 1999;134:1260-1262.

38. Naim JO, Pulley D and Scanlan K et al. Reduction of postoperative adhesions to Marlex mesh using experimental adhesion barriers in rats. J Laparoendosc Surg 1993, 3:187-190.

39. Baptista ML, Bonsack ME, Felemovicius I, Delaney JP. Abdominal adhesions to prosthetic mesh evaluated by laparoscopy and electron microscopy. J Am Coll Surg 2000;190:271-280.

40. Diamond MP. Reduction of adhesions after uterine myomectomy by seprafilm membrane (HAL-F): a blinded, prospective, randomized, multicenter clinical study. Fert Steril 1996;66:904-910.

41. Dinsmore RC, Calton WC, Harvey SB, Blaney MW. Prevention of adhesions to polypropylene mesh in a traumatized bowel model. J Am Coll Surg 2000;191:131-136.

42. Amid PK. Intraabdominal adhesions to prosthetic mesh. J Am Coll Surg 2000;191:342-3.

43. Amid PK. Expanded polytetrafluoro-ethylene patches Amer J Surg 1998;175342.

44. Klosterhalfen B, Klinge U. Biocompatibility of biomaterials: histologic aspects. In Schumpelink V and Kingsnorth AN, eds. Incisional Hernia. Berlin, Heidelberg, New York: Springer-Verlag; 1999:211.

45. Vrijland WW, Bonthius F, Steyerberg EW, Marquet RL, Jeekel J, Bonjer HJ. Peritoneal adhesions to prosthetic materials; choice of mesh for incisional hernia repair. Surg Endo 2000;14:960-963.

46. Devlin B. Polypropylene mesh repair of incisional hernia: Marlex and prolene. In Schumpelink V and Kingsnorth AN, eds. Incisional Hernia. Berlin, Heidelberg, New York: Springer-Verlag; 1999:294-302.

47. Chevrel JP, Rath AM. Polyester mesh for incisional hernia repiar. In Schumpelink V and Kingsnorth AN, eds. Incisional Hernia. Berlin, Heidelberg, New York: Springer-Verlag; 1999;327-333.

48. Wantz GE, Fischer E. Prosthetic incisional hernioplasty: Indications and results. In Schumpelink V and Kingsnorth AN, eds. Incisional Hernia. Berlin, Heidelberg, New York: Springer-Verlag; 1999: 303-311.

49. Toy FK, Bailey RW, Carey S, Chappuis CW, et al: Prospective, multicenter study of laparoscopic ventral hernioplasty. Surg Endo 1998;12:955-959.

50. Park A, Burch DW and Lovrics P. Laparoscopic and open incisional hernia repair: a comparison study. Surgery 1998;124:816-822.

51. Farrakha M. Laparoscopic treatment of ventral hernia. Surg Endo 2000;14:1156-1158.

52. Bellon JM, Contreras LA, Sabater C, Bujan J. Pathologic and clinical aspects of repair of large incisional hernias after implant of a polytetrafluoroethylene prosthesis. World J Surg 1997;21:402-407.

53. Bellon JM, Contreras LA, Bujan J, Pascual G, Carrera-San Martin A. Effect of relaparotomy through previously integrated polyupropylene and polytetraflouroethylene experimental implants in the abdominal wall. J Am Coll Surg 1999;188:466-472.

54. Gillion JF, Begin GF, Marecos C, Fourtanier G. Expanded polytetrafluoroethylene patches used in the intraperitoneal or extraperitoneal position for repair of incisional hernias of the anterolateral abdominal wall. Amer J Surg 1997;174:16-19.

55. Koller R, Miholic J, Jakl RJ. Repair of incisional hernias with ePTFE. Eur J Surg 1997;163:261-6.

56. Kyzer S, Alis M, Aloni Y, Charuzi I. Laparoscopic repair of postoperation ventral hernia. Early postoperation results. Surg Endo 1999 Sep;13:928-31.

57. Zuhle HV, Lorenz EMP, Straub EM, Savvas V. Pathophysiologie and klassifikation von adhasionen. Langenbecks Arch Chir Suppl II Verh Dtsch Ges Chir 1990;345:1009-1016.

CHAPTER 15

Methods of Fixation of the Prosthesis During Laparoscopic Incisional and Ventral Herniorraphy

K.A. LeBlanc

INTRODUCTION

Fixation of the prosthesis that is used is an integral component of the laparoscopic incisional and ventral herniorraphy (LIVH). While there are differences of opinion as to the most effective method of fixation, there will be some fixation device used in every case. Advancements in this technology has allowed for the development of this and many other minimally invasive procedures. Historically, the first fixation device that was described to repair hernias was the "Herniostat" described by Ger (1). He used this to fix a prosthesis in the inguinal area for the repair of inguinal hernias. Toy and Smoot later developed another device for the same purpose (Fig. 1). This was called the Nanticoke Hernia Stapler. Neither of these products became commercially available because of the development and introduction of other devices. Each was designed for use in the laparoscopic repair of inguinal hernias but ultimately the descendents of such devices have found a place in the laparoscopic repair of incisional and ventral hernias.

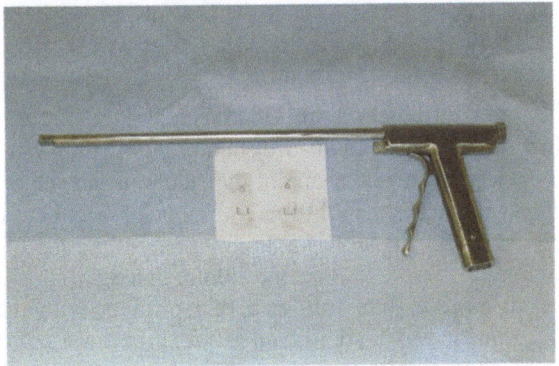

Fig. 1. Nanticoke Hernia Stapler and Staples

STAPLING INSTRUMENTS

The first stapling device that was mass-produced was the single fire stapler manufactured by Ethicon® Endosurgery, Inc. (Cincinatti, Ohio). This product fired a "box" type of staple that penetrated the biomaterial as it formed into the final shape. This was a good device but had the drawbacks of single usage and consequently required a reload of each staple after it was placed. This slowed down the operative procedure. Additionally, the shaft of the instrument was 10 mm and rigid. In such an early stage of laparoscopic herniorraphy, this did not represent a significant consideration as most instruments were 10 mm in diameter and did not "roticulate". Another aspect of the device that made it cumbersome was the fact that, on occasion, the staple would move from position just prior to firing the device, which resulted in poor placement and consequently poor fixation. In very limited areas, this product may still be available.

The next product that became available was the Endostapler® by United States Surgical Corporation (Norwalk, CN). It, too, was a 10mm instrument but it was a multi-fire device. Another feature that was particularly attractive was the articulating head that also rotated 360∞ (Fig. 2). The staple was also a "box" type in its final form. These improvements were seen as significant advancements for the laparoscopic inguinal hernia repair.

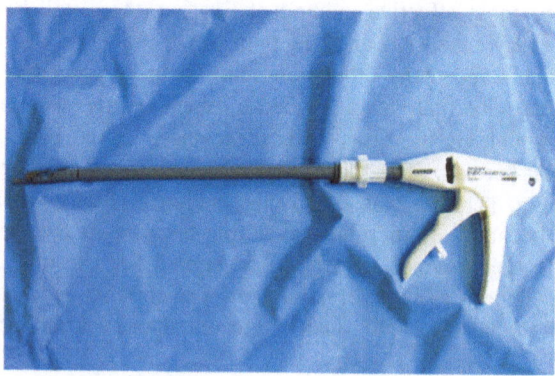

Fig. 2. United States Surgical Corporation Endostapler®

Shortly after the introduction by US Surgical of their device, Ethicon® Endosurgery, Inc. released their multi-fire stapler, the EMS device (Fig. 3). This continued with the same size and shape of the staple of the single fire device but this new instrument rotated and could fire several staples without reloading. The length of the crown of the staple was 5.3mm. The unfired leg of the staple was 3.7mm but once fired the staple leg became 2.0mm in length.

Ethicon® Endosurgery, Inc. followed this product with the Omni-tack® stapler. This instrument was a significant advance because not only could this device rotate 360∞ and articulate but also the final staple size could be altered, if necessary. This device has never been largely used due to the development of the helical tacks.

These stapling devices can be found in some limited areas and may still have
some application in the LIVH. Most investigators feel that the penetration of the
staple is not as secure as that of the newer tacks. In an unpublished study by this
author, the force required to remove the tacks and staples were compared. In
every aspect of comparison of these fixation devices, the staples were much less
secure than that of the tacks. Because of this, I discontinued the use of the staples.
However, in some areas of the abdomen such as the diaphragm, it may be found
that the staples may be preferable to the tacks. Few surgeons have chosen to do
so, however, and instead, will suture the prosthesis to the diaphragm, if this
becomes necessary.

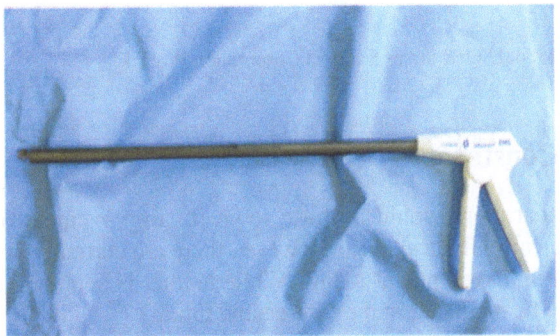

Fig. 3. Ethicon Endosurgery EAS® Stapler

Helical Tackers

These devices are the most commonly used method of fixation for the LIVH and
probably the laparoscopic inguinal hernia repair as well. These were first
introduced by Origin Medisystems, Inc. (Origin Medsystems, Inc., Menlo Park,
CA) The tack is a helical structure of titanium that is 5mm in length and 4mm in
diameter. This is fired through a 5mm device that is a marked improvement
because of the strength of fixation and the size of the delivery device. The tack
"screws" itself into the tissue and prosthesis as it is fired.

A similar product that functions as the above tacker is that of the Protack®
device and is manufactured by Tyco/United States Surgical Corporation (Fig. 4).
It, too, delivers a 5mm tack via a 5mm delivery device. The functional ease of this
instrument is superior to that of the Origin® product. Additionally, this instrument
allows for the removal of the tack. The end of the device can be placed onto the
inappropriately placed tack and rotated counterclockwise. This will "unscrew" the
tack upon which this is performed. The surgeon will unscrew the tack
approximately 2-3mm out of the tissue and then grasp it with an instrument for
removal. One must be careful during this maneuver that the offending tack is not
inadvertently dropped from the instrument and into the abdominal cavity. If this
occurs, the coil can sometimes be difficult to locate with the contents of the
abdomen.

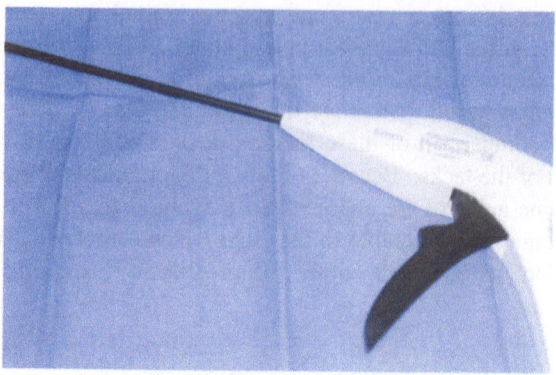

Fig. 4. United States Surgical Corporation Protack

Innovative "Constructs"

It would seem that there would be little room for improvement of the fixation methods that are currently available. However, there are currently at least two new products that are in development today. While neither is commercially available, both should soon be marketed in the foreseeable future.

Ethicon® Endosurgery, Inc. has sought to approach a new innovation by reportedly decreasing the size of the delivery shaft of the instrument that may be smaller than those previously released. This may be of benefit if the size of the trocars continues to decrease. The difficulty in the development of such a small diameter of this product will be the stiffness of the shaft and the resistance to deformation by the torque that will be applied by the operating surgeon. Firm fixation of the delivered fixation product will be the important component of the success of such a new product.

A totally new concept that has made itself more publicly known is that of the Salute™ product, manufactured by Onux Medical, Inc (Hampton, NH). This device is currently available to the clinician. This is an ingenious device that delivers a cylindrical "construct" of stainless steel. It is supplied via a spool that is within the handle of the instrument. Unlike the other fixation materials, this device is not preformed prior to the firing of the instrument. Upon the pulling of the "trigger" of the instrument the spool releases the wire that is then formed into the construct that will become the fixation product. The coil is in 90° rotation of that of the helical tacks that are so familiar today (Fig. 5). Based upon my own experience in the laboratory, it appears that this will be capable of securing the prosthetic biomaterial to the abdominal wall with sufficient strength that will allow appropriate in-growth of the biomaterial. The unique concept of this product is the fact that it will be the only non-disposable instrument that is a multi-fire device for the fixation of a prosthetic material.

Suture Fixation

Some surgeons dispute the use of sutures as an integral part of the fixation of the prosthetic biomaterial during the LIVH. Nevertheless, the majority of the published series have utilized this additional method of fixation. The suture choice is not critical but it must be a non-absorbable type of suture to provide permanent fixation.

It could be disputed that the use of the absorbable suture would provide for adequate fixation until such time that the in-growth of the product could support the fixation independent of the use of sutures. This has not been proven, however.

If sutures are to be used, they must be placed through the entire abdominal wall. The transfascial fixation of the biomaterial by the suture will tightly affix it. The surgeon must not allow the suture to become loosened during the knot tying process. This can be apparent after the knot is tied. The large amount of adipose tissue that is encountered in some patients may make this a cumbersome task but one that can be accomplished if careful technique is followed. If the suture is too loose, it must be cut and a new one must replace it.

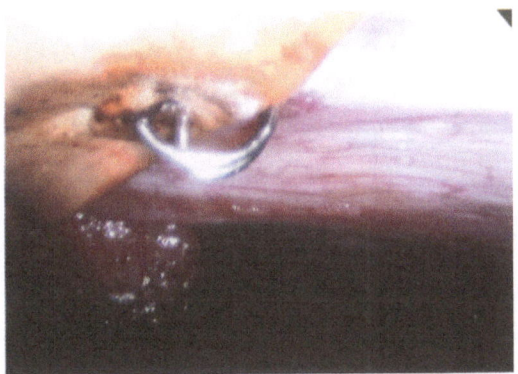

Fig. 5. "Construct" using the ONUX Medical Salute fixation device

CONCLUSION

The choice of the prosthetic that is used in the laparoscopic repair of the incisional and ventral hernia is important. Equally important is the choice of fixation. This must be firm enough to allow for the appropriate in-growth to occur. Currently, the most popular methods are the use of the helical tacker with or without sutures. Newer products are undergoing development. The surgeon must be familiar with the old products yet must be willing to seek out any improvement that may be seen in the future.

References

1. Ger R, Monro K, Duvivier R, et al. Management of Inguinal Hernias by Laparoscopic Closure of the Neck of the Sac. Am J Surg 1990;159:370-373.

CHAPTER 16

What have changed in Laparoscopic Ventral Hernia Repair: instruments, materials or technique? from the early 90s to nowadays

X. Feliu, E. Fernández-Sallent

INTRODUCTION

Incisional hernia is a relatively frequent complication of abdominal surgery, with an incidence rate of 11-20% in patients who undergo laparotomy (1-4). Although the condition occurs frequently and surgeons are quite familiar with such hernias, surgical treatment is not always successful. In fact, the recurrence and complication rates reported in the literature are around 30-54% (1, 3-6).

As a result, incisional hernias are a complex condition not always easy to treat and which frequently result in an unsatisfactory outcome that is disabling for the patient, with the attendant financial costs and morbidity rates (7, 8).

Once an incisional hernia has developed, the hernia tends to worsen steadily. In addition to the aesthetic defect, hemodynamic, respiratory and intestinal complications secondary to pressure changes produced by mechanical incompetence of the altered abdominal wall will occur (9).

Although the aesthetic defect is asymptomatic in some cases, most patients with incisional hernia present abdominal pain. Episodes of incarceration have been reported in 6-15% of cases (4, 6). As a result, a surgical solution to the problem should be recommended for these patients.

We still do not know exactly what causes an incisional hernia after a laparotomy. Most likely, no single factor is responsible for the condition and the etiology involves multiple factors that interact with each other to a lesser or greater extent. Some factors such as postoperative infection of the initial laparotomy and surgical repair techniques with tension appear to be particularly relevant (3). To a lesser extent, the size and site of the incisional hernia are important, as well as the number of previous surgeries, the type of material used to close the laparotomy, the surgeon's experience and the patient's co-morbidity (obesity, poor nutritional status, diabetes, constipation, corticotherapy, chronic cough, etc.).

In recent years the use of antibiotic prophylaxis and the widespread use of laparoscopic surgery have decreased the incidence of this condition, although other types of incisional hernias unknown until now have appeared (e.g., at post-laparoscopy trocar sites) and must be taken into account in the future.

INITIAL EVOLUTION OF LAPAROSCOPIC SURGERY FOR INCISIONAL HERNIA REPAIR

As occurred in inguinal hernias, surgical repair of incisional hernias has developed along with the technological advances and pathophysiological knowledge gained over time. In the years before prosthetic materials were developed, surgeons attempted to reconstruct the anatomy of the wall defect using the rectus muscles and their sheaths. A number of different techniques have been described, although all such techniques involved tension at the suture line, leading to an unacceptable recurrence rate of 20-54%, depending on whether the repair was primary or recurrent (3-6).

As the result of articles authored by Usher (10) in the 1960s, the appearance and popularization of prosthetic materials led to radical changes in the treatment of abdominal wall defects. The use of prostheses for the repair of incisional hernias has become steadily more widespread, causing a significant decrease in the rates of recurrences and postoperative complications, although some series still report high recurrence rates of 20-34% (4, 11, 12) and there are many discrepancies concerning the use, type, placement and fixation of prosthetic materials.

In addition to the appearance of prosthetic materials that allow tension-free repair, in the last decade abdominal wall defects have aroused further interest. The condition is no longer considered to be of secondary importance or used to fill surgical schedules and train new surgeons, with little interest for skilled high-level surgeons.

This led to the formation of groups specializing in abdominal wall defects, increasing the interest in the field.

This climate -characterized by major changes resulting in less invasive surgery and in patient expectations of reduced postoperative pain and shorter recovery periods- has led to a "boom" in laparoscopic surgery. Once they had begun to perform and standardize the use of laparoscopic cholecystectomy, pioneering surgeons in this technique took little time in applying their skills toward solving abdominal wall defects that could be visualized from a previously unheard-of intra-abdominal viewing point.

Initial publications on laparoscopic repair of abdominal wall defects were based on three precepts (1, 7, 8, 13, 14):

a) fewer disadvantages with respect to open surgery by preventing large incisions, parietal dissections and placement of drains, dissecting scar tissue handled in previous surgeries, thereby decreasing tissue damage and the subsequent development of hematomas and infection.

b) easier access to the abdominal wall defect for accurate diagnosis of the situation, by examining the status and integrity of the previous laparotomy; release of intestinal adhesions to the abdominal wall with less trauma to the wall and presumably, with a reduced subsequent capacity to form new adhesions.

c) placement of an intraperitoneal prosthesis. PTFE-e (1,7,8,14,15,16,17) has been used most often, since it results in a minimal adhesional reaction with intra-abdominal viscera. Good results have also been reported in laparoscopic repair of incisional hernias with polypropylene mesh in an intraperitoneal site with no prosthesis-related complications (9,13).

What has changed since the early years of laparoscopic surgery for incisional hernias?

Once the initial excitement had subsided, many groups questioned the continued use of the technique since the mid-term results were not exceptional in many cases and the technique had a high financial cost and expensive learning curve.

This slowed the standardization of the technique and most published series are non-randomized studies with few cases that generally report decreased hospitalization, less time away from work, reduced postoperative pain, and recurrence and wound infection rates below those of open techniques (1,18,19,20). Only one randomized study comparing this method with conventional open surgery and confirming the potential advantages of the laparoscopic technique has been published to date (15).

Most of these studies agree that the laparoscopic approach for the repair of incisional hernias is technically feasible and safe, has low complication and recurrence rates, and is particularly useful in obese and multirecurrent patients (1, 8, 13, 15, 19, 21).

In a literature review of published series with more than 50 cases, Leblanc recently reported infection and recurrence rates of 2% and 4%, respectively (range 0-11%) over a total of 1047 laparoscopic repairs of incisional hernia (20).

As in other laparoscopic procedures, surgeon training and standardization of the technique, and changes and improvements made in laparoscopic materials and instruments have led to a current climate very different from the early 1990s, as discussed below.

Laparoscopic instrument

One of the main points of discussion with regard to this technique has been secure fixation of the prosthesis to the wall and the role this procedure could play in the appearance of new recurrences.

Several options have been described, including running suture with nonabsorbable material, interrupted suture and fixation with staples.

Running intra-abdominal suture has the disadvantage that it is technically difficult and tedious, being used on a limited basis at present. Suture techniques using Reverdin needles or derived from such needles (Gore suture passer instrument®), which facilitate suture placement in the abdominal wall, have been described (22).

Staplers have improved significantly since the technique was first used. At the beginning of the technique Endo-Hernias were available. These devices used square staples that were often too short to attach the mesh thickness to the wall. Moreover, a 12-mm trocar was required to introduce the device in the abdomen (Fig. 1).

The appearance of the tack (ProTack, USSC®) was, in our opinion, one of the most significant improvements in the laparoscopic treatment of incisional hernias. The device is much thinner and can be inserted through a 5-mm trocar, thereby avoiding the need for 12-mm trocars (Fig. 2). In addition, the spiral shape allows deeper anchorage and removal if placement is not considered adequate.

At present most groups (including ours) have opted to use mixed techniques that combine tacks and sutures to ensure the fixation (20, 22).

New advances relating to coagulation such as harmonic scissors (Ultra-Shears, USSC®) based on the use of ultrasound or the argon laser terminal for laparoscopy have been shown to be useful for the release of parietal and intestinal adhesions (23), although we do not consider them essential to successful laparoscopic repair of incisional hernias.

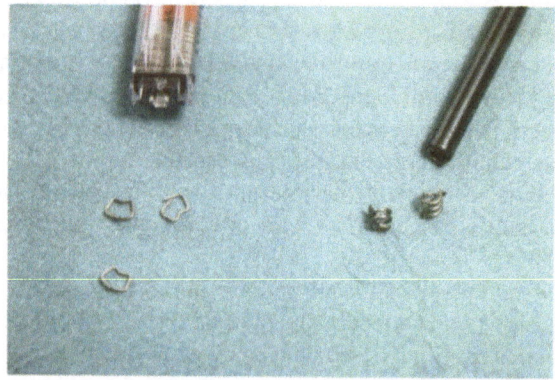

Fig. 1. Difference between the tack and the endo-hernia staple

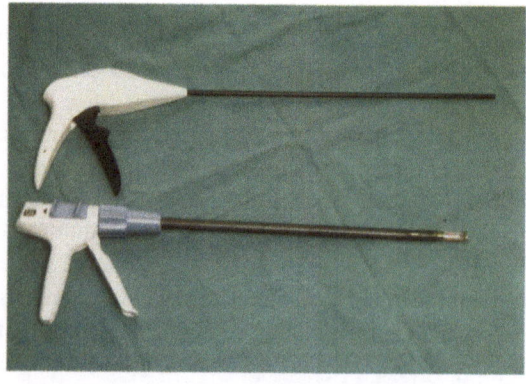

Fig. 2. Tacks and Endo-hernia

PROSTHETIC MATERIALS

In the 1950s Cumberland and Scales defined a series of criteria that are still valid, with the "ideal" material being one that combines the following:
1) chemically inert
2) no inflammatory, foreign body or allergic reactions
3) resistant
4) autoclavable
5) unchanged by body tissues or tissue fluids
6) non-carcinogenic
7) adequate clinical form

Most of the currently available materials have many of the desirable properties, however none of them can be considered ideal.

Numerous studies with experimental animals have been published, frequently with contradictory results and in which pressure from the pharmaceutical industry could play a key role. Morris-Stiff (24), author of an excellent review on non-absorbable prosthetic material, points out two surprising facts: first, there are no controlled long-term studies on hernia recurrence in humans that attempt to identify the actual advantages and results of prosthetic implants. The other interesting point he makes is that while most experimental studies invariably find peritoneal adhesions to the prosthesis to a lesser or greater extent, very few cases of late intestinal occlusion have been reported despite the high number of prosthetic repairs carried out. This is particularly important in the laparoscopic surgery of incisional hernias.

Generally speaking, the polypropylene prostheses have most of the desirable properties for a prosthetic material, although they produce a strong inflammatory foreign body response that causes dense, irregular adhesions between the intestine and the prosthesis, particularly in incisional hernias. As a result, several authors advise against their placement in contact with the intra-abdominal viscera (25).

The softness and flexibility of PTFE makes it easier to handle, and it has similar resistance and an inflammatory response well below other materials. Its capacity to form adhesions appears to be lower due to the chemical nature of PTFE and to the fact that the size of the pore (where the fibroblast will develop) is smaller (24-26).

Although some authors have reported good results in laparoscopic repair of incisional hernias with polypropylene mesh at intraperitoneal sites without the complications normally inherent to prostheses (13, 27), most surgeons experienced in this technique prefer using PTFE-e due to its lower adhesional response with intra-abdominal viscera and greater resistance to infection (1, 7, 8, 14, 15, 17).

Lastly, unlike earlier prostheses made of a single material, the new-generation meshes are characterized by the fact that each of the two surfaces has a different composition. The aim is to ensure as few adhesions as possible on the intra-abdominal side and to enhance wall fibrosis on the surface in contact with the abdominal wall.

PTFE Dual Mesh (WL Gore & Assoc®) has a low-porosity membrane on the intra-abdominal surface that hinders adhesion formation, whereas the surface in contact with the abdominal wall has a microstructure that allows fibroblast growth and fixation to the abdominal wall (22) (Fig. 3).

The Composix TM mesh (Bard®) is conceptually similar since it combines two different materials in a double surface. As in the previously mentioned mesh, it combines the advantages of PTFE-e on the intraabdominal side. The other surface is polypropylene, which encourages faster tissue growth and maximum adhesion. In addition, prostheses in which one half is polypropylene are less costly and have more memory, with a thickness more suitable for maneuvering in the abdominal cavity with laparoscopy, although they are harder to insert when a larger mesh is required. These facts make this mesh particularly useful in the laparoscopic repair of incisional hernia (Fig. 4).

Lastly, the Composite mesh (Sofradim®) is composed of polyester (a material not used very frequently in English-speaking countries but very popular in France) on the top and collagen on the intra-abdominal side.

Finally we agree with Seid (26), he thinks prosthetic materials have significantly contributed toward improving the results of hernia repair, nevertheless issues such as which material is best, in what type of hernia it should be used, and how and where it should be placed, etc. are not yet resolved.

Most likely, future materials, in addition to complying with the premises of Cumberland and Scales, should be completely resistant to infection, prevent adhesions to abdominal viscera and improve incorporation in tissues without causing encapsulation problems, issues not yet fully addressed in current materials.

▶ **Fig. 4.** Composix TM mesh (Bard®)

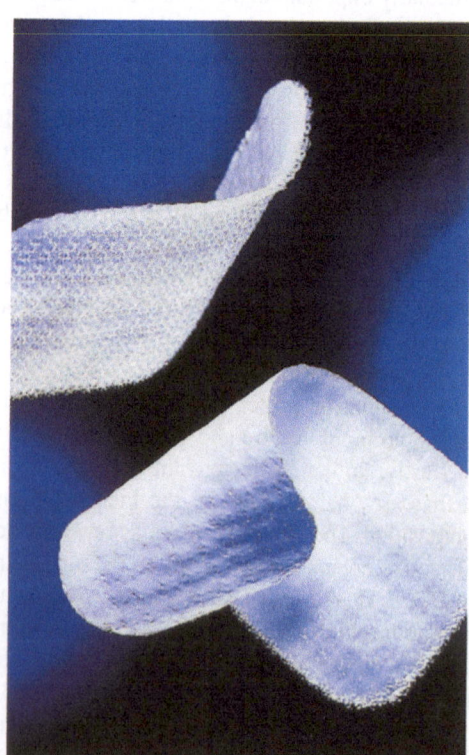

▼ **Fig. 3.** PTFE Dual Mesh (WL Gore & Assoc®)

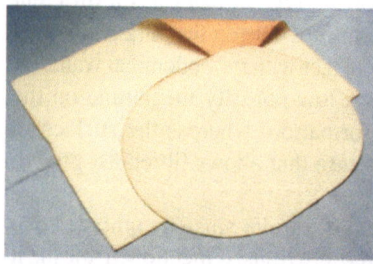

CHANGES IN THE SURGICAL TECHNIQUE

Improvements in prosthetic materials and laparoscopic instruments, along with the expertise gained in laparoscopic repair of abdominal wall defects have helped us to perfect the technique, which differs considerably from the technique described seven years ago (8).

No articles have been published on the learning curve in laparoscopic incisional hernia repair, although we feel this plays a key role in initial results and in consolidation of the technique. This factor has been studied in inguinal hernias, with most authors reporting learning curves of fifty hernia repairs, a period characterized by increased surgical time and higher conversion, complication and recurrence rates (28).

Most publications report early recurrence rates attributable to technical errors (small, poorly positioned or migrated prosthesis) during the learning curve. As a surgeon acquires more experience, this type of error does not occur and the conversion rate drops.

We have varied our initial technique in terms of number, site and caliber of the entry ports used. Four 10-12mm trocars located at the corners of the incisional hernia have been replaced with three trocars on the side flank (two 5-mm working trocars and one 10-mm trocar for the video camera). By doing so, we attempt to maintain the same orientation at all times. Since the tack can be introduced through a 5-mm trocar, larger trocars are not necessary (Fig. 5).

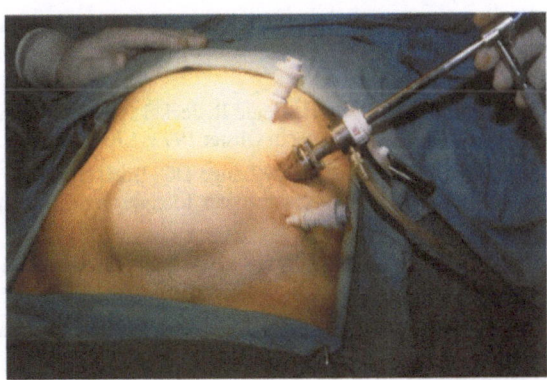

Fig. 5. Current placement of three trocars on the side flank, using two 5-mm working trocars and one 10-mm trocar for the scope

The prosthesis must extend 2-4 cm beyond the margins of the hernia defect, be properly secured and not display any tension (20, 22-23). Although there is no consensus on the use of fixation sutures in conjunction with tacks, most authors resort to this as a safety measure.

We place a pressure bandage on top of the hernia sac for 48 hours, in order to prevent residual seroma. When a seroma occurs, we do not use puncture.

A number of issues crucial to identifying the actual role of this technique in incisional hernia repair have yet to be resolved in the future:

1) Are the advantages of the laparoscopic approach over conventional surgery real and measurable?
2) Has medical industry pressure or the attractiveness of a "new procedure" influenced surgeons?
3) Standardization of the technique
4) Reduced learning curves
5) Universality-widespread use of the technique
6) Fixation, type and size of the prosthesis
7) Long-term results in randomized studies with a large number of cases
8) Lower financial cost for the material

Although we are still awaiting answers to the remaining questions, we feel that laparoscopic repair of incisional hernias is currently a safe, reproducible technique with a recurrence rate, complication rate, hospitalization time and surgical time below those obtained with conventional open surgery.

References

1. Toy FK, Bailey RW, Carey S, Chappuis CW, Gagner M, Josephs LG, Mangiante EC, Parks AE, Pomp A, Smoot RT, Uddo JF, Voeller GR. Prospective, multicenter study of laparoscopic ventral hernioplasty. Surg Endosc 1998; 12:955-959.

2. Utrera González A, de la Portilla de Juan F, Carranza Albarrán G. Large incisional hernia repair using intraperitoneal placement of expanded polytetrafluoroethylene. Am J Surg 1999. 177:291-293.

3. Hesselink VJ, Luijendijk RW, de Wilt JH, Heide R, Jeekel J. An evaluation of risk factors in incisional hernia recurrence. Surg Gynecol Obstet 1993; 176: 228-234.

4. Luijendijk RW, Hop WC, van den Tol MP, de Lange DC, Braaksma MM, Ijzermans JN et al. A comparison of suture repair with mesh repair for incisional hernia. N Engl J Med 2000; 343: 392-398.

5. Van der Linden FT, van Vroonhoven TJ. Long-term results after correction of incisional hernia. Neth J Surg 1988; 40: 127-129.

6. Read RC, Yoder G. Recent trends in the management of incisional herniation. Arch Surg 1989; 124: 485-488.

7. Leblanc KA, Spaw AT, Booth WT. Laparoscopic repair of ventral hernias using expanded polytetrafluoroethilene. Surg Laparosc Endosc 1993; 1:39-41.

8. Clavería R, Besora P, Basas J, Feliu X, Camps J, Viñas T, Codina J, Fernández E. Corrección de la eventración por vía laparoscópica. Experiencia inicial. Cir Esp 1994; 56:299-301.

9. Pareja Ciuró F, Galindo Galindo A, Domínguez Adame E, Ponce González JF, Morales Méndez S. Reparación de la pared del abdomen con material protésico. Hernias incisionales. Cir Esp 1996; 60:7-11.

10. Usher FC. A new plastic prosthesis for repairing tissue defects of the chest and abdominal wall. Am J Surg 1959; 97: 629-633.

11. Anthony T, Bergen PC, Kim LT et al. Factors affecting recurrence following incisional herniorrhaphy. World J Surg 2000; 24: 95-101.

12. Leber GE, Garb JL, Alexander AI, Reed WP. Long-term complications associated with prosthetic repair of incisional hernias. Arch Surg 1998; 133: 378-382.

13. Franklin ME, Dorman JP, Glass JL, Balli JE, et al. Laparoscopic ventral and incisional hernia repair. Surg Laparosc Endosc 1998; 8:294-299.

14. Toy FK, Smoot RT. Toy-Smoot laparoscopic hernioplasty. Surg Laparosc Endosc 1991; 3:151-155.

15. Carbajo MA, Martin del Olmo JC, Blanco JL, Cuesta C, Toledano M, Martin F, Vaquero C, Inglada L. Laparoscopic treatment versus open surgery in the solution of major incisional and abdominal wall hernias with mesh. Surg Endosc 1999; 13: 250-252.

16. Segura Movellán J. Cirugía laparoscópica en las eventraciones. En: JL Porrero. Cirugía de la pared abdominal. Ed Masson 1997; 282-285.

17. Morales Méndez S, Morales Conde S, Ponce JF, Barriga R, Gavilán F, Fernández V. Materiales protésicos en hernia incisional. Estudio experimental y clínico. En: JL Porrero. Cirugía de la pared abdominal. Ed Masson 1997; 257-268.

18. Rohr S, Vogt F, Thiry CL et al. Parietal prosthetic mesh in the treatment of large incisional hernias. J Chir (Paris) 1993; 130:37-40.

19. Park A, Birch DW, Lovrics P. Laparoscopic and open incisional hernia repair: a comparision study. Surgery 1998; 124:816-821.

20. Leblanc KA, Booth WV, Whitaker JM, Bellanger DE. Laparoscopic incisional and ventral herniorrhaphy in 100 patients. Am J Surg 2000; 180: 193-197.

21. Holzmann MD, Purut CM, Reintgen K, Eubanks S, et al. Laparoscopic ventral and incisional hernioplasty. Surg Endosc 1997; 11:32-35.

22. Heniford BT, Park A, Ramshaw BJ, Voeller G. Laparoscopic ventral and incisional hernia repair in 407 patients. J Am Coll Surg 2000; 190: 645-650.

23. Carbajo Caballero MA, Blanco Alvarez JI, Martín del Olmo JC, Martín Acebes F, Toledano Trincado M, de la Cuesta de la Llave C. Eventraciones y hernias ventrales: experiencia con 200 casos por abordaje laparoscópico. Técnica quirúrgica. Cir Esp 2001; 69: 18-21.

24. Morris-Stiff GJ, Hughes LE. The outcomes of nonabsorbable mesh placed within the abdominal cavity: Literature review and clinical experience. J Am Coll Surg 1998; 186: 352-367.

25. LeBlanc KA. Materiales bioprotésicos en la reparación por vía laparoscópica de los defectos de la pared abdominal. En: JL Porrero. Cirugía de la pared abdominal. Ed. Masson. Barcelona 1997; 156-162

26. Seid AS. Prosthetic biomaterials in hernia repair. En: Arregui ME and Nagan RF. Inguinal hernia. Advances or controversies? Radcliffe Medical Press. Oxford 1994; 505-510.

27. Bickel A, Eitan A. A simplified laparoscopic technique for mesh placement in ventral hernia repair. Surg Endosc 1999; 13: 532-534.

28. Feliu Palà X, Martín Gómez M, Morales Conde S, Fdez. Sallent E. The impact of the surgeon's experience on the results of laparoscopic hernia repair. Surg Endosc 2001; 15 (12): 1467-1470.

SECTION V

Technical Aspects of Laparoscopic
Ventral Hernia Repair

CHAPTER 17

Pre-operative Considerations of Laparoscopic Ventral Hernia Repair

J.R. Schwab, B.J. Ramshaw

Ventral abdominal hernias constitute a challenging problem for the practicing surgeon. Nearly 80% of ventral hernias in adults are incisional; other less common hernias include: umbilical, Spegalian and epigastric hernias (1, 5, 6). Controversy has existed regarding the best repair technique since long before the advent of the laparoscopic approach. Reports in the surgical literature estimate the recurrence rate of open primary ventral hernia repair to range from 25-52% (1-3). Performing open ventral hernia repair with mesh has reduced the recurrence rate to between 11-21% (1, 2, 4), but requires more extensive dissection and the raising of flaps. This more extensive dissection leads to increased wound infections and hematomas in open repair patients despite the routine use of drains with this approach.

The laparoscopic approach offers patients a reduced recurrence rate, decreased wound complications and other advantages over the open repairs; however, this approach may not be appropriate for all patients. This chapter reviews the pre-operative considerations in selecting patients for the laparoscopic approach for ventral hernia repair.

SELECTION OF THE LAPAROSCOPIC REPAIR

The Laparoscopic Approach

In order to realize which patients will benefit from a laparoscopic approach, it is important to recognize the differences between this approach and the open approaches for ventral hernia repair. The laparoscopic approach begins with the placement of a 10mm port and two 5mm ports, away from the area of the hernia defect, and a laparoscopic lysis of adhesions, if necessary. Next, mesh is fixed to the posterior side of the anterior abdominal wall with spiral tacks and full thickness permanent sutures. Although some sources have described hernia repair with polypropylene mesh, the authors use ePTFE dual mesh exclusively. Since the mesh is placed intrabdominally with direct exposure to the viscera, there is potential for ingrowth into the mesh. ePTFE has such small interstices (pores) that ingrowth is not possible and adherence is inhibited. A 3-5 cm overlap on all edges of the hernia defect is obtained and the hernia sac is not usually excised.

Indications for the Laparoscopic Approach (Table I)

The laparoscopic approach mimics the Stoppa open hernia repair, but the mesh is placed intraperitoneally requiring much less dissection. The minimal dissection and placement of incisions away from the hernia allows a decreased incidence of wound infections and hematomas (4). Early reports in the surgical literature have also shown a lower incidence of recurrence for the laparoscopic approach as opposed to the traditional open techniques (4,7).

Like many other minimally invasive procedures, laparoscopic ventral hernia repair potentially offers the patient decreased post-operative pain, decreased length of hospital stay, less operative blood loss and an earlier return to normal activities (4,7). Theoretically, patients unable to tolerate the trauma of an open hernia repair may benefit from a laparoscopic approach. Although the post-operative discomfort is significant from the laparoscopic approach, the authors' feel that it is less than that of a comparable open approach and therefore offers less chance of immobility or pulmonary complications post-operatively.

Laparoscopic ventral hernia repair is an excellent choice for primary repair of hernias greater than 4 cm in diameter. The laparoscopic approach is actually more applicable for larger, more complicated hernias than smaller uncomplicated hernias. When a large hernia is fixed by open repair or mesh on-lay, the fascia is reapproximated under tension. The laparoscopic approach, like the open Stoppa approach, allows for wide coverage of the fascial defect and a repair that is without tension. After experience with the laparoscopic approach was gained, it was applied to patients with complicated hernias at the authors' institution with excellent results (4).

Small ventral hernias, less than 4 cm in diameter, are usually adequately treated by primary repair. All patients treated laparoscopically require a general anesthetic and intraabdominal placement of mesh. Certainly, small umbilical hernias can be successfully treated without mesh and general anesthesia, and there may not be an advantage for the laparoscopic approach.

The laparoscopic approach is also well-suited for any patient who has undergone a previous ventral hernia repair and developed a recurrence. Approaching this hernia laparoscopically avoids dissection in the previous operative site and is potentially technically easier than approaching the hernia through the same site. Patients with a "Swiss cheese" hernia defect are optimally treated by the laparoscopic approach. This vantage point offers the clearest view of fascial defects, ensuring the maximum coverage of each with mesh.

For a recurrent hernia previously repaired with the open approach using mesh, caution must be utilized during a laparoscopic approach since bowel may be adherent to this mesh. The authors have encountered this in several cases, even if the mesh was initially placed above the rectus fascia. This situation requires advanced laparoscopic skills and experience and should be avoided if at all possible during a surgeon's early experience.

The lysis of adhesions is the most difficult and dangerous part of both open and laparoscopic ventral hernia repairs. Extensive laparoscopic lysis of adhesions should only be performed by experienced Laparoscopists and most experts avoid the use of energy sources during the majority of this dissection.

Obese patients are predisposed to the development of ventral hernias; therefore, it is not suprising that these patients represent a large portion of those who present for repair. Open ventral hernia repair in obese patients is associated with an increased incidence of wound infection and recurrence. The laparoscopic approach offers patients smaller wounds and therefore decreased wound complications (4). This makes the laparoscopic approach an ideal repair for obese patients, possibly even for small primary hernias.

Table I. Indications for Laparoscopic Ventral Hernia Repair

Hernias > 4 cm in diameter
Recurrent hernias- all sizes
Hernias < 4 cm in obese patients
Hernias < 4 cm in patients with other potential risk factors for recurrence
Hernias- all sizes: in patients who need to return to strenuous activity as soon as possible

Contraindications of the Laparoscopic Approach

Although the laparoscopic approach is well-suited for the majority of patients with ventral abdominal hernias there are some contraindications to a laparoscopic repair. As previously mentioned, primary hernias < 4 cm may be best treated by an open repair unless the patient is obese or has other characteristics increasing the likelihood of recurrence. Patients who cannot tolerate a general anesthetic should be operated upon by an open method or not at all since the laparoscopic approach requires general anesthesia. Also any patient with dense abdominal adhesions or a "frozen abdomen" may not be amenable to a laparoscopic repair, although this may not be known preoperatively. It is necessary to develop an adequate pneumoperitoneum in order to perform the operation.

The other limitations of the laparoscopic approach are mainly secondary to the requirement of mesh placement and its potential complications. Like any foreign body, mesh should not be placed in an infected field due to the subsequent risk of a post-operative infection, necessitating mesh removal. Therefore, mesh should not be placed in patients that have necrotic intestine for fear of bacterial seeding. The authors have used the laparoscopic approach for patients with incarcerated viscera that was not compromised and achieved good results. Mesh should be placed selectively when patients are undergoing a concurrent operation, which may jeopardize the sterility of the field and could lead to bacterial seeding of the mesh. For example, good intra-operative surgical judgement will determine whether it is possible to concurrently place mesh during a procedure such as a laparoscopic cholecystectomy. The surgeon must decide whether the level of infection of the gallbladder, amount of bile spillage during the operation and other factors prohibit the use of mesh for hernia repair. As with any operation, surgical judgement determines the most appropriate approach for hernia repair in patients needing concurrent procedures.

Children or childbearing age females with ventral abdominal hernias present a difficult problem. The likelihood of great increases in abdominal wall size in the future makes the placement of intraabdominal mesh less attractive. Likewise favorable results in ventral hernia repair of patients with cirrhosis and ascites are difficult to achieve with any approach.

A surgeon should initially perform laparoscopic ventral hernia repair in straightforward, uncomplicated cases in order to gain experience with the technique. Some patients suggested to be avoided would be those with "loss of domain", multiple abdominal surgeries, a history of dense abdominal adhesions, evidence of incarcerated contents, morbid obesity or multiple previous failed repairs, especially if previous mesh has been placed inside the abdominal cavity. This operation is conceptually easy and not technically demanding. Once the learning curve is passed the approach may be effective in more difficult cases.

PRE-OPERATIVE PREPARATION OF THE PATIENT

Psychological Preparation (Table II)

Like any operation, it is important that the patient's expectations and desired outcomes are discussed prior to the time of surgery. Several things should be specifically discussed regarding the ventral hernia repair operation, as well as, the laparoscopic approach.

As previously mentioned, nearly 80% of ventral hernias are secondary to incisional hernia, and the majority of the patients have had significant prior abdominal surgery. These patients usually have significant abdominal adhesions, and the possibility of enterotomy exists for any approach for repair. With the laparoscopic approach, the surgeon must be especially careful with adhesiolysis because enterotomies may be more difficult to recognize and repair. When these do occur, all is not lost. Reports exist in the literature of the successful laparoscopic closure of such enterotomies and the completion of mesh placement (7). Each patient must be individualized according to the significance of the injury and surgeon's comfort level with a successful outcome. If any question exists, the surgeon should use their best judgement for each situation. Another option is to open the patient, which should not be considered a complication, close the enterotomy and place the mesh or close the abdomen primary. Another strategy that has been utilized by the authors and others, is to finish the lysis of adhesions and repair the enterotomy then put the patient on antibiotics for a few days, the returning to the OR for delayed placement of mesh.

The patient should be made aware of the known risk of enterotomy and the possibility of abdominal sepsis or enterocutaneous fistula. The patient should be aware of that an encountered enterotomy might require conversion to an open procedure or the possibility of delaying mesh placement until a later operation. Prior knowledge of this risk assures that the patient and family will be more accepting of any potential complications.

The patient should also be counseled as to the risk of infection. As with any foreign body, mesh has an inherent risk in developing an infection that will become a significant problem. Although reports exist in the literature of conservative management of these infections, this is not always the case and infection may lead to re-operation and mesh removal. As previously mentioned, all necessary precautions should be exercised in order to prevent the development of such infections. One precaution is to use an Iodoform drape to cover the patient's skin during the operation. Also, surgery on patients with known active infections should be postponed until the infection is resolved. Prior counseling of the patient to the risk of such infections is necessary.

Although the laparoscopic approach may result in decreased postoperative discomfort, the patient will still have significant post-operative pain, especially for large hernia repairs. Theoretically this pain is from trauma and tension at spiral tack sites and full thickness suture sites. In addition, some full thickness sutures can cause pain in a dermatomal distribution related to cutaneous nerve entrapment. Although the use of such sutures increases the risk of postoperative pain, the authors and many others feel they are necessary for the structural stability of the repair. The pain related to nerve entrapment usually resolves within several weeks postoperatively. Occasionally, injection of local anesthesia may be required for timely resolution of this pain.

Another occurrence that should be discussed with the patient prior to surgery is the common incidence of seroma formation. After reduction of the hernia contents and mesh coverage within the abdominal cavity, the remaining subcutaneous space between the skin and mesh will fill with fluid and often be felt as a mass by the patient post-operatively. With reassurance, the patient will know that this is not a recurrence and this seroma will resolve with time. Most surgeons do not drain these seromas unless the patient has significant symptoms.

As with any hernia repair, the risk of recurrence should also be discussed with the patient. As outlined above, the laparoscopic approach, like any hernia repair, does have some inherent risk of complications. The risk of recurrence has been reported to be much less with this repair than others and is promising as the new standard in the treatment of this challenging problem.

Table II. Pre-operative points to discuss with the patient

Possibility of enterotomy and options for repair and mesh placement
Post-operative pain related to the size of the mesh that is placed
Seroma formation is common and to be expected
Infection of the mesh may require removal

Physiologic Preparation

All patients undergoing laparoscopic ventral hernia repair will require a general anesthetic, therefore the standard preoperative evaluation for such operations should be performed. This is usually an elective procedure that provides ample time for evaluation of the patient's medical condition and possible optimization for a surgical procedure. The patient's serum electrolytes and blood counts should be reviewed and any necessary therapy instituted.

In addition, the patient's cardiovascular status is important and the Goldman criteria, as well as any known coronary artery testing, should be investigated. Although, the laparoscopic approach may be less inhibitory to the pulmonary system than traditional approaches, this system still requires necessary review and preoperative questioning. Deep venous thrombosis should also be a standard preoperative concern and sequential compression devices should be placed on the lower extremities during the operation.

The potential to decrease post-operative infection is important and routine peri-operative antibiotics are important. Any skin ulceration overlying the hernia should be well-healed prior to the operative procedure and placement of mesh. As mentioned, an Iodoform drape may help prevent contamination of the mesh by skin flora. After experience with this procedure is gained, the surgeon will likely apply its usage to more difficult cases such as those patients with extensive abdominal adhesions. In these cases, it is wise to bowel prep the patient. In the event of enterotomy, there maybe less likelihood of complications.

Operative Preparation

The implementation of this new procedure for ventral hernia repair will be much more successful if the surgeon and his assistants are well-prepared. Obviously, the surgeon should be knowledgeable of the technique and familiar with advanced laparoscopic surgery.

Making sure the operative staff is prepared is also important. The majority of the equipment necessary for this procedure is used for laparoscopic cholecystectomy and is standard in most operating rooms. Some specific equipment is needed and the surgeon should assure its availability prior to the operative date. This equipment includes: (1) the suture passer, which is used to place full thickness abdominal wall sutures for securing of the mesh, (2) the laparoscopic tacker, which will fix the mesh to the abdominal wall, (3) mesh, specifically ePTFE dual mesh (4) permanent suture (5) Iodoform drape and (6) atraumatic graspers (for grasping bowel during adhesiolysis).

The surgeon should be prepared for all potential scenarios during the operation. Open procedure instruments should be available since conversion to an open procedure is always a possibility and especially in the event of an intra-operative emergency such as hemorrhage. Other non-standard equipment that should be readily available would include laparoscopic clip appliers or endoloops to be used to control bleeding. In the event of an enterotomy, laparoscopic suturing devices should be available if the surgeon desires to repair the enterotomy laparoscopically.

Although this procedure can appear to be complex and difficult, the learning curve is actually not long. In a short period of time the surgeon can implement it safely and effectively if appropriate training and patient selection are utilized. The reports of extremely low recurrence rates and complication rates from surgeons' intial experience with this procedure are encouraging. This minimally invasive approach of ventral hernia repair holds promise for the future treatment of this challenging surgical problem.

References

1. Hesselink VJ, Luijendijk RW, de Wilt JHW, et al. An evaluation of risk factors in incisional hernia recurrence. Surg Gynecol Obstet 1993; 176:228-234.

2. Stoppa RE. The treatment of complicated groin and incisional hernias. World J Surg 1989, 13: 545-554.

3. Linden van der FT, Vroonhoven van TJ. Long-term results after surgical correction of incisional hernia. Neth J Surg 1998; 40: 127-129.

4. Ramshaw BJ, Esartia P, Schwab JR, Mason EM, Wilson RA, Duncan TD et al. Comparison of laparoscopic and open ventral herniorrhaphy. Am Surg 1999;65(a): 827-832.

5. Larson GM, Vandertoll DJ: Approaches to repair of ventral hernia and full-thickness losses of the abdominal wall. Surg Clin North Am 1984; 64: 335-349.

6. Santora TA, Rosyln JJ: Incisional hernia. Surg Clin North Am 1993; 73:557-570.

7. Heniford BT, Park A, Ramshaw BJ, Voeller, G. Laparoscopic Ventral and Incisional Hernia Repair. J Am Coll Surg 2000; 6:645-650.

CHAPTER 18

Imaging Abdominal Wall Hernias

M.S. French, M.A. Arregui

REASONS FOR IMAGING ABDOMINAL WALL HERNIAS: WHY SHOULD WE BOTHER?

In general the diagnosis of abdominal wall hernia is straightforward. There are patients, however, in whom the diagnosis of a hernia is strongly suspected based on patient history or physical exam but a definitive diagnosis is not possible. Examples of these cases include: occult hernias (groin or abdominal pain without a palpable mass), recurrent groin pain after hernia repair, obese patients, patients with pain related to scars, patients with suspected bowel obstruction and those with an equivocal mass (mass of uncertain etiology). These patients require either further evaluation with radiologic studies or eventually undergo surgery for a presumed diagnosis. Accurate diagnosis and characterization of abdominal wall hernias is imperative in planning the most appropriate procedure for patients to hopefully improve the outcomes. The vast majority of the literature on this subject involves the diagnosis of inguinal hernias, however, the same approach can be used for ventral hernias.

TYPES OF ABDOMINAL WALL HERNIAS

Abdominal wall hernias consist primarily of *inguinal, femoral* and *ventral hernias*. Less commonly described hernias include *para-stomal, lumbar, obturator, sciatic, perineal* and *supravesicular* hernias. All of these lesions are related to defects in the abdominal wall fascia with resultant herniation of abdominal contents and protrusions of peritoneum. Herniated preperitoneal fat such as "lipoma" of the cord or round ligament may also be symptomatic (due to stretching of the abdominal wall fascia or impingement on nerves) even though it is not a true hernia that would allow bowel protrusion with its associated risk of incarceration or strangulation.

Sportsman's "hernia" is a diagnosis usually only considered in young athletes. The term is assigned to patients with chronic groin pain and no discernable bulge on physical exam. The most common etiology is thought to be weakness of the inguinal floor muscles or fascial strain secondary to overuse (1).

Ventral hernias, the focus of this text, include *epigastric, umbilical, Spigelian* and *incisional hernias*. *Umbilical hernias* make up about 10% of all abdominal wall hernias (2). They are generally considered congenital when discovered during childhood and acquired in adults. They are typically easy to diagnose and should be repaired when symptomatic. Imaging is rarely necessary.

Spigelian hernias occur along the lateral border of the rectus abdominis muscle at the semilunar line typically below the level of the umbilicus. In this region the aponeurosis of the transversus abdominus and internal oblique muscles run parallel, are thin and have multiple slit-like defects. If these defects correspond herniation is likely. Due to the overlying aponeurosis of the external oblique muscle the peritoneal protrusion does not enter the subcutaneous space. This makes diagnosis of these hernias on physical exam difficult, especially in obese patients (3). *Spigelian hernias* account for only 2% of all abdominal wall hernias (4). Due to frequent delays in diagnosis the complication rate associated with these hernias is relatively high (5).

Incisional hernias make up about 6% of abdominal wall hernias (2). Large hernias are easy to palpate, however, small lesions may not be apparent on physical exam. These hernias are suspected due to pain at incision sites. Trigger point injections are occasionally helpful in distinguishing hernias from nerve entrapment or adhesions. Included in this category are trocar site hernias following laparoscopic surgery.

Lumbar hernias (acquired hernias that occur at the site of previous flank surgery) and the female hernias *(obturator, perineal, sciatic and supravesicular)* are rare but can be the most difficult to diagnose, frequently requiring imaging studies. *Obturator hernias* typically occur in elderly women and can result in chronic pelvic pain or bowel obstruction (6). Occasionally they will present as a palpable mass of the inner thigh, however, usually there are no physical findings to suggest the diagnosis (7). *Perineal hernias* can be anterior or posterior. The anterior defects occur between the bulbocavernosus muscle medially, the ischiocavernosus laterally and the transverse perineal muscle posteriorly (image Nyhus 452).

DIAGNOSING HERNIAS ISN'T ALWAYS EASY

Machan reported that 70% of non-palpable femoral hernias were miss-diagnosed by the referring physician. Even more surprising was that 20-25% of patients undergoing emergency surgery for a femoral hernia had been miss-diagnosed by a surgeon (8). Distinguishing direct from indirect inguinal hernias can also be challenging. In 1994 Cameron et al. reported that the diagnosis of a direct inguinal hernia was correct only 56% of the time(9). Ralphs determined that physical exam was 69% accurate in distinguishing direct from indirect hernias (10). Spigelian hernias were only diagnosed with 52% accuracy as reported by Weis in 1974 (11) and obturator hernias were only diagnosed preoperatively in 20-38% of cases (12).

Occult hernias are typically identified in patients with pain but no palpable hernia on exam. Frequently they are discovered in women with groin pain. Spangen reported the results of 137 groin explorations performed on 125 women with groin pain and no palpable hernia. One hundred twenty-eight of the explorations revealed an indirect hernia (indirect sac in 92 and preperitoneal fat in 36). Seven patients had normal findings and no direct hernias were seen (13).

Groin pain is a frequent occurrence following repair of inguinal hernias. In one study 28.7% of patients complained of inguinal pain one year after surgery, 11% of whom said the pain interfered with work or leisure activity (14). Others have reported up to a 37% incidence of pain following hernia repair. Hamlin found that 18.5-42% of patients with post-operative pain actually had a hernia when examined with herniography (15).

Equivocal masses include; neoplasms (neurofibromas, schwanomas, lipomas, liposarcomas and lymphomas), cysts, vascular abnormalities (eg. pseudoaneurysms), and post-op masses (hematomas, seromas and hydroceles).

IMAGING TECHNIQUES

Imaging techniques include CT scan, MRI, herniography and ultrasound.

Other techniques have been used (barium enema, cystography) but are rarely employed in clinical practice. Of course there are advantages and disadvantages to all of the methods mentioned above and none can be considered the gold standard.

CT Scanning

CT scans are readily available and have a high positive predictive value. CT is probably the best overall imaging study in several clinical situations since it gives a look at the intra-abdominal contents in addition to the anterior abdominal wall (Fig.1). Good indications for CT include; patients with a suspected bowel obstruction, equivocal masses, abdominal pain, and suspected pelvic or perineal hernias (Fig. 2, 3). In evaluating equivocal masses Williams performed CT scans on 101 patients and made the correct diagnosis in 93% (16). In an evaluation of occult hernias in 24 patients (12 inguinal and 12 ventral) CT scans were correct 83% of the time with only one false positive and two false negative examinations. This resulted in a positive predictive value of .94 and a negative predictive value of .63 (17). CT has also been shown to be useful in patients with obturator hernias (Fig. 4). These patients are exceedingly difficult to diagnose by physical exam. Obstructive symptoms (nausea, crampy abdominal pain and emesis) are present in 80% of patients who are discovered to have an obturator hernia. The rate of strangulation ranges from 25-75% (18-22) leading to a mortality rate of up to 70% (18, 19, 21, 23). CT and ultrasound are able to make the diagnosis 75-100% of the time (12). Disadvantages of CT include the cost, radiation exposure, low negative predictive value and the fact that CT scans cannot be performed in real time. Newer spiral scanners are fast enough to evaluate patients holding their breath and performing a valsalva maneuver, however, they are still limited to performing evaluations in the supine position.

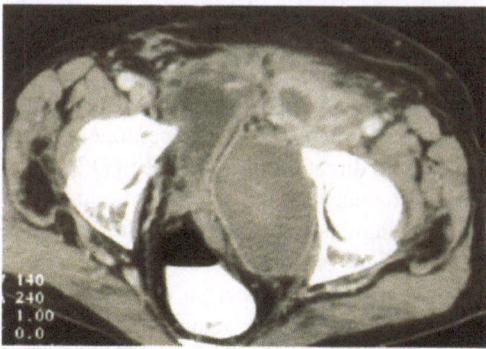

Fig. 1. CT scan showing a pelvic fluid collection. The study was ordered due to development of a right sided groin mass following laparoscopic preperitoneal inguinal hernioraphy. The collection was determined to be a hematoma by aspiration.

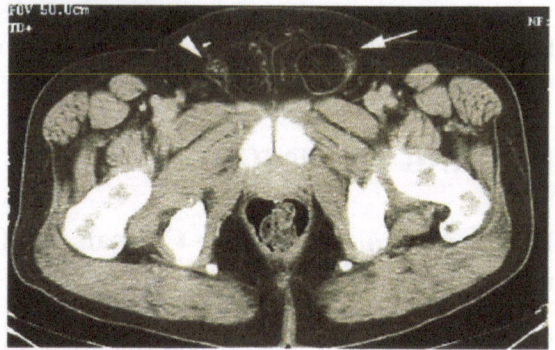

Fig. 2. Incidentally discovered left inguinal hernia. Note the enlarged inguinal canal on the left (arrow) compared to the normal canal on the right (arrowhead).

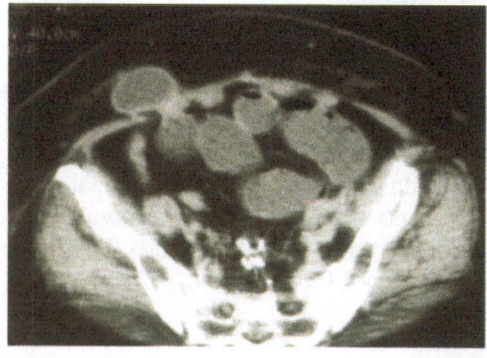

Fig. 3. CT scan showing bowel herniated through a fascial defect at a laparoscopic trocar site.

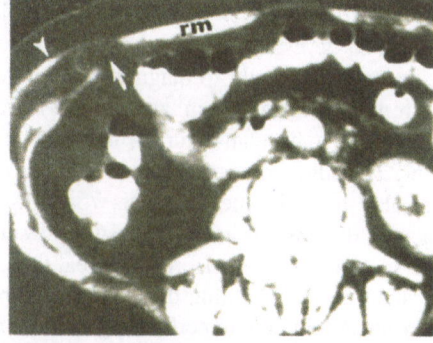

Fig. 4. CT scan showing a Spigelian hernia. (reprinted from Computed Body Tomography with MRI Correlation 2nd ed. Raven Press).

MRI

In general the indications for using MRI are the same as those listed above for CT. The anatomic detail of MRI is excellent. In a study by van den Berg he was able to identify the internal rings in all patients and the inferior epigastric vessels in 85% (Fig. 5, 6). Twenty patients were scanned half of whom had palpable hernias. A thirty minute exam was performed with the use of a body wrap-around coil centered at the pubic symphysis. Patients were asked to strain for 20 seconds during the dynamic portion of the study The diagnosis of a hernia was dependent upon visualizing a widened inguinal canal beyond the diameter of the spermatic cord or round ligament or when fat or bowel was imaged within the canal (24) (Fig. 7). Eleven of 13 hernias (85%) were accurately diagnosed (25). A subsequent study by the same author reported the sensitivity of MRI to be 94% in a similar patient population (26). Infusion of saline into the peritoneal cavity has been utilized in conjunction with MRI of the peritoneal cavity for the purpose of evaluating peritoneal surfaces in patients suspected of having tumor implants (27). This technique may improve the reliability of MRI in diagnosing abdominal wall hernias however, it would also subject the patient to a more invasive test with its inherent risks (24).

Advantages of MRI include better soft tissue imaging and better evaluation of the joint spaces (e.g. effusions). The prohibitive expense of performing MRI is the most significant disadvantage. In addition it is not possible to examine the patient in the upright position which can on occasion be the only way to identify a hernia. Most experience with MRI in diagnosing hernias involves hernias discovered incidentally and not in prospectively organized studies.

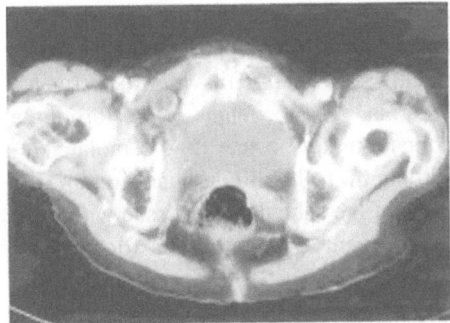

Fig. 5. CT scan of right sided obturator hernia. (reprinted from Southern Medical Journal).

Fig. 6. Open black arrows point to the fat entering the origin of the direct inguinal hernia medial to the inferior epigastric vessels (open white arrows). From : Toms AP, Dixon AK, Murphy JMP, Jamieson NV Illustrated review of new imagin techniqus in the diagnonsis of abdominal wall hernias (review) : Br J Surg, Volume 86 (10). October 1999.1243-1249.

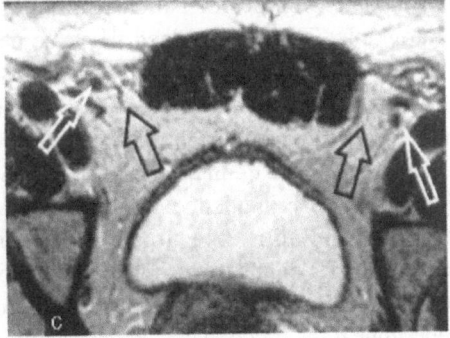

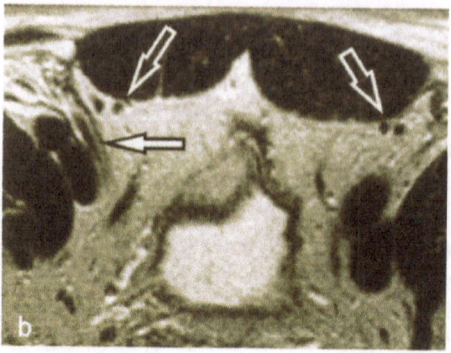

Fig. 7. Note the vas deferens and testicular vessels (solid whit arrow) medial to the external iliac vessels. Inferior epigastric vessels (open white arrows) are posterolateral to the rectus abdominis muscles. From : Toms AP, Dixon AK, Murphy JMP, Jamieson NV Illustrated review of new imagin techniqus in the diagonsis of abdominal wall hernia (review) : Br J Surg, Volume 86 (10). October1999. 1243-1249.

Herniography

Herniography was first described in the 1960s by Canadians attempting to diagnose contralateral hernias in the pediatric population (28). Today it is mainly used by physicians in Scandinavia and less frequently in the United Kingdom. This technique requires knowledge of the topography of the anterior peritoneal surface, specifically related to the umbilical folds (Fig. 8). Inguinal hernias are alternatively defined. Direct hernias protrude in the medial inguinal fossa, the space bounded by the medial and lateral umbilical folds, indirect hernias occur in the lateral inguinal fossa lateral to the lateral umbilical fold (Fig. 9) and femoral hernias arise from the lateral aspect of the medial inguinal fossa, at a right angle to the inguinal ligament (29). When read by experienced radiologist these studies have a low false negative and false positive rate. Indications for herniography include the following; patients with groin pain and no palpable hernia, chronic groin pain in women, obese patients, patients suspected of having a sportman's "hernia", obturator hernia or pelvic floor hernia. The technique for performing a herniagram is relatively simple yet complications do occur. Low osmolar non-ionic contrast is injected into the peritoneum following preparation of the abdomen below the umbilicus and infiltration of the subcutaneous tissue with local anesthetic. Fifty milliliters for women and seventy-five milliliters for men are injected under fluoroscopic guidance (Fig. 10). The patient is positioned in the prone position and can be asked to valsalva during the procedure if necessary (30). Macarthur found that when evaluating groin pain of uncertain origin with herniography 33-45% of patients had hernias discovered (31). In a review of herniography Toms determined the false negative rate of the procedure to be 2-7.9% and the false positive rate to be 0-18.7%. Herniography is more sensitive than CT, MRI and ultrasound for detecting a patent processus vaginalis (Fig. 11) and recurrent hernias which are non-palpable. In addition, like ultrasound, it is a real time study. The main disadvantage to this procedure is its invasive nature. There was a 6% incidence of minor complications which included; bleeding, hematoma, cellulitis, bowel or bladder puncture, scrotal swelling and allergic reaction to the contrast material. No major complications were reported (32). Additionally lipomas of the spermatic cord and ventral defects with herniated preperitoneal fat are not detected with herniography (33).

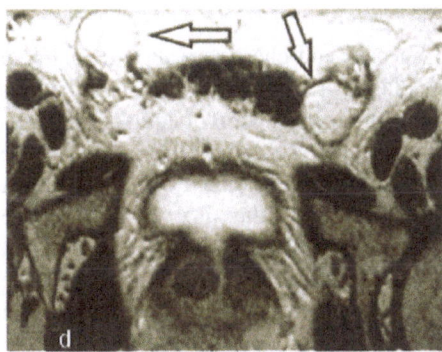

Fig. 8. Open black arrows point to direct inguinal hernias containing fat. The defect in the posterior wall of the inguinal canal is clearly seen on the right From : Toms AP, Dixon AK, Murphy JMP, Jamieson NV Illustrated review of new imagin techniqus in the diagonsis of abdominal wall hernias (review) : Br J Surg, Volume 86 (10). October 1999. 1243-1249.

Fig. 9. Normal inguinal fossae and peritoneal folds. The lateral and medial inguinal fossae are separated by the lateral umbilical fold (arrows), while the medial umbilical fold (arrowheads) divides the medial inguinal fossa into medial (supravesical) and lateral compartments. (reprinted from Bendavid).

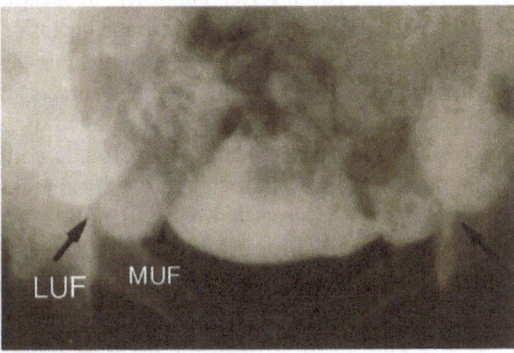

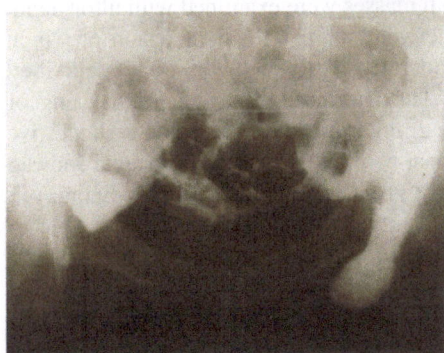

Fig. 10. Indirect left inguinal hernia. The lateral wall of the hernia sac continues without significant deviation from the lateral aspect of the abdominal wall. No intestinal loops were within the sac at the time of this exposure. (reprinted from Bendavid).

Fig. 11. Intraperitoneal injection of contrast material. Arcuate opaque lines are demonstrated as contrast material dispenses about loops of intestine. (reprinted from Bendavid).

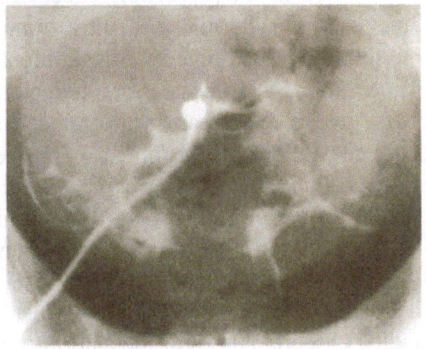

Ultrasound

Ultrasound is useful for evaluation of groin pain and characterization of inguinal hernias. It can also be very helpful in the diagnosis of uncommon ventral hernias (such as Spigelian and epigastric hernias) and in the evaluation of equivocal masses of the anterior abdominal wall. When evaluating the groin the following technique is used. The patient is positioned supine and is initially examined while relaxed. A linear array probe is used with the frequency set at either 7.5 or 10 MHz (the higher frequency provides better detail while the lower frequency is used when more penetration is needed). The examination begins with visualization of the femoral vessels in the femoral canal. The patient is then asked to cough and valsalva to look for a femoral hernia which is usually seen medial to the femoral vein (Fig. 12). The inferior epigastric vessels are then identified at either their takeoff from the femoral vessels or in the posterior aspect of the rectus muscle. The internal ring is found just lateral to the takeoff of the inferior epigastric vessel and the inguinal floor is just medial to these vessels. With the location of these in mind the inguinal floor is visualized and the patient is again asked to cough and valsalva (Fig. 13). During this process the spermatic cord is identified and followed from the internal ring to the pubic tubercle. Physiologic movement of the spermatic cord is normal, but an indirect hernia is identified when there is protrusion of bowel, from lateral to the inferior epigastric vessels, that travels with the cord structures. A lipoma of the cord which represents herniated preperitoneal fat moves in a similar fashion and is distinguished by its hypoechoic nature (Fig. 14). A direct hernia is noted as a protrusion through the inguinal floor, medial to the inferior epigastric vessels. In one series 95 patients with groin masses were examined with ultrasound. Seventy of these patients eventually underwent surgery for their lesion of which 95% were accurately diagnosed preoperatively (34). Chou et al described ultrasound in the pediatric population. He determined that an internal ring of greater than 4mm or one that increases by 2mm or more with valsalva is suggestive of a patent processus vaginalis or an inguinal hernia (35). Lilly and Arregui showed ultrasound to be 89% accurate in detecting groin pathology (hernia or lipoma) in patients with groin pain and no palpable bulge. In addition they were able to correctly identify the type of hernia (direct vs. indirect) in 87.7% of cases (33) which is a significant improvement over the 69% accuracy reported for physical exam alone (10). Evaluation of ventral hernias and anterior abdominal wall lesions also is performed using a linear probe set at 7.5MHz. The fascial around the lesion is identified as a hyperechoic sheet of tissue overlying the hypoechoic muscle. Diagnosis of a hernia with ultrasound is dependent upon demonstration of a muscular or fascial defect, exaggeration of the visualized lesion with straining of the abdominal wall muscles and reducibility of the lesion with pressure (except, of course in the case of an incarcerated hernia) (Fig. 15). Straining frequently will cause movement of peritoneal or pre-peritoneal contents into the subcutaneous tissue. Additionally a hernia can be confirmed by demonstration of peristalsis of the contents of the presumed hernia. Abdominal wall hernias have varied appearances when visualized with ultrasound depending on the contents of the hernia sac. Bowel loops and herniated mesenteric fat are highly echogenic and cast an acoustic shadow whereas herniated pre-peritoneal fat is typically hypoechoic. Lineaweaver studied obscure masses of the anterior abdominal wall and groin in 23 patients and found that ultrasound provided a clinically confirmed diagnosis in 91% of cases. In 39% of cases the ultrasound diagnosis was different from that suspected on physical exam. Of these patients 8 had confirmed hernias. The remaining lesions included lipomas, hematomas, suture granulomas and muscle diastases (36). In our own experience we have found that patients with pain at incision sites and no palpable hernias can sometimes have small fascial defects with herniated preperitoneal fat. These appear hypoechoic on ultrasound (Fig. 16).

One of the best uses of ultrasound in this context is with the evaluation of Spigelian hernias (Fig. 17). As previously stated almost half of all Spigelian hernias are miss-diagnosed. As a result 20 to 25% present emergently with associated complications. Spigelian hernias have been accurately diagnosed with high-resolution real-time ultrasound in patients presenting with non-specific lower abdominal pain (3). Multiple case reports exist in the literature in which diagnosis of these hernias by ultrasound was confirmed at surgery (3, 37).

The main disadvantage of ultrasound is its operator dependence. Few surgeons have extensive experience with ultrasound which is required to recognize the relatively subtle findings associated with hernias. Hernias can be mistaken for a variety of other lesions including lipomas, hematomas, abscesses and simple cysts due to their similar appearance on ultrasound (38).

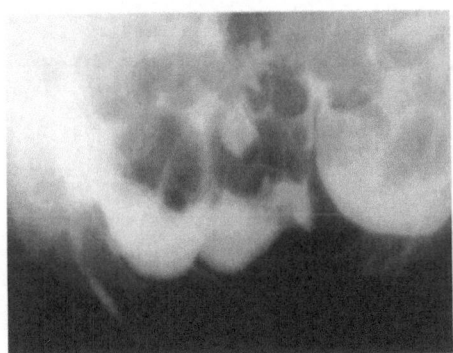

Fig. 12. Persistent patent processus vaginalis on the right, angled view. A slender extension of contrast material passes through the right internal inguinal ring and down the inguinal canal in a 34 year-old male with left groin symptoms. The diameter is less than 5mm and is therefore too small to admit intestine. (reprinted from Bendavid p 45.4).

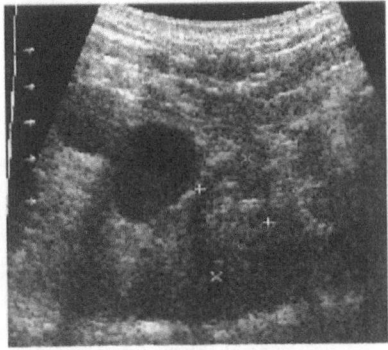

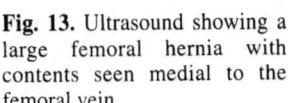

Fig. 13. Ultrasound showing a large femoral hernia with contents seen medial to the femoral vein.

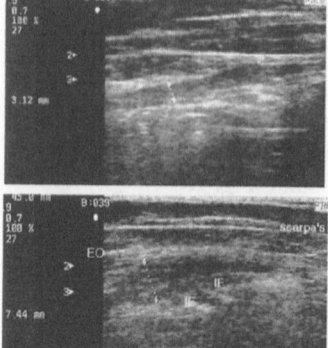

Fig. 14. Ultrasound showing widening of the inguinal canal due to herniation of intrabdominal or preperitoneal contents during valsalva.

Fig. 15. Ultrasound image showing the inguinal canal with a lipoma.

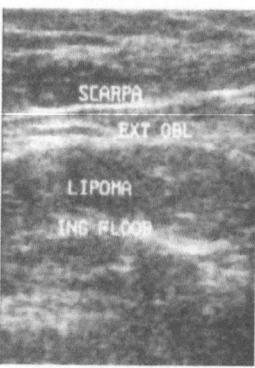

Fig. 16. Ultrasound image showing incisional hernia. The arrows point to the fascial edges and the dotted line traverses the neck of the hernia.

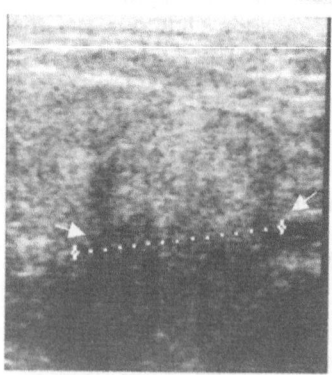

Fig. 17. Ultrasound showing herniated preperitoneal fat in a patient who was experiencing pain in the region of a prior surgical scar.

Fig. 18. Ultraound showing a Spigelian hernia. The arrows point to the fascial edges. Note that the herniated contents do not protrude through the external oblique fascia.

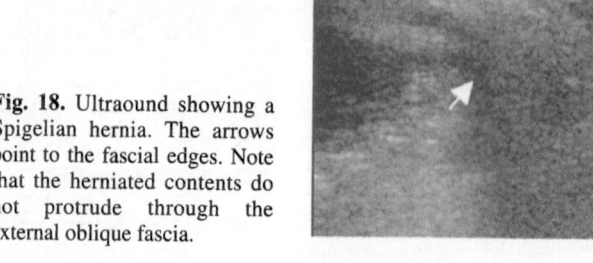

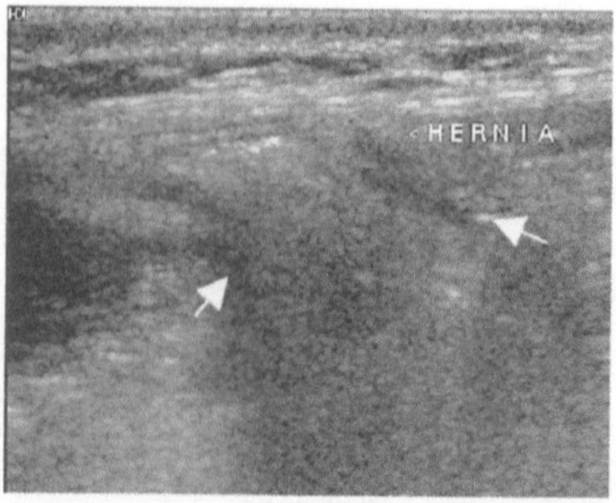

CONCLUSION

Since no trials have been performed to compare the accuracy of these studies it is impossible to declare one superior to the rest. When performed by an experienced physician ultrasound is safe, inexpensive and accurate. It is our procedure of choice for the evaluation of the anterior abdominal wall and groin in cases of suspected hernias.

References

1. Kavic MS. Chronic pelvic pain in women. In: Bendavid R, Abrahamson J, Arregui ME, Flament JB, Phillips EH, eds. Abdominal Wall Hernias: Principles and management. New York, Springer-Verlag, 2001:636.

2. Rutkow I. Epidemiologic, economic, and sociologic aspects of hernia surgery in the United States in the 1990's. Surg Clin North Am 1998; 78: 941-951.

3. Mufid MM, Abu-Yousef MM, Kakish ME, Urdaneta LF, Sl-Jurf AS. Spigelian Hernia: Diagnosis by high-resolution real-time sonography. Journal of Ultrasound in Medicine 1997;16:183-187.

4. Balthazar EJ, Subramanyam BR, Megibow A. Spigelian Hernia: CT and Ultrasonography Diagnosis. Gastrointestinal Radiology 1984;9:81-84.

5. Leis HP Jr., Mersheimer WL, Winfield JM. Spontaneous lateral ventral hernia. Surgery 1968; 43: 328-333.

6. Flament JB, Avisse C, Delatter JF. Anatomy of the Abdominal Wall In: Bendavid R, Abrahamson J, Arregui ME, Flament JB, Phillips EH, eds. Abdominal Wall Hernias: Principles and management. New York, Springer-Verlag, 2001: pp. 60-61.

7. Howship J, Practical remarks on the discrimination and appearances of surgical disease. London: John Churchill; 1840.

8. Machan L, Cooperberg PL. A femoral hernia diagnosed by ultrasonography and fine-needle aspiration biopsy. Journal of Ultrasound in Medicine 1984; 3(8): 379-80.

9. Cameron AEP. Accuracy of clinical diagnosis of direct and indirect inguinal hernia. The British Journal of Surgery 1994;81:250.

10. Ralphs DNL, Brain AJL, Grundy DJ, Hobsley M. How accurately can direct and indirect inguinal hernias be distinguished? BMJ 1980; 280:1039-1040.

11. Weiss Y., Lernan O., Nissan S.. Spigelian Hernia. Ann Surg 1974; 180: 836-839.

12. Green BT. Strangulated obturator hernia: still deadly. Southern Medical Journal 2001;94(1): 81-3.

13. Spangen L. Spigelian Hernia. In: Nyhus LM, Condon RE: Hernia, 4th edition. Philadelphia, J.B. Lipincott Company, 1995.

14. Bay-Nielsen M, Perkins FM, Kehlet H. Pain and functional impairment 1 year after inguinal herniography: a nationwide questionnaire study. Ann Surg 2001; 233(1): 1-7.

15. Hamlin JA, Kahn AM. Herniography in symptomatic patients following inguinal hernia repair. World Journal of Medicine 1995;162(1):28-31.

16. Williams MP, Scott IHK, Dixon AK. Computed Tomography in 101 Patients with a palpable abdominal mass. Clinical Radiology 1984;35:293-296.

17. Hojer AM, Rygaard H, Jess P. CT in the diagnosis of abdominal wall hernias: a preliminary study. European Radiology 1997;7:1416-1418.

18. Ziegler DW, Rhoads JE. Obturator hernia needs a laparotomy, not a diagnosis. Am Surg 1995; 170: 67-68.

19. Rogers FA. Strangulated obturator hernia. Surgery 1960; 48:394-403.

20. Yokoyama Y, Yamaguchi A, Isogai M, et al. Thirty-six cases of obturator hernia: does computed tomography contribute to postoperative outcome? World J Surg 1999; 23:214-217.

21. Yip AWC, AhChong AK, Lam KH. Obturator hernia: a continuing diagnostic challenge. Surgery 1993; 113:266-269.

22. Yokoyama T, Munakata Y, Ogiwara M, et al. Preoperative diagnosis of strangulated obturator hernia using ultrasonography. Am J Surg 1997; 174:76-78.

23. Hsu CH, Wang CC, Jeng LB, et al. Obturator hernia: a report of eight cases. Am Surg 1993; 59:709-711.

24. Van den Berg JC, de Valois JC, Go PM, Rosenbusch G. Groin Hernia: Can dynamic magnetic resonance imaging be of help? European Radiology 1998;8:270-273.

25. Van den Berg JC, de Valois JC, Go PM, Rosenbusch G. Dynamic Magnetic Resonance Imaging in the Diagnosis of Groin Hernia. Investigative Radiology 1997;32(10):644-647.

26. Van den Berg JC, de Valois JC, Go PM, Rosenbusch G. Detection of groin hernia with physical examination, ultrasound and MRI compared with laparoscopic findings. Invest Radiol 1999; 34:739-743.

27. Magre GR, Terk M, Colletti P, Muggia F, Boswell W. Saline MR Peritoneography. American Journal of Radiology 1996;167:749-751.

28. Ducharme JC, Bertrand R, Chacar R. Is it possible to diagnose inguinal hernia by x-ray? A preliminary report on herniography. Journal of the Canadian Association of Radiologists 1967; 18:448-451.

29. Ekberg O. Inguinal herniography in adults: technique, normal anatomy and diagnostic criteria for hernias. Radiology 1981; 138:31-36.

30. Hamlin JA. Imaging Hernias of the Abdominal Wall. In: Bendavid R, Abrahamson J, Arregui ME, Flament JB, Phillips EH, eds. Abdominal Wall Hernias: Principles and management. New York, Spinger-Verlag, 2001: pp. 335-340.

31. Macarthur DC, Grieve DC, Thompson AM, Greig JD, Nixon SJ. Short note: Herniography for groin pain of uncertain origin. The British Journal of Surgery 1997;84(5):684-685.

32. Toms AP, Dixon AK, Murphy JMP, Jamieson NV. Illustrated review of new imaging techniques in the diagnosis of abdominal wall hernias. The British Journal of Surgery 1999;86(10):1243-1249.

33. Lilly MC, Arregui ME. Ultrasound of the inguinal floor to evaluate hernias. Submitted and pending publication in Surg Endo 2001.

34. Deitch EA, Soncrant MR. Ultrasonic diagnosis of surgical disease in the inguinal femoral region. Surg Gyn Obst 1981; 152:319-322.

35. Chou TY, Chu CC, Diau GY, Wu CJ, Gueng MK. Inguinal hernia in children: Ultrasound versus exploratory surgery and intraoperative contralateral laparoscopy. Radiology 1996; 201:385-388.

36. Lineaweaver W, Vlasak M, Muyshondt E. Ultrasonic examination of abdominal wall and groin masses. Southern Medical Journal 1983; 76(5): 590-2.

37. Torzilli G, Carmana G, Lumachi V, Gnocchi P, Olivari N. The Usefulness of Ultrasonography in the Diagnosis of the Spigelian Hernia. International Surgery 1995;80(3):280-282.

38. Yeh HC, Lehr-Janus C, Cohen BA, Rabinowitz JG. Ultrasonography and CT of Abdominal and Inguinal Hernias. Journal of Clinical Ultrasound 1984;12:479-486.

CHAPTER 19

Anesthetic Considerations in Laparoscopic Repair of Ventral Hernias

A. Gutiérrez, M.A. Argüelles

INTRODUCTION

The rapid development of laparoscopic surgery in the last decade has posed a very real challenge for anesthesiologists, who are suddenly faced with a surgical technique of considerably different characteristics than conventional techniques. The aim of the new technique is rapid recovery of the patient. However, the technique itself affects normal function of the cardiocirculatory and respiratory systems and may present complications that are rarely observed in other type of surgeries. Over the years, it has been recognized that initial concerns about the "hazards" of laparoscopy were not entirely well founded and that the advantages of this technique greatly outweigh the risks when performed by experienced anesthesia-surgical teams. The proven benefits of minimally invasive surgery have caused a spectacular increase in the demand for this type of procedure, both by patients and health organizations. In fact, there are many conditions –cholelithiasis, splenectomy, gastroesophageal reflux, recurrent inguinal hernia– for which the surgical approach of choice is the laparoscopic procedure. Laparoscopic repair of ventral hernias is a technique that will probably end up being the initial indication for treatment of this type of defect.

PATHOPHYSIOLOGY OF THE PNEUMOPERITONEUM

Before discussing the management of anesthesia in laparoscopic procedures, an understanding of the pressure-based pneumoperitoneum and the pathophysiological changes it causes at the circulatory, respiratory and metabolic levels is required (Fig. 1). Laparoscopy techniques with a low-pressure pneumoperitoneum, in which cavity insufflation is replaced by suspension of the abdominal wall (gasless laparoscopy), have been developed. However, their application to ventral hernia repair is technically complex and they have not been used to date in this type of surgery. Therefore, they will not be discussed in this article.

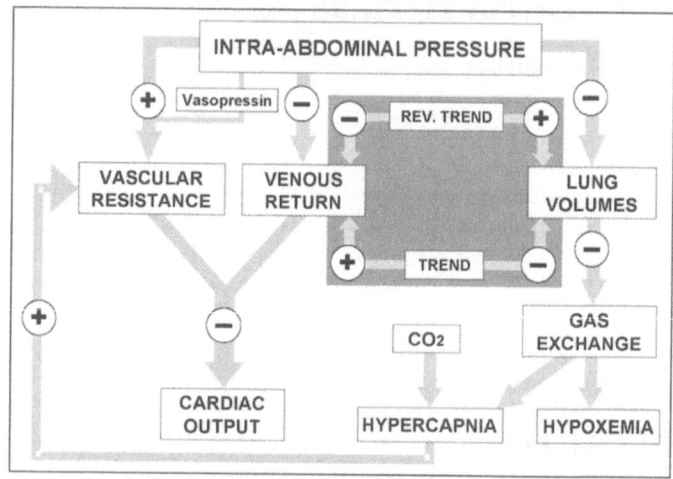

Fig. 1. Pathophysiology of pneumoperitoneum and position changes.

Pressure

To create the pneumoperitoneum, a gas is introduced into the abdominal cavity. This virtual cavity with zero pressure must distend, creating a chamber in which certain pressure is achieved, generally between 10 and 15 mmHg. With intra-abdominal pressures (IAP) below 10 mmHg, the hemodynamic changes are not very significant (1, 2) ; hence these levels are recommended for patients with little cardiocirculatory reserve, although visibility can be reduced. For incisional hernias we use the most commonly used pressure, between 10 and 12 mmHg.

Gas

The ideal gas for peritoneal insufflation is colorless, physiologically inert, nonflammable and highly soluble in plasma in order to ensure elimination and reduce the risks of a gas embolism. Several gases have been used for laparoscopy (Table I). Because of its high solubility and low cost, the most frequently used at present is carbon dioxide (CO_2), although it may affect the respiratory and circulatory physiology (see below). Buffered in the form of plasma bicarbonate, carbon dioxide is rapidly eliminated through pulmonary ventilation, hence the potential of causing severe hypercapnia when insufflated in the abdominal cavity is modest in patients with no severe respiratory pathology. In patients with a high risk of respiratory insufficiency, the use of nitrous oxide can be considered despite the risk of combustion (3).

Position

The dorsal decubitus is the most frequently used position for ventral hernioplasties, with the right arm at the side of the body and the left arm at a 70° angle. Modified lithotomy with the legs slightly separated is generally used for hiatal hernias. In order to displace the abdominal content from the surgical region, the Trendelenburg and inverted Trendelenburg positions are adopted for procedures in the lower and upper abdomen, respectively. Both positions compensate for some pneumoperitoneum-induced hemodynamic and respiratory changes and worsen others (Fig. 1), although the variations are not very significant unless the angle is greater than 15° (4).

Hemodynamic changes

An increase in cardiac output is observed when peritoneal insufflation is performed with low-pressure CO_2 (7 mmHg) (5). This can be explained by emptying at the splanchnic territory and the slight sympathetic stimulation induced by CO_2. As pressures above 10 mmHg are produced, the cardiac output decreases by 25-35% of its initial value, with this drop proportional to the increase in the IAP. When the effects of anesthesia, positive-pressure ventilation and the inverted Trendelenburg position are also considered, the reduction can be as high as 50% of the preoperative value (6, 7). The Trendelenburg position results in a slight increase in venous return and in cardiac output, but only partially corrects the hemodynamic effects of the pneumoperitoneum since the abdominal viscera move the diaphragm upward, increasing intrathoracic pressure (ITP) and hampering cardiac filling. From the physiopathological viewpoint, the drop in cardiac output is mediated by decreased preloading and increased postloading (Fig 1). The reduced preloading is due to a mechanical factor whereby the large abdominal vessels, particularly the inferior vena cava, are compressed, leading to a parallel decrease in venous return. Paradoxically, as the ITP increases due to diaphragm thrust and controlled ventilation, the cardiac filling pressures increase, although the right atrium transmural pressure (auricular pressure minus ITP), which is the actual expression of right ventricular filling, decreases slightly. The decrease in cardiac output is much greater than the decrease in transmural pressure, which suggests a shift in the ventricular function curve toward the right due to increased postloading. In effect, according to the literature (8, 9), an increase in systemic vascular resistance (SVR) of 36-95% of the previous values is observed from the start of peritoneal insufflation, which explains the rise in blood pressure parallel to the drop in output. The SVR increase appears to be the cause rather than the result of this drop, since vasodilation induced by anesthesia or specific drugs improves cardiac output even when preloading does not vary (6). The cause of this sharp rise in SVR, which is the most important hemodynamic alteration resulting from the pneumoperitoneum with CO_2, is multifactorial. There is a mechanical factor from compression of the aorta and the splanchnic vascular bed associated with humoral factors, among which, elevated levels of catecholamines or prostaglandins, activation of the renin-angiotensin system (6, 8) and release of vasopressin have been cited (10). The release of these mediators is related to the adrenergic stimulus caused by peritoneum distention with elevation of the IAP, absorption of CO_2 (11) and increased pressure of the right auricula (10).

The severity of the hemodynamic deterioration induced by the pneumoperitoneum and the position changes depends, to a large extent, on the patient's volemia and cardiac reserve, hence, comprehensive preoperative assessment and optimization of cardiocirculatory function is mandatory (see below).

Respiratory changes

The main problem observed during CO_2-based pneumoperitoneum is hypercapnia, which arises in conjunction with alterations in the gas exchange and diffusion of intra-abdominal CO_2. Gas exchange alterations result from increases in the IAP which reduce diaphragm mobility and limit ventilation, decreasing total lung compliance (Ct) and functional residual capacity, and increasing the intrapulmonary shunt (12,13). These changes can be partially offset with increased ventilation support, although the use of positive-end expiratory pressure (PEEP) is not advisable since the hemodynamics are noticeably worsened (14). The inverted Trendelenburg position helps to recover pulmonary volumes restricted by the pneumoperitoneum, but does not significantly improve the Ct, and the Trendelenburg position leads to further reductions of the Ct (15). Airway pressure inevitably increases when insufflating the abdominal cavity, due to this reduction in pulmonary distensibility. This elevation in insufflation pressures distends the alveoli and compromises perfusion, increasing the dead space. These imbalances in the ventilation-to-perfusion ratio promote the development of hypercapnia, but do not generally compromise oxygenation in healthy patients (6). CO_2 is directly absorbed from the abdominal cavity into the blood during laparoscopy. This is influenced by the duration of the pneumoperitoneum, the degree of pressure, the speed of the insufflation and the presence of small holes in the peritoneum. The pattern of CO_2 absorption is seen as a sharp, sudden rise, which after a few minutes is followed by a reduction and a maintained stability throughout the procedure. This stability is probably due to the pressure of the pneumoperitoneum on the splanchnic capillaries, which reduces CO_2 uptake by the blood. When the cavity is emptied and the pressure is released, there is a sudden increase in uptake as the residual CO_2 is absorbed (16), a factor that must be taken into account when discontinuing ventilation support at the end of surgery.

Renal and metabolic changes

Perfusion of the intra-abdominal organs is sensitive to pneumoperitoneum pressure. When the IAP reaches 15 mmHg, the renal cortical blood flow drops 60% (17), glomerular filtration decreases by 25% and diuresis decreases (18). Perfusion also decreases in the remaining organs, with a drop sharper than that of cardiac output. Due to this hypoperfusion, tissue oxygenation in the splanchnic territory decreases, detectable by a drop in the gastric intramucosal pH (19), and this can lead to a certain degree of metabolic acidosis (20). These alterations are not very significant if the IAP is kept below 12 mmHg and baseline values are recovered within a short period after exsufflating the abdominal cavity (18, 19). The only reported case of renal insufficiency possibly related to the pneumoperitoneum occurred in a patient in whom renal function had been previously affected (21). Another factor to take into account is that the insufflation of dry gas at room temperature causes a decrease in body temperature directly proportional to the duration of pneumoperitoneum (0.3 to 0.5° C per hour) and to the amount of gas used (22, 23). Since a significant amount of heat is lost to evaporation when the gas is humidified in the abdomen, the use of heated insufflators has been shown to be effective in preventing this hypothermia (23).

Table II contains a summary of the precautions that should be taken in all laparoscopic procedures to minimize the adverse physiological effects of the pneumoperitoneum and prevent some of the potential complications of this technique.

Table I. Gases used for pneumoperitoneum

Agent	Solubility (ml/100 ml H_2O)	Combustion	Risk of embolism
CO_2	171	-	Minimum
N_2O	130	++	Moderate
Air	2.92	++	High
Helium	0.97	-	High
Argon	5.6	-	High

Table II. Measures to decrease the effects of the pneumoperitoneum

1. Insufflate slowly, without exceeding 1L/min.
2. Limit the pressure to 10-12 mmHg (6-8 in patients at risk)
3. Tilt the position slowly.
4. Limit the tilt to 15°.
5. Minimize the duration.
6. Minimize gas leaks.
7. Use heaters-humidifiers

ASSESSMENT AND SELECTION OF PATIENTS

The preoperative assessment of patients who will undergo laparoscopic surgery does not differ substantially from that of any other conventional surgery with moderate associated risk. The basic lines of the assessment are summarized in Tables III and IV (24). Laparoscopy is associated with two special factors, namely pressure-based pneumoperitoneum and positioning, both of which can affect the cardiocirculatory and respiratory systems, as discussed earlier in this article. Thus it is essential to assess the functional status of these systems by performing all necessary additional tests whenever any sign of a cardiovascular or respiratory condition is observed in the clinical history or physical examination. Since a comprehensive review of these tests goes beyond the scope of this article, we recommend two recent reviews on this topic (25, 26).

Frequent pathologies

Most patients who experience incisional hernias share a series of common characteristics. Except for patients with congenital defects, these are typically overweight individuals with one or more concomitant disease, including diabetes, hypertension and/or chronic obstructive pulmonary disease (27). Moderate or severe obesity and chronic bronchial disease significantly alter respiratory function and can be associated with cardiovascular pathology (26, 28). Diabetes and uncontrolled hypertension are associated with a higher probability of coronary disease, which may be asymptomatic (27), as well as a certain degree of autonomic nervous system dysfunction (29). The implications of each of these pathologies on anesthesia management will be presented throughout this article. However, due to their importance from the standpoint of intraoperative hemodynamic complications caused by neurovegetative dysfunction (30), autonomic nervous system function should be assessed prior to surgery. This can be carried out using relatively simple tests (31).

Contraindications

The initial reviews on anesthesia in laparoscopic procedures outlined a full series of limitations and contraindications for the practice of this type of surgery, particularly in high-risk patients (32). Advances in anesthesia and monitoring techniques, along with the growing expertise of surgical teams, have led to progressive changes in this scenario and we can now affirm that contraindications for anesthesia are the exception. The unquestionable advantages of this approach in high-risk patients reside in the minimal surgical trauma, which significantly reduces postoperative complications, particularly respiratory problems and infection, and shortens the hospital stay (33). To obtain these advantages we must deal with a series of disadvantages that can be classified into two groups: hemodynamic and ventilation overload caused by the pressure-based pneumoperitoneum and the almost inevitable need for general anesthesia. The alterations induced by the pneumoperitoneum can be offset by the use of low insufflation pressures and by various circulatory and respiratory support techniques, which will be discussed below. Therefore, the only *a priori* contraindication for anesthesia is the impossibility to use general anesthesia, due to either the patient's physical condition or refusal to accept it. In our opinion, the idea that should remain in the anesthesiologist's mind when assessing patients proposed for laparoscopic surgery is not *whether or not* they can withstand laparoscopy, but rather *how to ensure* that they withstand laparoscopy. From the surgical point of view, clotting disorders and generalized peritonitis are still contraindications.

Preparation (Table V)

Patients with chronic respiratory disease should continue on medication until the time of surgery. The benefits of quitting smoking are only obvious if the patient stops at least eight weeks before the procedure. In fact, more pulmonary complications are reported in patients who quit smoking less than four weeks before than in patients who continued smoking (34). Nevertheless, cigarette smoking should cease at least 48 hours before to decrease carboxyhemoglobin levels and lessen the cardiovascular effects of nicotine. A respiratory physiotherapy program to promote the elimination of secretions will help to control coughing, a decisive factor in achieving a successful outcome in hernioplasties.

In general, antihypertensive and cardiological medications should also be maintained, although there is some controversy concerning diuretics and renin-angiotensin system inhibitors. Diuretics reduce the intravascular volume during the first six months of therapy, and patients treated with angiotensin-converting enzyme inhibitors (ACEIs) or angiotensin-receptor antagonists (ARAs) adapt poorly to reduced venous return and can experience severe hypotension and bradycardia crises during anesthesia (35, 36). Due to the difficulties in venous return that can occur during laparoscopy, discontinuation of these drugs 24 hours prior to surgery should be considered and vascular filling should be optimized in all cases before anesthesia is administered (see below). Postponement of the procedure is advisable when diastolic blood pressure values are above 110-120 mmHg. Hypotensive therapy should be started -preferably without diuretics or ACEIs/ARAs- and continued for several days or weeks until systemic vascular resistance is reduced and the relative hypovolemia of the hypertensive patient is offset.

The indications and guidelines for thromboembolism prophylaxis in laparoscopic surgery are not yet well defined. According to several studies, the risk of deep venous thrombosis is lower than in open surgery (37), whereas others find a similar risk (38). The concern for bleeding complications related to the use of low molecular weight heparins (LMWH) and the possibility of early ambulation has led to more conservative approaches such as mechanical methods that compress the lower extremities and the intraoperative use of dextran, which appear to be equally effective in clinical practice (39, 40). If ambulation is scheduled during the first 12 hours of the postoperative period, we do not believe that the protocol calls for LMWHs, unless the patient has several risk factors (Table V).

The prophylactic use of antibiotics in laparoscopic surgery has also been questioned due to its poor cost-benefit ratio. Studies performed with cholecystectomies have provided contrasting results for (41, 42) and against (43) antibiotic prophylaxis, with no studies on its usefulness in abdominal hernia repairs. Nevertheless, if the hernioplasty involves implantation of a prosthetic mesh, prophylaxis (preferably with 1st or 2nd-generation cephalosporins) seems to be advisable.

Lastly, optimal preoperative preparation must consider two important aspects related to successful laparoscopy outcome. The first is prevention of postoperative nausea and vomiting, which can be the cause of delays in hospital discharge and even compromise the result of the surgery (44). The most effective drugs for this purpose are anti-serotoninergic agents, (ondasetron, granisetron) droperidol and dexamethasone, alone or in combination. Reduced gastric volume and acidity is another objective, given the risk of regurgitation associated with pressure-based pneumoperitoneum and increased acidity of the gastric juice, which can cause hypercapnia during laparoscopy (45). For this purpose, treatment with H_2 antihistamines or proton pump inhibitors is indicated in the hours prior to the surgery.

Table III. Preoperative assessment

GENERAL CLINICAL HISTORY
Systematic medical history by organs and systems
Allergies or adverse reactions

ANESTHESIOLOGICAL CLINICAL HISTORY
Family history
Previous incidents or accidents

PHYSICAL EXAMINATION
Special attention to airways

ADDITIONAL TESTS (Table II)

LATEST REPORTS
Diagnosis, functional degree and treatment of associated diseases

---

Table IV. Additional tests (for ASA 1 patients*) (1)

AGE	MEN	WOMEN
Children	Hb or Hemato	Hb or Hemato
<45 years	EKG	EKG Hb or Hemato Pregnancy test**
45-65 years	EKG	EKG Hb or Hemato Pregnancy test**
>65 years	EKG Chest x-ray Hb or Hemato Glucose Creatinine	EKG Chest x-ray Hb or Hemato Glucose Creatinine
Obesity and smoking >20 cigarettes/day: Chest x-ray Alcohol intake >60 g/day: Prothrombin time, platelets and gamma-GT		

* ASA Class 1 is assigned to healthy patients who will undergo scheduled surgeries.
** If the patient cannot completely rule out the possibility of pregnancy.
Hb= Hemoglobin; Hemato= Hematocrit; EKG= Electrocardiogram

Table V. Preoperative preparation

PREVIOUS PATHOLOGIES
    COPD*: Stop smoking (48 hours)
             Respiratory physiotherapy
             Continue medication
  Hypertension: Control of blood pressure
             Continue medication (except diuretics,
             ACEIs and ARAs)
    Diabetes: Ordinary subcutaneous insulin dosage

ANTITHROMBOTIC PROPHYLAXIS
  Pressure bandaging of lower extremities
  HBPM (if risk factors exist)
      History of pulmonary thromboembolism
      Obesity
      Varicose veins
      Oral contraceptives
      Smoking
      Thrombocytosis

ANTIBIOTIC PROPHYLAXIS (hernioplasty with mesh)
  1st or 2nd-generation cephalosporin

ANTIEMETIC PROPHYLAXIS
  Droperidol/anti 5-HT/dexamethasone

REDUCTION OF GASTRIC VOLUME
  Anti H_2/omeprazole

* Chronic obstructive pulmonary disease.

PRACTICAL ASPECTS

Laparoscopic surgery in general and hernia repair in particular involves a number of special characteristics of which the anesthesiologist must be aware. Our discussion includes a series of important technical details and practical questions that are key to obtaining a favorable surgical outcome (Table VI).

Anesthesia technique

Although there are a few isolated reports of laparoscopies performed with epidural anesthesia (46), the anesthesia alternatives for extensive laparoscopic surgery are limited to one of the variations of general anesthesia. All the drugs and techniques currently in use can be employed safely, although several characteristics unique to surgery for abdominal wall repair must be taken into account. Although initial insufflation of the pneumoperitoneum is extremely reflexogenic due to irritation of the peritoneal surface, the rest of the hernioplasty technique is generally less painful than conventional surgery, hence, the use of opiates at the end of the procedure should be reduced to limit postoperative nausea. The administration of nonsteroidal anti-inflammatory drugs such as diclofenac or ketorolac at the end of the operation will help to control postoperative pain. The use of nondepolarizing muscle relaxants is indicated since laparoscopic repair of both ventral and esophageal hiatal hernias requires immobilization and broad, clear visualization that only can be obtained with potent relaxation of the abdominal cavity. Patients with hypertension and diabetes who have some degree of autonomic dysfunction are particularly prone to hypotension crises after induction of anesthesia (30), hence, the anesthetic must be administered slowly and gradually. There is some controversy surrounding the use of nitrous oxide since it would increase postoperative nausea and cause distention of the intestinal loops, hindering visualization. Nevertheless, these effects have not been proven in clinical practice with laparoscopic surgery (47) and there seems to be no contraindication to its use at present.

Ventilation support

Due to the respiratory overload produced by the pneumoperitoneum and the exogenous supply of CO_2, endotracheal intubation and ventilation support is generally required. The limitations of thoracopulmonary distensibility imposed by increased intra-abdominal pressure make the use of volume-controlled ventilation advisable, with volume adjustment based on expired CO_2 ($EtCO_2$) values. Generally an increase of 15-20% in current volume over normal figures and maintenance of the respiratory rate are sufficient, although occasionally the latter must also be increased to control hypercapnia. The CO_2 absorption rate tends to stabilize after the initial rise (see above) and does not usually represent a major problem. Nevertheless, in patients with severe pulmonary disease CO_2 retention may occur. In the case of sudden, extreme hypercapnia, a gas leak to the subcutaneous tissue, pleural space or mediastinum must be ruled out (48) (see Complications). Insufflation of the pneumoperitoneum and the resulting abdominal thrust on the pulmonary parenchyma can produce endobronchial intubation, with increased airway pressure and hypoxemia (Fig. 2).

In order to help prevent hypothermia observed in laparoscopic procedures of some duration (22, 49), the use of closed or semi-closed circuit ventilation systems with low flow rates and humidifying filters is advisable.

Hemodynamic support

The drastic reduction in venous return caused by the pneumoperitoneum can be offset by prior vascular filling with crystalloid solutions at 10 to 20 ml/kg of body weight, depending on the positioning to be used (the inverted Trendelenburg requires more aggressive filling), although certain patients with a low cardiac reserve may need the help of inotropic drugs to adequately manage this volume load. The adoption of measures to counteract blood trapping in the lower extremities, e.g. elevation and pressure bandages on the legs, helps to offset hemodynamic deterioration due to the inverted Trendelenburg position (6). The SVR increase observed at the start of abdominal cavity CO_2 insufflation can be controlled by short-acting vasodilators (urapidil, nitroglycerine), which reduce hemodynamic deterioration and re-establish circulatory function in patients with severe cardiovascular disease (50). By combining the use of inotropic drugs, vasodilators and invasive monitoring, these procedures can be successfully handled in patients at high cardiocirculatory risk (51).

Abdominal decompression

In order to prevent abdominal viscera lesions while inserting the needles and trocars, the use of a nasogastric tube and bladder catheter is indicated. Nasogastric intubation in an already anesthesized patient can pose difficulties in large hiatal hernias and, therefore, insertion while the patient is awake should be considered, in order to take advantage of the swallowing mechanism and esophageal peristalsis. In short procedures, the bladder catheter can be avoided by telling the patient to urinate before entering the surgical theater.

Monitoring

The basic guidelines for monitoring and supervision do not differ from the general guidelines for all anesthesia, although several special considerations are necessary (Table VII). Electrocardiography, pulse oximetry and blood pressure measurements are mandatory, as well as airway and intra-abdominal pressure measurements. $EtCO_2$ measurement is effective for detecting complications (Fig. 2), but is only a guideline. Moreover, although healthy patients maintain a good correlation with arterial CO_2 values ($PaCO_2$) (52), the variations in $PaCO_2$ may not be reflected in $EtCO_2$ (53) in patients with cardiopulmonary disease. As a result, blood gas analysis should be considered in high-risk patients or in intraoperative situations of hypoxemia, elevated airway pressure or sudden changes in $EtCO_2$. Lateral flow spirometry can be used to detect changes in lung compliance and in ventilation flow and pressure curves, parameters of use for diagnosing respiratory complications. During insufflation of the pneumoperitoneum, close monitoring of hemodynamic parameters is necessary in all patients for early detection of catastrophic complications, such as vascular puncture or gas embolism (see Complications). A physical inspection should also be performed to rule out the possibility of subcutaneous emphysema. Insufflation and the position changes must be performed gradually in patients with high cardiocirculatory risk, and hemodynamic variables should be monitored before, during and after the changes. In patients with limited cardiac function, direct, continuous measurement of arterial and central venous pressures must be considered, possibly with the insertion of a pulmonary artery catheter to control hemodynamic changes (50). During the entire procedure, one should be alert to the surgical movements and carry out regular inspections of the abdomen, since the surgeons are focused on a specific area of the monitor and may not notice a problem in another area.

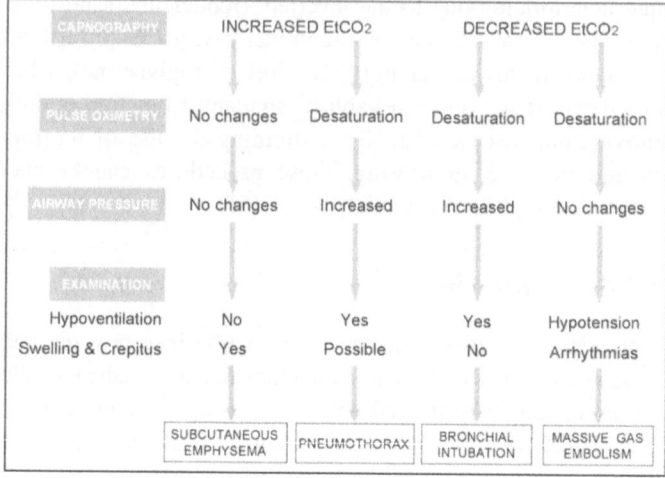

Fig. 2. Acute respiratory complications: diagnostic algorithm. (Modified from Wahba RW et al. (59)).

Table VI. Anesthesia management

ANESTHESIA TECHNIQUE
General anesthesia
Opiate restriction
Effective relaxation
Postoperative analgesia with NSAIDs
VENTILATION SUPPORT
Controlled volume
Increase Vt by 20%
Adjust frequency until achieving normocapnia
Low flow rates
HEMODYNAMIC SUPPORT
Initial load: 10-20 mL/kg of crystalloids
Bandaging and elevation of lower extremities
Inotropics
Vasodilators
ABDOMINAL DECOMPRESSION
Nasogastric tube
Bladder catheter

Table VII. Monitoring

ESSENTIAL
EKG
Pulse oximetry
Blood pressure
Airway pressure
Intra-abdominal pressure
Exhaled CO_2
RECOMMENDED
Lateral flow spirometry
Diuresis
Arterial gasometry
OPTIONAL (according to previous pathologies)
Direct blood pressure
Central venous pressure
Pulmonary capillary pressure
ST analysis
Transesophageal echocardiography

COMPLICATIONS

Most complications presenting during laparoscopic surgery are caused by problems resulting from the surgical technique itself, and are not due to patient characteristics or anesthesia technique. The incidence of complications is higher while the technique is being learned. The most serious complications, vascular or visceral lesions and gas embolism, are inherent to the laparoscopic approach and do not occur in open surgery. The risk of these complications meant that laparoscopy was originally considered a potentially hazardous technique only useful in reasonably healthy patients. Its multiple advantages were subsequently demonstrated and the complication rate obtained by experienced teams was shown to be similar or lower than that of open surgery (54, 55), thereby helping it to become the technique of choice for various surgical processes. The complications of laparoscopic surgery can be divided into two major groups: those resulting from the pneumoperitoneum and those related to the surgical technique.

Complications related to the pneumoperitoneum

Apart from the hemodynamic and respiratory alterations normally caused by pressure-based pneumoperitoneum (see above), the insufflation of CO_2 in the abdominal cavity can cause arrhythmias in up to one third of patients (56, 57), generally tachyrhythmias and ventricular extrasystoles attributable to adrenergic stimulation induced by CO_2 absorption. On other occasions, the excessively sudden distention of the peritoneum during insufflation triggers a vasovagal reflex with bradycardia that can even become asystolic (57, 58). The maintenance of $PaCO_2$ at normal limits and gradual insufflation of the abdominal cavity can reduce the incidence of these arrhythmias.

The entrance of CO_2 outside the abdominal cavity creates areas of emphysema, which can be located in the subcutaneous tissue or preperitoneal space. The opening of anatomic communications between the peritoneal cavity and the pleural cavity due to the IAP permits the development of a pneumothorax (59). In patients with esophageal hiatal hernia, the potential for direct passage of CO_2 to the mediastinum during the surgical procedure, causing pneumomediastinum and pneumothorax, must be taken into account (60). The gas can also pass to the mediastinum through the retroperitoneum (61). All these situations tend to cause considerable hypercapnia due to massive absorption of CO_2 (62). If hypoxemia with increased airway pressure also occurs, the presence of a pneumothorax should be suspected. A physical examination of the patient, along with palpation and auscultation, will aid the diagnosis (Fig. 2). The impossibility of controlling hypercapnia by increasing ventilation or the presentation of a pneumothorax under tension are indications that laparoscopy should be suspended and the surgery should be converted to a conventional procedure. The pneumothorax can be drained from the abdominal cavity, although the simple application of positive end-expiratory pressure can solve the problem (60).

One of the most serious complications of laparoscopic surgery is massive gas embolism. Nevertheless, cases of clinically significant embolism are infrequent since CO_2 is easily soluble in blood and the quantity needed to cause a fatal embolism is high, compared to other gases (63). Isolated cases with fatal results have been reported, generally in conjunction with an inadvertent vascular lesion that allowed massive entrance of gas in circulation (64, 65). The use of an elevated IAP and the inverted Trendelenburg position creates a pressure gradient between the abdomen and thorax that favors the introduction of CO_2 into the circulatory system (59), which shows up as a decrease in $EtCO_2$, hypoxemia, arrhythmias and arterial hypotension (Fig. 2). Transesophageal ecocardiography is extremely sensitive in detecting gas embolisms (66), although its routine use is not justified. Treatment includes immediate discontinuation of the pneumoperitoneum, placement in left lateral decubitus, aspiration through a central venous catheter and cardiocirculatory support measures.

Complications related to the surgical technique

Although laparoscopy is a minimally invasive technique, blind insertion of needles and trocars in the abdominal cavity can result in punctures of intracavity vessels and organs. The frequency of this type of lesion ranges from about 1/1,000 for visceral punctures to 0.5/1,000 for retroperitoneal vessel punctures (67, 68). Despite careful technique, intestinal lesions may go unnoticed and trigger peritonitis with fatal results if not diagnosed in time (67). Vascular punctures, in contrast, tend to be recognized at the time they occur, particularly if due to a trocar. Nevertheless, a small vascular puncture can cause a retroperitoneal hematoma that goes unnoticed for several hours until hemodynamic deterioration becomes significant. The mortality from the retroperitoneal vessel punctures can be as high as 15% of cases (67, 69), hence immediate hemostasia is essential. Lesions to abdominal wall vessels, particularly epigastric arteries, can also cause hematomas if not diagnosed, although bleeding through the inlets is usually obvious. Certain abdominal hernioplasty techniques rely on percutaneous suture of the mesh, which can increase the risk of lesion to wall vessels.

The location and extension of visceral or vascular lesions varies considerably. Since some lesions can be repaired by a laparoscopic procedure, the decision to convert to open surgery must be discussed and agreed between the surgeon and anesthesiologist; in all cases, the anesthesiologist must watch the vital signs of patient closely and indicate immediate suspension of the procedure and emptying of the cavity if the patient presents severe hemodynamic deterioration. Once the cause has been determined and cardiovascular stability has been restored with adequate support measures, conversion is evaluated in conjunction with the surgical team. The potential causes of cardiovascular collapse during laparoscopy are shown in Table VIII (70).

Table VIII. Cardiovascular collapse. Causes

Adverse drug reaction to anesthetic drugs
Vasovagal reflex
Excessive IAP
Excessive tilt
Arrhythmias
Myocardial ischemia
Hemorrhaging
Pneumothorax under tension
Gas embolism

SUMMARY

The approach to anesthesia for any surgical laparoscopic technique requires an in-depth understanding of the pathophysiology of the pressure-based pneumoperitoneum. In most patients, even those with cardiocirculatory and respiratory risk factors, the hemodynamic and ventilation changes occurring in the procedure can be offset with individualized preoperative treatment. Nevertheless, the anesthesiologist handling this type of surgery must keep in mind that a minimally invasive procedure is not necessarily a low-risk procedure. Hence, the combination of suitable preparation, careful surgical technique and strict monitoring are essential to significantly decreasing the incidence of serious complications and the repercussion of such complications for the patient.

References

1. Ishizaki Y, Bandai Y, Shimomura K, Abe H, Ohtomo Y, Idezuki Y. Safe intraabdominal pressure of carbon dioxide pneumoperitoneum during laparoscopic surgery. Surgery. 1993; 114(3): 549-54.

2. Wallace DH, Serpell MG, Baxter JN, O'dwyer PJ. Randomized trial of different insufflation pressures for laparoscopic cholecystectomy. Br J Surg. 1997; 84(4): 455-8.

3. Menes T, Spivak H. Laparoscopy. Searching for the proper insufflation gas. Surg Endosc. 2000; 14(11): 1050-6.

4. Berg K, Wilhelm W, Grundmann U, Ladenburger A, Feifel G, Mertzlufft F. Laparoscopic cholecystectomy-effect of position changes and CO_2 pneumoperitoneum on hemodynamic, respiratory and endocrinologic parameters. Zentralbl Chir. 1997;122(5): 395-404.

5. Dexter SP, Vucevic M, Gibson J, Mcmahon MJ. Hemodynamic consequences of high- and low-pressure capnoperitoneum during laparoscopic cholecystectomy. Surg Endosc. 1999; 13(4): 376-81.

6. Joris JL, Noirot DP, Legrand MJ, Jacquet NJ, Lamy ML. Hemodynamic changes during laparoscopic cholecystectomy. Anesth Analg. 1993;76(5):1067-71.

7. Hirvonen EA, Poikolainen EO, Paakkonen ME, Nuutinen LS. The adverse hemodynamic effects of anesthesia, head-up tilt, and carbon dioxide pneumoperitoneum during laparoscopic cholecystectomy. Surg Endosc. 2000; 14(3): 272-7.

8. Torrielli R, Cesarini M, Winnock S, Cabiro C, Mene JM. Hemodynamic changes during celioscopy: a study carried out using thoracic electric bioimpedance. Can J Anaesth. 1990; 37(1): 46-51.

9. Girardis M, Broi UD, Antonutto G, Pasetto A. The effect of laparoscopic cholecystectomy on cardiovascular function and pulmonary gas exchange. Anesth Analg. 1996; 83(1): 134-40.

10. Viinamki O, Punnonen R. Vasopressin release during laparoscopy: role of increased intra-abdominal pressure. Lancet. 1982 Jan 16;1(8264):175-6.

11. Ho HS, Saunders CJ, Gunther RA, Wolfe BM. Effector of hemodynamics during laparoscopy: CO_2 absorption or intra-abdominal pressure?. J Surg Res. 1995; 59(4): 497-503.

12. Hasnain JU, Matjasko MJ. Systemic changes during laparoscopic surgery. Respiratory system. Surgical Laparoscopy. Ed. Karl A. Zucker. Quality Medical Publishing Inc. 1991.

13. Wahba RW, Beique F, Kleiman SJ. Cardiopulmonary function and laparoscopic cholecystectomy. Can J Anaesth. 1995; 42(1): 51-63.

14. Kraut EJ, Anderson JT, Safwat A, Barbosa R, Wolfe BM. Impairment of cardiac performance by laparoscopy in patients receiving positive end-expiratory pressure. Arch Surg. 1999; 134(1): 76-80.

15. Makinen MT, Yli-Hankala A. Respiratory compliance during laparoscopic hiatal and inguinal hernia repair. Can J Anaesth. 1998; 45(9): 865-70.

16. Blobner M, Felber AR, Gogler S, Feussner H, Weigl EM, Jelen G, Jelen-Esselborn S. The resorption of carbon dioxide from the pneumoperitoneum in laparoscopic cholecystectomy. Anaesthesist. 1993 May;42(5):288-94.

17. Chiu AW, Chang LS, Birkett DH, Babayan RK. The impact of pneumoperitoneum, pneumoretroperitoneum, and gasless laparoscopy on the systemic and renal hemodynamics. J Am Coll Surg. 1995; 181(5): 397-406.

18. Mcdougall E, Monk T, Wolf J et al. The effect of prolonged pneumoperitoneum in an animal model. J Am Coll Surg. 1996; 186(4): 317-28.

19. Schilling MK, Redealli C, Krahenbuhl L, Signer C, Buchler MW. Splanchnic microcirculatory changes during CO_2 laparoscopy. J Am Coll Surg. 1997; 184(4): 378-82.

20. Gandara V, De Vega DS, Escriu N, Zorrilla IG. Acid-base balance alterations in laparoscopic cholecystectomy. Surg Endosc. 1997; 11(7): 707-10.

21. Ben-David B, Croitoru M, Gaitini L. Acute renal failure following laparoscopic cholecystectomy: a case report. J Clin Anesth. 1999; 11(6): 486-9.

22. Castillo V, Gutiérrez-Crespo A, Suarez F, Luis-Navarro JC, Gómez-Arguelles MA. Variación de la temperatura corporal en relación con la insuflación de CO_2 en el curso de la colecistectomía laparoscópica. Rev Esp Anestesiol Reanim. 1996; 43(6): 201-203.

23. Jacobs VR, Morrison JE JR, Mettler L, Mundhenke C, JONAT W. Measurement of CO_2 hypothermia during laparoscopy and pelviscopy: how cold it gets and how to prevent it. J Am Assoc Gynecol Laparosc. 1999; 6(3): 289-95.

24. Guía De Práctica Clínica en Anestesiología y reanimacíon. Sociedad Española de Anestesiología, Reanimación y Terapia del Dolor. Rev Esp Anestesiol Reanim 1995; 42(6): 218-21.

25. Smetana GW. Preoperative pulmonary evaluation. N Engl J Med. 1999; 340: 937-40.

26. Eagle K, Brundage B, Chaitman B et al. Guidelines for preoperative cardiovascular evaluation of the non-cardiac surgery. A report of the American Heart Association / American College of Cardiology. Task Force on Assessment of Diagnostic and Therapeutic Cardiovascular Procedures. Circulation. 1996; 93: 1278-1317.

27. Sanders LM, Flint LM, Ferrara JJ. Initial experience with laparoscopic repair of incisional hernias. Am J Surg. 1999; 177: 227-31.

28. Shenkman Z, Shir Y, Brodsky JB. Perioperative management of the obese patient. Brit J Anaesth. 1993; 70 (3): 349-60.

29. Charlson ME, Mackenzie CR, Gold JP. Preoperative autonomic function abnormalities in patients with diabetes mellitus and patients with hypertension. J Am Coll Surg. 1994; 179: 1-10.

30. Latson TW, Ashmore TH, Reinhardt DJ et al. Autonomic reflex dysfunction in patients presenting for elective surgery is associated with hypotension after anaesthesia induction. Anesthesiology. 1994;80: 326-37.

31. Ziegler D, Dannehl K, Muhlen H, Spuler M, Gries FA. Prevalence of cardiovascular autonomic dysfunction assessed by spectral analysis, vector analysis, and standard tests of heart rate variation and blood pressure responses at various stages of diabetic neuropathy. Diabet Med. 1992; 9(9): 806-14.

32. Pannen F, Frangenheim H. "Surgical" laparoscopy: indications and value. Chirurg. 1975; 46(9): 405-10.

33. Bacher A, Andel H, Grabner V, Twrdy T, Zadrobilek E, Lackner F. Laparoscopic cholecystectomy as a suitable procedure for patients with cardiopulmonary risk factors?. Wien Klin Wochenschr. 1994; 106(4): 97-102.

34. Warner MA, Divertie MB, Tinker JH. Preoperative cessation of smoking and pulmonary complications in coronary artery bypass patients. Anesthesiology. 1984; 60: 380-3.

35. Coriat P, Ricker C, Douraki T et al. Influence of chronic angiotensin converting enzyme inhibition on anesthetic induction. Anesthesiology 1994; 81: 299-307.

36. Colson P, Ryckwaertf F, Coriat P. Renin angiotensin system antagonists and anesthesia. Anesth Analg. 1999. 89(5):1143-55.

37. 14: Lindberg F, Bergqvist D, Rasmussen I. Incidence of tromboembolic complications after laparoscopic cholecistectomy: review of the literature. Surg Laparosc Endosc. 1997; 7(4): 324-31

38. Catheline JM, Gaillard JL, Rizk N et al. Risk factors and prevention of thromboembolic risk in laparoscopy. Ann Chir. 1998; 52(9): 890-5

39. Baca I, Schneider B, Kohler T, Misselwitz F et al. Prevention of thromboembolism in minimally invasive interventions and brief inpatient treatment. Results of a multicenter, prospective, randomized, controlled study with a low molecular weight heparin. Chirurg. 1997; 68(12): 1275-80.

40. Lindberg F, Rasmussen I, Siegbahn A, Bergqvist D. Coagulation activation after laparoscopic cholecystectomy in spite of thromboembolism prophylaxis. Surg Endosc. 2000;14(9): 858-61.

41. Lippert H, Gastinger J. Antimicrobial prophylaxis in laparoscopic and conventional cholecystectomy. Conclusions of a large prospective multicenter quality assurance study in Germany. Chemotherapy 1998; 44(5): 355-63.

42. Tocchi A, Lepre L, Costa G et al. The need for antibiotic prophylaxis in elective laparoscopic cholecystectomy: a prospective randomized study. Arch Surg. 2000; 135(1): 67-70.

43. Higgins A, London J, Charland S et al. Prophylactic antibiotics for elective laparoscopic cholecystectomy: are they necessary?. Arch Surg. 1999; 134(6):611-3.

44. Soper NJ, Dunnegan D. Anatomic fundoplication failure after laparoscopic antireflux surgery. Ann Surg. 1999; 229(5): 669-76.

45. Baraka A, Jabbour-Khoury S, Karam V et al. Correlation of the end-tidal PCO_2 during laparoscopic surgery with the pH of the gastric juice. J Soc Laparoendosc Surg. 1998; 2(2):163-7.

46. Pursnani KG, Bazza Y, Calleja M, Mughal MM. Laparoscopic cholecystectomy under continuous epidural anesthesia in patients with chronic respiratory disease. Surg Endosc. 1998;12(8):1082-4.

47. Taylor E, Feinstein R, White PF, Sopor N. Anesthesia for laparoscopic cholecystectomy: is nitrous oxide contraindicated?. Anesthesiology. 1992; 76: 541-43.

48. Hall D, Goldstein A, Tynan E, Braunstein L. Profound hypercarbia late in the course of laparoscopic cholecystectomy: detection by continuous capnometry. Anesthesiology. 1993; 79(1): 173-4.

49. Rose DK, Cohen MM, Soutter DI. Laparoscopic cholecystectomy: the anaesthetist's point of view. Can J Anaesthesiol. 1992; 39: 809-15.

50. Feig BW, Berger DH, Dougherty TB et al. Pharmacologic intervention can reestablish baseline hemodynamic parameters during laparoscopy. Surgery. 1994; 116(4): 733-41.

51. Hein HA, Joshi GP, Ramsay MA et al. Hemodynamic changes during laparoscopic cholecystectomy in patients with severe cardiac disease. J Clin Anesth. 1997; 9(4): 261-5.

52. Mckinstry LJ, Perverseff RA, Yin RW. Arterial and end-tidal carbon dioxide in patients undergoing laparoscopic cholecistectomy. Anesthesiology. 1992; 77 A108.

53. Yamanaka MK, Sue DY. Comparison of arterial-end-tidal PCO_2 difference and dead space/tidal volume ratio in respiratory failure. Chest. 1987; 92(5):832-5.

54. Shea JA, Healey MJ, Berlin JA, Clarke JR, Malet PF, Staroscik RN, Schwartz JS, Willimas SV. Mortality and complications associated with laparoscopic cholecystectomy. A meta-analysis. Ann Surg. 1996; 224(5): 609-20.

55. Chung RS, Rowland DY, Li P, Diaz J. A meta-analysis of randomized controlled trials of laparoscopic versus conventional appendectomy. Am J Surg. 1999; 177(3): 250-6.

56. Scott DB, Julian DG. Observations on cardiac arrhythmias during laparoscopy. Br Med J. 1972; 1: 411-13.

57. Myles PS. Bradyarrhythmias and laparoscopy. A prospective study of heart rate changes during laparoscopy. Am J Obstet Gynecol. 1973; 31: 173-73.

58. Harris MNE, Plantevin OM, Crowther A. Cardiac arrhythmias during anaesthesia for laparoscopy. Br J Anaesth. 1984; 56: 1213-16.

59. Wahba RW, Tessler MJ, Kleiman SJ . Acute ventilatory complications during laparoscopic upper abdominal surgery. Can J Anaesth. 1996; 43(1): 77-83.

60. Joris JL, Chiche JD, Lamy ML. Pneumothorax during laparoscopic fundoplication: diagnosis and treatment with positive end-expiratory pressure. Anesth Analg. 1995; 81(5): 993-1000.

61. Chein GL, Soifer BE. Pharyngeal emphysema with airway obstruction as a consequence of laparoscopic inguinal herniorraphy. Anesth Anal. 1995; 80(1): 201-3.

62. Murdock CM, Wolff AJ, Van Geem T. Risk factors for hypercarbia, subcutaneous emphysema, pneumothorax, and pneumomediastinum during laparoscopy. Obstet Gynecol 2000; 95(5): 704-9.

63. Graff TD, Arbegast NR, Phillips OC et al. Gas embolism: a comparative study of air and carbon dioxide as embolic agents in the systemic venous system. Am J Obstet Gynecol. 1959; 78: 259-65.

64. Blaser A, Rosset P. Fatal carbon dioxide embolism as an unreported complication of retroperitoneoscopy. Surg Endosc. 1999; 13(7): 713-4.

65. Lantz PE, Smith JD. Fatal carbon dioxide embolism complicating attempted laparoscopic cholecystectomy-case report and literature review. J Forensic Sci. 1994; 39(6):1468-80.

66. Couture P, Boudreault D, Derouin M, et al. Venous carbon dioxide embolism in pigs: an evaluation of end-tidal carbon dioxide, transesophageal echocardiography, pulmonary artery pressure, and precordial auscultation as monitoring modalities. Anesth Analg. 1994; 79(5): 867-73.

67. Deziel DJ, Millikan KW, Economou SG, Doolas A, Ko ST, Airan MC Complications of laparoscopic cholecystectomy: a national survey of 4,292 hospitals and an analysis of 77,604 cases. Am J Surg. 1993; 165(1): 9-14.

68. Champault G, Cazacu F, Taffinder N. Serious trocar accidents in laparoscopic surgery: a French survey of 103,852 operations. Surg Laparosc Endosc. 1996; 6(5): 367-70.

69. Nordestgaard AG, Bodily KC, Osborne RW JR, Buttorff JD. Major vascular injuries during laparoscopic procedures. Am J Surg. 1995; 169(5): 543-5.

70. Crist DW, Gadacz TR. Complications of laparoscopic surgery. Surg Clin North Am. 1993; 73(2): 265-89.

CHAPTER 20

Trocar Placement and Access for Laparoscopic Ventral Hernia Repair

S. Morales-Conde, J.M. Pacheco, M. Bustos

INTRODUCTION

The laparoscopic approach to the abdominal cavity involves the use of various sizes of trocars through which instruments are introduced to perform surgical procedures for diagnostic and/or therapeutic purposes. Trocar placement and patient position are key factors in laparoscopic surgery, since the relative position determines the angle of vision and the access to the various structures, thereby affecting the ease and convenience with which the surgeon handles the procedure. Thus, the positioning of the trocars, both those used for visualization and as working channels, must be clearly described for proper laparoscopic repair of ventral hernias. There is no standard for patient and trocar positioning in laparoscopic repair of this type of hernia. Unlike other procedures, such as cholecystectomy –where the gall bladder is always in the same position–, this pathology involves several locations and sizes varying greatly in extension. Determining the optimum placement of the trocars depends on these factors and on the physical characteristics of the patient.

Before discussing trocar positioning, however, we should analyze how and where the pneumoperitoneum must be performed, as this is another key issue in this technique. Generally speaking we encounter previously operated patients who have had several incisions. The frequent presence of adhesions to the anterior wall of the abdomen in these patients increases the risk of lesion to the intestinal loops. This requires a comprehensive approach to the pneumoperitoneum and the insertion of the initial trocar.

ENTERING THE ABDOMEN: LAPAROSCOPIC ACCESS FOR VENTRAL HERNIA REPAIR

The unique characteristics of any analysis of how and where to create the pneumoperitoneum are determined by the existence of adhesions from previous operations. In fact, in our series of laparoscopic ventral hernia repair, 3.75% of hernias were primary while the rest were incisional hernias. This shows that previously operated patients have a tendency to adhesions, a fact that must be kept in mind. The adhesions are determined by previous incisions and the procedure used for the prior surgery, factors that must also be taken into account. This aspect is important, as it will allow us to avoid cases with a large number of adhesions where both adhesiolysis and access to the abdominal cavity are more complex. One case in our series required conversion precisely due to dense adhesions, in this case we had expected difficult access to the cavity even before starting surgery since the patient had been previously operated for tuberculous peritonitis. Creation of the pneumoperitoneum in this case was very difficult and conversion was subsequently required because of the presence of numerous, tightly attached adhesions.

The first question to be solved when performing the pneumoperitoneum concerns the incision site for insertion of the Hasson trocar or positioning of the Veress needle followed by the first trocar. Most authors agree (and we share their opinion) that the best place for initial access to the cavity is the left upper quadrant (Fig. 1). There is seldom intraabdominal pathology in this area and inflammatory processes are infrequent; hence it usually has few adhesions. In cases with incisions in the left upper quadrant or displacement of the hernia toward the patient's left hemiabdomen, we create the pneumoperitoneum in the right upper quadrant. For creation of the pneumoperitonium, some authors such as Park (1) have defended use of the Veress needle at the suprapubic level for supraumbilical incisional hernias in patients with no infraumbilical incisions. In this situation, our group still prefers access from the left upper quadrant, although somewhat farther toward the side. Park's access would involve placing a bladder catheter in these patients to prevent bladder lesions, a procedure we normally avoid in patients with hernias at this site.

The next point of discussion concerns how to access the cavity in order to create the pneumoperitoneum. Many lesions occurring in this procedure are due to blind placement of the initial trocar rather than to insertion of the Veress needle. Several methods are used to access the abdominal cavity in order to create the pneumoperitoneum and insert the initial trocar. There are three main access approaches:
- Open technique with Hasson trocar
- Veress needle with blind trocar insertion
- Veress needle with direct visualization of trocar insertion

The decision about which system to use depends on several factors, including the surgeon's usual technique in other laparoscopic procedures, his/her experience with each method and the specific characteristics of the patient and the hernia being repaired.

Open technique with Hasson trocar

The open technique with Hasson trocar is supported by many authors (1-6) as the safest technique since entry into the cavity is performed under direct vision. The method consists in making a mini-incision, sectioning the various layers under direct vision until arriving to the abdominal cavity, then opening the peritoneum, placing a Hasson trocar or sealing trocar, insufflating the cavity and creating the pneumoperitoneum.

The theoretical advantages of this method reside in its safety when creating the pneumoperitoneum and placing the initial trocar, since access to the cavity under direct vision reduces the risk of intestinal lesion. Intestinal loop lesions due to the use of this access method have, however, been described.

The use of this method also has several drawbacks which include the following:

- Difficult access in obese patients, since placement of the initial trocar is usually on the side of the abdomen with the greatest amount of fatty tissue. In an obese patient, placement of a Hasson trocar at the umbilical level poses fewer difficulties since there is less fat in this area and extensive dissection of the fat is not necessary. On the flanks, however, fatty tissue tends to be more abundant and a much larger incision than the initial trocar hole would be required. We should also keep in mind that obesity is one of the risk factors for the development of incisional hernias, hence the population of patients operated for this condition have a body mass index above the average for patients operated for other conditions. The body mass index in our serie of ventral hernias was above 30, an level indicative of excess weight.

- Gas leak at the Hanson site, since placement of this trocar involves performing an incision of larger diameter than the trocar. This often results in a sustained CO_2 leak, which can produce poor insufflation and difficult visualization throughout the process. In order to prevent these gas leaks, the use of balloon-tipped trocars to produce better sealing of the trocar opening and minimize pneumoperitoneum leaks from the cavity has been proposed.

- The need to select the initial trocar access site with the abdominal cavity desufflated; this may mean that the trocar site is not the most convenient site for the surgery once the cavity is insufflated, since the size and distance of the initial incision to the margin of the hernia defect may change once the abdominal cavity is insufflated.

Veress needle with blind trocar insertion

In this technique the pneumoperitoneum is created with use of Veress needle (figure 1) followed by blind trocar insertion. This method has been criticized since both accesses are blind, although the two systems (Veress needle and trocar) are equipped with safety shields. We have systematized the use of this procedure in all patients, regardless of the surgery being performed or the presence of previous incisions. In fact we have performed more than 4,000 laparoscopies with a Veress needle and blind trocar insertion without producing lesions and, therefore, feel comfortable using this approach. We have also employed this method of access in all ventral hernias treated by laparoscopic repair with no lesions; this has been the experience of several other authors (7, 8) who also use this approach.

The benefits of this method for accessing the abdominal cavity and creating the pneumoperitoneum include the fact that initial trocar insertion is performed with an insufflated abdominal cavity, which gives us a better idea of the area where the trocar must be inserted and where we can work most easily, thereby avoiding one of the disadvantages mentioned above as being associated with the Hasson trocar. Direct insertion of the initial trocar prevents problems of gas leakage and also provides more convenient access in obese patients.

Veress needle with direct optical trocar insertion

We could consider this system to be a method "half-way" between the two previous methods that combines the advantages of both systems and is, therefore, supported by several authors (9-10). The pneumoperitoneum is initially performed with the Veress needle, then an access zone is selected for the first trocar, which will be an optical trocar. This allows visualization as the trocar passes through the various layers of the abdominal wall, allowing access under direct vision and decreasing the risk of intestinal lesion. This access system minimizes the theoretical risk of lesion due to initial blind trocar insertion. It does not prevent potential lesions from the insertion of the Veress needle but does avoid the disadvantages of open access (e.g., leaks, access in obese patients and selection of the access site with desufflated abdomen).

One of the major drawbacks associated with this system is related to its cost since the system can only be used once, a factor that increases the total cost of the surgical procedure.

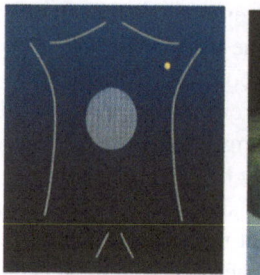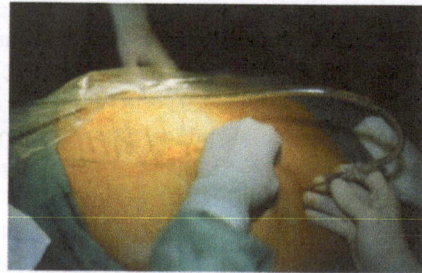

Fig. 1. Pneumoperitoneum being created using a Veress needle in the left upper quadrant of the patient.

TROCARS

As mentioned earlier, trocar placement during laparoscopic repair of ventral hernias depends basically on three factors: the defect site, the hernia size and the physical characteristics of the patient, although the diameter of the trocars to be used should be discussed first.

Trocar size

A variety of trocar sizes are commercially available including 2, 3, 5, 10, 11 and 12-mm trocars, with specific instruments for each trocar size and telescopes of 2, 3, 5 and 10 mm; the 5 and 10-mm are zero, thirty-degree and forty five-degree telescopes. A series of factors should be considered when choosing the trocars:

- A trocar of at least 10 mm is required for introducing a mesh. We prefer to introduce the mesh through a trocar since contamination of the mesh due to microorganisms on the wall can easily occur when attempting to introduce the mesh through the incision of the trocar once it is removed, maneuver supported by some authors (11) that allows three 5-mm trocars with a telescope of this caliber to be used. As a result, we select the trocar on the basis of the size of the expanded polytetrafluoroethylene mesh (PTFE-e; Gore-tex Dual-mesh corduroy plus with holes; WL Gore & Associates, Flagstaff, AZ, USA); the most frequently used sizes in this type of procedures are 10 x 15cm and 15 x 19cm, as well as others of larger size. We use a 10-mm trocar when expecting to use a 10 x 15cm mesh and an 11-mm trocar when expecting to use a 15 x 19cm mesh, since this last measure does not easily enter through the 10-mm trocar. For larger mesh sizes, we use a 10-mm trocar and insert the mesh through the incision of the trocar after it is removed, since larger meshes cannot be passed through any of the trocars. In these cases the mesh to be inserted is wrapped in plastic to prevent contamination from microorganisms on the wall; this plastic is subsequently removed from the abdominal cavity.

- We prefer to use 10-mm 30-degree telescopes which requires a trocar of at least 10 mm since the visualization available with 5-mm 30-degree telescopes is not as good, mainly due to the lack of light.

- A 5-mm trocar is used for introducing the tacks. Before this fixation system appeared, this step was performed using an endo-stapler with a diameter of 12 mm that required the use of 12-mm trocars.

Under these premises, we believe a 10 or 11-mm trocar (depending on mesh size) should be used for laparoscopic repair of ventral hernias, as they accommodate a 10-mm thirty-degree telescope and can be used to introduce the mesh. A 5-mm trocar should be used to introduce the tacks that attach the mesh and another trocar should be used as another working channel. This can be 3 or 5-mm, although we prefer 5-mm as it provides a different angle for placing the tackers. Some authors support the systematic use of three 10-mm (12) or 11-mm trocars (13) to change the position of the telescope and obtain different angles of vision during the adhesiolysis process and to position and fix the mesh.

Trocar placement

Our current series of ventral hernias by laparoscopic repair includes surgeries performed from November 1998, when we began to systematize the technique we presently use. In 1995 we made two attempts to repair two centroabdominal hernias. In addition to the difficulties encountered with the material (mesh and fixation system) available at the time, we placed the trocars in an position that required conversion in both cases since the technique was difficult and complicated. During this period we used four 10-mm trocars arranged in a square around the centroabdominal defect, as this had the theoretical advantage of allowing the surgeon to approach the defect from the four insertion points. Our current trocar placement system is based on three trocars in line on the patient's left flank (figure 2). The interrelation between hernia size and site allows us to establish the exact location of the trocars for each specific case, while still adhering to this premise. Most authors use this trocar layout, although several authors, such as LeBlanc (11), prefer to locate the scope at the midline whenever possible to prevent mirror imaging.

The first factor that must be taken into account when placing the trocars is that the initial trocar must be laterally as far away as possible from the defect, particularly in midline hernias. This will provide sufficient distance to obtain correct visualization of the defect margin closest to the trocar and the expected mesh fixation region, with the mesh extending at least 3cm overlaping the margins of the defect.

Trocar distribution and patient position on the operating table are as follows:
- Defects of the midline (Fig. 3) or in right abdomen (figure 4): supine decubitus position with three trocars in line in the left abdomen
- Defect in left abdomen (Fig. 5): supine decubitus with three trocars in line in the right abdomen
- Small subxiphoid defects (the defect size is assessed on the basis of the patient's physical characteristics) (Fig. 6): Working between the patient's legs with the patient in the gynecological position, one 10-mm trocar would be placed at the umbilical level and one 5-mm trocar on each side.
- Large subxiphoid defects (Fig. 7): supine decubitus with three trocars in the left flank, although the lowest trocar would be farther forward than the others (i.e., closer to the midline), tracing a straight line with the caudal margin toward the midline.
- Small suprapubic defects (the defect size is assessed on the basis of the patient's physical characteristics) (Fig. 8): one 10-mm trocar is placed at the umbilical level and one 5-mm trocar is placed on each side with the patient in supine decubitus.
- Large suprapubic defects (Fig. 9): in supine decubitus with three trocars in the left flank although the uppermost trocar would be farther forward than the others and closer to the midline.
- Lumbar defects (Fig. 10): the patient is placed in semi-lateral supine decubitus with the three trocars in line away from the defect, at a suitable distance to reach the most distal point with the instruments and to maneuver adequately at the hernia margin closest to the trocars.

In certain cases an additional trocar is necessary, usually to fix the mesh in the area closest to the scope, in these cases the angle needed to securely attach the mesh to the wall cannot be achieved when the trocars are arranged in a line. In these cases a 5-mm trocar is placed in the opposite hemiabdomen, or a 10-mm trocar if we also want to visualize the final appearance of the fixed, extended mesh from another angle. The visualization through this trocar is complex due to mirror imaging if we only have one monitor, but it is necessary for more secure mesh attachment.

Normally the monitor faces the surgeon and the assistant stands next to the surgeon in order to assist with the camera.

Naturally the characteristics described here varies somewhat, depending on the surgical team and its experience with other pathologies. However we have attempted to analyze the opinions and conclusions we have reached regarding the most suitable procedure for laparoscopic repair of ventral hernias.

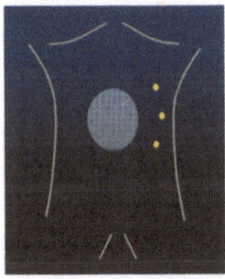 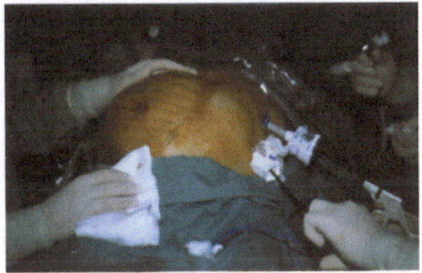

Fig. 2. Trocar placed on the patient's left flank.

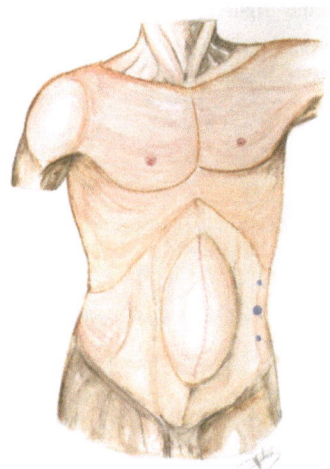

Fig. 3. Defects of the midline: patientes should be placed in supine decubitus position with three trocars in line in the left abdomen.

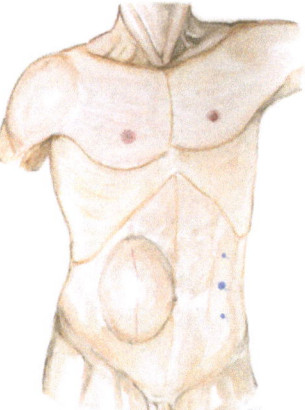

Fig. 4. Defects in right abdomen: patientes should be placed in supine decubitus position with three trocars in line in the left abdomen.

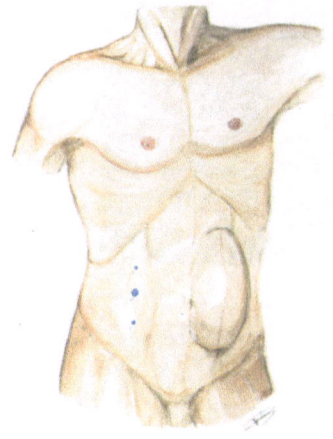

Fig. 5. Defect in left abdomen: patientes should be placed in supine decubitus with three trocars in line in the right abdomen.

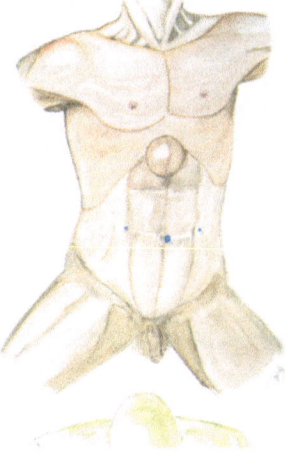

Fig. 6. Small subxiphoid defects: working between the patient's legs with the patient in the gynecological position, one 10-mm trocar would be placed at the umbilical level and one 5-mm trocar on each side.

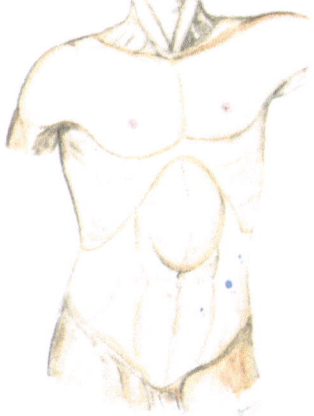

Fig. 7. Large subxiphoid defects: patientes in supine decubitus with three trocars in the left flank, although the lowest trocar would be farther forward than the others, closer to the midline.

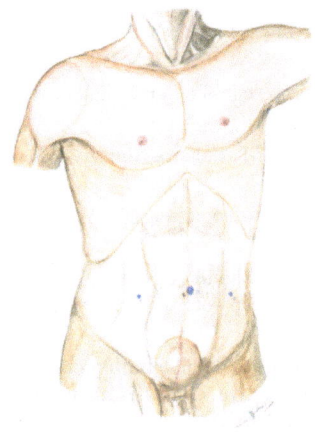

Fig. 8. Small suprapubic defects: one 10-mm trocar is placed at the umbilical level and one 5-mm trocar is placed on each side with the patient in supine decubitus.

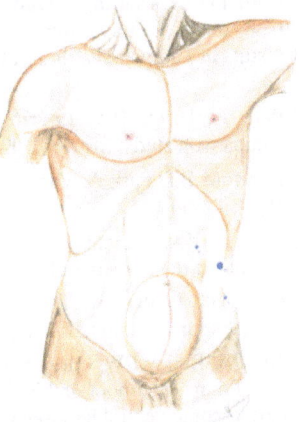

Fig. 9. Large suprapubic defects: in supine decubitus with three trocars in the left flank, although the uppermost trocar would be farther forward than the others and closer to the midline.

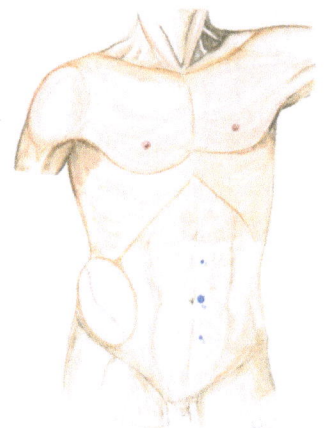

Fig. 10. Lumbar defects: the patient is placed in semi-lateral supine decubitus with the three trocars in line away from the defect.

References

1. Park A, Gagner M, Pomp A. Laparoscopic repair of large incisional hernias. Surg Laparosc Endosc 1996; 6(2):123-128.

2. Heniford BT, Park A, Ramshaw BJ, Voeller G. Laparoscopic ventral and incisional hernia repair in 407 patients. J Am Coll Surg 2000; 190(6):645-650.

3. Costanza MJ, Heniford BT, Arca MJ, Mayes JT, Gagner M. Laparoscopic repair of recurrent ventral hernias. Am Surg 1998; 64(12):1121-1127.

4. Sanders LM, Flint LM, Ferrara JJ. Initial experience with laparoscopic repair of incisional hernias. Am J Surg 1999; 177:227-231.

5. Koehler RH, Voeller G. Recurrences in laparoscopic incisional hernia repairs: a personal series and review of the literature. Journal of the Society of Laparoendoscopic Surgeons 1999; 3:293-304.

6. DeMaria EJ, Moss JM, Sugerman HJ. Laparoscopic intraperitoneal polytetrafluorethylene (PTFE) prosthetic patch repair of ventral hernia. Prospective comparison to open prefascial polypropylene mesh repair. Surg Endosc 2000; 14:326-329.

7. Kyzer S, Alis M, Aloni Y, Charuzi I. Laparoscopic repair of postoperation ventral hernia. Surg Endosc 1999; 13:928-931.

8. Carbajo MA, Martín del Olmo JC, Blanco JI, de la Cuesta C, Martín F, Toledano M, Perna C, Vaquero C. Laparoscopic treatment of ventral abdominal wall hernias: preliminary results in 100 patients. Journal of the Society of Laparoendoscopic Surgeons 2000; 4:141-145.

9. Park A, Birch DW, Lovrics P. Laparoscopic and open incisional hernia repair: a comparison study. Surgery 1998; 124(4):816-822.

10. Heniford BT, Park A, Voeller G. Laparoscopic ventral hernia repair. Surgical prospectus 1999; 1:1-11.

11. LeBlanc KA. Current considerations in laparoscopic incisional and ventral herniorrhaphy. Journal of the Society of Laparoendoscopic Surgeons 2000; 4(2):131-139.

12. Ritter DR, Paulsen JK, Debord JR, Estes NC. Five-year experience with the "four-before" laparoscopic ventral hernia repair. Am Surg 2000; 66(5):465-469.

13. Toy FK, Bailey RW, Carey S, Chappuis CW, Gagner M, Josephs LG, Mangiante EC, Park AE, Pomp A, Smoot Jr RT, Uddo Jr JF, Voeller GR. Prospective, multicenter study of laparoscopic ventral hernioplasty. Preliminary results. Surg Endosc 1998; 12: 955-959.

CHAPTER 21

Laparoscopic Adhesiolysis

S. Morales-Conde, I. Poves, C. Ballesta

INTRODUCTION

One of the problems associated with laparoscopic repair of ventral hernias is the need to perform proper release of adhesions in order to adequately identify the hernia defect and repair it by placing a mesh intraperitoneally. This adhesiolysis process is a major issue as it is sometimes the source of serious complications for the patient. Included among these is the appearance of missed perforations of the intestinal wall during the postoperative period, a potentially life-threatening situation (1). This complication will require another operation to suture the perforation or performance of an ostomy. Additionally the mesh implanted will have to be removed, increasing the possibility of recurrence of the original hernia. Hence the importance of this chapter, since we consider adhesiolysis to be a key component of laparoscopic ventral hernia surgery. Because of the potentially disastrous consequences for the patient, it is important to discuss the proper performance of the adhesiolysis process and to take into consideration the necessary precautions and management of possible complications that may arise.

CURRENT STATUS: POSTOPERATIVE ADHESIONS

Postoperative adhesions occur when scar tissue joins two structures or organs. This event, which may occur in all body tissues handled surgically, is particularly important after intra-abdominal surgery since the adhesions typically involve the intestinal bowel. Estimates have indicated that up to 93% of patients who have undergone abdominal surgery develop adhesions (2). In most cases they do not have clinical consequences; however on occasion they do produce symptoms. Thirty-five per cent of patients who undergo abdominal and/or pelvic surgical procedures must be readmitted at some time for problems resulting from adhesions (3).

Postoperative adhesions after abdominal surgery generally present in two forms: as frank episodes of occlusive crises of abdominal pain or as intercurrent episodes of chronic abdominal pain. Although it cannot be considered a clinical manifestation of adhesion syndrome, up to 20% of cases of infertility are reported to be the result of postoperative adhesions (4). Adhesions can present in various forms, ranging from single strips to multiple adhesions. They may develop between several intestinal loops, between intestinal loops and solid organs, or between the abdominal wall and the intestine. Some authors believe that surgical examination of the abdominal cavity is indicated in patients with chronic abdominal pain and a history of prior abdominal and/or inguinal surgery, once neoplastic disease has been ruled out. By this method, adhesion syndrome is identified as the organic cause of the pain in more than 60% of cases, and the clinical condition will improve with adhesiolysis (5).

Adhesion syndrome is considered to be a major postoperative complication and is the leading cause of intestinal occlusion in patients operated on in developed countries (6). It is a serious social and health problem with a significant financial cost. Postoperative adhesions account for 1% of all hospital admissions and 3.3% of all laparotomies (7). In 1994 a total of 303,836 adhesiolysis procedures were performed in the United States, accounting for an expenditure of 1.3 billion dollars (8). It has been postulated that the use of laparoscopic techniques will lead to decreased hospital admissions for intestinal occlusion and fewer surgeries for chronic abdominal pain in the future. However, this assertion has not yet been verified and it is suggested that other, more important mechanisms are involved in adhesion formation (8).

In the early years of laparoscopy, prior abdominal surgery was thought to be an incontrovertible contraindication for laparoscopic abdominal surgery. These criteria have changed over time and it is now considered a relative contraindication only in certain cases. The advances in the technique are so significant that laparoscopy is even considered the approach of choice for adhesiolysis. In cases of elective surgery, the laparoscopic approach can be used successfully in up to 80% of patients, whereas in emergency surgery this decreases to 59% (6). The conversion rate to laparotomy in this type of surgery is between 5.4% and 16%, depending on the group (2, 6). The conversion rates are higher in the case of emergency surgery versus elective surgery, being 36% and 7%, respectively. At present laparoscopic adhesiolysis can be considered a safe, effective technique in patients who must undergo elective or emergency surgery for adhesion syndrome (2). We believe that any patient can benefit from the laparoscopic approach for adhesiolysis. It is suitable in surgery for any condition in which adhesiolysis is necessary to perform the specific procedure, in chronic abdominal pain directly related to the adhesions, or in laparoscopic repair of an incisional hernia accompanied by the presence of numerous adhesions, which is the subject addressed in this chapter.

PREOPERATIVE ASSESSMENT OF ADHESIONS

Factors associated with the presence of adhesions

When considering laparoscopic repair of a ventral hernia, it is difficult to determine how many adhesions may be present in the abdominal cavity before the actual operation. Therefore, surgical indications cannot be established on the basis of the number and type of adhesions that are expected within the abdominal cavity. For groups that are beginning with this surgical technique, however, there are some indirect data that can indicate the presence of a larger than usual number of adhesions, which may make adhesiolysis more difficult. A medical history of one or more of the following is often associated with a large number of adhesions (Table I):

- Type of process for which the previous surgery was performed: in diffuse peritonitic abdominal processes, particularly those with purulent material, the formation of adhesions is more frequent because the inflammatory process occurs in both the parietal and visceral peritonea (9). Adhesions are stronger and more frequent in patients who have had surgery for tuberculous peritonitis. In fact, the only case we had to convert in our series involved a young patient who developed an incisional hernia after emergency surgery through a supra-infraumbilical midline laparotomy for acute abdomen that turned out to be of tuberculous origin.

- Type of surgery: surgery involving extensive dissection of tissues, considerable manipulation of intestinal loops and the need for abundant irrigation of the cavity with irritating substances such as betadine can lead to larger numbers of adhesions.

- Type of incision during the previous surgery: surgery carried out through an infraumbilical midline laparotomy is associated with a greater number of adhesions (10).

- Evolution of previous surgery: complications of previous surgery at both the intra-abdominal and the abdominal wall level are also associated with an increased number of adhesions.
  • Intra-abdominal complications: several complications can be associated with the development of numerous adhesions; these include:
  • intra-abdominal abscess, in which resolution was either spontaneous with conservative treatment or by percutaneous drainage;
  • intestinal fistula, with stronger adhesions in the area where the fistula occurred due to the surrounding inflammatory response, particularly the firm adhesion formed between the intestinal loop where the fistula originated and the abdominal wall.
  • the need for another operation in the immediate postoperative period, regardless of the cause.
  • Complications related to the abdominal wall:
  • deep infection of the abdominal wall leads to the appearance of a greater number of adhesions, and this is also one of the predisposing factors for the development of an incisional hernia. Thus, in a high percentage of cases what we find is a combination of incisional hernias and previous wall infections, a situation in which there is a much higher probability that adhesions will be present.
  • evisceration, both well-contained evisceration and evisceration that requires surgical repair during the immediate postoperative period, are also associated with an increased number of adhesions.

- Type of previous repair in the case of recurrent hernias: Our experience has shown that patients with recurrent ventral hernia in which the previous repair consisted of conventional open surgery with placement of a polypropylene mesh have a larger number of associated adhesions (9). Moreover, in these patients the adhesions produce intestinal fistulas (11-15) that are more severe than those found in patients in whom the previous repair was performed by simple suture or using a PTFE-e mesh. In large series with long-term follow-up of this latter technique, there were no complications related to the formation of intestinal fistulas or occlusive adhesions (16). In these cases, an increased number and strength of the adhesions was observed despite the fact that the polypropylene mesh was not placed in an intraperitoneal position and was always covered by the peritoneum, at the minimum.

- Inherent properties of the hernia being repaired:
  • Ethiology of the hernia: incisional hernias are associated with a larger number of adhesions that are more difficult dissected than those occurring in primary hernias.
  • Hernia site: those found in the upper abdomen usually present omental adhesions, which are more conducive to dissection and less dangerous than adhesions associated with hernias of the lower abdomen. In this region adhesions of the small intestine are more frequent and they require greater precaution in dissection .
  • Incarcerated hernias: chronically incarcerated hernias can also present associated adhesions that are harder to dissect. Once the incarcerated content is reduced, there are often adhesions within the sac that tend to be very prominent and can hinder visualization of the proper area for dissection.

Table I. Procedures usually associated with the presence of a larger number of adhesions.

1.- Process causing the previous surgery
Diffuse peritoneal abdominal processes
2.- Type of surgery
Significant dissection of tissues
Extensive manipulation of intestinal loops
Irrigation of cavity with irritating substances
3.- Type of previous incision
Midline infraumbilical laparotomy
4.- Evolution of the previous surgery
Intra-abdominal complications
Intra-abdominal abscess
Intestinal fistula
Re-operation
Wall complications
Deep infection
Evisceration
5.- Type of previous repair in hernia recurrence
Use of polypropylene mesh
6.- Inherent properties of the hernia being repaired
Ethiology of the hernia: incisional rather than primary
Hernia site: infraumbilical rather than supraumbilical
Incarcerated hernias

Detection of adhesions during the preoperative period

Even though there is some possibility of predicting the presence and type of adhesions based on the factors described, it is quite difficult to identify the cases with the largest number of adhesions and, therefore, the ones involving the greatest difficulty for the surgeon. In fact, our predictions have failed on many occasions. Cases expected to be simple can be associated with processes involving dense adhesions that might even require conversion to open surgery. The opposite situation can also occur, that is, one in which the need for extensive adhesiolysis is expected but the abdomen actually shows almost no adhesions. One of the problems resulting from the difficulty in predicting the number and type of adhesions is the inability to properly anticipate the time required for surgery in order to conform with operating room availability and to plan its use for the other surgeries. Based on the foregoing, the need to identify the difficulty associated with the surgery according to the number and the type of adhesions has led several authors to attempt to predict the presence of adhesions on the basis of results from different imaging techniques.

Various imaging techniques have been studied in this context in an attempt to identify intra-abdominal adhesions prior to the surgery. In fact, an attempt has been made to create an imaging map of the abdominal cavity before performing laparoscopic procedures other than ventral hernia repair in patients who have previously undergone open surgery, in order to detect adhesion-free areas and thereby minimize the risk of lesions with the Veress needle used to create the pneumoperitoneum or with the insertion of the initial trocar. In published studies sonography has shown a diagnostic accuracy of 88.5% with a specificity of 31.8% to 90% and a sensitivity of 90% to 100% in the detection of adhesions during the preoperative period in patients who will undergo laparoscopic surgery (17,18). Magnetic resonance (19) has also been used to create a map of intraperitoneal adhesions during the preoperative period in patients scheduled for laparoscopic surgery, showing a sensitivity of 87.5% and a specificity of 92.5%.

MANAGEMENT OF ADHESIONS

Creation of pneumoperitoneum and introduction of trocars

Due to the presence of adhesions in the abdominal cavity, surgeons recognize that there is a risk of intra-abdominal lesion when creating the pneumoperitoneum or introducing the initial "blind" trocar. This has led some authors to recommend open laparoscopy using a Hasson trocar in patients with previous surgeries who will undergo laparoscopy, e.g., patients who are being considered for repair of a ventral hernia by this approach (20). We, however, are not of this opinion. We systematically use the Veress needle to create the pneumoperitoneum in these patients and there has been no case of intra-abdominal lesion in our series due to the Veress needle or the introduction of the first trocar.

In addition, a high number of patients presenting ventral hernias are obese, this factor being associated with the appearance of incisional hernias and with their recurrence (21). In these patients, performing an incision on the side of the abdomen (where trocars for laparoscopic repair of this type of hernia are normally inserted) in order to place a Hasson trocar often involves performing a minilaparotomy, since the panniculus adiposus is generally thicker at the sides than at the midline. This larger incision can result in pneumoperitoneum leaks and other complications such as infections, incisional hernias, etc.

We generally use the Veress needle to create the pneumoperitoneum in all cases. The needle is usually inserted in the left hypochondrium since this is the area of the abdomen where we are likely to find fewer adhesions because of the lower frequency of inflammatory processes at this level.

Once the pneumoperitoneum has been created, we usually place the initial trocar in the patient's side (normally, the left abdomen) away from the proximal border of the hernia in this area. Use of a Visiport or Optiview would be indicated in these cases, since they provide good visualization while the initial trocar is introduced, thereby reducing possible lesions (22). Perforations are often associated with blind insertion of the initial trocar rather than with the Veress needle itself.

Once the trocar and the scope are inserted, we may encounter the first problems related to the presence of adhesions:

- On the one hand, we might find that the entire greater omentum has adhered to the anterior wall of the abdomen, as if it were a part of it. The loops of the small intestine would be seen below and the greater omentum in the upper position, through which the trocar was inserted. In order to solve the problem in this case, the trocar is withdrawn under direct vision until the area between the peritoneum and the greater omentum is reached. We then attempt to insert the trocar and the telescope into this plane and thereby perform blunt dissection with the tip of the laparoscope. If this is not possible, we remove the trocar, and introduce a finger in the hole in order to locate this area and then perform blunt dissection. Once the greater omentum is dissected and the pneumoperitoneum properly created, the surface of the omentum is checked for bleeding before inserting the remaining trocars.

- On the other hand, we may encounter dense adhesions that must be released to obtain the space needed to introduce the remaining trocars. The first step will be to perform blunt dissection of the adhesions with the tip of the scope, aided by pressure exerted from the outside. If this is not possible, a 5-mm trocar should be placed in the adhesion-free existing space (even though this is not the site where we originally intended to place the second trocar) in order to perform adhesiolysis with scissors on the area where the remaining trocars are to be placed.

Adhesiolysis process

As mentioned earlier, we believe that this is the most important process of laparoscopic repair of ventral hernias, due to the enormous consequences associated with complications resulting from incorrect adhesiolysis. Adhesiolysis complications are not only associated with laparoscopic surgery. Cases of intestinal perforation have also been reported after open surgery, with consequences similar to those occurring after laparoscopic surgery (23). In fact, in studies comparing laparoscopic and open surgery for the treatment of ventral hernias, higher rates of intestinal perforation due to adhesiolysis were reported in the open surgery group than in the laparoscopic group (15, 24).

The first controversial point concerns the extent of adhesiolysis. At present, it appears evident that when undertaking laparoscopic repair of an incisional hernia, adhesiolysis must cover the entire area of the previous incision in order to identify possible wall defects at this level, other than those originally destined to be repaired. This is precisely one of the advantages of laparoscopy over traditional open repair. Defects that were not identified during the clinical examination and that were the cause of recurrence or appearance of a new defect after open repair, can be detected and repaired in the same surgical procedure(25).

At the start of our series, we thought that the ultrasonic scalpel would be helpful when performing adhesiolysis since it would avoid possible complications derived from the use of electrocoagulation. These include the transmission of energy to the surrounding structures, with resulting intestinal lesions or the production of necrotic tissue that could become detached after the operation and produce a peritonitis requiring another operation in the immediate postoperative period. Our expectations regarding this instrument lessened with experience. The adhesiolysis process often requires fine dissection with the tip of the scissors in order to properly identify the dissection plane, and the tip of the ultrasonic scalpel is much too blunt for this purpose. In our experience, therefore, use of this instrument is relegated to cases with intense omental adhesions. One should ensure that there are no intestinal loops behind the greater omentum during dissection, since the temperature occasionally attained by the vibratory blade (although less than the traditional electroscalpel) could damage their walls.

As we acquired experience (26) in laparoscopic repair of ventral hernias, we encountered many kinds of adhesions (Table II). Depending on the type of adhesions and the circumstances encountered, the following factors should be taken into consideration :

1. Adhesions of small intestine and colon: when performing adhesiolysis of the intestinal loops one should remember that:
- The loops adhering to the wall tend to experience episodes of dilation, which in some cases is due to pseudo-occlusive conditions. One must assume that the walls of these loops experience periods of stress that weaken them; hence they should be handled with extreme care.
- It is sometimes hard to distinguish between the walls of the intestinal loops and the tissue that forms the hernia sac, and it may be difficult to determine whether or not an intestinal loop has been perforated. Naturally, if there is any doubt, the procedure should be converted or a small laparotomy should be performed by lengthening one of the trocar holes in order to ensure that none of the loops have been injured.

With these considerations in mind, adhesiolysis of the intestinal loops should be performed as follows:
- Use non-traumatic surgical instruments for manipulation of the intestinal loops

- Avoid traction, performing it gently only when strictly necessary
- Avoid excessive force in the case of blunt dissection
- Handle the intestinal loop from different angles in order to mobilize it from the best side
- Visualize the dissection plane adequately, particularly in the case of adhesions within the hernia sacs, by exposing the adhesions with external pressure and lateral views with the 30-degree telescope
- Maintain close, clear, clean vision of the dissection plane
- Adequately present the right dissection plane by means of external pressure, for better control and greater solidity of the cutting plane
- Use fine dissection with the scissors, properly identifying the plane between the loop and the wall
- Use the scissors with the curved part toward the abdominal wall in order to adequately control the section.
- Dissect the peritoneum with the loop whenever there are very firm adhesions due to severe scar entrapment
- Try to avoid coagulation between the loop and the wall during fine dissection, since the loop could be injured or necrotic material could remain. Later, once the loop wall is at a distance, the abdominal wall can be coagulated if necessary
- At the end of the procedure, thoroughly examine the intestinal loops affected by dissection and the parietal dissection to detect possible lesions

2. Greater omentum adhesions: in these cases we perform adhesiolysis with the assistance of traction, blunt dissection and the use of the energy we deem appropriate, electrocoagulation or ultrasonic energy. The following precautions, however, should be taken into account:
- The most important aspect to consider when dissecting adhesions of the greater omentum is to ensure at all times that there are no intestinal loops behind the dissection plane that could be injured. The dissection must be performed carefully, always maintaining close surveillance by lateral traction of the greater omentum and lateral views with the 30-degree telescope, to ensure that there are no loops behind the dissection plane.
- In obese patients, the existence of thick mesenteries can mask the presence of the transverse colon since they may be confused with the greater omentum. Thus, lesions can be inadvertently produced to both the colon wall and the mesocolon with the resulting compromise of vascularization in these structures.
- The most frequent complication associated with adhesiolysis of the greater omentum is bleeding; hence hemostasis should be checked constantly along the way, using the various available tools: electrocoagulation, ultrasonic energy, clips, endoloops or sutures.

3. Adhesions to solid organs: sometimes adhesions to solid organs are encountered, particularly to the liver. When performing adhesiolysis, we must try not to break Glisson's capsule since we would enter the liver parenchyma, causing active oozing of blood. Therefore, as in the case of firm intestinal adhesions due to severe scar entrapment, the peritoneum must be sectioned with the liver capsule to prevent

bleeding. Absorbable hemostatic materials are very useful for inhibiting bleeding of the liver parenchyma when it cannot be achieved with simple electrocoagulation.

Regardless of the circumstances mentioned above, one of the difficulties we may encounter when starting adhesiolysis is the presence of a hernia with incarcerated content that is not reduced after creating the pneumoperitoneum. If the content is greater omentum, traction on the omentum from inside and pressure from the outside, together with sectioning of the fibrous bands joining the greater omentum to the margin of the hernia defect, is usually sufficient to reduce the omentum from the sac without difficulty. If, however, the content consists of intestinal loops, we should not perform excessive traction or press too much from the outside, since perforation of the bowel could occur. In these cases, what we do is move about one or two centimeters away from the margin of the defect and section the wall toward the sac margin at that level, in order to open the sac and release the bowel from the ring of the defect that held them inside the sac and then continue with the adhesiolysis process. In addition, in these cases (which usually present a large sac), once the incarcerated content is reduced, adhesiolysis tends to be more difficult since hard-to-visualize adhesions are often present within the sac, making it necessary to exert constant pressure from the outside to adequately expose the dissection plane. Moreover, care must be taken with the use of electrocoagulation since the sac wall and the skin tend to be very thin in this area and a skin burn is possible.

Table II. Type of adhesions found in the first 91 cases of our series *(S. Morales-Conde, M. Martín, S. Morales-Méndez)* (26) who underwent laparoscopic repair of primary and incisional hernias

TYPE OF ADHESIONS	
Omentum	44
Small bowel (SB)	4
SB + omentum	28
Colon	1
Colon + omentum	2
Colon + omentum + liver	1
Liver + omentum	1
None	10

COMPLICATIONS OF ADHESIOLYSIS

Intraoperative complications of adhesiolysis

Intestinal perforation

As is true with lesions of the main biliary tract during laparoscopic cholecystectomy, the importance of this complication lies in its intraoperative detection, due to the fatal consequences it may have in the postoperative period if it is missed, being necessary a reoperation that involves a major risk of sepsis that may be life-threatening (1). All intestinal loops implicated in the adhesiolysis process must be meticulously examined before continuing the procedure and introducing the mesh. If there is any suspicion of perforation, the indication is conversion to open surgery or performance of a minilaparotomy by lengthening one of the trocar holes to check the loop and then continue by laparoscopy to repair the hernia.

Once the adhesiolysis is completed the loops that were adhered to the wall are carefully checked. If we found a tear of the serosa of the bowel, we must ensure that there are no leaks and assess the need for suturing. This can be done by laparoscopy. If a perforation is detected, its extension should be determined, since a puncture or small perforation can be sutured by laparoscopy. As described earlier, when the perforation is larger, we usually perform a minilaparotomy at the site used for the largest trocar in order to repair the loop. Then we continue by laparoscopy after closing the minilaparotomy.

When intestinal perforation occurs, a decision must be made as to whether or not to place an intraperitoneal mesh, in light of the potential contamination of the cavity as a consequence of the bowel injury. In our experience, we believe that each case must be assessed individually. Nevertheless, the usual fasting period of 8-12 hours required before surgery under general anesthesia is enough for the loops of the small intestine to be empty of significant intestinal content that could spill into the cavity in the case of perforation. Thus, contamination of the cavity would be minimal, with mesh placement being possible inside the abdomen, in contrast to the recommendations of some authors for open surgery (23). If there is significant intestinal content inside the small intestine or the colon opening, hernia repair during a second procedure should be considered. Surgery would be concluded once the perforation was repaired and the cavity cleaned.

Bleeding

This usually occurs after dissection of greater omentum adhesions and is stopped in most cases with simple electrocoagulation. Sometimes the use of clips or endoloops is also necessary. In the case of hepatic parenchyma bleeding due to rupture of Glisson's capsule, electrocoagulation should be attempted, as explained earlier. If bleeding continues, placement of a absorbable hemostatic materials will generally control it.

Wall bleeding after completing adhesiolysis is usually stopped with simple electrocoagulation. Adequate hemostasis is extremely important since it helps to decrease the size of possible seromas and the creation of hematomas which, if they grow and create significant tension, could displace the mesh. We usually perform coagulation of the wall of the entire area of adhesiolysis in order to coagulate small foci of bleeding and thereby, help to minimize the appearance of seromas.

Conversion

Conversion is another of the complications of adhesiolysis. Open surgery may be required when there are numerous adhesions, when adhesions are so tightly attached to the abdominal wall that intense scar sectioning would make progress impossible or when the risk of injuring the intestinal loop is extremely high. On the other hand, conversion may be needed because of one of the complications described above, e.g., perforation or uncontrollable bleeding during the adhesiolysis process that requires repair by open surgery.

Postoperative complications of adhesiolysis

Intestinal perforation

This has been reported as one of the most serious complications of this type of surgery (9) and it should be taken into account, although it is not unique to the laparoscopic approach since it has also been reported after open surgery (27). If a patient who has undergone laparoscopic repair of a ventral hernia develops fever and abdominal pain with signs of a peritonitis, missed perforation of the bowel should be immediately suspected. Early detection is key to preventing a life-threatening septic condition. For this reason, if there is any suspicion of this condition, the patient should be operated on again by open surgery. In the event that the diagnosis is unclear because of the clinical and analytical condition of the patient or the imaging findings, laparoscopy should be performed followed by laparotomy if confirmed, since abundant irrigation and suction of the cavity plus resection of the affected segment will be necessary. Depending on the intra-abdominal situation, an ostomy or primary anastomosis should be performed and the prothesis should be removed, since it has been exposed to a septic environment. The abdominal wall can then be closed by simple suturing without the use of prosthetic materials.

Bleeding

Although it has been also described as a complication of adhesiolysis (28), bleeding is a rather infrequent fact after this type of surgery. However, it may require the performance of another laparoscopic, or open, procedure to suck blood from the cavity and to identify and inhibit the focus of bleeding. The mesh does not need to be removed in the cases performed by laparoscopy but in cases of performing an open procedure should be considered in each individual case.

Complications associated with adhesiolysis in our series

Complications associated with the presence of adhesions during other laparoscopic procedures (data from the C. Ballesta and I. Poves series)

The results of 225 patients operated on by laparoscopy between January 1992 and June 1997 who had previously undergone some kind of open surgery (28% supramesocolic and 72% inframesocolic) are presented. The surgeries carried out were 164 cholecystectomies, 45 anti-reflux procedures, 4 partial gastrectomies, 4 adhesiolysis procedures, 3 cholecystectomies with choledochotomy, 2 gastroenteroanastomoses, 2 left colectomies and 1 colotomy with polypectomy. A 0-degree telescope was used in all cases.

Although adhesiolysis as such was only carried out in four cases, all these surgeries were undertaken after performing extensive release of adhesions (to one degree or another), and the adhesions were one of the main reasons for conversion to laparotomy. The conversion rate to laparotomy in our series was 1.3%. Three patients were converted, one because it was impossible to continue due to dense adhesions and another two due to uncontrollable bleeding (Table III).

Complications associated with the presence of adhesions during laparoscopic repair of ventral hernias (data from S. Morales-Conde, M. Martín-Gómez and S. Morales-Méndez series)

Between November 1998 and November 2001, 91 laparoscopic ventral hernia repairs were performed in 88 patients, specifically five cases for primary hernias (three umbilical and two epigastric) and 86 incisional hernias (two after laparoscopy and 84 after laparotomy or recurrence of primary hernias) (26).

There were three intraoperative complications (3.3%) resulting directly from the adhesiolysis: one conversion (1.1%) in a young patient previously operated on for acute abdomen of tuberculous origin in whom dense intra-abdominal adhesions make necessary to convert to open surgery to complete the process of adhesiolysis; and two intestinal perforations (3.3%), one of them sutured by laparoscopic approach and the other two requiring a minilaparotomy in which one of the trocar holes was lengthened to perform resection and anastomosis in order to continue with the hernia repair by laparoscopy .

In terms of postoperative complications, our series had only one case (1.1%) directly related to the adhesiolysis process. This case corresponded to a missed perforation that produced acute peritonitis during the immediate postoperative period requiring reoperation and resection and anastomosis of the bowel along with abundant irrigation of the cavity and removal of the mesh that had been in a septic environment (Table III).

Table III. Intraoperative and postoperative complications related to adhesiolysis in our series

	Series 1* *(225 cases)* *(C Ballesta, I Poves)*	*Series 2** (91 cases)* *(S Morales-Conde, M Martín,* *S Morales-Méndez)*
INTRAOPERATIVE COMPLICATIONS	*5 (2.22%)*	*4 (4.4%)*
Conversion	3 (1.33%)	1 (1.1%)
Intestinal perforation	-	3 (3.3%)
Bleeding	2 (0.88%)	-
POSTOPERATIVE COMPLICATIONS	*0*	*1 (1.1%)*
Intestinal perforation	-	1 (1.1%)
Bleeding	-	-

* Series 1.- 225 laparoscopic procedures in patients with previous laparotomies
** Series 2.- 91 ventral hernias repaired by laparoscopy (S Morales-Conde, M Martín, S Morales-Méndez) (26)

References

1. Koehler RH, Voeller G. Recurrences in laparoscopic incisional hernia repairs: A personal series and review of the literature. JSLS 1999; 3: 293-304.
2. Schenk C, Scheuerecker H, Glaser F. Laparoscopic adhesiolysis: results following prospective surveillance. Chirurg 2000; 71 (1): 66-71.

3. Ellis H, Moran DJ, Thompson JN et al. Adhesion – related hospital readmissions after abdominal and pelvic surgery: a retrospective cohort study. Lancet 1999; 353: 1476.

4. Holmdahl L, Risberg B, Beck D et al. Adhesions: pathogenesis and prevention – panel discussion and summary. Eur J Surg 1997; Suppl 577: 56-62.

5. Lavonius M, Gullichsen R, Laine S, Ovaska J. Laparoscopy for chronic abdominal pain. Surg Laparosc Endosc 1999; 9 (1): 42-44.

6. Chosidow D, Johanet H, Montariol T, Kielt R, Manceau C, Marmuse JP, Benhamou G. Laparoscopy for acute small bowel obstruction secondary to adhesions. J Laparoendosc Adv Surg Tech A 2000; 10 (3): 155-159.

7. Menzies D, Ellis H. Intestinal obstruction from adhesions – how big is the problem? Ann R Coll Surg Engl 1990; 72: 60-63.

8. Ray NF, Denton WG, Thamer M, Henderson SC, Perry S. Abdominal adhesiolysis: inpatient care and expenditures in the United States in 1994. J Am Coll Surg 1998; 186 (1): 1-9.

9. Kyzer S, Alis M, Alón Y, Charuzi I. Laparoscopic repair of postoperation ventral hernia. Surg Endosc 1999; 13:928-931.

10. Ray NF, Denton WG, Thamer M, Henderson SC, Perry S. Abdominal adhesiolysis: inpatient care and expenditures in the United States in 1994. J Am Coll Surg 1998; 186(1):1-9.

11. Leber GE, Garb JL, Alexander AI, Reed WP. Long-term complications associated with prosthetic repair of incisional hernias. Arch Surg 1998; 133:378-382.

12. Kaufman Z, Engelberg M, Zager M. Fecal fistula: a late complication of Marlex mesh repair. Dis Colon Rectum 1981; 24:543-544.

13. Scheider R, Herrington JL Jr, Granda AM. Marlex mesh in repair of a diaphramatic defect later eroding into the distal esophagus and stomach. Am Surg 1979; 45:337-339.

14. Nagy KK, Fildes JJ, Mahr C. Experience with three prosthetic materials in temporary abdominal wall closure. Am Surg 1996; 62:331-335.

15. Park A, Birch DW, Lovrics P. Laparoscopic and open incisional hernia repair: a comparison study. Surg 1998; 124(4):816-822.

16. Bauer JJ, Harris MT, Kreel I, Gelernt IM. Twelve-year experience with expanded polytetrafluoroethylene in the repair of abdominal wall defects. The Mount Sinai Journal of Medicine 1999; 66(1):20-25.

17. Borzellino G, De Manzoni G, Ricci F. Detection of abdominal adhesions in laparoscopic surgery. A controlled study of 130 cases. Surg Laparosc Endosc 1998; 8(4):273-276.

18. Kolecki RV, Golub RM, Sigel B, Machi J, Kitamura H, Hosokawa T, Justin J, Schwartz J, Zaren HA. Accuracy of viscera slide detection of abdominal wall adhesions by ultrasound. Surg Endosc 1994; 8(8):871-874.

19. Lienemann A, Sprenger D, Steitz HO, Korell M, Reiser M. Detection and mapping of intraabdominal adhesions by using functional cine MR imaging: preliminary results. Radiology 2000; 217(2):421-425.

20. Park A, Gagner M, Pomp A. Laparoscopic repair of large incisional hernias. Surg Laparosc Endosc 1996; 6(2):123-128.

21. Hesselink VJ, Luijendijk RW, de Wilt JHW, Heide R, Jeekel J. An evaluation of risk factors in incisional hernia recurrence. Surgery, Ginecology and Obstetrics 1993; 176:228-234.

22. LeBlanc KA. Current considerations in laparoscopic incisional and ventral herniorrhaphy. JSLS 2000; 4(2):131-139.

23. Koller R, Miholic J, Jakl RJ. Repair of incisional hernias with expanded polytetrafluoroethylene. Eur J Surg 1997; 163:261-266.

24. Carbajo MA, Martín del Olmo JC, Blanco JI, de la Cuesta C, Toledano M, Martín F, Vaquero C, Inglada L. Laparoscopic treatment vs open surgery in the solution of major incisional and abdominal wall hernias with mesh. Surg Endosc 1999; 13:250-252.

25. Condon RE, DeBord JR. Expanded polytetrafluoroethylene prosthetic patches in repair of large ventral hernia. In: Nyhus LM, Condon RE eds. Hernia (4th edition). Philadelphia: Lippincott Willians & Wilkins 1995; 20:328-336.

26. Morales-Conde S, Martín-Gómez M, Morales-Méndez S. Double Crown Technique for laparoscopic ventral hernia repair. Personal communication during the International Surgical Week and 39th World Congress of Surgery. Brussels, Belgium August 26-30, 2001.

27. Ramshaw BJ, Esartia P, Schwab J, Mason EM, Wilson RA, Duncan TD. Comparison of laparoscopic and open ventral herniorraphy. Am Surg 1999; 65:827-832.

28. García Moreno F, Ots Gutierrez JR, Gutierrez Romero JR, Cuevas del Pino D, López Díez S. Repair of incisional hernias by laparoscopy: technique and results. Cir Esp 2001; 70(supl1):89.

CHAPTER 22

Management of Mesh and Sutures during Laparoscopic Ventral Hernia Repair : a lesson learned from an experimental model

S. Morales-Conde, I. Cadet, S. Morales-Méndez.

INTRODUCTION

Conventional surgery repair of incisional hernias requires wide dissection and mesh placement, often with drains (1, 2). It also often involves a lengthy postoperative stay and a delay of several weeks in the return to normal activities. Laparoscopic hernia repair has been used successfully to repair inguinal hernias as well as some ventral hernias, either primary or incisional hernias (3, 4). The laparoscopic approach for ventral hernias is performed by placing a mesh intraperitoneally, covering the defect of the abdominal wall. One of the main concerns of surgeons performing this technique by the laparoscopic approach is the production of adhesions and fistulas by placing the mesh in contact with the bowel, but it is difficult to determine if the adherences are produce to the mesh itself, to the sutures used to fix the mesh to the abdominal wall, to the edges of the mesh, or if they are due to the inflammatory response of the anterior abdominal wall after realising the intrabdominal adherences to the sac of the hernia or to previous scar.

We have developed an experimental model to analyze what factors may influence on the presence of adhesions to the material we are using (e-PTFE), and if these adhesions depend on the material or on the surgical technique. We also try to determine a macroscopic evaluation of mesh integration and how to manage the mesh and the tacks to avoid recurrences and adhesions formation.

MATERIAL AND METHOD

We have develop an experimental study in 20 pigs to compare the differences between two mesh of e-PTFE, *Micro-mesh* and *Dual-Mesh plus with holes (W.L. Gore and Associates, Flagstaff, AZ, USA)*, carrying on a macroscopic evaluation of the integration of both meshes implanted, and how different factors, such as the tacks used to fix the mesh to the abdominal wall, the edge of the mesh, the surgical technique and the inflammatory response of the peritoneum after releasing adherences, may influence on mesh integration and on adhesion formation. The variables we use were three: the sutures of fixation, choosing the tacks because we thought they were an excellent method to fix the mesh to the abdominal wall, and that there was no place for the old endostapler; the mesh, comparing the differences between the *Micro-mesh* and *Dual-Mesh plus with holes*; and the characteristic of the hernia related to the presence or absence of adhesions, because we thought there were two types of hernias, the one in which there are multiple adhesions, being necessary a process of adhesiolysis with the subsequent inflammatory response of the peritoneum, and those hernias with no adhesions in which no adhesiolysis is needed and no reaction of the peritoneum is expected to influence in the integration of the mesh and in the formation of adhesions to the mesh or to the abdominal wall.

The macroscopic parameters analyzed were: the size of the mesh, the formation of adhesions, and the presence or absence of fistulas, seromas, hematomas, granulomas, infection, and abscesses, all related to the center of the mesh and to the edge, were the tacks were placed. The type of adherences were classified in type 1 (when adhesions are separated from the mesh only with traction), 2 (when blunt dissection is needed) and 3 (dissection of adherences is done with scissors).

Pigs were divided into two groups of ten: group A, those that were sacrificed one week after the implantation of the mesh; and group B, pigs sacrificed after five weeks. All pigs were operated under general anaesthesia through an infraumbilical laparotomy (Fig. 1), placing in the upper abdominal wall of each pig four four by four centimetres meshes, two *Micro-mesh* and two *Dual-mesh plus with holes*, one of each mesh in one side of the pig, being fixed intraperitoneally by four tacks, one in each corner. An abrasion of the peritoneum (Fig. 2) of the left upper quadrant of the abdominal wall was performed to create an inflammatory responses, similar to the process of cicatrisation that occurs after adhesiolysis, this abrasion was performed before to place the meshes (Fig. 3 and 4). Five different areas were determine in the upper abdomen of the pig were the mesh were attached: 1. a four by four *Micro-mesh* was placed, 2. *Micro-mesh* with previous abrasion of the peritoneum, 3. *Dual-mesh plus with holes*, 4. *Dual-mesh plus with holes* with abrasion, and 5. only with tacks without any type of mesh. Once the pigs were sacrificed macroscopic parameters were analysed.

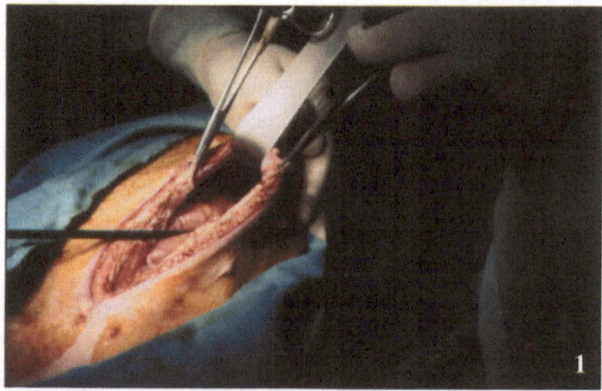

Fig 1. Infraumbilical incisión in a pig before to implant the mesh.

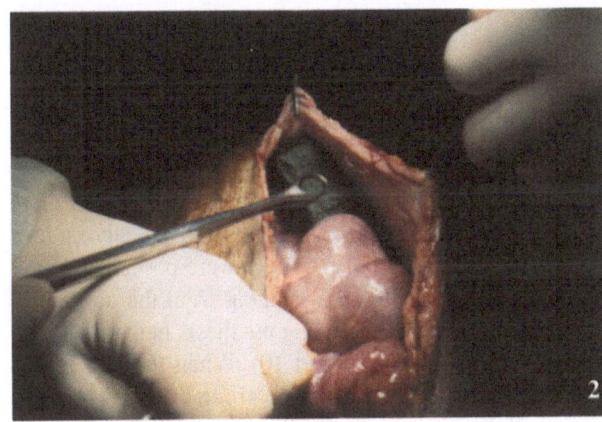

Fig. 2. Abrasion of the peritoneum before to implant the meshes.

Fig. 3. Implantation of the mesh with the tack in the left upper quadrant of the pig.

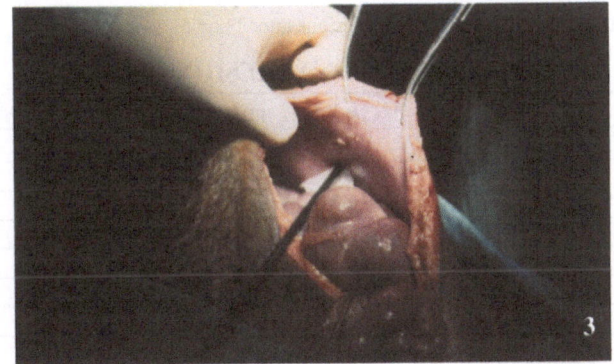

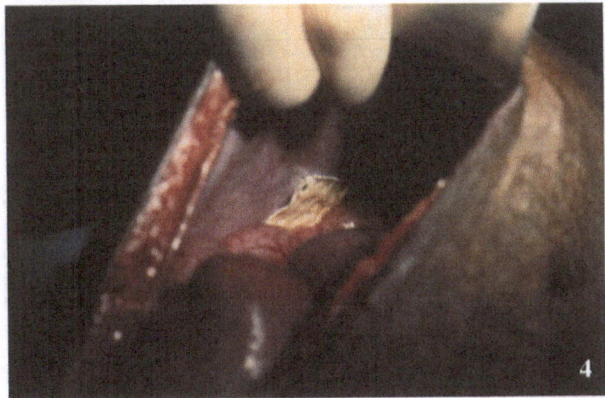

Fig. 4. *Dual-mesh* plus with holes implanted in the rigth upper quarant of the pig.

RESULTS

There were no cases of fistulas, seromas, hematomas, granulomas, infection or abscesses. The presence of adhesions are described in Table I and II, these ones were more important to *Micro-mesh* than to *Dual-mesh* (Fig. 5 and 6) and to the meshes placed in an area with the abrasion of the peritoneum, being also observed more adhesions to the edge of the mesh than to the center of them. We have analyzed how in most of the cases where adhesion to the edge of the mesh were observed (Fig. 7 and 8), the tacks or the edge of the mesh itself were hanging from the abdominal wall. We have also observed a new mesothelium covering the mesh, being thicker in the case of the *Dual-mesh plus with holes* (Fig. 9 and 10). When the adherences were classified in type 1, 2, or 3, in most of the cases of the group of *Dual-mesh* this new mesothelium came with the adherences when we pulled of them (Fig. 11).

On the other hand, we have observed how the size of the mesh decreased as is shown in table III and 4 (Fig. 12 and 13), specially the *Dual-mesh plus with holes* in those pig sacrified five weeks later after the mesh was implanted, with a reduction of a medium of 1.63cm out of the 4cm of the initial measure.

Table I and II. Results of adhesions after 1 and 5 weeks.

ADHESIONS - 1 week

Number	Micro-Mesh	MM with A	Dual-Mesh	DM with A	Tacks
1	-/-	-/-	-/-	-/-	2
2	-/-	3/3	-/-	1/1	-
3	-/-	-/2	-/-	-/2	-
4	3/3	-/-	-/-	-/-	-
5	2/3	2/3	-/1	1/1	2
6	-/-	-/2	-/1	-/2	2
7	-/2	2/2	-/-	1/1	-
8	-/1	2/2	-/1	1/1	-
9	-/2	2/2	-/-	1/1	-
10	2/2	-/-	-/-	-/-	-

ADHESIONS - 5 weeks

Number	Micro-Mesh	MM with A	Dual-Mesh	DM with A	Tacks
11	-/-	-/-	-/-	-/-	-
12	-/-	-/-	-/-	-/-	-
13	1/1	3/3	-/-	-/-	-
14	-/-	-/-	-/-	-/-	-
15	-/-	3/3	-/-	3/3	-
16	-/-	-/-	-/-	-/-	-
17	-/3	-/-	-/-	-/-	3
18	3/3	2/2	-/2	2/2	-
19	2/3	2/2	-/-	3/3	2
20	-/-	-/-	1/1	-/-	-

MM = Micro- Mesh - A = Abrasion - DM = Dual-Mesh plus with holes - number/number = adherences to the center of the mesh/adherences to the edge of the mesh or tacks
- = no adherences - 1 = adherences are dissected only with traction - 2 = adherences are dissected with blunt dissection - 3 = adherences are dissected with scissors

Table III. Size of the mesh (centimetres) after 1 week.

Number	Micro-Mesh	MM with A	Dual-Mesh	DM with A
1	2.8 x 2.7	2.5 x 2.6	2.8 x 2.8	2.9 x 2.9
2	3.0 x 3.0	3.3 x 3.1	3.1 x 3.2	3.2 x 3.3
3	3.5 x 3.4	3.1 x 3.2	3.3 x 3.3	3.5 x 3.4
4	3.0 x 2.9	3.3 x 3.2	2.9 x 2.8	3.0 x 3.0
5	3.6 x 3.5	3.5 x 3.5	3.4 x 3.4	3.5 x 3.4
6	3.0 x 3.1	2.9 x 3.1	3.3 x 3.2	3.4 x 3.3
7	3.3 x 3.4	3.3 x 3.3	2.8 x 3.0	3.1 x 3.1
8	3.3 x 3.3	3.2 x 3.2	3.4 x 3.4	3.4 x 3.6
9	3.3 x 3.2	3.3 x 3.2	3.5 x 3.4	3.5 x 3.5
10	3.3 x 3.3	3.2 x 3.3	3.2 x 3.3	3.6 x 3.5
	3.21 x 3.18	*3.16 x 3.17*	*3.17 x 3.18*	*3.31 x 3.3*

Table IV. Size of the mesh (centimetres) after 5 week.

Number	Micro-Mesh	MM with A	Dual-Mesh	DM with A
1	3.0 x 3.1	2.9 x 2.8	2.5 x 2.4	2.7 x 2.6
2	3.0 x 3.0	3.1 x 2.9	2.2 x 2.3	2.3 x 2.4
3	2.8 x 2.7	3.1 x 3.2	2.4 x 2.4	2.7 x 2.7
4	2.8 x 2.8	3.1 x 3.0	2.3 x 2.1	2.4 x 2.3
5	2.5 x 2.5	3.0 x 3.1	2.6 x 2.4	2.7 x 2.8
6	2.7 x 2.8	3.1 x 3.1	2.5 x 2.5	2.7 x 2.7
7	3.0 x 2.9	3.0 x 2.9	2.3 x 2.5	2.5 x 2.6
8	2.8 x 2.9	3.0 x 3.0	2.5 x 2.6	2.8 x 2.8
9	2.5 x 2.7	3.3 x 3.2	2.1 x 2.2	2.2 x 2.3
10	2.8 x 2.7	3.0 x 2.8	2.3 x 2.3	2.5 x 2.5
	2.79 x 2.81	*3.06 x 3.0*	*2.37 x 2.37*	*2.55 x 2.57*

MM = Micro- Mesh
A = Ablation
DM = Dual-Mesh plus with holes

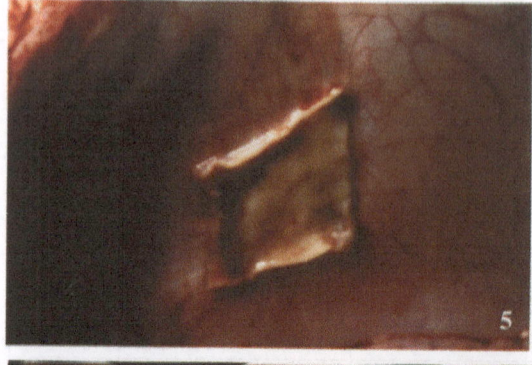

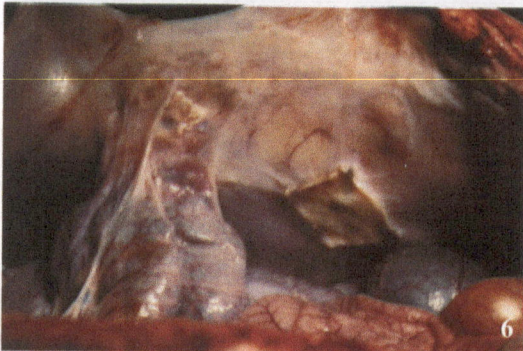

Figs. 5 and 6. In figure 5 (on the left) we observed a *Dual-mesh plus with holes* with no adhesions, while the differences between the *Dual-mesh plus with holes* and the *Micro-mesh* is observed in figure 6 (on the right).

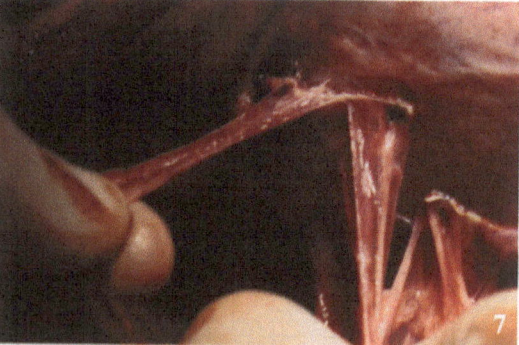

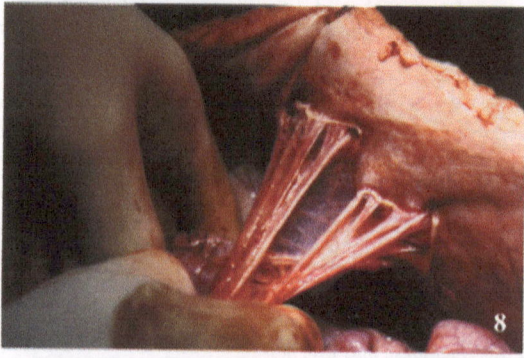

Figs. 7 and 8. Adherences to the edges of the mesh, being observed in figure 7 (on the left) the absence of adhesions to the center of the mesh.

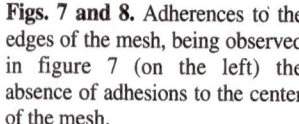

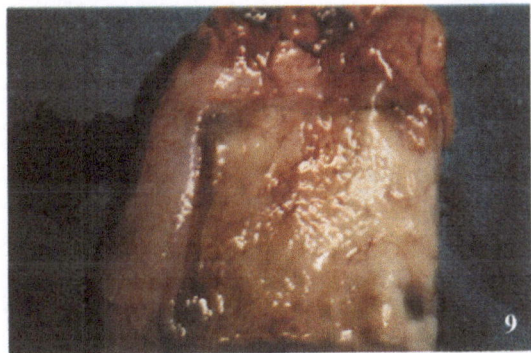

Figs. 9 and 10. New mesothelium covering a *Dual-mesh plus with holes* removed after 5 weeks.

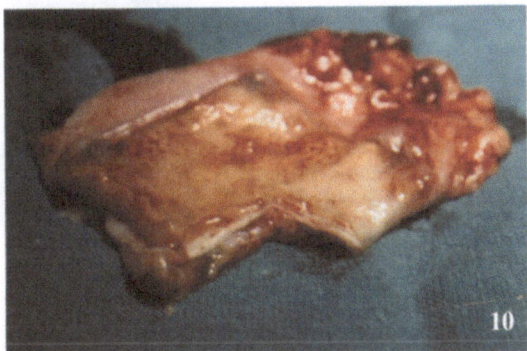

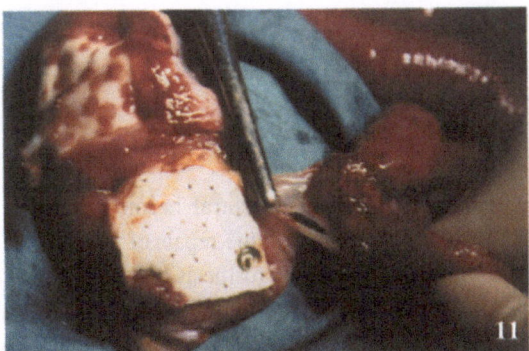

Fig. 11. The new mesothelium created covering the *Dual-mesh plus with holes* came with the adherence when we pulled of the bowel easier than when the adherence was created to the *Micro-mesh*.

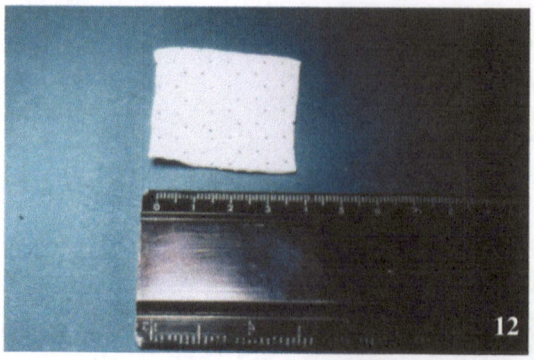

Figs. 12 and 13. We have observed how the size of the mesh decreased in all cases, specially the *Dual-mesh plus with holes*, as it is observed in these figures.

DISCUSSION OR HOW TO MANAGE MESH AND SUTURES DURING LAPAROSCOPIC VENTRAL HERNIA REPAIR

Thirty per cent of the patients undergoing repair of a ventral hernia without a prosthetic patch will have a recurrence (5), for that reason the repair of this type of hernias requires, in most of the cases, the use of synthetic prosthesis to avoid tension. While small defect (< 3-4cm) can be performed with minimal dissection on an outpatient basis (6), conventional repair of larger hernias requires a large incision, wide dissection to obtein adequate fascial margin, the subsequent need for drains, postoperative disconfort, and long hospitalisation. The laparoscopic approach offers the possibility to carry out the necessary adhesiolysis to clear the abdominal defect to repair the abdominal wall without tension by placing a mesh. As the mesh is placed intraperitoneally, one of the main concerns is the possibility of creating adhesions, that can then lead to bowel obstruction or migration of the mesh into the intestinal lumen and formation of intestinal fistulas. The presence of adhesions decreases by the use of e-PTFE better than polypropylene (7-10), and by the use of *Dual-mesh* better than *Micro-mesh*, as we can see in our results. But in this study we can observe how there are other factors that may influence on the production of adhesions: the dissection of abdominal adhesions prior to place the mesh produces an inflammatory response that determines the presence of adhesions to the mesh and to the area where it is placed, as we see in this study with the meshes placed in the area where the peritoneum has been previously abrased; on the other hand, the surgical technique also influences on the creation of adhesions, because we have seen that most of these adhesions appear at the edge of the mesh, and it was observed that there was more adhesions when the tacks or the edge of the mesh were left hanging from the wall, so the transition between the mesh and the anterior abdominal wall should not leave the mesh hanging and the tacks should be stacked all the way into the mesh to avoid the creation of adhesions, and to avoid the possibility of creting a fistula by these tacks to the lumen of the intestinal loop (Fig. 14 and 15). We have also observed how most of the adhesions created at one week to the *Dual-mesh* plus with holes are type 1, and how four weeks later there are less adhesions and these are type 2 or 3, what means that the initial response of the organism to the mesh when they are placed intraperitoneally is the creation of labile adhesions that either will disappear or will become stronger. We have also observed the new mesothelium created over the mesh and how this was more important in the *Dual-mesh plus with holes*, we have also observed how when we pull of the adherences these were attached to the mesh itself in the cases of Micro-mesh, but in those cases of *Dual-mesh* this new mesothelium comes with the mesh when we pull of the adhesions, as if the mesothelium were protecting the bowel from the mesh, and the adherence were attached to this layer of mesothelium and not to the mesh itself.

Another consideration is that the laparoscopic approach to repair ventral hernia decrease the risk of infection of the prosthetic patch, because this one is placed distant from the incision, the potential portal of infection, and there is no dissection over the patch superficial to the peritoneum. In our study we have not observed infection of the meshes implanted what lead us to believe that the risk of infection decrease using this approach, what is considered one of the reasons of recurrences in many cases (11).

We also have observed in this study a decrease of the size of the meshes, this retraction is more important after 5 weeks in the group of *Dual-mesh plus with holes*, where we have seen a reduction of the patch of 1.7 centimetres. In recent studies, computed tomography after the treatment of large incisional hernias with e-PTFE prostheses has showed the e-PTFE mesh encapsulated by newly formed tissue (12), this new tissue is more important with the *Dual-mesh plus with holes*, what could be the reason of the greater retraction of this mesh compared with the *Micro-mesh*. So, this newly formed tissue and the scar reaction surrounding the mesh produce a decreases of the size of the prostheses what lead us to recommend that the mesh used for the laparoscopic ventral hernia repair should overlap the defect of the hernia at least 3cm in order to avoid recurrences.

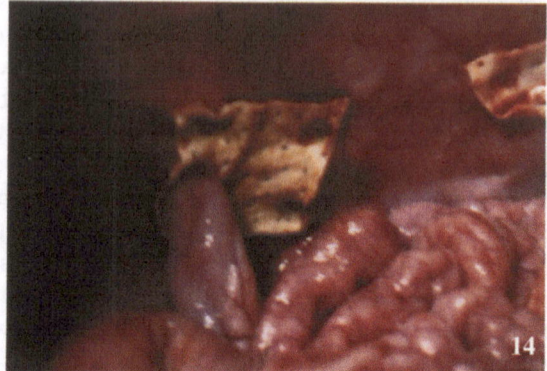

Figs. 14 and 15. Creation of adhesions of the bowel to a tack left hanging from the wall (on the left), being observed the erosion produced on the wall of the intestinal loop (on the right).

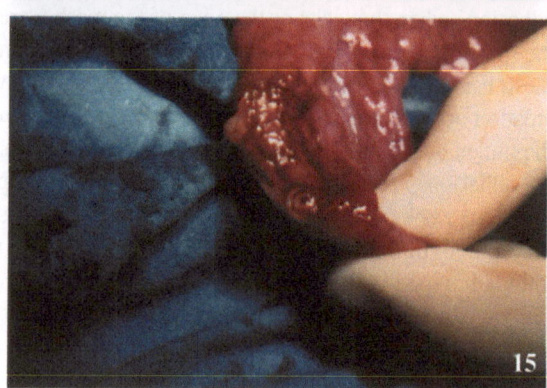

References

1. Ellis H. Management of the wound. In: Schartz SI, Ellis H, eds. Maingot's abdominal operations. Norwalk, Connecticut: Appleton & Lange, 1990:210-213.

2. Abrahamson J Hernias. In: Schartz SI, Ellis H, eds. Maingot's abdominal operations. Norwalk, Connecticut: Appleton & Lange, 1990:273-296.

3. Sanders LM, Flint LM, Ferrara JJ. Initial experience with laparoscopic repair of incisional hernias. Am J Surg 1999; 177:227-231.

4. Park A, Gagner M, Pomp A. Laparoscopic repair of large incisional hernias. Surg Laparosc Endosc 1996; 6(2):123-128.

5. Bauer JJ, Salky BA, Gelernt IM, Kreel I. Repair of large abdominal wall defects with expanded polytetrafluoroethylene (PTFE). Ann Surg 1987; 206:765-769.

6. Hesselink VJ, Luijendijk RW, de Wilt JHW, Heide R, Jeekel J. An evaluation of risk factors in incisional hernia recurrence. Surg Gynecol Obstet. 1993; 176:228-234.

7. Ponce González JF, Barriga Beltrán R, Martín Zurita I, Morales Conde S, Morales Méndez S. Prosthetic materials in incisional hernias. Experimental study. Cir Esp 1998; 63:189-194.

8. Le Blanc KA, Booth WV. Laparoscopic repair of incisional abdominal hernias using expanded polytetrafluoroethylene: preliminary findings. Surg Laparosc Endosc 1993; 3:39-41.

9. Law NW. A comparison of polypropylene mesh, expanded polytetrafluoroethylene patch and polyglycolic acid mesh for the repair of experimental abdominal wall defects. Acta Chir Scand 1990; 156:759-762.

10. Christoforoni PM, Kim YB, Preys Z, Lay RY, Montz FJ. Adhesion formation after incisional hernia repair: a randomised porcine trial. Am Surg 1996; 62(11):935-938.

11. Bucknall TE, Cox PJ, Ellis H. Burst abdomen and incisional hernia: a prospective study of 1129 major laparotomies. B M J 1982; 284:931-933.

12. Bellon JM, Contreras LA, Sabater C, Bujan J. Pathologic and clinical aspects of large incisional hernias after implant of a polytetrafluoroethylene prosthesis. World J Surg. 1997; 21(4):402-406.

7. ...
8. ...
9. ...
10. ...

CHAPTER 23

Consideration regarding Concomitant Operations during Laparoscopic Ventral Hernia Repair: indications, management and trocar position

S. Kyzer, I. Charuzi

INTRODUCTION

The patient undergoing laparoscopic ventral hernia repair may suffer from other surgical pathologies. These pathologies can be symptomatic prior to the repair of the ventral hernia or their symptoms can be manifested at a later stage. Theoretically, the surgical treatment of these concomitant pathologies, either by the laparoscopic or the open approach, can be postponed to a later time. However, this delay may complicate the previously performed ventral hernia repair by causing infection of the mesh or development of recurrent hernia. In addition, when laparoscopic treatment of concomitant intraabdominal pathologies are done at a later stage, severe intraabdominal adhesions can be encountered. For these reasons, we think that the surgeon must strive to treat associated pathologies simultaneously with ventral hernia repair. However, the surgeon's decision whether or not to perform concomitant procedures must take into account the circumstances of each individual case. Some crucial points for consideration are: (1) whether the patient is symptomatic or not; (2) can the patient tolerate the concomitant procedure which means longer operation time and increased surgical injury; and (3) whether performance of the concomitant procedure may increase the likelihood for mesh infection.

POSSIBLE CONCOMITANT PROCEDURES

Taking into consideration the above mentioned points, there are several pathologies that can be treated simultaneously during laparoscopic repair of ventral hernia. Theoretically, every procedure that is not associated with opening of a contaminated viscus can be performed. However, according to our literature survey, the concomitant procedures that were performed included: cholecystectomy (1-4), inguinal herniorrhaphy (2, 4, 5), antireflux procedure (2, 4), peritoneal catheter manipulation (1,4) and tubal ligation (5). In the following paragraphs, we will discuss separately some of these concomitant procedures, the indications and the surgical techniques.

LAPAROSCOPIC CHOLECYSTECTOMY

As the incidence of gallstones among the "healthy" population is about 20%, it is essential before repair of ventral hernia to be informed about their presence. This is important because subsequent development of biliary colic, acute cholecystitis or other complications of gallstones may necessitate performance of laparoscopic cholecystectomy at a later stage. This can result in infection of the mesh due to the inflammatory process and/or puncture of the previously laid mesh by the trocars. For these reasons, we think that the surgeon must endeavor, in the presence of uncomplicated gallbladder disease, to remove the gallbladder simultaneously with the laparoscopic repair of the ventral hernia. Laparoscopic cholecystectomy must be performed very carefully in order to prevent spillage of bile. In case gross contamination of bile occurs with a finding of acute cholecystitis, the hernia repair must be postponed. For most of the cases before approaching the gallbladder, it is essential to release the hernia content and the adhesions to the peritoneal layer. When planning the operation, the trocar sites must be located outside the anticipated borders of the mesh. For this reason in the presence of midline incisional hernia, we prefer to introduce the first trocar at the left anterior axillary line halfway between the costal margin and the anterior superior iliac crest (Fig. 1). After lysis of the hernia's contents and the surrounding adhesions, the gallbladder can be easily viewed by introducing a 30° scope through this trocar. The epigastric trocar can be introduced at its usual location unless in the presence of an epigastric hernia. In this case, the scope can be introduced at the usual subumbilical site, and the dissection is performed through the trocar at the left anterior axillary line. In most of the cases, the two 5 mm trocars for grasping the gallbladder (trocars Nos. 3 and 4) can be introduced at their usual locations (Fig. 1).

It is essential to leave a drain at the subhepatic space in order to prevent mesh infection by small bile leakage from the gallbladder bed. If bile leakage is excluded, this drain has to be removed as early as possible. It must not be forgotten that the patient must receive a perioperative antibiotic. If no bowel injury occurred during the repair of the ventral hernia, oral feeding can be resumed in most cases on the first or second postoperative day, and the patient can be discharged accordingly under the usual postoperative management.

LAPAROSCOPIC INGUINAL HERNIA REPAIR

Laparoscopic repair of ventral hernia located in the lower abdomen may prevent the ability for laparoscopic repair of inguinal hernia by the preperitoneal as well as the intraperitoneal approach in the future. In addition, the postoperative increase of the intraabdominal pressure may cause incarceration of the inguinal hernia shortly after closure of the abdominal wall defect. For these reasons, we think that concomitant repair of inguinal hernia is recommended if the ventral hernia repair is not complicated with bleeding or bowel injury. We think that, for most of the patients, addition of laparoscopic inguinal hernia repair does not significantly increase the surgical stress in terms of operative tissue injury and postoperative pain.

We recommend the use of the transabdominal preperitoneal (TAPP) approach because it prevent any manipulation through the scarred abdominal wall. If the ventral hernia is located in the upper abdomen and the abdomen below the umbilicus is free from any surgical scars, the totally extraperitoneal (TEP) approach can be also used.

For the TAPP approach, two 10mm trocars are introduced at the anterior axillary line above the anterior superior iliac crest in the contralateral side of the hernia (Fig. 2). The trocar for the 45° scope is introduced in the subumbilical area or into the anterior axillary line at the level of the umbilicus on the other side.

If performance of the TEP approach is feasible, positioning of the trocars can be performed in the usual manner.

LAPAROSCOPIC HIATAL HERNIA REPAIR

In patients suffering from gastroesophageal reflux disease due to sliding hernia or from paraesophageal hernia, we recommend its concomitant laparoscopic repair. With this approach, we prevent the need for subsequent repair of the hernia with the sequelae mentioned above or from aggravation of the symptoms caused by the hiatal hernia due to the increased intraabdominal pressure. It is essential to release initially the hernia's content and the surrounding adhesions before repair of the hiatal hernia. Then the needed trocars for the repair of the hiatal hernia are introduced. As the initial proper trocar placement is important for success of the hiatal hernia repair, their position should not have to be changed, even if they are located just inside or very close to the hernia's sack. In the presence of a large hiatal defect which its proper closure cannot be achieved, we recommend facilitating the closure with the use of Gore-Tex® patch. This technique that we adapted for the repair of hiatal hernia is also very useful on the concomitant repair of ventral hernia and hiatal hernia because it may prevent early recurrence of the hiatal hernia. In case the release of the ventral hernia content and its surrounding adhesions is very tenuous and associated with significant bleeding, prolonged operation time or there is doubt about the integrity of the bowel, the repair of the hiatal hernia must be postponed. In most cases, the nasogastric tube can be removed on the first postoperative day, and oral feeding can be resumed gradually.

ACKNOWLEDGMENT
We thank Ms. Judy Brandt for her English editing,
word processing and contributions.

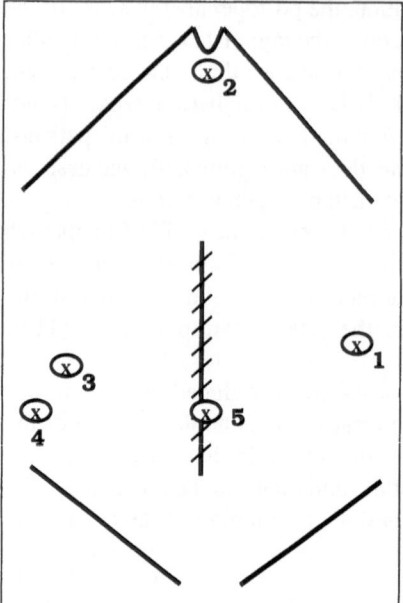

Fig. 1. Trocar positions for laparoscopic
P.O.V.H. repair and laparoscopic
cholecystectomy - 1. Scope or dissection site
in presence of epigastric hernia - 2.
Dissection site (If there is no epigastric
hernia.) - 3.,4. 5 mm trocars for grasping the
gallbladder - 5. Scope site in presence of
epigastric hernia.

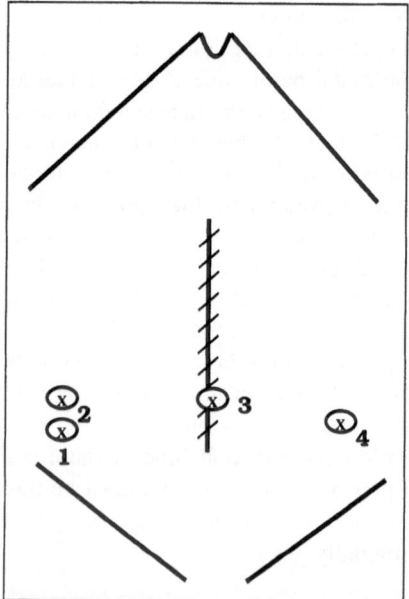

Fig. 2. Positions of trocars during
P.O.V.H. repair and transabdominal inguinal
hernia repair - 1.,2. Working trocars - 3.,4.
Possible locations of the scope.

References

1. Szymanski J, Voitk A, Joffer J, Alvarez C, Rozenthal G. Technique and early results of outpatient laparoscopic mesh onlay repair of ventral hernia. Surg Endoscopy 2000;14:582-584.

2. Franklin ME, Dorman JP, Glass JL, Balli JE, Gonzalez JJ. Laparoscopic ventral and incisional hernia repair. Surg Laparoscopy and Endoscopy 1998;8:294-299.

3. Kyzer S, Alis M, Aloni Y, Charuzi I. Laparoscopic repair of postoperation ventral hernia. Early postoperation results. Surg Endos 1999;13:928-931.

4. Reitter DR, Paulsen KJ, Debord JR, Estes NC. Five-year experience with the "four-before" laparoscopic ventral hernia repair. Am Surg 2000;66:465-469.

5. Heniford BT, Ramshaw BJ. Laparoscopic ventral hernia repair. A report of 100 consecutive cases. Surg Endos 2000;14:419-423.

References

SECTION VI

Techniques and Results of Laparoscopic Ventral Hernia Repair

CHAPTER 24

Laparoscopic Percutaneous Repair of Incisional Hernia: Indications, technique and results

A. Al Dohayan, M. Al Sebayel, A. Al Abdul Kareem, A. Al Otiaby, T. Jaber

INTRODUCTION

Incisional hernia is a well-known complication of abdominal surgery. As high as 4% of patients who undergo abdominal surgery develop incisional hernias. Procedures for repair of these hernias include the standard open suturing technique, with as without the use of a mesh. However, several complications have been reported following the open technique such as long skin scars, hernia recurrence (Recurrence rate of upto 40%), infection, hematoma, rejection of the mesh, bowel injury and fistula formation.

The introduction of laparoscopic surgery has opened a new field in the management of incisional hernias. Advantages of the laparoscopic technique include small incisions, a well know decrease in the rate of wound complications which may lower hernia recurrence and the ability to release bowel adhesions under magnification. Recently, a pure laparoscopic technique using gortex (PTFE) mesh has been reported. In that technique the fascial edges are not approximated and the mesh is fixed to the fascial defect from the inner (Peritoneal) rather than the outer (Subcutaneous) surface.

We have developed a new laparoscopic technique to repair incisional hernias and labeled it "The percutaneous laparoscopic technique". Through 3 ports the laparoscopic is used and release bowel adhesions. With the help of small incision, the sac is excised and fascial edges are then approximated, by sutures. Finally a marlex mesh is sutured on the outer (Subcutaneous) surface to augment the fascial repair. This "Percutaneous" technique has been used successfully in 18 patients at our institution.

TECHNIQUE

The patient is placed in supine on the operating table with arms tucked at the side. Extending the arms may not allow enough room for the surgeon to operate comfortably. The trendenburg and, antitrendenburg position allows the bowel to fall away from the laparoscopic field. The surgeon stands on the patient's side (with the monitor positioned at the head of the table) for upper midline hernias, and at the foot of the table for lower midline hernias. The assistant stands opposite to the surgeon. Preoperative bowel preparation is carried out with prophylactic antibiotics. The placement of trocars depends on the site of the hernia. For midline hernia the is placed 2-3 inches away from the lower edge of the hernia (Fig. 1). A O Degrees 5 mm scope is introduced after insuflation of CO_2 inside the peritoneal cavity. After inspection of the hernia and the site of the adhesions, the surgeon will decide about for insertion for the two 5 mm trocor on the lateral side of the hernia (Fig. 1). On the other, hand for lower abdominal hernia the camera's trocar placed below the costal margins and 2 working port placed lateral to the hernia (Fig. 2). A third trocar may placed at the opposite site for additional help. The scope can be placed at any port for better view. A non-crushing grasper is used and scissor for holding and cutting the adhesion at the peritonium of the abdominal wall. After sepration of the adhesion. Two incisions are made at the lower end and upper end, of the hernia 1 inch distal to lower edge and 1 inch proximal to the upper edge. For dissection of the hernia sac and the neck of the sac is tranfixed with suture. Alkhwiteer, Al Dohayan needle (A.A. NEEDLE) Fig. 3 is mounted with a nonabsorbable synthetic suture passed through healthy fascia 1.5cm distal the lower edge Fig. 3 and retrieved from at 1.5 cm proximal to the healthy upper edge. The same procedure is applied for the other end This step is repeated several times to cover the defect with sutures. Usually 4-7 sutures are applied. The pneumperitoneum is evacuated and sutures are tied percautaneousely. A marlex mesh is applied perecautaneously to cover the defect 4 cm away from it. The mesh is fixed, to the fascia, using a non absorbable synthetic suture is passed and retrieved passed through the mesh and fascia. A nonabsorbabel synthetic suture mounted to Alkhwiteer – Al Dohayan. Needle and retrieved by needle forceps and suture tied. This step is repeated several times for securing the mesh percautaneously. The wound is washed and closed. Occasionally a drain is used for 24 hours only. Patients use an abdominal binder for 9 months.

RESULTS

A total of 18 patients underwent repair of incisional hernia using this technique. All patients tolerated oral fluid within 24-hour surgery and could move the next day. No wound infection occurred and all patients were discharged average hospital stay of 2.8 days the follow up period averaged 20 months and no hernia recurrence was observed.

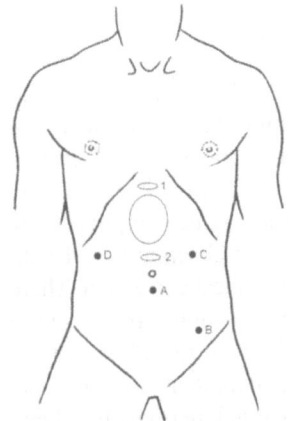

Fig. 1

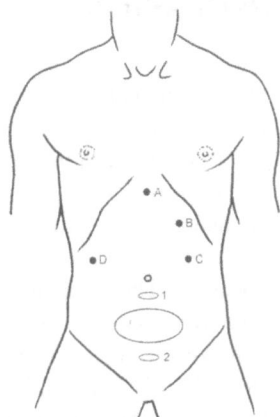

Fig. 2

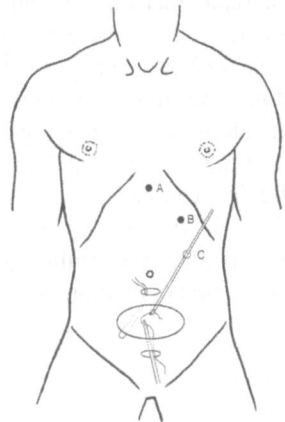

Fig. 3

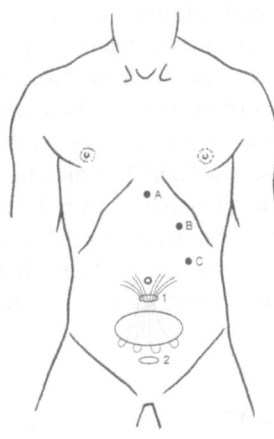

Fig. 4

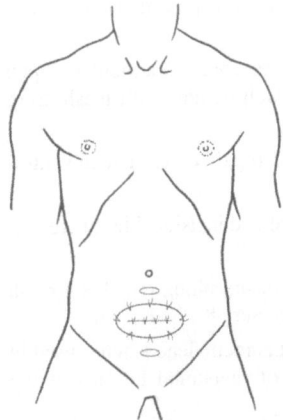

Fig. 5

Fig. 1. Site of the ports (ABC) & 1.2 are the places for percautoneous surgery for upper midline hernia.

Fig. 2. The arrangement for ports as site (A,B,C) and percautoneous surgical incisions (1,2) for lower midline hernia.

Fig. 3. The gasper is holding the sitch from Alkhwiteer A Al-Dohayan needle.

Fig. 4. The final suture pattern for percautoneous taying.

Fig. 5. The final appearance of the repair with percautoneous mesh fixation.

DISCUSSION

Upto 5% of patients who undergo abdominal surgery develop Incisional hernias which are unique in that they are the only abdominal hernias that are considered to be iatrogenic. The Incisional hernias may be associated with pain and discomfort, loss of time from productive employment, and may lead the patient to change his life style and daily activities. Additionally, incisional hernias may be complicated by serious morbidity such as incarceration, strangulation and ischaemic bowel with perforation. Therefore incisional hernias need obligatory surgical correction. There are many techniques in repairing incisional hernias such as using primary suture repair with or without mesh augmentation. However the recurrance rate ranges from 24 to 45 percent. The need of proper technique is important. Recently, the introduction of laparoscopy in management of incisional hernias has been reported. As expected, the laparoscopic approach has several advantages over the open technique which includes a decreased risk for trauma and other wound complications such as wound infection as well as a rapid recovery. In our percutaneous laparoscopic technique, the laparoscope is used to dissect the adhesions under magnification and hence reducing the risk of bowel injury. First approximation of the edges of the fascial defect is done with non absorbable synthetic suture to form a net over the defect and tied percaucaneously. Secondly a non absorabable synthetic, mesh is applied and fixed to musculo fascial layer percautoneously. Our technique is economic, easy effective can be utilized by surgeons with laparoscopic surgery experience. It is well known that 50% recurrences of incisional hernias occur in the first year. Our preliminary results are encouraging with no recurrence over the average follow-up period of 20 months.

References

1. Al-Dohayan A, Al-Sebayel M. Laparoscopic Percutaneous Repair of Incisional Hernia (Initial Report) Proceeding the 7th World Congress of Endoscopic Surgery 413-415, 2000.
2. Bickel A, Eiten A. A simplified laparoscopic technique for mesh placement in ventral hernia repair. Surg Endosc 13:532-534, 1999.
3. Carbajo MA, Martin del Oimo JC, Blanco JT, et al. laparoscopic treatment vs open surgery in the solution of major incisional and abdominal wall hernias with mesh. Surg endosc 13:250-252, 1999.
4. Costanza MJ, Heniford BT, Arca MJ et al.; laparoscopic repair of recurrent ventral hernias. Am surg 64:1121-1127, 1998.
5. Franklin ME, DormanJP, Glass JL, et al.; laparoscopic ventral and incisional hernia repair, surg Laparosc Endosc 8:294-299, 1998.
6. Gersin KS, ponsky JL, Heniford BT. Simplified technique for untrolling prosthetic mesh during laparoscopic ventral hernia repair. J Laparoendosc Adv Surg 8:79-81, 1998
7. Gillion JF, Begin GF, Marecos C, et al. expanded polytetraflueoroethylene patches used in the intraperitoneal or extraperitoneal position for repair of incisional hernias of the anterolateral abdominal wall. Am J Surg 174:16-19, 1997.
8. Hesselink VJ, Luijendi RW, deWilt JHW, et al. An evaluation of risk factors in incisional hernia recurrence. Surg Gynecol Obstet 176:228-234, 193.

9. Holzman MD, Purut CM, Reintgen K, et al. Laparoscopic ventral and incisional hernioplasty. Surg endosc :32-35, 1997.

10. Larson GM. Lapaoscopic repair of ventral hernia. In scott-conner CEH (ed). The society of American Gastrointestinal Surgeons Manual: Fundamentals of Laparoscopy and Gastrointestinal Endoscopy. New York, springer 1998, 314-325.

11. Larson GM, Harrower HW; Plastic mesh repair of incisional hernia. Am J Surg 135-559-563, 1978.

12. Laron GM, Vandertoll DJ. Approaches to repair of ventral hernia and full-thickness losses of the abdominal wall, wurg clin North Am 64:33-349, 1984.

13. Leblanc KA, Booth WV. Laparoscopic repair of incisional abdominal hernias using expanded polytetrafluoroethylene: preliminary findings. Surg Laparosc Endosc 3:39-41, 1993.

14. Park A, Birch DW, Lovrics p, et al. Laparoscopic and open incisional hernia repair. A comparison study. Surgery 124:816-22, 1998.

15. Santora TA, Roslyn JJ: Incisional hernia. Surg Clin North Am 73:557-570, 1993

16. Toy FK, Bailey RW, Carey S, et al. Prospective, multicenter study of laparoscopic ventral hernioplasty. Surg Endosc 12:955-959 1998.

17. Usher FC. A new plastic prosthesis for repairing tissue defect of the chest and abdominal wall. Am J Surg 97:629-633, 1959.

18. Usher FC. The surgeon at work: The repair of repair of incisional and inguial hernias. Surg Gynecol Obstet 131:525-530 1970.

19. Voyles CR, Richardson JD, Bland KL, et al. Emergency abdominal wall reconstruction with polypropylene mesh. Ann Surg 194:219-223, 1981.

CHAPTER 25

Endoscopic totally Preperitoneal Ventral Hernia Repair: indications, technique and results

M.Miserez

INTRODUCTION

The use of prostheses has dramatically reduced the recurrence rate in incisional and primary ventral hernia repair (1). In open surgery, extraperitoneal sublay mesh implantation is generally preferred versus intraperitoneal placement (2), following the same principles as in "giant prosthetic reinforcement of the visceral sac", described for inguinal hernia repair (3). Endoscopic surgery is a tool to obtain the same operative end-result by minimal invasive means compared to open surgery. Laparoscopic ventral hernia repair (LVHR) with intraabdominal mesh placement has been reported with excellent results, but does not take advantage of immediate mesh fixation by a peritoneal sac. Furthermore, transabdominal laparoscopic incisional hernia repair may lead to various complications due to adhesiolysis and accidental enterotomy (4, 5) and due to late intestinal erosion by the mesh and/or the fixating devices (6). In an attempt to combine the advantages of extraperitoneal mesh implantation with a minimally invasive approach, we describe the technical aspects and our initial clinical experience of a endoscopic totally preperitoneal approach for the treatment of incisional and primary ventral hernias.

SURGICAL TECHNIQUE

After installation of the patient in supine position, the hernial orifice(s) ("inner circle") and surface to be covered by the mesh with an overlapping of 5 cm circumferentially ("outer circle") are marked with a pencil since this allows optimal identification of all hernia orifices with maximal collaboration of the patient due to abdominal wall muscle contraction. No other specific preoperative measures are necessary. The operation is performed under general anaesthesia. A second generation cephalosporin is administered as antibiotic prophylaxis at the time of induction in a single dose. After full muscle relaxation and before draping the lining of the "inner circle" and "outer circle" is verified. After desinfection, the operative field is covered with an adhesive drape (Fig. 1).

The position of the surgeon and the insertion of the first trocar is of utmost importance for adequate exposure of the operative field and depends on the location and the size of the hernia and on the course of the residual scar. Three trocars are used: one 12 mm trocar for the scope and insertion of the mesh and two 5 mm trocars as working channels. They are best placed on one imaginary line (vertical or horizontal), with the first trocar in the middle at the level of the hernia orifice. In most cases, the surgeon is standing on the patient's side with the ipsilateral arm along the body of the patient or elevated ensuring unrestricted surgical manipulations. In this case, the trocars can be placed on a vertical line (longitudinal approach; LONG) (Fig. 2). This approach can be used in most midline hernias and in lateral hernias (e.g. parastomal hernia, spigelian hernia, lumbar hernia). It is much easier than the transversal approach because in the latter, a larger part of the dissection is done with only one working trocar, as will be clear from the description below. A transversal approach (TRANS) with all trocars placed on a horizontal line (Fig. 2) is preferred for a subxyphoidal incisional hernia (e.g. poststernotomy). In this case, the surgeon may stand between the legs of the patient, as in the french approach for laparoscopic cholecystectomy. Table I shows the different steps chronologically in both the longitudinal and transversal approach.

The first trocar (12 mm Blunt balloon-tipped trocar, Tyco) should be placed at least 3 cm away from the "outer circle". In TRANS the first trocar is introduced under direct view via a small paramedian transverse incision of the anterior rectus sheath and luxation of the rectus muscle to visualize the posterior rectus sheath. The trocar can then be inserted retromuscularly (above the arcuate line) (step TRANS 1). In LONG, the first trocar is best introduced under direct view in the retromuscular plane just medial to the lateral border of the rectus muscle by splitting the latter up to the posterior rectus sheath where the trocar is inserted (step LONG 1). For midline hernias, this can be done either from the left or the right side whereas for laterally extending hernias, a contralateral approach is mostly used. Care should be taken not to damage the epigastric vessels by inserting the trocar (Fig. 3).

After endoscopic control of the exact position of the first trocar in the retromuscular plane, insufflation is started up to a pressure of 15 mm Hg. Initial ipsilateral retromuscular dissection is done bluntly with the tip of the scope. A 0° scope might be used for this, but a 30° degree scope is necessary when the other trocars are placed and for the rest of the procedure (step TRANS/LONG 2).

In the longitudinal approach, two additional 5 mm trocars are placed outside the "outer circle" mostly in a vertical line slightly triangular to the first trocar, one cephalad and one caudal (Fig. 3). This can be done after inserting a long intramuscular needle percutaneously to check the position (step LONG 3). In the transversal approach, one additional lateral trocar is inserted ipsilaterally on the

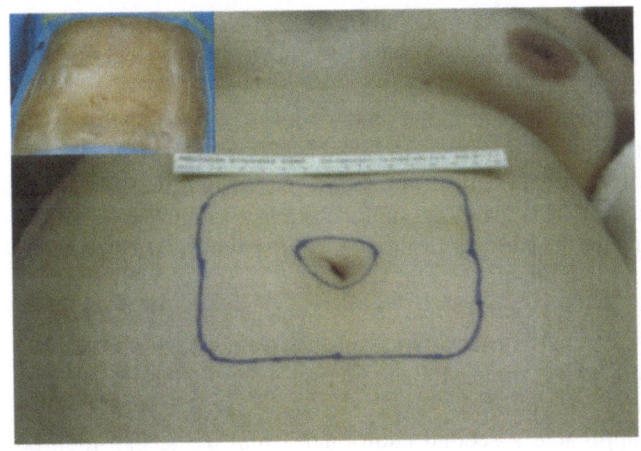

Fig. 1. Installation of the patient in supine position with preoperative marking of hernia orifice ("inner circle") and circumferential overlapping of 5 cm ("outer circle"); the operative field is covered with an adhesive drape (inset).

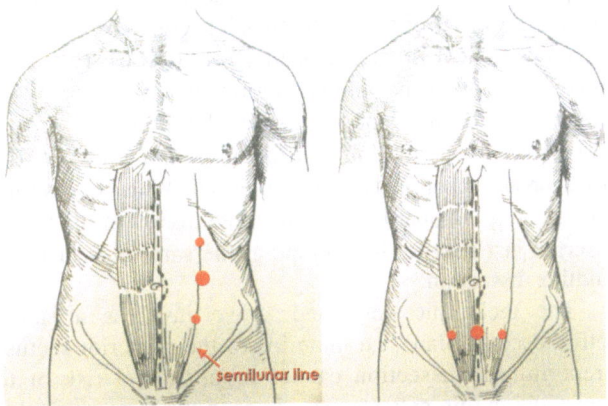

Fig. 2. Example of trocar positioning for mesogastric ventral hernia in longitudinal approach (left) and transversal approach (right); the large dot indicates the position of the 12 mm trocar; the smaller dots indicate the positions of the 5 mm trocars.

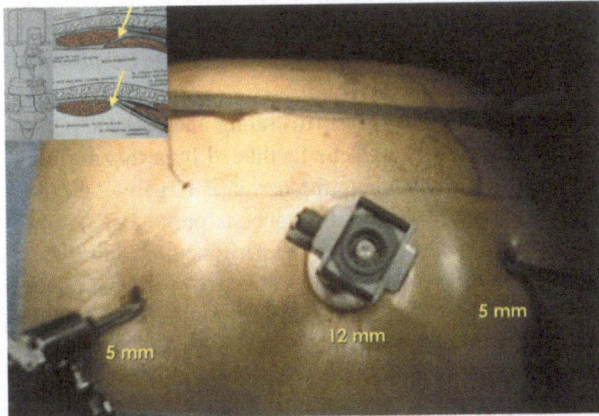

Fig. 3. Intraoperative view of trocar positioning in longitudinal approach: two 5 mm working channels and 12 mm trocar for the endoscope in between at the lateral border of the left rectus muscle. The marker on the midline shows the length of the mesh to be inserted. Detailed picture of the anatomic retromuscular plane of insertion of the first trocar 12mm balloon-tipped trocar above (upper) and below (lower) the arcuate line (inset).

same horizontal line (step TRANS 3). An atraumatic grasping forceps and/or endoscissors (with unipolar coagulation) are used for further blunt retromuscular dissection up to the midline.

Because of the presence of the linea alba on the midline, the medial border of the ipsilateral posterior rectus sheath needs to be incised (step TRANS/LONG 4) in order to perform a true preperitoneal dissection on the midline (with later dissection of the hernia sac). This leaves a small longitudinal rim of preperitoneal fat on the midline with the hernia sac in the center. Especially after previous surgery via a midline incision, this dissection is not easy. A good landmark is the contralateral rectus muscle which can be reached by opening the medial border of the contralateral posterior rectus sheath as soon as possible (step TRANS/LONG 5). This allows to continue retromuscular dissection at the contralateral side around the hernia sac.

In the transversal approach, a second additional 5 mm trocar can then be inserted contralaterally on the same horizontal line to facilitate further dissection more cephalad (step TRANS 6). In lateral hernias, a true *preperitoneal* dissection (i.e.posterior to the posterior rectus sheath) is done lateral to the semilunar line: the lateral border of the rectus sheath needs to be opened to continue dissection in the preperitoneal Bogros' space (step LONG 6). This dissection can be continued fairly easy up to the lumbar region. In order to prevent damage to the motor innervation of the anterolateral abdominal wall and to proceed easily with dissection, the exact preperitoneal plane between the peritoneum and the transversalis fascia needs to be cleaved. When the hernia orifice is located very laterally (e.g. lumbar hernia), the three trocars of the longitudinal approach can be inserted just next to the midline at the same side of the hernia in order to avoid midline dissection.

The technique described above involves a standard dissection in the retromuscular plane, i.e. anterior to the posterior rectus sheath, because a true preperitoneal dissection carries a substantial risk of tearing the peritoneum, especially in thin patients, exactly as in the open surgical technique (2). Below the arcuate line however, preperitoneal dissection is much more easily achieved in Bogros' and Retzius' space, as in endoscopic totally preperitoneal (TEP) inguinal hernia repair. This advantage can be used by inserting the first trocar and/or performing the initial dissection in the lower abdomen where the posterior rectus sheath is absent. Extending the dissection more cephalad involves then opening of the posterior rectus sheath at the arcuate line to continue with retromuscular dissection (Fig. 4).

The dissection of the hernia sac is often the most frustrating and delicate part of the procedure (step TRANS/LONG 7). This might be facilitated by a maximum of dissection of the surrounding tissue. In cases where the hernia is largely composed of preperitoneal fat without or with only a small subcutaneous peritoneal sac, full reduction of the hernia without or with minimal tearing the peritoneum is fairly easy. No attempt should be made to dissect out a sac firmly attached in the superficial subcutaneous tissue because of the danger for accidental perforation or secondary ischemic necrosis of the skin. This can be appreciated with a visual control of the abdominal wall by transillumination with the endoscope. When reduction is not possible, the peritoneum is incised at the hernia neck, leaving a circumferential perforation of the peritoneum at this site. This stage of the procedure should be performed with extreme caution because of the risk for damage to intestinal loops in the hernia sac. After reducing the hernia contents, the abdominal cavity can be entered with the scope in order to confirm the absence of intestinal damage due to the dissection. Adequate dissection is continued in all directions and can be verified by applying external compression at the hernia orifice and inserting an intramuscular needle along the "outer circle" percutaneously. If further dissection in the extraperitoneal space becomes too tedious due to the intraabdominal pressure, a Veress needle can be placed in the left subcostal region. In most cases, no attempt is made to close the hernia neck. On the other hand, the edges of the lacerated/incised peritoneum are approximated whenever possible with clips or sutures. Hemostasis is carefully performed before insertion of the mesh.

The choice of the mesh depends on the integrity of the peritoneum. In the cases with no or only a minimal defect of the peritoneum or with the intestinal loops covered by omentum, a polypropylene mesh is used. In the other cases, where at least part of the mesh is in direct contact with the intestines, a specially designed mesh for maximal tissue ingrowth in the abdominal wall and minimal adhesion formation at the visceral side is used. The mesh is cut ensuring a minimal circumferential overlapping up to the "outer circle". Before insertion, the mesh is marked with a pencil or a small slit in the middle upper or lower border to facilitate orientation after implantation. The mesh is rolled along its longest axis and introduced under direct view with an endoscopic grasping forceps through the incision of the 12 mm trocar, which is temporarily removed and then reinserted (Fig. 5). This needs to be a smooth manoeuvre in order to maintain the pneumoperitoneum. The mesh is unrolled in the retromuscular space and fixed into the abdominal wall with titanium helicoidal tackers (Protack®, Tyco) on the "outer circle" circumferentially, starting in the upper corner on the contralateral side of the trocars and continuing along the borders every 3-4 cm all around, to obtain flat application under slight tension, ensuring tension-free application after desufflation. Fixation of the mesh is performed under continuous control with a long intramuscular needle inserted percutaneously along the "outer circle" (Fig. 5). During the tacking, counterpressure from outside is applied, ensuring the absence of skin retraction due to a too superficial tacker insertion. If needed, a tacker can easily be removed using a Maryland curved dissector. No transcutaneous sutures are used. In some cases, a fourth 5 mm trocar can be inserted for adequate mesh fixation.

In larger hernias, a closed suction drain is inserted in the space underneath the mesh. Removal of the trocars and desufflation is performed under direct view. The fascia at the 12 mm site is closed with interrupted Vicryl® 1 sutures (Ethicon). The skin is closed with interrupted Monocryl® 3/0 sutures (Ethicon) intracutaneously. A pressure dressing is not applied systematically (Fig. 6).

Oral intake is started the next day. Nonnarcotic analgesics are generally sufficient for pain relief, although the tackers may cause some prolonged pain on mobilisation. The suction drain is removed when draining ≤ 10cc over 24 hours. Patients are discharged after a few days with the advice to restrict heavy physical activity (lifting, weight bearing) during the first three weeks postoperatively.

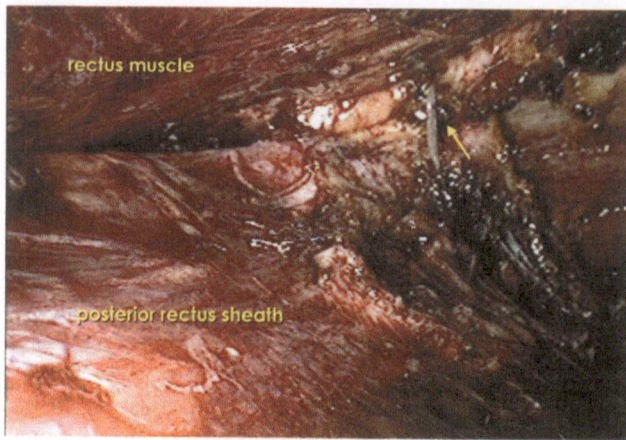

Fig. 4. View of the retromus-cular plane with the intact peritoneum below. The arrow shows an intramuscular needle inserted percutaneously to verify adequate dissection.

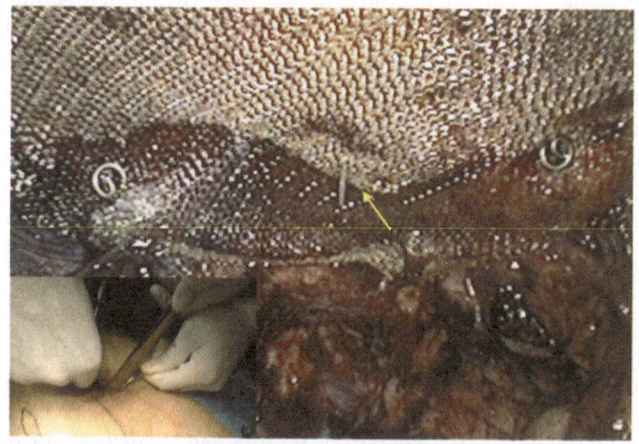

Fig. 5. Polypropylene mesh introduced (inset) and fixed with helicoidal tackers; in the middle of the picture an intramuscular needle is inserted percutaneously to verify adequate mesh covering in the right upper corner.

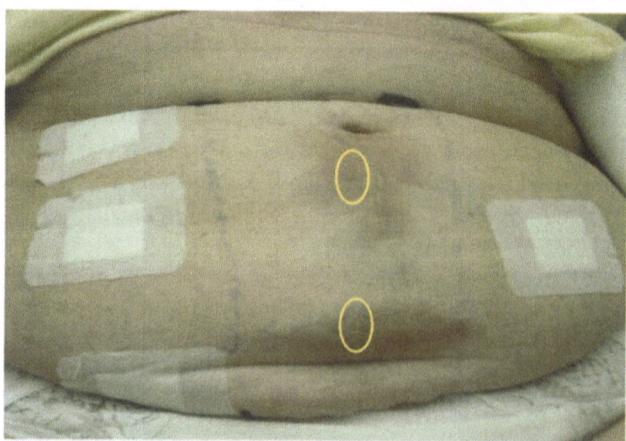

Fig. 6. Postoperative view on day 1 with minimal bruising at the two hernia orifices (ellipse subumbilical and suprapubic). In this patient one additional trocar was inserted contrala-terally for adequate mesh fixation.

Table I. Different steps in endoscopic totally preperitoneal ventral hernia repair

<u>**Longitudinal approach (LONG)**</u>

1. first trocar at semilunar line
2. ipsilateral retromuscular dissection
3. two additional trocars on the same vertical line (one cephalad, one caudal to the first trocar)
4. midline preperitoneal dissection after opening of the medial border of the ipsilateral posterior rectus sheath
5. contralateral retromuscular dissection after opening of the medial border of the contralateral posterior rectus sheath
6. in lateral hernias: opening of the lateral border of the contralateral posterior rectus sheath + preperitoneal dissection
7. dissection of hernia sac

<u>**Transversal approach (TRANS)**</u>

1. first trocar just next to the midline (paramedian)
2. ipsilateral retromuscular dissection
3. one additional lateral trocar on the same horizontal line (ipsilateral)
4. midline preperitoneal dissection after opening of the medial border of the ipsilateral posterior rectus sheath
5. contralateral retromuscular dissection after opening of the medial border of the contralateral posterior rectus sheath
6. second additional lateral trocar on the same horizontal line (contralateral)
7. dissection of hernia sac

RESULTS

During a period of 9 months (September 2000 – May 2001) we operated 15 patients with an incisional or ventral hernia who underwent an extraperitoneal mesh repair by endoscopic approach. Complete reduction of the hernia without peritoneal laceration could be accomplished in one third of our patients. Three of these 5 patients had an epigastric hernia, either primary or incisional. In two patients (13%), one epigastric and one umbilical incisional hernia, full reduction of the sac was possible, but with damage of the peritoneum. In the 8 other patients (53%) the peritoneum was incised at the hernia neck. A Veress needle was only necessary in one patient. In order to minimise postoperative seroma formation, a large subcutaneous sac was retracted and fixed with a suture to the fascia edge in one patient and in another patient with a lumbar incisional hernia, the elongated transversalis fascia was reefed onto the abdominal wall next to the hernia orifice. In a patient with a paracolostomy hernia, the fascial edges were approximated with an Ethibond® 0 suture (Ethicon). In all other cases, no attempt was made to close the hernia orifice. On the other hand, the edges of the peritoneal sac were reapproximated whenever possible, once with clips and once, in the parastomal hernia, with a Vicryl® 2/0 suture (Ethicon). The average width of the hernia orifice was 3 ± 0.93 cm (median ± 95% confidence interval; range 1.5-9 cm). A polypropylene mesh (Marlex®, Bard) was used in six cases. In the other patients, expanded polytetrafluoroethylene (ePTFE) (DualMesh plus with holes®, Gore; n=4) or a composite mesh of polypropylene and ePTFE (Composix®, Bard; n=5) was used. The median surface area of the meshes used was 285±51 cm^2 (range

143-552 cm^2). In two cases, a fourth 5 mm trocar was inserted during fixation. A closed suction drain was inserted in the retromuscular space in 9 patients (60%). Four patients developed minimal subcutaneous bruising/ecchymosis, but none of the patients without a suction drain developed a seroma or hematoma. The median duration of postoperative hospital stay was 5±1 days (range 3-13 days). The prolonged hospital stay of one patient (13 days) was due to a cerebrovascular accident in the postoperative period. Patients were only discharged when drainage had ceased and the suction drain was removed, except in our first patient. He developed a postoperative ileus and was discharged 10 days postoperatively with the drain in situ because of prolonged drainage of serous fluid. This drain was removed 4 days after discharge. He was readmitted on the 25th postoperative day with fever and a local subcutaneous infection (2 x 2 cm) with total regression after IV antibiotics and local incision. One other patient developed fever and local cellulititis signs (20 x 15 cm) after discharge. A third patient had postoperative fever without a clear focus. Both were also successfully treated with antibiotic. The further course in all patients was uneventfull with a median follow-up period of 126±37 days (range 13- 276 days). Apart from the postoperative ileus in our first patient, no other intraabdominal complications (hematoma, intestinal perforation, abcess formation) were encountered. One patient has a small palpable painless and nonreducible subcutaneous nodule, possibly a reaction on a tacker. One recurrence was seen 5.5 months postoperatively (6.7%). This was the fourth patient in the series with the fourth largest defect (epigastric eventration with three hernia orifices in a transverse incision) in whom a large mesh (28 x 12 cm) was inserted preperitoneally.

DISCUSSION

A recently published randomized trial has confirmed the superiority of mesh repair versus suture repair in the treatment of incisional hernias (7). However, the combined use of synthetic material and an extensive dissection in the abdominal wall implicates a substantial risk for local abdominal wall complications such as prolonged postoperative pain, wound infection and seroma or hematoma formation (8). These drawbacks might be counteracted by a laparoscopic approach. Advantages of laparoscopy such as minimal postoperative pain and decreased rate of wound complications resulting in an early recovery with shorter hospital stay and faster return to daily activities have been related to the minimal surgical trauma to the abdominal wall. Therefore, it is not surprising that LVHR with intraabdominal placement of a mesh (without abdominal wall dissection) was reported for the first time early in the nineties (9). This technique has been reported to be safe and efficacious with excellent results on the short- and long-term in some larger, but not randomized, series (10, 11). Length of hospital stay was shown to be a major advantage in two prospective nonrandomized series comparing laparoscopic versus open repair, but the difference in postoperative abdominal wall complications was less obvious. On the contrary, the reoperation rate for major complications was higher in the laparoscopy groups (6, 12). The only randomized trial available in literature, showed, apart from a significantly lower length of hospital stay, also less postoperative and late complications in the laparoscopy group. Reoperation rate was comparable in both groups. The number of recurrences after a mean follow-up period of 27 months was 0% for the laparoscopic group vs. 6.7% in the open group (13).

Though apart from the minimal invasive approach, LVHR differs in three major ways from the basic principles of the widely accepted french technique of extraperitoneal (retromuscular) mesh implantation in open surgery (2, 3, 14, 15).

Firstly, the extraperitoneal localization ensures adequate abdominal wall reinforcement due to immediate firm fixation of the prosthesis with the intrabdominal pressure exerted via the peritoneal envelope (16). Also tissue ingrowth might be more extensive than in the intraabdominal position. This might have an effect on the recurrence rate, the major outcome parameter in hernia surgery. In large series of open mesh repair with long follow-up, recurrence rates are around 5-6% (17). Recent reports of LVHR show recurrence rates comparable with or superior to the open technique (5, 10, 13, 18). It may be that the exact position of the mesh, extra- versus intraperitoneal is not that relevant, as long as the mesh is placed in the sublay position, i.e. underneath the hernia orifice, taking advantage of the intraabdominal pressure. Nevertheless, a follow-up of at least three to five years is necessary to determine the long-term recurrence rate (19). The longest follow-up in laparoscopic incisional hernia repair available in the literature is more than 4 years (mean 51 months), with a recurrence rate of 9.3% (11). These authors clearly state that in order to minimize the recurrence rate (due to mesh migration or shrinkage) adequate overlapping of the defect and fixation of the mesh with full thickness transparietal sutures is necessary.

Although the use of foreign material inside the peritoneal cavity has been discouraged before in open surgery (20, 21), a new generation of meshes with different surfaces and/or materials for intraperitoneal implantation have been developed in recent years in order to promote tissue ingrowth on the parietal side and to minimize the formation of intestinal adhesions on the visceral side, resulting in a diminished risk for intestinal occlusion, erosion and fistulisation at the site of the mesh or at the site of the staples used to fix the mesh (6). However, as in endoscopic inguinal hernia repair, a polypropylene mesh (22) may be used when positioning the mesh in the extraperitoneal plane as described, precluding the use of these more expensive new meshes. Together with the use of reusable instruments (only the 12 mm trocar is a disposable instrument in our technique) this may be a more cost-effective solution. In addition, extraperitoneal mesh implantation may reduce the need for extensive surgical fixation (2) and therefore not only avoid complications related to the intraperitoneal position of the mesh but also of the fixating devices, especially in the suprapubic or subxyphoidal region (bleeding, bladder trauma, nerve entrapment with prolonged postoperative pain, pericardial effusion...). Most late complications of mesh implantations occur with a delay of several months or even years and are thus being neglected by most of the present reports (23).

Secondly, in contrast to Flament and Rives (15), we believe that in most cases in open surgery, the peritoneum does not need to be opened or only to a minimal extent, thus avoiding adhesiolysis, potential intestinal damage and prolonged postoperative ileus. The transabdominal route in LVHR however carries a small but inherent risk for postoperative peritonitis due to delayed intestinal perforation (after coagulation trauma) or nonrecognised enterotomy during adhesiolysis (4, 5). This makes laparoscopic incisional or ventral hernia repair a procedure reserved for experienced laparoscopic surgeons.

Thirdly, in LVHR and in our technique, a mesh is inserted tension free without reconstruction of the abdominal wall. The posterior or anterior rectus sheath are not approximated and thus, the hernia orifice is not closed. The latter does not seem to be a major problem in terms of tensile strength of the abdominal wall, as in some cases in open mesh repair, the abdominal wall cannot be reconstructed either without undue tension (2, 15). As long as the inserted mesh is sufficiently overlapping the hernia defect and fixed within the abdominal wall, approximation of the posterior and/or anterior rectus sheath is probably not necessary in order to prevent hernia recurrence. With regard to the risk for local skin complications in case of direct contact between the mesh and the skin (in patients with a thin subcutaneous fat layer), the presence of a retained subcutaneous hernia sac will cover the prosthesis at the hernia orifice and may prevent subsequent superficial erosion due to the mesh.

We developed this new technique, mimicking the open surgical procedure and following the principles of the TEP repair for inguinal hernia, thus combining the advantages of mesh positioning in the retromuscular plane, but avoiding the potential complications related to the transabdominal approach of LVHR and the more traumatic incision of the open repair. Apart from one case report of a patient who underwent an endoscopic retroperitoneal fixation of a mesh to the iliac crest for a lumbar hernia following iliac bone crest harvesting (24), there are no reports in the literature using this technique for the repair of ventral hernias. These results are of course very preliminary and need further long-term evaluation, but our short-term results show that endoscopic totally preperitoneal ventral hernia repair is feasible with minimal morbidity. Three patients developed postoperative fever and/or signs of superficial infection treated by antibiotics, although this might have been overshooting in our patient with fever of unknown origin. Preperitoneal dissection, with more surgical trauma to the abdominal wall than in LVHR, postoperative drainage is advocated in case of extensive retromuscular disection because blood and exudates can easily accumulate and cause postoperative haematoma and seroma formation. This may cause postoperative discomfort and be a substrate for infection. In case of prolonged wound drainage (more than 4-5 days), vacuum suction can be changed into passive drainage before removing the drain. Taking these measures and restricting the administration of intravenous antibiotics would definitely decrease hospital stay further. With a median follow-up period of only 4 months, no conclusions can be drawn concerning the recurrence rate. One may argue that the opening of the medial border of both posterior rectus sheath around the hernia orifice in our technique is a point of weakness in the abdominal wall, because both sides are not approximated. This argument seems of minimal importance from experiences in open mesh repair (15) and because there is no posterior rectus sheath at all beneath the arcuate line. Adequate overlapping of at least 5cm circumferentially seems to be the key for recurrence prevention. In contrast to LVHR, fixation of the mesh with sutures or tackers might be of lesser importance.

Another important topic is the fact that most reports of LVHR come from so-called centers of excellence with a wide experience in laparoscopic surgery (efficacy studies). Since ventral hernia surgery is a very common procedure, the new technique should be as safe on the short- and long-term as the open procedure. Our approach is technically definitely more demanding than LVHR, at least in the beginning of the learning curve period, with longer operative times at least for the first ten interventions. Later on, operative time is drastically reduced and the surgery does not take longer than the open procedure. In order to get familiar with endoscopic dissection in the extraperitoneal space of the anterior abdominal wall, we advocate to carefully select the first patients and to start with a longitudinal approach for a hernia in the lower or upper abdomen with a hernia orifice not larger than 5 x 5 cm. This would allow a prosthesis to be inserted of maximum 15 x 15 cm. For midline hernias, this fits exactly within the rectus sheath with the trocars inserted at the level of the semilunar line in most patients. A suprapubic incisional hernia or incisional hernia postappendectomy has the advantage that dissection in the preperitoneal space is rather straightforward, as in TEP inguinal hernia repair. A epigastric hernia has the advantage that in many cases a lot of preperitoneal fat is protruding superficial to the hernia sac. Together with the absence of a previous midline incision in case of a primary hernia, this will substantially facilitate the dissection at the hernia orifice and further on the midline. Here also, preperitoneal dissection is possible far above the subcostal margin and consequently, mesh positioning is easier with minimal fixation. A slightly obese patient with some more preperitoneal fat is therefore a more suitable candidate than a very thin patient because of easier dissection and lower risk for accidental perforation of the peritoneum.

The strategy in our department for primary ventral and incisional hernia mesh repair at the moment is a preperitoneal endoscopic approach in most cases, except for giant hernias (more than 10 cm in width), recurrence after previous open preperitoneal mesh repair and previous multiple laparotomies, although the extent of intraabdominal adhesion formation is only of minimal relevance. If dissection is cumbersome and takes too long, e.g. due to difficulty to find the right plane of dissection, bleeding or extensive damage to the peritoneum, the repair is continued by a classical open approach. In these cases, the time consumed for dissection is not lost, since essentially the same plane can be used for open mesh repair. In some selected cases, we do use a true laparoscopic approach with an intraabdominal mesh. In our view, the optimal patient for the latter procedure is a patient with a rather small hernia (e.g. umbilical hernia) and several risk factors for recurrence (obesity, pulmonary disease...) which support the use of a prosthesis. In most of these cases, no major adhesiolysis needs to be performed and adequate overlapping is easily obtained. Another good indication is a recurrence after extraperitoneal mesh repair. Mesh fixation is performed with helicoidal tackers and four full thickness transparietal nonabsorbable sutures. These staples need to be fixed deeply in the mesh and the abdominal wall to minimize the risk for late intestinal erosion.

In conclusion, the potential advantages of endoscopic totally preperitoneal ventral hernia repair are comparable with those for TEP inguinal hernia repair. For the reasons pointed out below (Table II), and a condition that the long term results are (at least) comparable to those of open surgery, we believe the endoscopic total preperitoneal technique deserves to be compared in future studies with open incisional hernia repair on one hand and LVHR on the other hand.

Table II. Comparison between endoscopic totally preperitoneal and laparoscopic ventral hernia repair (LVHR)

Totally preperitoneal repair	LVHR
more difficult dissection (longer duration of surgery)	easier dissection (shorter duration of surgery)
no extensive adhesiolysis required	extensive adhesiolysis eventually required
retromuscular mesh position (mesh covered by peritoneum)	intraperitoneal mesh position (mesh not covered)
adequate overlapping of the defect necessary	adequate overlapping of the defect necessary
minimal mesh fixation necessary (?)	maximal mesh fixation necessary
postoperative drainage advocated in selected cases	postoperative drainage not required (?)

References

1. Stoppa R. The treatment of groin and incisional hernias. World J Surg 1989; 13: 545-554.

2. Wantz GE. Incisional hernias of the abdomen. In Atlas of hernia surgery. Raven Press, New York 1991, pp 179-216.

3. Stoppa R, Quintin M. Les déficiences de la paroi abdominale chez le sujet âgée – colloque avec le practicien. Sem Hop Paris 1969; 45: 2182-2185.

4. Koehler RH, Voeller G. Recurrences in laparoscopic incisional hernia repairs: a personal series and review of the literature. JSLS 1999; 3: 293-304.

5. Kyzer S, Alis M, Aloni Y, Charuzi I. Laparoscopic repair of postoperation ventral hernia. Surg Endosc 1999; 13: 928-931.

6. DeMaria EJ, Moss JM, Sugerman HJ. Laparoscopic intraperitoneal polytetrafluoroethylene (PTFE) prosthetic patch repair of ventral hernia. Surg Endosc 2000; 14: 326-329.

7. Luijendijk RW, Hop WCJ, van den Tol MP, de Lange DCD et al. A comparison of suture repair with mesh repair for incisional hernia. N Engl J Med 2000; 343: 392-398.

8. Leber GE, Garb JL, Alexander AI, Reed WP. Long-term complications associated with prosthetic repair of incisional hernias. Arch Surg 1998; 133: 378-382.

9. LeBlanc KA, Booth WV. Laparoscopic repair of incisional abdominal hernias using expanded polytetrafluoroethylene: preliminary findings. Surg Laparosc Endo 1993; 3(1): 39-41.

10. Heniford BT, Park A, Ramshaw BJ, Voeller G. Laparoscopic ventral and incisional hernia repair in 407 patients. J Am Coll Surg 2000; 190: 645-650.

11. LeBlanc KA, Booth WV, Whitaker JM, Bellanger DE. Laparoscopic incisional and ventral herniorraphy : our initial 100 patients. Hernia 2001 ; 5 : 41-45.

12. Balique JG, Alexandre JH, Arnaud JP, Benchetrit S et al. Intraperitoneal treatment of incisional and umbilical hernias: intermediate results of a multicentric prospective clinical trial using an innovative composite mesh. Hernia 2000; 4 (Suppl): S10-S16.

13. Carbajo MA, Martin del Olmo JC, Blanco JI, de la Cuesta C et al. Laparoscopic treatment versus open surgery in the solution of major incisional and abdominal wall hernias with mesh. Surg Endosc 1999 ; 13 : 250-252.

14. Rives J, Lardennois B, Pire JC, Hibon J. Les grandes éventrations. Importance du « volet abdominal » et des troubles respiratoires qui lui sont secondaires. Chirurgie 1973 ; 99 : 547-563.

15. Flament JB, Rives J. Major incisional hernia. In Hernias and Surgery of the Abdominal Wall. Edited by JP Chevrel. Springer-Verlag, Berlin Heidelberg New York 1998, pp 128-158.

16. Stoppa R, Henry X, Odimba E, Verhaeghe P et al. Traitement chirurgical des éventrations post-opératoires. Utilisation des prothèses en tulle de Dacron et de la colle biologique. Nouv Presse Med 1980 ; 9 : 3541-3545.

17. Alexandre JH, Aouad K, Bethoux JP, Bouillot JL. Recent advances in incisional hernia treatment. Hernia 2000; 4 (suppl): S1-S2.

18. Chowbey PK, Sharma A, Khullar R, Mann V et al. Laparoscopic ventral hernia repair. J. Laparoendosc Adv Surg Tech 2000; 10: 79-84.

19. Hesselink VJ, Luijendijk RW, de Wilt JHW, Heide R, Jeekel J. An evaluation of risk factors in incisional hernia recurrence. Surg Gynecol Obstet 1993; 176: 228-234.

20. Stoppa R, Louis D, Henry X, Verhaeghe P. Les éventrations postopératoires. A propos d'une série de 247 opérés. Chir (Paris) 1985 ; 111 : 303-305.

21. Stoppa R. Errors, difficulties and complications in hernia repairs using the GPRVS. Prob Gen Surg 1995; 12: 139-145.

22. Amid PK, Silulman AG, Lichtenstein IL. Selecting synthetic mesh for the repair of groin hernia. Postgraduate Gen Surg 1992; 150-155.

23. Klinge U. Congress report on "Incisional Hernia, Aachen, Germany, September 17-18, 1999. Hernia 1999; 3: 241-242.

24. Woodward AM, Flint LM, Ferrara JJ. Laparoscopic retroperitoneal repair of recurrent postoperative lumbar hernia. J Laparoendosc Adv Surg Tech A 1999; 9: 181-186.

CHAPTER 26

Laparoscopic Transabdominal Prepritoneal Ventral Hernia Repair: indications, technique and results

S. Roll, W.C. Marujo

INCISIONAL HERNIAS

Incidence

Incisional hernias represent one of the more common complications of abdominal surgical procedures. The true incidence of incisional hernias has not been well defined, although a number of reports suggest that 3 to 13% of patients undergoing laparotomy will develop a fascial defect in their abdominal scar (1). The majority of incisional hernias occur within the first postoperative year. However, the limited follow-up of most series may underestimate late hernia occurrence.

Diagnosis

Most patients with small and uncomplicated incisional hernias are asymptomatic or have only minor or intermittent complains. However, these postoperative hernias may be a significant source of morbidity. Patients with incisional hernias alter their lifestyles so as not to exacerbate their abdominal wall hernia and often report an aesthetic appearance or suffer from discomfort, pain, or, occasionally, intestinal obstruction.

Predisposing factors

Predisposing factors for the development of incisional hernias include patient characteristics such as advanced age; male gender; prostatism; radiotherapy; steroid therapy; and systemic diseases such as obesity, cancer, chronic hepatic and cardiopulmonary failures, severe anemia, and malnutrition (2, 3). The underlying pathologic process and operative technical factors are also fundamental factors. Although the clinical experience seems to suggest that vertical celiotomy and the type of suture used, e.g., continuous suture and mass tissue closure, may increase the risk of incisional hernias, randomized studies have failed to show that any of these factors significantly alters the incidence of postoperative incisional hernia. Wound infection is associated with a fivefold increase in the risk of developing hernia (1, 4).

PRINCIPLES OF TREATMENT

The classical principles of ventral hernia repair are wound closure with no excessive tension, sutures placed in healthy tissue, and the use of strong material to support the wound through the critical period of healing. In many cases of incisional hernia with small-size defects, fascial closure can be achieved by apposing the fascial edges, closing the wound. When the fascial defect is large, a number of techniques have been proposed, including relaxing incisions, internal retention sutures, muscle or fascial flaps, fascial grafts, and the mesh repair (5). However, the results have been often disappointing. Primary repair with suture only has been associated with 25 to 52% failure rates (6). The use of a prosthetic material to cover the hernia defect has substantially reduced the incidence of recurrence. In a multicenter randomized trial enrolling 100 patients on each arm, Luijendijk et al. compared the results of suture alone to mesh repair for incisional hernias (7). After a follow-up of 36 months, the three-year cumulative rates of recurrence among patients who had suture only and those who had mesh repair of a primary hernia were 43% and 24%, respectively. The recurrence rates were 58% and 20% for repair of the first recurrence. The risk factors for recurrence were suture repair, infection, prostatism, and previous surgery for abdominal aortic aneurysm. The size of the hernia did not affect the rate of recurrence. The majority of the recurrences occurs in the first two years after the repair. The same factors involved in the genesis of these incisional hernias may contribute to these results.

Prosthesis materials

The use of prosthetic materials to assist in incisional hernioplasty usually demands a more extensive dissection and may slightly increase the risk of wound healing complications (5, 8). The synthetic material should be physically unmodified by tissue fluid, chemically inert and non-carcinogenic. It should also induce no inflammatory or foreign body-reaction, no allergy and no hypersensitivity (9, 10). Finally, it should be capable to resist mechanical stress, to be tailored in the form required and to be easily and fully sterilized. The most popular prosthesis materials are made of polypropylene (PP), polyester (POL) and expanded polytetraflourethylene (ePTFE). They are all non-absorbable and there is no clear evidence from the literature that supports a preference for the clinical use of any one of the three main materials (11). PP showed a relatively small inflammatory response with a far lesser degree of foreign-body reaction than does the POL mesh. Expanded PTFE elicits less chronic inflammatory-cell reaction but greater foreign-body reaction. Mesh infection rates in selected laparoscopic series for repair of ventral and incisional hernias varies from 0.5 to 12% (12). Despite different characteristics regarding fibroblastic reaction and time of incorporation, all these prosthetic materials are associated with a high incidence of dense adhesions and the reported low risk of adhesions and fistula formation by placing the mesh in contact with the peritoneum is not undisputable (13). On the basis of current data, it seems that cost should be the deciding factor.

Repair strategies

Although the modern era of hernia repair began more than a century ago, controversies continue about the optimal surgical technique to repair incisional hernias. Open techniques involve a large incision, an extensive subcutaneous and intrabdominal dissection and often necessitate the placement of drains. Complication rates range from 8 to 19% after open ventral repair (14, 15). Fistula rates after elective open hernia mesh repair varies from 2 to 5% (6). Moreover, the infected prosthesis should be taken off, demanding a further more complicated repair. Transabdominal approaches carry the risk of injuring the viscera adherent to the undersurface of the scar. The basic strategy of the open repair is based on the Stoppa technique: the peritoneal cavity should not be entered and the mesh is secured to the fascial edges in the preperitoneal space (16). However, the risk of reentering the site of a previous incision is an inadvertent enterotomy. The open repair allows the concomitant excision of a usually wide, irregular and aesthetic scar. If this is the case, it is not unusual to enter the abdominal cavity.

Surgical laparoscopy has become an increasingly popular mode of treatment for many diseases because it potentially offers cost savings as a result of shorter hospital stays, less postoperative pain and more rapid return to work (17). Laparoscopic hernioplasty has been reported to be a safe and feasible technique with low morbidity and low rates of early recurrence. LeBlanc and Booth first reported the laparoscopic approach to repair incisional hernias in 1993, and several series have now demonstrated the efficacy of minimally invasive surgery in incisional hernia repair (18). The laparoscopic repair involves no long incision, no wide fascial dissection or flap creation, and usually no drains. It also minimizes the manipulation of a potentially contaminated site because the trocars are placed far distant from the original wound (19). Moreover, the pneumoperitoneum facilitates the necessary adhesionlysis in order to identify the edges of the defect and the hernia sac. Enterotomy rates in selected laparoscopic series of ventral hernia repair, including incisional hernias and many with previous open mesh repair, vary from 0 to 14% (Table I). Mesh infection rates vary from 0.5 to 12% (12). One of the drawbacks of the laparoscopic approach is that it does not allow a aesthetic reconstruction of the abdominal wall since the old scar that covers the hernia defect is left untouched. The need for an overall aesthetic result cannot be underestimated because this is frequently demanded by the patient.

Table I. Comparison studies of laparoscopic versus open repair of ventral/incisional hernia

Study	Repair		Defect	Surg.	Complications			Hosp.			
	Type	Patients	Size (n)	Time (cm2)	Intraop. (min)	Postop.	Reop.	Stay (days)	Follow-up (months)	Recurrence	Cost (US$)
Holzman et al (25)	Open	16	148	98	0	5	2	4.9	18	2	7.299
	Lap	21	105	128	1	4	0	1.6	20	2	4.395
Park et al (26)	Open	49	105	78	1	17	0	6.5	53	17	–
	Lap	56	99	95	0	10	2	3.4	24	6	–
Carbajo et al* (27)	Open	30	141	111	0	35	1	9	27	2	–
	Lap	30	139	87	0	5	1	2	27	0	–

Prospective Trial

INDICATIONS FOR LAPAROSCOPIC REPAIR

The size of the defect and the characteristics of a particular patient should dictate the best technical strategy. Patient selection for laparoscopic incisional hernioplasty is usually based on a demonstrable fascial defect over a previous abdominal incision or a highly suspected abdominal wall defect in a very obese patient such as seen in Spigelian hernia. The patient must be able to tolerate general anesthesia and abdominal insufflation (20). Patient size is not a prohibiting factor, nor is the history of previous abdominal explorations or previous attempted repairs with or without placement of prosthetic material. A massive incisional hernia with the protrusion of a substantial portion of the abdominal viscera might be a contra-indication for a laparoscopic approach. A significant loss of the abdomen domain by the intestine might preclude the placement of the functional trocars because of insufficient lateral space. A densely scarred abdomen, inability to safely establish a pneumoperitoneum and the presence of infected material in the abdomen may also contra-indicate the laparoscopic approach. It should be noted that intensity and extension of the adhesion formation is unpredictable. This way, multiple previous abdominal operations do not preclude laparoscopy since an entry port for the first trocar can be obtained. The so-called "Swiss cheese" hernia is a good indication for the laparoscopic approach since it allows a very clear delineation of the wall defects and a more precise repair. Hernias very close to the costal margin may be difficult to treat through an open approach since they usually lack a good rim of strong tissue to secure the mesh. In this situation, the laparoscopic approach is more appropriate, considering the mesh can be easily tacked to the internal face of the abdominal cavity. Moreover, full-thickness stitches around this area are usually followed by pain.

LAPAROSCOPIC TRANSABDOMINAL PREPERITONEAL REPAIR

Patient preparation and room setup

A thorough preoperative evaluation is performed. The patient is fully informed about the risks of recurrence and the chances for conversion into an open procedure. Educative handouts are given in order to help convalescence, emphasizing pain control. Factors that might increase the recurrence rate are corrected if at all possible in the preoperative period. Special attention is given to respiratory care before admitting the patient to the hospital. In-hospital standard guidelines to prepare patients for abdominal surgery are followed. Mechanical bowel preparation is not usually necessary. The patient is asked to void just before leaving the ward.

The patient is placed on the operating table in a dorsal recumbent position with the arms padded along the body. It is important that the patient be securely belted to the operating table in order to permit the extremes of table positioning, occasionally necessary for visceral retraction. General anesthesia is instituted and an orogastric tube is inserted for gastric decompression. Patients are given prophylactic antibiotic, usually a first-generation cephalosporin.

For most midline hernias, the surgeon stands on either the patient's left or right side. The video monitor is positioned on the opposite side, so the surgeon's view on the screen is parallel and in line with the laparoscopic repair of the hernia within the abdomen. The assistant stands opposite the surgeon, and a second monitor is placed in a suitable position.

Operative technique

Good laparoscopic skills are mandatory, since each anatomical situation may be unique. The surgeon must always keep a low threshold for conversion to an open repair. Access to the abdominal cavity is obtained in an area away from the hernia using the Veress needle or, more frequently, by the open technique. Pneumoperitoneum is established by insufflating the abdomen to 12-mm Hg with carbon dioxide. A 30-degree laparoscope is introduced through the initial trocar, and the abdomen is explored. The hernia defect and any associated adhesions are identified. Usually two or three additional trocars are inserted under direct vision. The ultimate number and the exact site of the trocars depend on each individual case. For an optimal view and exposure, it is better to place the working ports as far away from the hernia defect as possible. Since the mesh will overlap the defect by about 3 cm, a very lateral or inferior position of the trocar sites maximizes the view and the efficiency of the instruments.

The repair technique is based on the Stoppa technique utilized in the open surgical procedure, in which the prosthetic material is placed posteriorly to the anterior fascia (21). An adhesionlysis is performed to free the bowel off the abdominal wall and the margins of the hernia defect are clearly defined. External manual pressure on the abdominal wall helps to delineate the edges of the hernia defect. It also changes the angles of vision and usually facilitates the dissection. Once the entire abdominal wall is cleared up and any incarcerated omentum or bowel reduced, the hernia defect is measured by introducing a sterile ruler into the peritoneal cavity. The surgeon must be very cautious when dissecting the bowel wall or omentum off the hernia sac, which typically encompasses attenuated fascia and peritoneum. The adhesionlysis is almost always the most challenging part of this procedure, especially if a previous mesh repair has already been attempted. Any energy source is capable of causing a full-thickness injury to the bowel wall.

A harmonic scalpel may obviate the chances of an inadvertent injury. The standard approach in the advent of an enterotomy is the immediate simple suture. If this injury is complicated by a significant spillage of luminal fluids, an open primary repair might be performed or a staged laparoscopic mesh placement be devised.

The hernia sac contents are reduced and the peritoneal sac is now opened, followed by the precise delineation of the fascial defect, with at least 4-cm of healthy tissue surrounding it. Whenever possible, small-size fascial defects can be primarily closed by simply suturing the edges of the defect without tension. The suture is then covered by a mesh to reinforce de herniorrhaphy. This procedure may prevent the annoying sensation of the mesh just underlying the skin.

Dissecting within the preperitoneal plane in attempting to develop an intact layer to separate the mesh from the abdominal contents might be extremely difficult in some patients. If unsuccessful, this might result in a large peritoneal defect, leaving the mesh internally exposed. This is especially true in those patients with only a thin layer of subcutaneous fat and skin overlying the hernia. In this case, some authors recommend interfacing the omentum between the mesh and the bowel. However, we struggle to interface the sac layer between the mesh and the abdominal contents. (Fig. 1) Some particular hernias are easier to dissect out the healthy fascial edges within the preperitoneal space, including incisional hernias secondary to extra-peritoneal surgical incisions, such as lumbotomies or Pfannenstiel's, and defects away from the midline. If the preperitoneal technique is deemed impossible, the hernia sac is neither reduced, ressected nor opened and the mesh is positioned intraperitoneally according to the onlay technique (22).

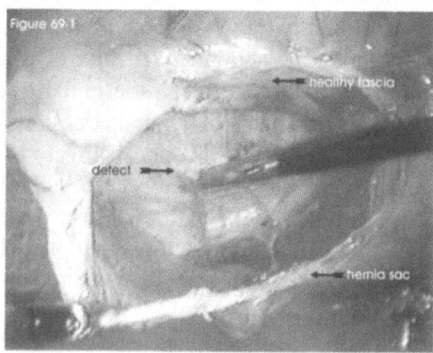

Fig. 1. The hernia sac is opened and the healthy fascia along the defect rim is clearly defined.

Prosthetic materials have been used with increasing confidence in direct contact with the abdominal contents. Complications have been few but may reflect selective reporting of good results. We always attempt to perform a transabdominal preperitoneal repair that uses mesh prosthesis to cover and close the hernia defect. The mesh, under some tension, should be secured to the abdominal wall using a hernia stapler or a tacking device, or sutured into position with full thickness transabdominal stitches buried in the subcutaneous tissues. The stitches along the outer border of the mesh should leave a 3 cm margin lateral to the edges of the fascial defect (Fig. 2). Drains are not used. The trocar sites are then closed in the usual fashion (23).

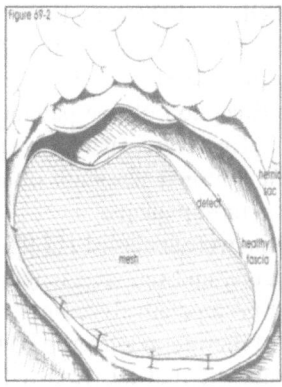

Fig. 2. The mesh is positioned into the preperi-toneal space and secured to the abdominal wall. The stitches along the outer border of the mesh must overlap the rim of the hernia defect by at least 3 cm.

The most common early complications after the laparoscopic repair are suture site pain, when using the transabdominal stitches, and seroma. The former is probably related to some muscular ischemia and nerve entrapment. The development of seroma is secondary to the creation of a dead space and a secretory reaction to the prosthetic material. Only large and symptomatic collections should be aspirated.

Immediate postoperative care

Postoperatively, patients are given narcotics for appropriate analgesia. Liquid diet is started on the same day, and patients are encouraged to ambulate as soon as possible. Bowel function usually resumes very early on (24). Selected patients may go home on the same day but most are discharged on the first postoperative day. Most patients develop an area of induration at the previous hernia site, but this resolves without complications or treatment within 4 to 6 weeks. In general, the patient is oriented to return to work at his convenience and heavy physical activities are allowed 2 to 4 weeks later.

PERSONAL SERIES RESULTS

From January 1997 to December 2000, 31 patients underwent attempted laparoscopic incisional hernia repair. We excluded from this series Spigelian hernias and incisional hernias which ended up requiring the intraperitoneal onlay technique. Total hernia repairs were 32 (one patient with 2 incisional hernias) and one required conversion to an open repair because of dense adhesions and an inadvertent intestinal injury. Thirteen were females and 18 males. The defect size ranged from 64 to 225 cm^2. The original surgical procedures were: hysterectomy (3), appendectomy (10), prostatectomy (5), gastrectomy (2), nephrectomy (5), laparotomy (2), epigastric herniorrhaphy (4), and umbilical herniorrhaphy (1). In all cases, except one (two incisional hernias), the defect was covered with a single large piece of mesh. In all but 3 patients (POL mesh), we used a PP mesh for the repair. The average operating time was 60 minutes (range: 30 – 240 minutes), varying in relation to the degree of adhesionlysis required. All patients were discharged in the first 24 hours, with the exception of one patient who had an enterotomy recognized during the procedure. The mean length of hospital stay was 1.2 days (1 to 4 days). Patients required minimal amounts of post surgical analgesia. Bowel function returned quickly in most patients.

There were no deaths. Four complications were recorded (12.9% of patients), most of them minor: 2 seromas. 1 hematoma, and one accidental small bowel enterotomy. Patients were closely followed postoperatively from 1 to 47 months (mean: 36 months), with no evidence of hernia recurrence. Most patients developed an area of induration at the hernia site, but this resolved without any treatment within 4 to 6 weeks. Apart from this transient induration, we have encountered no complications as a result of excising the hernia sac.

COMPARATIVE STUDIES OF OPEN VERSUS LAPAROSCOPIC REPAIR

Two retrospective studies and only one prospective study were designed to compare the results of the open surgery technique versus the laparoscopic approach for the repair of ventral hernias, which mostly included incisional defects (Table II). In 1997, Holzman et al. compared 21 patients with ventral / incisional hernias repaired laparoscopically with a group of 16 patients who had undergone the conventional open mesh repair. The mean follow-up was similar and two recurrences occurred in each group. The investigators concluded that the advantages of the laparoscopic approach seem to be a reduced rate of postoperative complications and wound healing problems, and more rapid recovery after surgery (25). In 1998, Park et al. compared 56 laparoscopic prosthetic repairs of large incisional hernias with 49 open surgical procedures. (26). The mean follow-up was 24 months for the laparoscopic group and 53 months for the open procedure. The hernia recurred in 6 patients in the laparoscopic group (11%) and in 17 patients in the open repair group (34%), but the investigators could not make a meaningful comparison of the recurrence rates because of the large difference in the follow-up period. They founded that the laparoscopic procedure took longer to perform but it was associated with fewer complications and shorter postoperative hospital stay. In the only prospective randomized study of laparoscopic repair versus open repair, Carbajo et al. randomized 60 patients over a 3-year period into two homogeneous groups to be operated on for major ventral hernias using mesh (27). Two recurrent hernias occurred in the open repair group and none in the laparoscopic group, with an average follow-up of 27 months. They concluded that laparoscopic repair reduces complications and the recurrence rate and offers several advantages over the classic surgical repair of abdominal wall defects.

Table II. Comparative results of laparoscopic ventral/incisional hernioplasty serices

Study**	Patients (n)	Complications Intraop.	Hosp. Postop.	Stay (days)*	Follow-up (months)*	Recurrences (n)
Toy(24)	193	4	28	2.0	22	9
Franklin(33)	176	0	9	2.2	30	2
Costanza(14)	31	0	2	2.0	18	1
Sanders(34)	12	0	3	3.5	12	1
Scott Roth(20)	73	2	14	2.9	17	7
Roll(35)	28	1	3	1.2	36	0
Heniford(6)	415	5	48	1.8	23	14

*Mean

**Ref.:

ADVANTAGES AND DISADVANTAGES OF DIFFERENT LAPAROSCOPIC TECHNIQUES

The critical assessment of the reported results is difficult and potentially misleading due to the significant variations in terminology, patient selection and operative techniques (28). There are no available data to unequivocally support an overt advantage of any particular technique to repair incisional hernias. Clinical judgment, previous experience and team surgical skills should guide the decision of which technique to apply to a particular patient. Despite the pitfalls of the availale data, mainly from retrospective studies of selected patients, recurrence and complication rates do not seem to be much different, regardless the technique employed: open versus laparoscopic, laparoscopic intraperitoneal versus preperitoneal.

The most popular laparoscopic technique of incisional hernia repair proposes a transperitoneal approach using a composite mesh prosthesis in intraperitonel location (29, 30). Biomaterials have become an important tool because they can permanently replace the defective transversalis fascia and permit the creation of a true tension-free hernioplasty. However, utilization of biomaterials is associated with four major concerns: rejection, infection, early adhesion and fixation and host tissue incorporation. It is well known that a peritoneal defect or the presence of a foreign body in the abdominal cavity creates adhesions (13). This in turn may result in major complications, including intestinal obstruction, migration of the foreign body and erosion into the bowel, fistula and infection. In general, complications resulting from intraperitoneal adhesions account for 1% of all emergency surgical admissions and 3% of emergency abdominal operations (7). These concerns have prompted the development of a further refinement in the transabdominal laparoscopic approach: the preperitoneal laparoscopic mesh repair. Dissecting within the preperitoneal plane in order to create an anatomical room for the mesh may sometimes be extremely difficult. On the other hand, our own experience shows that this approach is technically feasible in many circumstances and, indeed, this procedure is an extension of our current laparoscopic techniques for repairing inguinal hernias (31). However, we should also underscore the fact that even the preperitoneal repair of inguinal hernias have not been free of adhesions and associated bowel complications. Only a longer follow-up will be able to determine if the theoretical advantages of positioning the mesh in the preperitoneal location will overcome the possible disadvantages of a more tedious procedure that usually demands a longer operative time (32).

SUMMARY

The laparoscopic route has made possible the introduction of new surgical techniques for the repair of major abdominal wall defects. The laparoscopic surgeon is able to minimize the great degree of tissue traumatism involved in the classic surgery, typically associated with large fascial dissections, tense sutures, and postoperative drainages.

Laparoscopic repair of incisional hernias is a promising but still new technique that may be seen as a further refinement of the current surgical armamentarium to treat this common problem in general surgery. As with any new operation, we should initially be more careful about patient selection before embarking in a broader application of this technique. Adequate training and judicious indication can certainly ensure good surgical outcomes.

Up to now, patients in several series have tolerated the procedure well and had shorter postoperative hospitalizations in comparison to open procedures. Accordingly, given the potentially lower morbidity due to the smaller abdominal wall incisions, the overall hospital cost may be reduced, making this a more attractive approach to incisional hernias. Moreover, laparoscopy allows a comprehensive exploration of the abdominal cavity, an adequate assessment of the adherences in the hernia process, and a clear delineation of the topography.

Laparoscopic incisional hernia repair can be safely performed with no increased morbidity or mortality. It may be the procedure of choice in patients who develop recurrence following a prior open hernia repair. The ultimate outcome in assessing the success of any hernia repair must be the rate of recurrence. The literature suggests that the laparoscopic approach, regardless where the mesh is placed, has a mid-term recurrence rate at least as good as that seen after the open operation. However, long-term assessment from large and well-controlled prospective studies is needed to confirm the expected advantages of the laparoscopic approach.

References

1. Santora TA, Roslyn JJ. Incisional hernia. Surg Clin North Am 73:557, 1993.

2. Maekelae JT, Kivinieme H, Juvonen T, et al. Factors influencing wound dehiscence after midline laparotomy. Am J Surg 170:387, 1995.

3. Niggebrugge AH, Hansen BE, Trimbos JB, et al. Mechanical factors influencing the incidence of burst abdomen. Eur J Surg 161:655, 1995.

4. Meissner K, Jirikowski B, Szecsi T. Repair of parietal hernia by overlapping onlay reinforcement or "gap-bridging" replacement polypropylene mesh: preliminary results. Hernia 4:29, 2000.

5. Larson GM. Ventral hernia repair by the laparoscopic approach. Surg Clin North Am. 80:1329, 2000.

6. Heniford BT, Park A, Ramshaw BJ, et al. Laparoscopic ventral and incisional repair in 407 patients. J Am Coll Surg 190:645, 2000.

7. Luijendijk RW, Hop WCJ, Tol P, et al. A comparison of suture repair with mesh repair for incisional hernia. NEJM 343:392, 2000.

8. Leber GE, Garb JL, Alexander AI, et al. Long-term complications associated with prosthetic repair of incisional hernias. Arch Surg 133:378, 1998.

9. Amid PK. Classification of biomaterials and their related complications in abdominal wall hernia surgery Hernia 1:15, 1997.

10. Amid PK, Shulman G, Lichtenstein I, et al. Preliminary evaluation of composite materials for the repair of incisional hernias. Ann Chir 49:539, 1995.

11. Morris-Stiff H. The outcomes of nonabsorbable mesh. J Am Coll Surg 186:352, 1998.

12. Koehler RH, Voeller G. Recurrences in laparoscopic incisional hernia repairs: A personal series and review of the literature. JSLS 3:293, 1999.

13. Marchal F, Brunaud L, Sebbag H, et al. Treatment of incisional hernias by placement of an intraperitoneal prosthesis: a series of 128 patients. Hernia 3:141, 2000.

14. Costanza MJ, Henniford BT, Arca MJ, et al. Laparoscopic repair of recurrent ventral hernias. Am Surg. 64:1, 1998.

15. Luijendijk RW, Lemmen MHM, Hop WCJ, et al. Incisional hernia recurrence following "vest-over-pants" or vertical Mayo repair of primary hernias of the midline. World J Surg 21:62, 1997.

16. Stoppa R. The treatment of complicated groin and incisional hernias. World J Surg 13:545, 1989.

17. Park A, Gaguer M, Pomp A. Laparoscopic repair of large incisional hernias. Surg Laparosc Endosc 6:123, 1996.

18. Le Blanc KA, Booth WV. Laparoscopic repair of incisional abdominal hernias using expanded polytetrafluoroetilene: preliminary findings. Surg Laparosc Endosc 3:39, 1993.

19. Hashizume M, Migo S, Tsugawa Y, et al. Laparoscopic repair of paraumbilical ventral hernia with increasing size in a obese patient. Surg Endosc 10:933, 1996.

20. Roth JS, Park AE, Witzke d, et al. Laparoscopic incisional / ventral herniorrhaphy: a five-year experience. Hernia 4:209, 1999.

21. Wants GE. Incisional hernioplasty with Mersilene. Surg Gynecol Obst 172:129, 1991.

22. Barie PS, Mack CA, Thompson WA. A technique for laparoscopic repair of herniation of the anterior abdominal wall using a composite mesh prosthesis. Am J Surg 170:62, 1995.

23. Larson GM: Laparoscopic repair of ventral hernia, in Scott-Conner CEH (ed): The SAGES Manual. New York, Springer, 1998; p 379.

24. Toy FK, Bailey RW, Carey S, et al. Prospective multicenter study of laparoscopic ventral hernioplasty. Surg Endo 12:955, 1998.

25. Holzman MD, Purut CM, Reintgen K, et al. Laparoscopic ventral and incisional hernioplasty. Surg Endosc 11:32, 1997.

26. Park AE, Birch DW, Lovrics P. Laparoscopic and open incisional hernia repair: A comparison study. Surgery 124:816, 1998.

27. Carbajo MA, Martín del Olmo JC, Blanco JI, et al. Laparoscopic treatment vs open surgery in the solution of major incisional and abdominal wall hernias with mesh. Surg Endosc 113:250, 1999.

28. Chevrel JP, Rath AM. Classification of incisional hernias of the abdominal wall. Hernia 4:7, 2000.

29. Alexandre JH, Aouad K, Bethoux JP, et al. Recent advances in incisional hernia treatment. Hernia 4:1, 2000.

30. Balique JC, Alexandre JH, Arnaud JP, et al. Intraperitoneal treatment of incisional and umbilical hernias: intermediate results of a multicenter prospective clinical trial using an innovative composite mesh. Hernia 4:10, 2000.

31. Roll S, DePaula AL, Miguel P, et al. Laparoscopic transabdominal inguinal hernia repair with a preperitoneal mesh. Surg Endosc 8:484, 1994.

32. Saiz AA, Willis IH, Paul DK, et al. Laparoscopic ventral hernia repair: A community hospital experience. Am Surg 62:336, 1996.

33. Franklin ME, Dorman JP, Glass JL, et al. Laparoscopic ventral and incisional hernia repair. Surg Lap Endosc 8:294, 1998.

34. Sanders LM, Flint LM. Initial experience with laparoscopic repair of incisional hernias. Am J Surg 177:227, 1999.

35. Roll S, Benatti M, Roncada, P, et al. Laparoscopic incisional preperitoneal hernioplasty. Poster Presentation in 7th World Congress of Endoscopic Surgery, Singapore, 2000.

CHAPTER 27

Laparoscopic Intraperitoneal Ventral Hernia Repair with Sutures

F.R. Abiad, G.R. Voeller

INTRODUCTION

With the resounding success of the laparoscopic cholecystectomy, a similar panacea for the difficult problem of ventral/incisional hernia was sought beginning in the early 1990s. The stimulus for success in this area occurred when the laparoscopic investigators adopted the retrorectus repair using a prosthetic mesh, as described by Rives/Stoppa. The senior author's first attempt at laparoscopic repair of a ventral/incisional hernia involved a Spigelian hernia. This was prior to the development of automatic hernia staplers and a reloadable hernia stapler was used to affix a piece of mesh to the abdominal wall. While aesthetically pleasing, the hernia soon recurred. When evaluated laparoscopically it could be seen that the prosthetic mesh had simply migrated with the peritoneum into the hernia defect. We thus realized that suture fixation as in the Rives/Stoppa approach would be critical to long term success in these often times large patients. During the following decade, our technique has been modified by our and other surgeons' growing experience, along with new improved tacking devices and prosthetic material. In this chapter, we present the current technique we use for the laparoscopic repair of ventral hernia.

PATIENT PREPARATION

The indications for laparoscopic ventral/incisional hernia repair have been well described in the previous section. In open ventral hernia repair, weight loss in the obese patient is something that is desirable. Over the years, we have tried to do the same but without much success. Most of our patients with ventral/incisional hernias are large and weight loss prior to repair has been modest at best. It is probably idealistic to assume that these patients will be able to lose significant amounts of weight. One advantage of the laparoscopic approach, however, is that the wound complications in these obese patients are not seen as frequently as with the open repair. Thus weight loss prior to surgery may not be as critical laparoscopically as it is in the open approach.

The patient who has had several previous surgeries with what is thought to be densely adherent or incarcerated viscera will undergo a formal bowel preparation. The patients are always told that if it is not safe to lyse adhesions or reduce the bowel then an open repair will be done. It is also explained to them that if an enterotomy occurs, then we may or may not proceed with repair based on the type of injury, contamination, and ease of repair.

Foley catheters and nasogastric tubes are not routinely used. A Foley catheter is placed if it is likely that it will be a prolonged operation or if the hernia being repaired lies low close to the pubic bone. In this latter instance, the mesh may have to be anchored to Cooper's ligament and this will require making a peritoneal flap and assuring the bladder is out of harms way. The Foley allows decompression of the bladder, and in addition can be used to instill normal saline to distend the bladder to aid in identification during dissection. A nasogastric tube is only used if the stomach is distended or in the way during the dissection.

The surgeon and assistant will need to approach the patient from all angles and this means being able to operate from any direction. In order to do so it is ideal if the arms can be "tucked" to the side of the patient. If this can not be done, one should move the operating table away from the anesthesiologist and drape out above the arm boards to allow the surgeon and/or assistant to position themselves properly. All patients have sequential pneumatic compression boots placed on their legs and these are left on until the patient is ambulating. One dose of prophylactic antibiotics is administered at the time of induction of anesthesia.

EQUIPMENT

The majority of ventral/incisional hernias can be repaired with two video monitors similar to a laparoscopic cholecystectomy. However, as the hernia moves more caudad, the monitor(s) will need to be moved caudad so the surgeon works in the same direction the camera is viewing.

An up-to-date video endoscopic camera, monitor and light source are absolutely essential. A 30° degree or 45° degree angle view laparoscope is optimal to perform the operation. The angle telescope allows one to evaluate the anterior abdominal wall and then can be turned over to inspect the abdominal cavity, etc. One 10mm port is used for the initial access; the rest of the working ports are either 5mm or needlescopic ports. This requires the use of a 5mm angle telescope at times and it is beneficial to have one available for this procedure. The newer 5mm telescopes have an excellent field of vision, as well as light transmission.

Atraumatic bowel graspers and sharp scissors are required for proper dissection and prevention of bowel injury. The most difficult part of the dissection has to deal with lysing adhesions and reducing viscera from the hernia. Energy sources should be used at a bare minimum. Monopolar cautery is acceptable as long as it is used far away from the viscera and again used sparingly. If the proper planes are maintained, minimal blood loss is expected. The harmonic scalpel has been advocated for lysis of adhesions by some surgeons, but one must be cautious since this instrument gets very hot at the tip. Even though there is minimal thermal spread, the tip of the instrument can damage the viscera and this may not be apparent at the time of surgery. We do not use the harmonic scalpel routinely.

As will be mentioned, suture fixation of the mesh is critical for long-term good results. We initially selected polypropylene type sutures due to their monofilament nature; however, we found that they were difficult to work with through the laparoscope due to their memory. We now use the Gore CV-0 suture since it is nonabsorbable, has no memory, and it is quite easy to use through the laparoscope. The suture passer developed by Toy and Smoot is ideally suited for passing the suture through the abdominal wall (Fig. 1). A Keith needle and other instruments can also be used for this purpose. The 5mm spiral tackers are used to prevent internal hernia formation between the mesh and the peritoneal cavity. These allow good apposition of the edges of the mesh to the peritoneum and work much better than the staplers that were more common prior to the tacking devices being available.

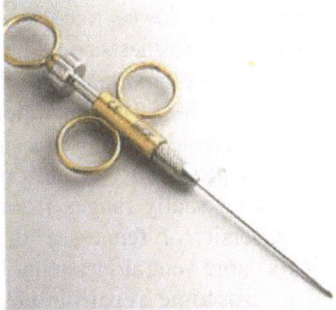

Fig. 1. The Toy Smoot suture passer.

With respect to the mesh used for laparoscopic repair, it is becoming apparent that polytetrafluroethylene (PTFE) meshes are probably the best suited for this repair. The mesh will have to be placed intraperitoneally and there is extensive documentation showing that polyester and polypropylene meshes cause a severe inflammatory response with dense adhesions. This carries the risks of bowel obstruction and/or fistula formation. It also leads to an extremely difficult re-operation if required. Over the past years as this procedure has evolved, W. L. Gore has developed a Dual-Mesh Plus® which is meant for intraperitoneal placement (Fig. 2). One side of the mesh has very small size pores that inhibit tissue ingrowth; this side is placed against the viscera. On the other side, the pore size is large enough that tissue ingrowth can occur; this side is placed next to the peritoneal surface. In addition, the newer mesh is impregnated with chlorhexadine and silver salts thus providing additional guard against infection.

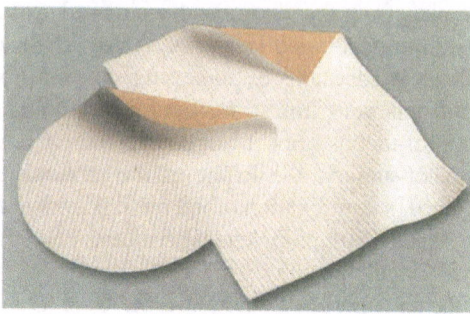

Fig. 2. The Gore Dual-Mesh Plus®.

TECHNIQUE

The American Hernia Society has declared that the Rives/Stoppa open repair for large ventral/incisional hernias should be the standard of care. It has been well documented that this repair, which places the prosthesis behind the rectus muscle and behind the fascial defect leads to the lowest rates of recurrence. This technique was specifically developed so that the prosthesis could be placed behind the hernia defect but kept off of the viscera. This is important since the technique is described using polypropylene or polyester meshes. This operation is a large undertaking with wide skin and soft tissue flaps created leading to a significant amount of dead space and a high rate of wound problems. In addition to the complications described above, the hospital stay usually ranges from 5-8 days and recovery requires 6-8 weeks. At the University of Tennessee, the Rives/Stoppa approach became the method of repair for large ventral/incisional hernias. As we began to develop the technique for laparoscopic repair it became apparent that the technique done laparoscopically should try to mimic this open approach that leads to such low recurrence rates.

The indications for the laparoscopic repair of ventral/incisional hernias are the same as those for the open repair. Hesselink has shown that any hernia larger than 4cm, if not repaired with mesh, leads to a high recurrence rate. In addition, there is evidence to suggest that hernias that are recurrent, even if smaller than 4cm, or in the morbidly obese patient are candidates for the mesh repair.

The patient is prepped from xiphoid to pubis, and as far laterally as possible. The draping should also be done very laterally to allow access with trocars. It is critical that sterile technique is not compromised. The skin is covered with an Ioban® protective skin drape to avoid any contact between skin flora and the prosthetic.

Access

An open access technique is used on almost all patients. The access site is at either costal margin as far lateral as possible, while staying anterior to the colon. Hasson

"S" shaped retractors are absolutely essential to perform this step in order to retract each fascial and muscle layer as it is incised and separated. Once the peritoneum is visualized, it is incised with an #11 scalpel blade and a balloon-tipped blunt Hasson trocar can then be easily placed. The angle endoscope is then introduced and the abdominal cavity assessed. The hernia is inspected and if possible its contents reduced. The density of adhesions between the viscera and the abdominal wall is noted in addition to the presence of unsuspected hernia defects. The angle endoscope is helpful since it allows the inspection to be performed from different angles. Additional trocar placement depends on the size and location of the hernia (Fig. 3).

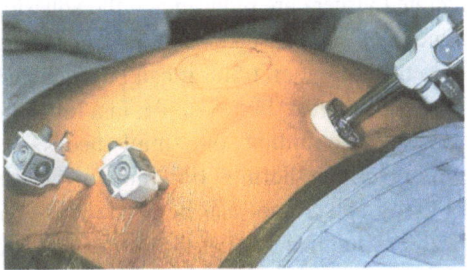

Fig. 3. Trocar placement. Note the Ioban® protective skin drape.

Adhesionlysis

This is the most critical step in the operation. Following placement of the Hasson port, one or two 5 mm ports are placed on the same side. The trocars are placed laterally to leave space for the later placement of the mesh. The division of adhesions is done in an avascular plane of fibrous tissue that is formed between the viscera and the abdominal wall. The use of atraumatic graspers and proper retraction allow adequate visualization of this plane, and we prefer to take these adhesions down using sharp scissors and no energy source. If these adhesions are flimsy however, they can be taken down with blunt dissection. These patients are usually quite large and often times it is easier to simply use an instrument through one 5mm port with the dominant hand, while the non-dominant hand compresses the abdominal wall to bring it down to the scissor tip or the grasper tip for dissection. Some hernias can be quite adherent and not easily reduced. In these patients, we have found the best approach is to make a small incision over the hernia through which these adhesions are taken down and the hernia reduced. The incision is then closed and the procedure completed laparoscopically. In our experience, the patients who had the laparoscopically assisted repair had a similar postoperative course to patients who had the repair done totally laparoscopic.

The entire abdominal wall should be cleared of all adhesions to evaluate every area for possible hernia defects. It is common to see defects that are not appreciated preoperatively on examination. If at any time viscera cannot be safely reduced or if there is some concern about bowel injury that cannot be appreciated the patient should be opened and a safe repair undertaken of either the viscera or the hernia. If an enterotomy is created, the safest thing to do is to repair the enterotomy laparoscopically or through a very small incision and then come back another day to repair the hernia. We have on occasion repaired a small bowel enterotomy laparoscopically and continued with the hernia repair and these patients have don fine. However, we must emphasize that safety is critical and if there is any question then open surgery should be considered.

Hernia defect assessment

Once all of the incarcerated viscera are reduced and the adhesions taken down, the next step is to determine the fascial borders and the extent of the defect. There are several techniques to do this and often times it can be evaluated by looking at the abdominal wall and the hernia defect. For example, in a long midline incision with multiple defects up and down the midline, one simply needs to look at the old scar to determine the borders of the hernia. For more accurate assessment, the technique described by Toy and Smoot can be used. This consists of passing a spinal needle through the abdominal wall at the estimated borders and watching where it comes out in the peritoneal cavity in relation to the hernia defect. As the cephalad, caudad and lateral borders are determined, these are diagrammed on the abdominal wall with a marking pen. The mesh should cover the defect and overlap 3-5cm of healthy fascia on each side. Therefore, the diagram of the mesh is drawn by adding 3-5cm to the dimensions of the defect on all sides. This gives us the diagram of the fascial defect and of the prosthesis that needs to be used (Fig. 4). The abdominal cavity is then deflated and the measurements of the actual size of the defect and the required mesh are made using a ruler. It is important to make the measurements with the abdominal cavity deflated, otherwise the size of the defect will be overestimated and the mesh will come out redundant.

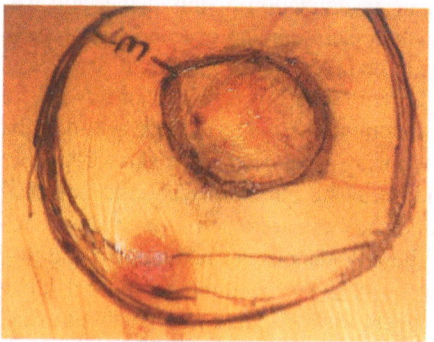

Fig. 4. The diagram showing an inner circle representing the fascial defect, and an outer circle representing the required mesh with 3cm of overlap with healthy fascia.

Mesh Preparation

The mesh is marked to designate its top; in addition, "X's" are made on the mesh and on the skin at corresponding sites, usually at the midpoint of each side. These "X's" indicate the location of the initial stay sutures that will be placed to hold the prosthesis against the abdominal wall when they are tied. Gore CV-0 suture is then used to place "U" stitches at each of these "X's" on the prosthesis. The sutures are tied leaving the tails long enough to be brought up through the abdominal wall once the mesh is place intraperitoneally. A medium hemoclip is placed on each suture tail; this facilitates grasping and passing the sutures with the suture passer. Five or six stay sutures are used for large patches and 4 stay sutures are used for smaller patches (Fig. 5). The mesh is then rolled from each edge towards the middle. If the mesh is rolled in one continuous fashion from one side to the other, it becomes difficult to unroll once it is placed in the peritoneal cavity. Smaller pieces of mesh can be placed through the 10mm Hasson port directly, but most large pieces require introduction through the open access site after removal of the balloon-tipped trocar. To do this a grasper is placed through the Hasson port using a 5mm port placed on the opposite side. The grasper is directed out through the Hasson cannula; the Hasson cannula is then removed and the pneumoperitoneum evacuated. This leaves the tip of the grasper protruding through the fascial defect of the Hasson port. The mesh is grasped and the grasper is drawn into the abdominal cavity bringing the mesh with it. Once the mesh is entirely inside the abdominal cavity, the Hasson port is reinserted and pneumoperitoneum reestablished. The laparoscope is then turned with the view looking down onto the viscera. This allows one to view the mesh and unfurl the mesh using two graspers placed in the middle of the mesh and pushing in opposite directions.

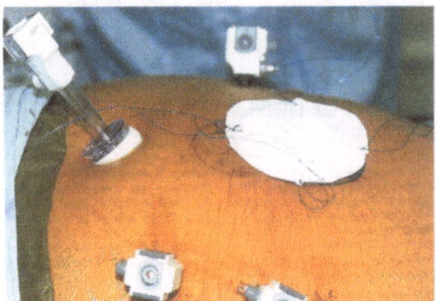

Fig. 5. The mesh with four stay sutures, one on each side. A larger mesh requires more stay sutures.

Mesh Fixation

At each "X" marked on the skin, small skin punctures are then made. The Toy-Smoot suture passer is then used to bring each suture pair out through the entire thickness of the abdominal wall (Fig. 6). Both suture tail-ends come out through the same skin puncture, but through a separate fascial puncture such that there is at least a 1cm bridge between each suture tail-end. This is simply done by redirecting the suture passer as it penetrates the fascia. Once all the sutures are brought out through the entire thickness of the abdominal wall they are then tied with the knots residing in the subcutaneous tissue. These sutures thus have anchored the mesh to the entire thickness of the abdominal wall. One must understand that the sutures are the main strength of this repair. The spiral tacks are then used to tack the edges of the mesh to the peritoneal surface between the stay sutures. These tacks are simply to prevent internal hernia formation. One must tack in the direction of the camera. Counter pressure on the abdominal wall is very important for good accurate tacking. The mesh should be stretched very tightly so that when the pneumoperitoneum is evacuated there is a good solid tension free repair without protrusion of the mesh into the hernia defect (Fig. 7). Once tacking is complete, additional stay sutures can now be placed, using the suture passer, at every 5-7cm intervals. In very large hernias, sutures can be placed at even more frequent intervals if need be. The 10mm Hasson port can be closed laparoscopically. A drain is not routinely used.

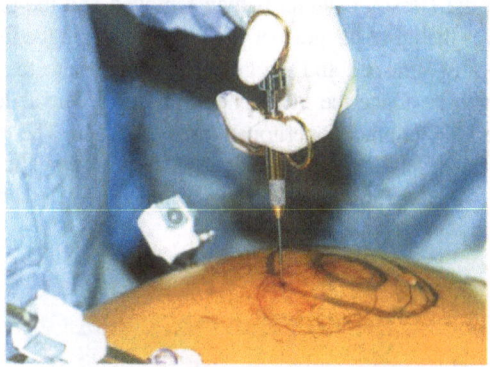

Fig. 6. The suture passer is used to extrude the suture tail.

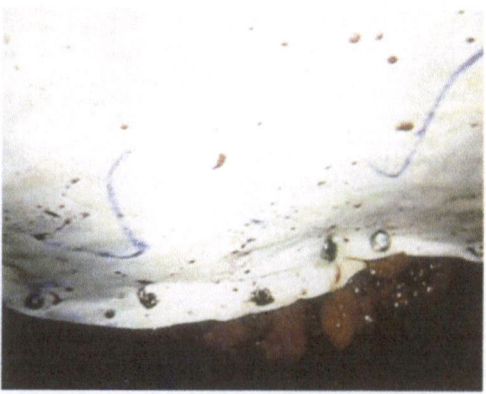

Fig. 7. The finished mesh.

POST OPERATIVE INSTRUCTIONS TO PATIENT

Immediately post operatively, the peritoneal tacking and "U" stitches cause significant discomfort and narcotic analgesia is required. If the patient is to stay overnight, we use patient controlled analgesia by the intravenous route. The pain dissipates quite quickly, however, and on the first post-operative day oral medications are all that are required to control the pain. We routinely start liquids post operatively and advanced the diet as the patient tolerates. If there is a significant fascial defect that has been repaired or one large hernia with significant soft tissue excess, then we place a large compression bandage over the area. This compression bandage is left in place for 7-10 days. The patient is allowed to shower and activity is not restricted. The discomfort that the patient experiences will limit his or her activities for approximately two weeks and this is all that is required.

We believe all patients get a seroma between the patch and the peritoneal sac. Not all of these become clinically evident, however, some do. Most surgeons will leave the seroma, since most all of them "disappear". We, however, do aspirate large seromas. This makes the patient more comfortable. To date we have yet to cause a single mesh infection. We have, on few patients, injected fibrin glue into this hernia cavity to prevent seroma formation.

References

1. Heniford BT, Park A, Ramshaw BJ, Voeller G. Laparoscopic ventral and incisional hernia repair in 407 patients. J Am Coll Surg 2000 Jun;190(6):645-50.

2. Hesselink VJ, Luijendijk RW, de Wilt JH, Heide R, Jeekel J. An evaluation of risk factors in incisional hernia recurrence. Surg Gynecol Obstet 1993 Mar;176(3):228-34.

3. Koehler RH, Voeller G. Recurrences in laparoscopic incisional hernia repairs: a personal series and review of the literature. JSLS 1999 Oct-Dec;3(4):293-304.

4. Rives J, Pire JC, Flament JB, Convers G. Treatment of large eventrations (apropos of 133 cases). Minerva Chir 1977 Jun 15;32(11):749-56.

5. Stoppa RE. The treatment of complicated groin and incisional hernias. World J Surg 1989 Sep-Oct;13(5):545-54.

6. Toy FK, Bailey RW, Carey S, et al. Prospective, multicenter study of laparoscopic ventral hernioplasty. Preliminary results. Surg Endosc 1998 Jul;12(7):955-9.

7. Wantz GE. Incisional hernioplasty with Mersilene. Surg Gynecol Obstet 1991 Feb;172(2):129-37.

CHAPTER 28

Laparoscopic Intraperitoneal Ventral Hernia Repair without Sutures: "Double crown" technique

S. Morales-Conde, S. Morales-Méndez

INTRODUCTION

Laparoscopic surgery continues to advance in achieving further benefits over the conventional approach for certain pathologies. Although not originally considered to be a pathology that could benefit from this approach, laparoscopic repair of ventral hernias has attained wide acceptance in recent years because of the significant advantages afforded by improvements in prosthetic materials and in attachment methods, as well as in the surgical technique used. The laparoscopic procedure offers greater comfort during the postoperative period, reduced hospitalization time and lower complication rates. Even though many series still have a limited follow-up, the technique has shown lower recurrence rates, making it a procedure that solves a longstanding challenge for the surgeon.

EVOLUTION OF THE TECHNIQUE IN OUR SURGICAL TEAM

In 1991, LeBlanc et al. carried out the first laparoscopic repairs of ventral hernias (1). Initially, there was little interest in the technique worldwide, since the instruments, mesh, and suturing materials did not allow much improvement in the procedure, and the surgery itself was tedious and had very limited application. In 1995 our group made an initial attempt at repairing ventral hernias, using the technique described by various authors at the time, which basically consisted in placing four trocars, one at each corner of the defect. This system resulted in failure and conversion was required in the two cases we performed. By 1998, technical guidelines had been established by various surgeons and numerous improvements had been made in materials and instrumentation, including the use of tacks and the new e-PTFE mesh. In the light of these advances, we decided to perform the procedure again, with significant success and excellent results.

Various surgical techniques have been described for the repair of ventral hernias using the laparoscopic approach, the majority of which are described herein. Our group usually implants an intraperitoneal mesh in contact with the abdominal loops to cover the defect in the anterior wall of the abdomen. We believe this is technically more feasible and reproducible than other procedures and we have obtained excellent results with it. Basically it involves introducing a mesh with optimal properties for placement in contact with the bowel inside the abdomen. The benefits of such material have been shown in various experimental studies, such as the one we conducted comparing different prosthetic materials (2).

Regardless of the technique chosen, laparoscopic repair of ventral hernias is a procedure that is clearly advancing and gaining acceptance worldwide. It is now being standardized in various centers as the technique of choice for the treatment of this pathology. Nevertheless, there are certain points of controversy that should be clarified, starting with the simple fact of establishing more precise indications for the use of this approach. In addition, a multitude of more specific technical details should be discussed, including how to perform adhesiolysis, how to manage the hernia sac, how to choose the type and size of the mesh, and how to insert and secure the mesh inside the cavity. Moreover the surgeon has to know how to deal with intraoperative complications, such as intestinal perforation, and postoperative complications, including the management of seromas. One of the most interesting points currently being debated is whether or not it is necessary to use sutures and tacks or tacks alone.

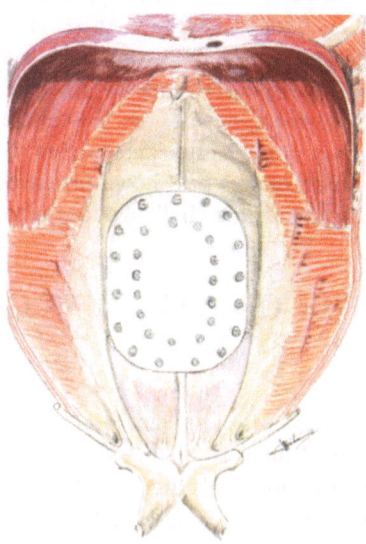

Fig. 1. "Double Crown" technique for laparoscopic ventral hernia repair. External sutures are avoided and the mesh is fixed with a double crown of tacks alone.

Our surgical team has developed a laparoscopic procedure for the repair of ventral hernias from the start which uses a technique we have come to call the "double crown" technique. This system basically consists in avoiding the use of external sutures by fixing the mesh with a double crown of tacks alone (Fig. 1). This ensures proper anchorage of the mesh, decreasing surgery time, diminishing postoperative pain at this level and retaining the same recurrence rate as described in the literature by groups using transmural sutures.

SURGICAL TECHNIQUE: "DOUBLE CROWN" TECHNIQUE

Indications

Basically all ventral hernias can be repaired by laparoscopy as the standard procedure, whereas emergency operations performed in cases of strangulated hernias must be analyzed on an individual basis to assess whether or not laparoscopy should be used. However, various factors place limits on the indications for laparoscopic repair such as size of the defect (both very small and very large) and the site where it has occurred. Subxiphoid, suprapubic, lumbar and parastomal hernias require special considerations for laparoscopic repair and several technical details must still be surmounted. At the lower end of the size spectrum, hernias that can be repaired with local anesthesia, encompassing those under 3-4 cm, are naturally excluded. However, in patients requiring laparoscopic surgery for other concomitant conditions and in obese patients, laparoscopic repair would be indicated despite the small size of the hernia. Regarding the upper end of the hernia size spectrum, our team has performed many successful repairs of massive abdominal wall defects. We therefore conclude that until the limits are clearly established, the degree of difficulty in managing the instruments within the cavity is the only actual limit to the technique, as far as large hernias are concerned. Definitive guidelines will have to be elaborated on the basis of results from prospective studies comparing open and laparoscopic approaches for major defects.

Preoperative considerations

Basing our discussion on the repair of primary or incisional ventral hernias at the midline and about three centimetres from the xiphoid and suprapubic area, we will now describe the technique we generally use. We usually place the patient in supine decubitus, with the surgeon and the assistant to the patient's left and the monitor in front of them to the patient's right. Urethral catheters are only used in patients with suprapubic hernias or hernias located at the middle third below the midline. We use a nasogastric tube to decompress the stomach in patients with subxiphoid hernias or hernias in the third above the midline.

We start antibiotic prophylaxis in all cases with a preoperative dose of a second-generation cephalosporin. If the patient has any risk factor such as diabetes, prophylaxis is continued with two doses during the postoperative period.

Creation of pneumoperitoneum and placement of trocars

In all cases we start by creating the pneumoperitoneum using a Veress needle in the left hypochondrium. We do not use the Hasson trocar in any case, regardless of the number of previous laparotomies the patient has undergone. Our group has performed more than 4,000 laparoscopies for a variety of pathologies and there has never been a lesion from the use of the Veress needle. Hence, we feel confident when creating the pneumoperitoneum with this technique, even in patients with a history of multiple operations.

Once the pneumoperitoneum is created, we generally approach the cavity from the patient's left side, placing three trocars in line (one 10-mm trocar for the scope and two 5-mm trocars as working channels), introducing the 10-mm trocar first and then placing the other trocars under direct vision. Several authors have described the use of initial trocars under direct vision in order to ensure that no intrabdominal structure sustains a lesion (3). An important thing to remember when placing the trocars is to stay as far as possible away from the defect margin closest to the surgeon. This will provide proper visualization of the margin, making it easier to achieve ample overlap with the mesh and perform any maneuvers needed to secure the prosthesis. When it is not possible maintain a suitable distance from this margin, we introduce another 5-mm trocar in the patient's opposite flank in order to adequately fix the mesh on the margin closest to the trocar used for the scope. If necessary, a contralateral 10-mm trocar can be inserted to help anchor the mesh more securely.

Adhesiolysis

Once the trocars are introduced, the adhesions are evaluated. We consider adhesiolysis to be a key point of this procedure, since incorrect performance of the adhesiolysis process can have extremely serious consequences for the patient. The aspects to be considered when performing adhesiolysis are analysed in other chapters of the book and will not be discussed in this section. Nevertheless, any doubts regarding the possibility of intestinal perforation are grounds for conversion, or at least for lengthening one of the trocar incisions to check the bowel. Missed perforation of the abdominal bowel is associated with high morbidity and mortality.

Preparation of the surgical field and mesh

Once the adhesiolysis process is completed, we proceed to identify the defect and the sac (Fig. 2). Depending on the author, several approaches to the sac have been proposed in order to avoid postoperative seroma. These range from conservative management (i.e., no action) to burning the entire sac with an electroscalpel or argon scalpel. The middle-ground (what we use) consists of complete coagulation with electroscalpel of the area where adhesiolysis has been performed, without touching the area where there were no adhesions.

Once the hernia is identified, the actual defect presented by the patient must be delimited by drawing the margin of the hernia (not the sac) on the skin (Fig. 3). In this case we use one of the working instruments under laparoscopic vision to exert pressure on the margin, feeling the pressure from the outside and drawing the entire defect on the patient's skin. In obese patients it is difficult or impossible to feel the gras per on the outside. In these cases we insert an intramuscular needle in the skin, visualizing the needle tip inside the cavity under laparoscopic vision to detect and trace the hernia defect on the patient's skin.

Once the exact measurements of the defect have been determined, we proceed to choose the mesh. We systematically use Gore-tex PTFEe mesh *Corduroy dual-mesh plus with holes (W.L. Gore & Associates, Flagstaff, AZ, USA)* having dimensions that overlap at least 3cm beyond the hernia orifice in all directions to ensure broad coverage of the defect. Once the mesh is selected, several marks are traced on the patient's abdomen and on the mesh surface that will be placed in contact with the viscera, in order to facilitate orientation of the prosthesis within the cavity. A circular mark is traced at the craniad end of the mesh, drawing the same mark on the patient's abdomen where the mesh will be anchored within, i.e., at least 3cm above the margin of the defect drawn earlier. A triangle is then drawn at the caudad end of the mesh and the abdominal wall, followed by a line that passes through the triangle, starting at the lower limit of the tracing of the hernia defect. This is the line where the caudad tack will be positioned, since the outside measurements are different from the internal measurements. Once the craniad tack is placed internally, the distance will not correspond exactly to the triangle drawn on the patient's abdomen when the mesh is tensed. The second (caudad) tack will be placed at the level of the line that passes through the middle of the triangle. A cross is then drawn on the left side of the patient's abdomen and on the mesh and two crosses are drawn on the right in order to extend the mesh in both directions properly (Fig. 4). These drawings must be done on the mesh and on the patient with the abdomen desufflated so the internal measurements are closer to the external measurements. If the hernia sac is distended, correct placement of these reference points will be significantly more difficult.

Afterwards, we roll the mesh along its long axis, leaving the mesh side that will be in contact with the bowel rolled toward the inside (Fig. 5). This will make it easier to perform the maneuvers needed to extend the mesh once attachment is begun. We are in favor of introducing the mesh through one of the trocars to prevent potential contamination that can occur when it is inserted through the skin, a strategy which is preferred by some authors (Fig. 6). A 10 x 15cm mesh can be introduced through a 10-mm trocar without difficulty. When a 15 x 19cm mesh is required, a 11-mm trocar can be used to insert it. If larger prostheses are needed, we prefer to remove the trocar and insert the mesh wrapped in sterile plastic through the trocar hole, and then remove the plastic from inside the cavity. This decreases the possibility of mesh contamination.

Placement and fixation of the mesh

Once the mesh is inside the cavity and unrolled properly (Fig. 7a and 7b), it must be oriented by using the circle drawn on the mesh. Then the area where we want to fix the mesh must be located by pushing on the abdominal wall in this area. If the patient is extremely obese, identification of this area may be significantly more difficult. In this case we insert a needle at the level of the circle of the abdomen in order to locate the area where the most craniad tack should be placed. When the first tack is placed (Fig. 8a and 8b), we stretch the mesh in the caudad direction and perform the same maneuver, placing the second tack in the line that intersects the triangle traced earlier (Fig. 9). Subsequently, the lateral tacks are placed following the same system with the crosses, avoiding the tendency of the mesh to move in the opposite direction from the point where scope is introduced (Fig. 10a and 10b).

Once the mesh is fixed in the four cardinal points, we proceed to extend it adequately, adding an outer crown of tacks that are placed right on the margin of the mesh (Fig. 11). These tacks are separated from each other by a distance of one centimeter, an adequate distance to ensure that the bowel do not slip between the tacks and cause acute incarceration. While the crown is being placed, the surgeon must exert strong pressure against the tacker from the outside to ensure that the mesh is attached to the surfaces closest to the wall surface, thereby reaching the muscle fascia. Once the mesh is adequately extended with the tacks of the outer crown, we check for any mesh areas that may not be adequately extended and adhered to the anterior wall of the abdomen; adhesions would occur at the hanging sections of the mesh (4). We then add the necessary tacks at this level to extend the mesh adequately and prevent these adhesions.

Once the outer crown is finished, we add the inner crown of tacks. Since this level contains a smaller amount of preperitoneal fat, the inner crown is placed at the margin of the hernia sac to ensure better attachment of the mesh (Figure 12a and 12b). Similarly, to identify the sac margin, we draw the defect on the abdomen of the patient before inserting the mesh inside the cavity. Pressure can then be exerted from the outside or a needle can be introduced at this level in obese patients and we can identify the area where the inner crown of tacks should be placed. These are also executed while exerting pressure from the outside to ensure good anchorage at this level. As in the case of the tacks used for the outer crown, the inner crown tacks are placed about 1cm apart.

Once all the tacks are placed (Fig. 13), we proceed to identify any that are left hanging from the wall or that are improperly placed, and insert them through the entire thickness of the mesh. Poorly positioned tacks will lead to adhesions, as we have shown in our experimental study (4), and could cause major complications in the future, such as fistulas or occlusions.

Finishing the procedure and immediate postoperative period

Once the procedure is completed, the abdomen is desufflated, the 10-mm and 11-mm trocars are removed, and the orifices and skin are closed. A compressive bandage is placed at the level of the hernia sac to reduce the space between the mesh and the sac and to prevent seroma. This bandage is kept on for 1 week and is withdrawn at the 7-day follow-up visit to remove the skin sutures.

Once the procedure is completed, we start the patient on fluid intake about 6 to 8 hours after the surgery, continuing to solid foods as tolerated. The patient is normally discharged within 24 hours of the surgery. In terms of physical activity, we do not establish any limitation for the patient and only recommend gradual resumption of regular daily activities based on the patient's progress during postoperative recovery. Patient follow-up is carried out at one month, three months, six months and one year, with yearly visits thereafter.

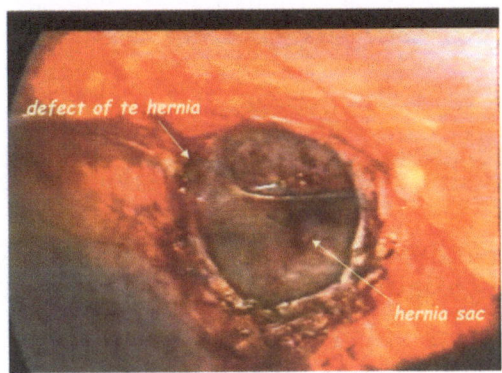

Fig. 2. Defect of the hernia that need to be cover, once the adhesiolysis process is completed.

Fig. 3. The defect presented by the patient is delimited by drawing the margins on the skin of the patients, being most of the time the sac larger than the real defect. These margins will indicate the line where the inner crown of tacks will be placed.

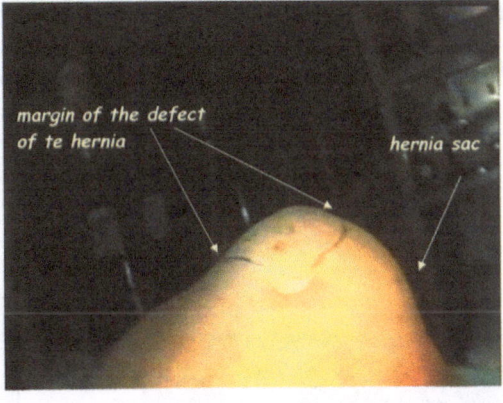

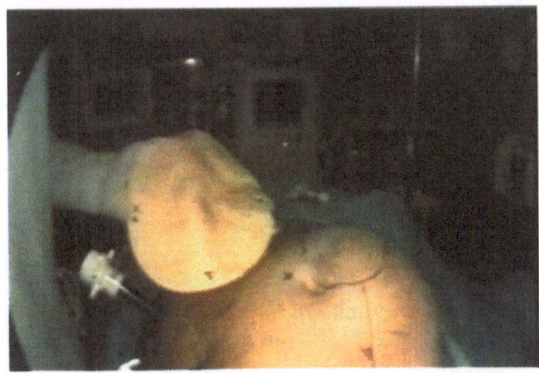

Fig. 4. Drawings on the mesh and on the skin of the patients will help to orientate the prothesis once is introduced inside the abdominal cavity.

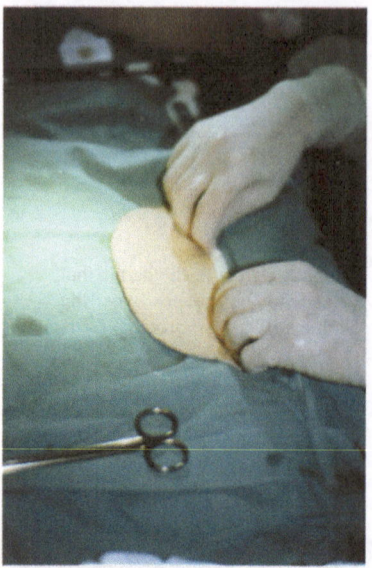

Fig. 5. Mesh is rolled along its long axis.

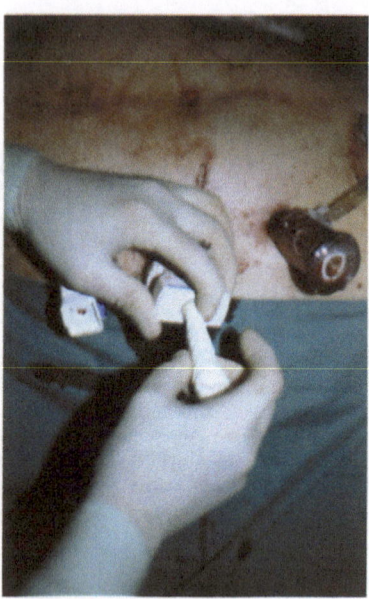

Fig. 6. Mesh is introduced through one of the trocars to prevent potential contamination.

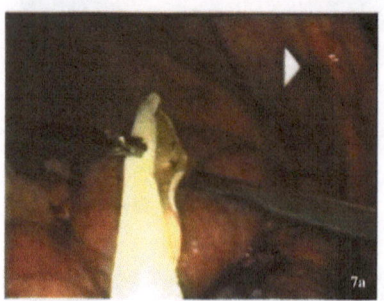

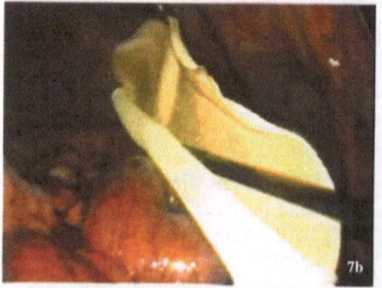

Figs. 7a and 7b. Mesh is unrolled properly inside the abdominal cavity.

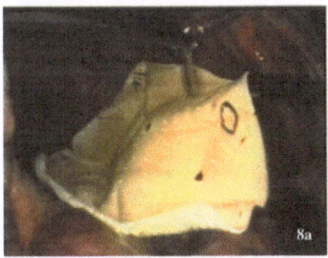 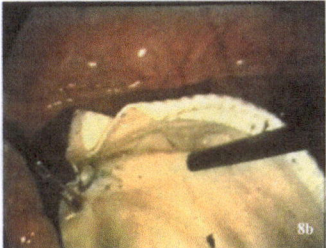

Figs. 8a and 8b. The circle is identified (8a). The first tack is placed where the the circle was drawn on the mesh and on the skin of the patient (8b).

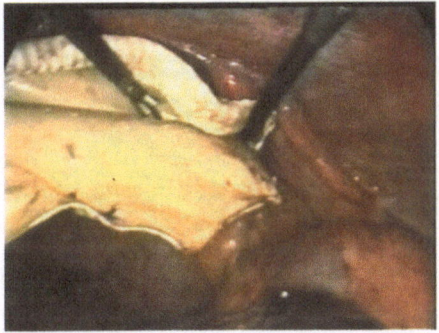

Fig. 9. Second tack is placed in the opposite position where the first tack was placed, where the triangle was drawn on the mesh.

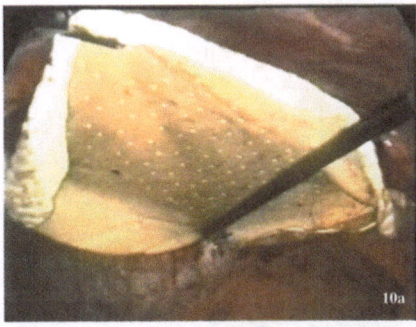 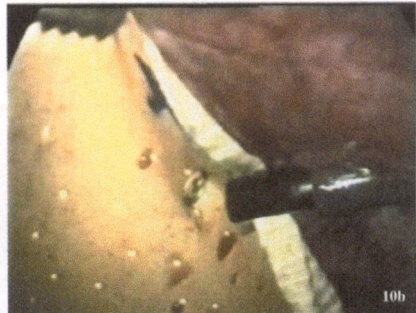

Figs. 10a and 10b. Lateral tacks are placed, so the four cardinal points extend the mesh properly to start tacking the mesh all around.

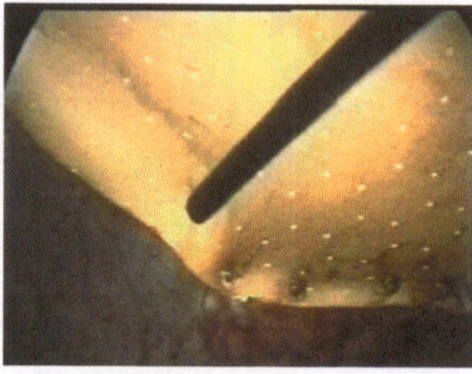

Fig. 11. The outer crown of tacks are placed rigth on the margin of the mesh.

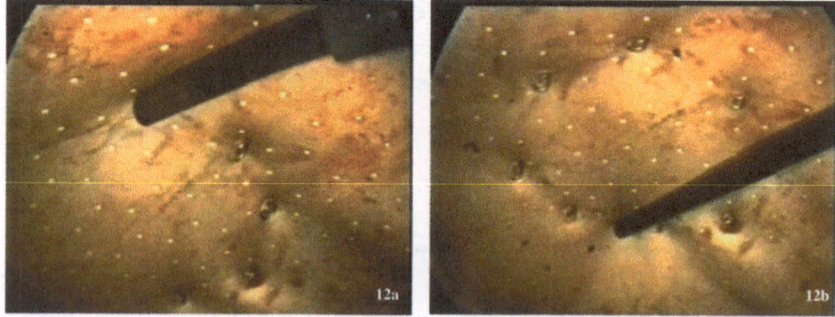

Figs. 12a and 12b. The inner crown of tacks are placed at the margin of the hernia sac to ensure better attachment.

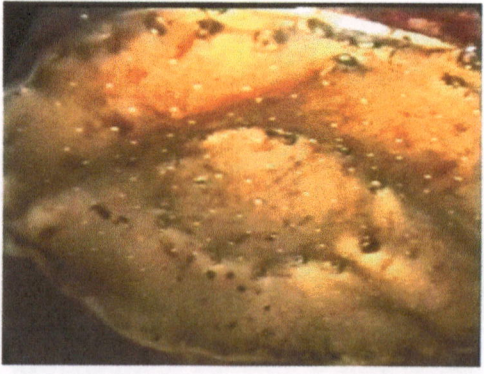

Fig. 13. The double crown of tacks is completed.

SUTURES VS NO SUTURES: CURRENT UPDATE

There is evidence of the enormous advantages offered by laparoscopic versus open surgery for the repair of ventral hernias during the immediate postoperative period, with clearly lower morbidity than that associated with the open technique (5, 6) and lower general costs of this surgery (7, 8). Despite these excellent results, however, we should clearly establish the indications for laparoscopic repair of ventral hernias and perform long-term follow-up to compare recurrence rates. Patients who were operated on by laparoscopy appear to have lower recurrence rates (5, 6), within an acceptable follow-up time. Recurrence in the laparoscopic group generally occurs earlier than in patients undergoing conventional open surgery (10-12).

Despite the lower recurrence rate, various authors have made efforts to analyze the causes for recurrence in order to adequately define the laparoscopic technique and thereby achieve an even lower recurrence rate. In this context there is a current debate concerning the need for transmural sutures to anchor the mesh and prevent hernia recurrence.

Initial laparoscopic ventral hernia repair series established a direct correlation between recurrence and the absence of external sutures (6, 9, 13). In fact they demonstrated that one of the essential factors to avoid recurrence is the use of these transmural sutures (14). Analysis of the data derived from these early series of patients operated on for ventral hernias by laparoscopic approach, data which were later the basis for recommendations on the use of sutures, shows that there could have been other factors involved in the development of recurrence in these patients besides the use or not of transmural sutures. The prostheses initially recommended were small, overlapping the defect by only 2 (10, 15) to 2.5cm (11) in all directions, and not the minimum of 3cm currently recommended. Recurrence was due mainly to the smaller size of the e-PTFE mesh as we have shown in our experimental study (4), probably because of the scar tissue reaction and the encapsulation process experienced by the mesh. The attachment method was also inadequate, since tack sutures were not yet available and mesh patches were anchored with the old endostaplers that did not ensure secure attachment of the material to the most superficial layers of the abdominal wall. This problem was particularly important with the e-PTFE mesh because of its thickness. Thus, the use of transmural sutures was necessary in these cases, and the real purpose of the endostaplers was to prevent the bowel from slipping between the sutures rather than to anchor the mesh (10, 15, 16). Lastly, the learning curve is more directly related to the appearance of recurrences than the placement or not of transmural sutures.

In addition to a supposed decrease in the recurrence rate after laparoscopic repair of ventral hernias with the use of sutures as compared to the "double crown" technique, sutures have also been defended as a way of reducing the number of tacks needed. Clinical (7) and experimental (4) studies have reported reductions in costs and in the danger associated with tack use. However, the above-mentioned experimental study showed that the potential risk of the tacks is more likely to be related to incorrect usage rather than to the actual number. If the tacks are placed properly and inserted completely into the wall and the mesh and not left hanging, the risk of adhesions (and consequently, fistulas and occlusions) disappears. Apart from this, the use of sutures does not necessarily result in a decrease in the number of tacks used in comparison with the "double crown" technique. Based on an analysis of the suture procedures reported in the literature, in addition to transmural sutures every 3-5 cm, the recommendation is to use tacks every 1 cm as an outer crown (as in our technique). Authors using sutures recommende tack placement in the innermost area to avoid dead spaces at this level and, hence, the actual savings in tacks is not substantial (9, 16).

Surgeons advocating the use of transmural sutures affirm that they facilitate orientation of the mesh inside the cavity. This is largely accomplished by the four first sutures, which are typically placed at the four corners. Since we do not use sutures, we have solved this initial problem in orienting the mesh by marking the mesh (described earlier) and the abdomen. This tactic makes it much easier to position the prosthesis. On the other hand, some authors consider that it is difficult to initially place sutures for positioning the mesh. They believe that the mesh cannot be adequately extended when sutures are used since the external and internal measurements are different, and that subsequent repositioning will be required for proper placement of the mesh, lengthening the surgery time. For this reason, these authors recommend fixing the mesh first with tacks and then adding the transmural sutures (17). We only use sutures (without tying) to position the mesh in large hernias where we are using prostheses larger than 15 x 19cm, since these prostheses tend to be difficult to manage inside the cavity due to their size.

We do not believe that these sutures are needed to reduce the recurrence rates as reported by several authors; nevertheless, they are associated with a number of disadvantages: longer surgery time, more incisions, worse cosmetic results, higher infection rate and more pain during both the early and late postoperative period.

- *Longer operating time:* Surgery times associated with transmural suture placement are longer because sutures are recommended every 5 cm (16), 4-5cm (11), or even every 3-4cm (14), in addition to the four corners. The operating time in our series is around 79 minutes. The time in the other published series that uses only tacks and no sutures is 87 minutes (5). The operating times for groups using sutures were between 82 (6) and 210 minutes (18), with a mean of 120 minutes (6, 11, 18-20), showing a significant increase in surgery time due to the maneuvers needed to place these sutures.

- *More incisions in the skin:* Transmural suture placement involves incisions of 2-3 mm at a pre-established distance of 3 to 5 cm, depending on the author, as mentioned earlier. These incisions determine the cosmetic results and are associated with greater pain during the immediate postoperative period.

- *Poorer aesthetic results:* because of the incisions which, although small, are needed to place the sutures. The incisions only require a steri-strip and typically leave a small scar, however, they do contribute to a higher number of scars in the abdominal wall.

- *Greater infection rate:* In our series, the mesh infection rate was 0%, in keeping with results reported by other authors who do not use these sutures (5). The infection rate reported by groups using transmural sutures was as high as 11.1% (7), with a mean of 4.87% (6, 7, 21). In addition to mesh infection, the sutures can become infected subcutaneously and superficially in the small incisions in the skin. In fact, in the only case in our series where we used sutures, the patient presented superficial infection in the skin at the site of the incisions made to place two of the sutures.

- *Pain during the early postoperative period:* Regardless of these factors, even more importantly, the use of transmural sutures involves taking 1 to 2 cm of tissue, trapping it and compressing it by tying at the subcutaneous cell tissue level. This is associated with greater pain during the immediate postoperative period and in the longer-term. In the short-term, some authors defending the use of these sutures recognize that there is more pain during the immediate postoperative period than after laparoscopic cholecystectomy (14) and that this pain could extend the hospitalization. There may also be discomfort at the suture level during the first two weeks of the postoperative period (20).

- *Long-term postoperative pain:* Even more important is the pain at long term, whether continuous or associated with movement, and the pulling sensation at the site of the through-and-through sutures. In some cases, oral narcotics, non-steroid anti-inflammatory drugs (21) or even repeated injections of local anesthetics at the suture site have been required, perhaps due to nerve entrapment (20, 21). Re-laparoscopy has been recommended to assess the condition of the mesh and the sutures and to section them if necessary (3).

Irrespective of the above disadvantages associated with sutures, if the recurrence rate in our series were higher than the series using transmural sutures, their use would be warranted. In series that advocate the use of sutures, the recurrence rate ranges anywhere from 0% (15) to 8.3% (18), with a mean of 3.98% (6, 7, 10, 14-16, 18-20, 21). The recurrence rate of our series is 3.33 % with a mean follow-up of 26 months. As we saw earlier, recurrence after laparoscopic repair of ventral hernias tends to appear more frequently during the first few months of the postoperative period. An analysis of our recurrences shows that they were not directly related to the use of sutures: one case was due to use of a short mesh at the begining of our series and the other two cases were two suprapubic hernias with recurrence at the inferior margin. Recurrence in these two cases resulted from inadequate exposure of the pubis and Cooper's ligament after taking down the peritoneum in order to anchor the mesh more securely at this level, a complicated area presenting difficulty when placing transmural sutures. Even authors who advocate the use of sutures do not recommend them at this level.

RESULTS OF OUR SERIES

Between November 1998 and November 2001 we operated on 91 ventral hernias using the "double crown" technique. Our series included 54 women and 37 men, with a mean age of 57.74 years (range: 26 to 80 years). The ventral hernias we operated on included 5 primary hernias, 3 umbilical and 2 epigastric hernias, and 86 incisional hernias. The hernia site varied considerably, with 74 midline hernias and 17 lateral hernias. The mean size of the defect repaired was 121.17cm^2.

Only one case was converted to open surgery, a patient with extremely dense adhesions who had been operated on previously for acute peritonitis resulting from acute abdomen of tuberculous origin. Intraoperative complications included three intestinal perforations; one was sutured by laparoscopy and the other two required enlarging one of the trocar incision to perform resection and anastomosis, later continuing by laparoscopy. The following complications were encountered during the postoperative period: three clinical seromas that required drains, one hematoma at the level of the abdominal wall, one prolonged paralytic ileus, and three reoperations. One of the reoperations was for missed bowel intestinal perforation during the surgery that caused peritonitis requiring emergency laparotomy, suture of the perforated bowel and removal the mesh. The other reoperations was in a patient who had fever of 45 days' duration. The seroma fluid was drained repeatedly, but cultures were negative. It was assumed that the patient had a foreign body reaction and the mesh was removed. The last one was due to a small bowel is chemia.

Hospitalisation was 1.84 days, with a mean of 2.48 days in our first 45 cases and dropping to 1.11 days in the last cases of our series. There were three recurrences accounting for 3.3 % of all our cases, with a mean follow-up of 22 months. These recurrences corresponded in one case to a patient in our initial series in which a too-small mesh was implanted and to two cases of suprapubic hernias in which the pubis and Cooper's ligament were not adequately exposed for suitable anchoring of the mesh.

CONCLUSIONS

Our results indicate that the use of transmural sutures are not necessary and that the "double crown" technique described using only tacks offers a number of clear advantages over the combined suture-and-tack method. When using the technique described, we obtained a similar recurrence rate versus series that use sutures, while also reducing the hospital stay and short-, medium- and long-term postoperative pain. Hence, we consider the "double crown" technique to be a valid alternative to ventral hernia repair with sutures.

References

1. LeBlanc KA, Booth WV. Laparoscopic repair of incisional abdominal hernias using expanded polytetrafluoroethylene: preliminary findings. Surg Laparosc Endosc 1993; 3 (1): 39-41.

2. Ponce JF, Barriga R, Martín I, Morales-Conde S, Morales-Méndez S. Prosthetic materials in incisional hernia: experimental study. Cir Esp 1998; 63(3): 189-194.

3. LeBlanc KA. Current considerations in laparoscopic incisional and ventral herniorrhaphy. JSLS 2000; 4(2):131-139.

4. Morales-Conde S, Cadet I, Tutosaus JD, Carrasco P, Palma F, Morales-Méndez S. Macroscopic evaluation of mesh incorporation placed intraperitoneally for laparoscopic ventral hernia repair. Experimental model. Proceedings of the 7th World Congress of Endoscopic Surgery (Singapore June 1-4, 2000). Monduzzi Editore. Bologna, Italy. 2000: 455-460.

5. Carbajo MA, Martín del Olmo JC, Blanco JI, De la Cuesta C, Toledano M, Martín F, Vaquero C, Inglada L. Laparoscopic treatment vs open surgery in the solution of major incisional and abdominal wall hernias with mesh. Sur Endosc 1999; 13:250-252.

6. Ramshaw BJ, Esartia P, Schwab J, Mason EM, Wilson RA, Duncan TD et al. Comparison of laparoscopic and open ventral herniorrhaphy. Am Surg 1999; 65(9):827-832.

7. DeMaria EJ, Moss JM, Sugerman HJ. Laparoscopic intraperitoneal polytetrafluoroethylene (PTFE) prosthesis patch repair of ventral hernia. Sur Endosc 2000; 14:326-329.

8. Morales-Conde S, López F, Tutosaus JD, Cadet H, Ortega Jm, Cantillana J, Martín M, Morales S. Cost-effectiveness of "Double Crown" technique for laparoscopic ventral hernia vs open repair. 9th International Congress of he European Association for Endoscopic Surgeons. Maasctricht.13-16 June 2001:66.

9. Koehler RH, Voeller G. Recurrences in laparoscopic incisional hernia repairs: a personal series and review of the literature. JSLS 1999; 3:293-304.

10. Park A, Gagner M, Pomp A. Laparoscopic repair of large incisional hernias. Surg Laparosc Endosc 1996; 6(2): 123-128.

11. Park A, Birch DW, Lovrics P. Laparoscopic and open incisional hernia repair: a comparison study. Surgery 1998; 124(4):816-822.

12. Carbajo MA, Martín del Olmo JC, Blanco JI, de la Cuesta C, Martín F, Toledano M, Perna C, Vaquero C. Laparoscopic treatment of ventral abdominal wall hernias: preliminary results in 100 patients. JSLE 2000; 4:141-145.

13. Chari R, Chari V, Eisenstat M. A case controlled study of laparoscopic ventral hernia repair. Surg Endosc 1998; 12(suppl):S09.

14. Costanza MJ, Heniford BT, Arca MJ, Mayes JT, Gagner M. Laparoscopic repair of recurrent ventral hernias. The American Surgeon 1998; 64(12):1121-1127.

15. LeBlanc KA, Booth W, Whitaker JM. Laparoscopic repair of ventral hernias using an intraperitoneal onlay patch: report of current results. Comtemporary Surgery 1994; 45(4)

16. Toy FK, Bailey RW, Carey S, Chappuis CW, Gagner M, Josephs LG, Mangiante EC, Park AE, Pomp A, Smoot Jr RT, Uddo Jr JF, Voeller GR. Prospective, multicenter study of laparoscopic ventral hernioplasty. Preliminary results. Sur Endosc 1998; 12:955-959.

17. Phillips E, Dardano AN, Saxe A. Laparoscopic repair of abdominal hernias using an ePTFE patch. A modification of a previously described technique. JSLS 1997; 1(3): 227-279.

18. Sanders LM, Flint LM, Ferrara JJ. Initial experience with laparoscopic repair of incisional hernias. The American Journal of Surgery 1999; 177:227-231.

19. Reitter DR, Paulsen JK, Debord JR, Estes NC. Five-year experience with the "four-before" laparoscopic ventral hernia repair. The American Surgeon 2000; 66(5):465-469.

20. Heniford BT, Ramshaw BJ. Laparoscopic ventral hernia repair: a report of 100 consecutive cases. Surg Endosc 2000; 14:419-423.

21. Heniford BT, Park A, Ramshaw BJ, Voeller G. Laparoscopic ventral and incisional hernia repair in 407 patients. J Am Coll Surg 2000; 190(6):645-650.

CHAPTER 29

Results of Laparoscopic Intraperitoneal Ventral Hernia Repair with Sutures

F.R. Abiad, G.R. Voeller

The short and long term results of open repair of incisional/ventral hernia have been reported extensively in the literature. Despite the use of a variety of procedures, the recurrence rate has remained significant. In a well conducted study, Hesselink et al. (4) found a 36 percent recurrence rate with a mean follow-up period of 34.9 months. Other recurrence rates reported after primary repair of ventral and incisional hernia range from 25% to 52% (4,17). In a multicenter randomized trial, Luijendijk et al. (10) compared the recurrence rate following primary suture repair with that following mesh repair; they found the latter to be superior with regard to the recurrence of hernia, regardless of the size of the hernia. In this study, the recurrence rate following mesh repair was 24 percent. It has been well documented that the Rives/Stoppa repair leads to the lowest rates of recurrence. For this reason, the American Hernia Society has declared that this open repair for large ventral/incisional hernias should be the standard of care. The use of prosthetic material in the repair of ventral and incisional hernias has reduced the rate of recurrence; however, more important wound complications were seen with this technique. The laparoscopic repair of ventral and incisional hernia achieves the same result as the Rives/Stoppa open repair. Since the wounds are smaller and the abdominal wall soft tissue is manipulated minimally, the wound complications are expected to be less. Early in our experience, the mesh was fixed to the abdominal wall by staples. We soon discovered that this was not adequate, and we converted to the suture mesh repair. Below is a summary of our results as well as those published by surgeons using a similar technique.

RESULTS

The earliest prospective multi-center study of laparoscopic ventral hernia repair was originated by Toy and Smoot (18). The vast majority of patients included in this study underwent a laparoscopic sutured mesh repair. The preliminary data was published in 1998 and consisted of 144 patients. Various types of ventral hernias were repaired with the majority being incisional. The findings in this study were encouraging, and showed the laparoscopic repair to be feasible and safe. The mean operative time (120 min) was acceptable, and the postoperative hospital stay (2.3 days) was short. Although the mean follow-up period was not long (7.4 months), the recurrence rate was low (4.2%). In another large study, the laparoscopic repair of ventral and incisional hernia was performed on 407 patients (3). The patients were large with a mean BMI of 32kg/m^2 .The vast majority of patients (89%) had previous surgery, and 136 of the hernias were recurrent. In this study, the mean follow-up period was longer (23 months). There has been other studies that looked at the results of laparoscopic repair of ventral and incisional hernia (3, 8, 12, 18); these studies have confirmed the findings by Toy et al. The results are summarized in Table II. In another study, Reiter et al. (14) looked into the patient satisfaction rate and found that 90 percent of their patients were "satisfied" with their operation and results.

Table II. Complications in 407 Patients Who Underwent Laparoscopic Ventral Hernia Repair

Complications	n	%
Prolonged ileus	9	2.21
Seroma>6wk	8	1.97
Suture site pain>8wk	8	1.97
Intestinal injury	5	1.23
Cellulites of Trocar site	5	1.23
Mesh infection	4	0.98
Hematoma or post op bleeding	3	0.74
Urinary retention	3	0.74
Fever of unknown origin	3	0.74
Respiratory distress	2	0.49
Intraabdominal abscess	1	0.25
Trocar site herniation	1	0.25
Total	**53**	**13.0**

COMPLICATIONS

Multiple studies have documented that open repair of ventral hernia has significant morbidity. Leber et al. (7) reported a 27% long term complication rate including infection, hematoma and seroma, chronic sinus tract formation, mesh extrusion, fistula formation as well as soft tissue problems such as non-healing wounds.

White et al. (20) reported that 34% of 250 open ventral hernia repairs had wound related complications. The wide dissection of soft tissue that is required for a Rives/Stoppa type repair or the flaps raised for an anterior type repair often lead to wound related problems. Since the laparoscopic repair avoids these dissections, it is hoped that many of these complications can be avoided.

In our study of 407 patients that underwent the laparoscopic repair, the incidence of complications was 13% (Table II).The majority of these complications were minor. The wound and soft tissue problems so often seen with the open repair were infrequent (2%). Robins et al. (16) found that only 3% of patients undergoing laparoscopic repair of ventral hernia had a major wound complication as compared with 22% of patients undergoing open herniorrhaphy. This is not unexpected , since the laparoscopic approach avoids the long incision and the wide flaps seen with the open repair. We saw only four cases of mesh infection (1%). One of these cases showed no bacterial growth when the mesh was later removed. The senior author in his own personal series of over 250 laparoscopic ventral/incisional hernia repairs has yet to have a single case of mesh infection.

Early seroma formation is common. The patient usually develops a fluid collection between the mesh and the abdominal wall; this collection is usually not apparent to the patient and will eventually resolve (9). In our study, the seroma, in 8 patients (2%), persisted for more than six weeks. The management of seromas depends on the surgeon's preference. We have occasionally aspirated these collections without any adverse effect. However, with patient reassurance and understanding, these seromas resolve on their own if given time. We recently have used fibrin glue prophylactically to obliterate the dead hernia space in four patients with large ventral hernias. Only one of the four developed a seroma.

The most dreaded complication that has been seen with the laparoscopic approach is bowel injury. These bowel injuries can be missed, with catastrophic consequences. Enterotomy is a well-documented complication during open hernioplasty (7, 20). It usually occurs during lysis of adhesions with either sharp or blunt dissection. When noted, it can be repaired through the incision. The procedure then can be completed if a primary repair is planned. With the laparoscopic approach, the enterotomy can occur at different stages of the procedure. It can occur initially when an access is being established. More frequently though, it occurs during adhesiolysis. A limited field of vision and aggressive dissection are important culprits. However, the magnification and high-intensity light source allow good visualization of the adhesions. With proper and careful technique, the adhesions can be taken down safely. Bowel injury secondary to thermal spread is more commonly seen with the laparoscopic repair. Monopolar cautery has the problem of current spread. This is not present with the use of the ultrasonic or high frequency dissection. However, the tip of this instrument remains very hot after use, and that can cause unrecognized injury. For this reason, we believe that the use of energy source at the time of dissection should be avoided or kept to a minimum. In our study, an enterotomy occurred in five patients (1.2%). All were recognized and repaired.

RECURRENCE

The true incidence of recurrence following the repair of incisional and ventral hernia depends on the duration of follow-up. Hesselink et al. (4) found that the vast majority of recurrences occurred during the first three post-operative years. The recurrence rates reported after primary repair of ventral and incisional hernia range from 25% to 52% (4,17). Open mesh repair have a lower incidence of recurrence. One of the advantages of the laparoscopic repair is that it allows a thorough inspection of the abdominal wall for clinically undetected hernias. These can be missed with the open repair, especially with the anterior approach, and do present later as "recurrences". Most of the laparoscopic repair series have a relatively short mean follow-up period (Table I). In the majority, the recurrence rate is small, less than 6%. One series, however, showed a 9.3% recurrence rate (8). This series had the longest mean duration of follow-up (51 months). The authors noted that all the recurrences occurred in patients where the mesh was stapled but not sutured. This has been our experience as well. For this reason, we believe that suture fixation should be an integral part of the operation. We have recently operated on patient with a recurrent incisional hernia post a laparoscopic repair. The mesh was sutured to the abdominal wall. However, the mesh size was too small and there was minimal overlap between the edges of the mesh and healthy fascia. In our experience, the two main technical causes for early hernia recurrence are the non-suture fixation of the mesh and the use of a small mesh (6). If the principles of the repair mentioned in the previous chapter are adhered to, we believe the recurrence rate will be small.

Table I. Laparoscopic Ventral Hernia Repair

Study	No of patients	Mean size of defect (cm²)	Mean length of operation (min)	Mean hospital stay (days)	Mean Follow-up period (month)
LeBlanc KA et al.	100	155	-	1-2	51
Heniford BT et al.	407	100	97	1.8	23
Park A et al.	28	104	108	4.3	18
Toy F et al.	144	98	120	2.3	7.4

COMPARISON OF OPEN VERSUS LAPAROSCOPIC REPAIR

Early results of the laparoscopic repair of ventral and incisional hernia compared favorably to the published results of the open repair. Several studies have reported direct comparison between open and laparoscopic repair of ventral and incisional hernia (1, 2, 5, 11, 13). The studies differed with respect to operative times, with some reporting the laparoscopic repair to take longer, while other studies reporting the opposite. However, the hospital stay and rate of complications were significantly less with the laparoscopic repair. Holzman et al. (5) and Demaria et al. (2) compared the total hospital costs between the two approaches and found them more with the open repair. In all of the studies, the recurrence rate following the laparoscopic repair was the same or less than following the open repair. Although none of these studies was a randomized prospective study, the trends are apparent.

CONCLUSION

The laparoscopic repair of ventral and incisional hernia is feasible. It is associated with less wound complications than with the open repair. If performed properly, the incidence of major complications can be minimized. The total hospital costs are comparable or even less than the open repair. We believe suture fixation of the mesh to be an integral part of the procedure and has implications on the recurrence rates. Results with long term follow-up are needed, but the data we have do suggest a trend towards less recurrences and higher rates of patient satisfaction with the laparoscopic repair of ventral hernia.

References

1. Chari R, Chari V, Eisenstat M, Chung R. A case controlled study of laparoscopic incisional hernia repair. Surg Endosc 2000 Feb;14(2):117-9.

2. DeMaria EJ, Moss JM, Sugerman HJ. Laparoscopic intraperitoneal polytetrafluoroethylene (PTFE) prosthetic patch repair of ventral hernia. Prospective comparison to open prefascial polypropylene mesh repair. Surg Endosc 2000 Apr;14(4):326-9.

3. Heniford BT, Park A, Ramshaw BJ, Voeller G. Laparoscopic ventral and incisional hernia repair in 407 patients. J Am Coll Surg 2000 Jun;190(6):645-50.

4. Hesselink VJ, Luijendijk RW, de Wilt JH, Heide R, Jeekel J. An evaluation of risk factors in incisional hernia recurrence. Surg Gynecol Obstet 1993 Mar;176(3):228-34.

5. Holzman MD, Purut CM, Reintgen K, Eubanks S, Pappas TN. Laparoscopic ventral and incisional hernioplasty. Surg Endosc 1997 Jan;11(1):32-5.

6. Koehler RH, Voeller G. Recurrences in laparoscopic incisional hernia repairs: a personal series and review of the literature. JSLS 1999 Oct-Dec;3(4):293-304.

7. Leber GE, Garb JL, Alexander AI, Reed WP. Long-term complications associated with prosthetic repair of incisional hernias. Arch Surg 1998 Apr;133(4):378-82.

8. LeBlanc KA, Booth WV, Whitaker JM, Bellanger DE. Laparoscopic incisional and ventral herniorraphy: our initial 100 patients. Hernia 2001 Mar;5(1):41-5.

9. Lin BH, Vargish T, Dachman AH. CT findings after laparoscopic repair of ventral hernia. AJR Am J Roentgenol 1999 Feb;172(2):389-92.

10. Luijendijk RW, Hop WC, van den Tol MP, et al. A comparison of suture repair with mesh repair for incisional hernia. N Engl J Med 2000 Aug 10;343(6):392-8.

11. Park A, Birch DW, Lovrics P. Laparoscopic and open incisional hernia repair: a comparison study. Surgery 1998 Oct;124(4):816-21.

12. Park A, Gagner M, Pomp A. Laparoscopic repair of large incisional hernias. Surg Laparosc Endosc 1996 Apr;6(2):123-8.

13. Ramshaw BJ, Esartia P, Schwab J, Mason EM, Wilson RA, Duncan TD, Miller J, Lucas GW, Promes J. Comparison of laparoscopic and open ventral herniorrhaphy. Am Surg 1999 Sep;65(9):827-31.

14. Reitter DR, Paulsen JK, Debord JR, Estes NC. Five-year experience with the "four-before" laparoscopic ventral hernia repair. Am Surg 2000 May;66(5):465-8.

15. Rives J, Pire JC, Flament JB, Convers G. Treatment of large eventrations (apropos of 133 cases). Minerva Chir 1977 Jun 15;32(11):749-56.

16. Robbins SB, Pofahl WE, Gonzalez RP. Laparoscopic ventral hernia repair reduces wound complications. Am Surg 2001 Sep;67(9):896-900.

17. Stoppa RE. The treatment of complicated groin and incisional hernias. World J Surg 1989 Sep-Oct;13(5):545-54.

18. Toy FK, Bailey RW, Carey S, et al. Prospective, multicenter study of laparoscopic ventral hernioplasty. Preliminary results. Surg Endosc 1998 Jul;12(7):955-9.

19. Wantz GE. Incisional hernioplasty with Mersilene. Surg Gynecol Obstet 1991 Feb;172(2):129-37.

20. White TJ, Santos MC, Thompson JS. Factors affecting wound complications in repair of ventral hernias. Am Surg 1998 Mar;64(3):276-80.

CHAPTER 30

Results of Laparoscopic Intraperitoneal Ventral Hernia Repair without Sutures

M.A. Carbajo, F. Martin-Acebes, M. Toledano

INTRODUCTION

Laparoscopic repair of primary and incisional hernias was first performed by several surgical groups following an article published by K.A. LeBlanc in 1993 (1). The mesh was placed with external sutures tied subcutaneously and completed using conventional peripheral stapling with minimal tissue penetration.

Our initial experience used a similar technique and encountered some of the problems associated with the mesh fixation procedure, including prolonged surgery time due to technical difficulties resulting from placing and tying the sutures, the need to insert the suture removal instrument in two different positions in order to "entrap" a sufficient amount of parietal tissue, the risk of vascular lesion in the muscle layer and postoperative pain due to tension of the external knots on the abdominal wall. In addition, the intraperitoneal stapling instruments available at that time provided a flat staple with minimal penetration and consistency that occasionally did not perforate the PTFE mesh properly. Due to these and other problems, the initial enthusiasm faded and some groups stopped using the technique.

Between 1995 and 1996, a new mesh fixation instrument for preperitoneal laparoscopic repair of inguinal hernias became available. This instrument applied tacks with sufficient pressure to attach the mesh in the periosteum of the pubis.

Although the manufacturer originally designed the tacker to treat inguinal hernias, our group began using it immediately to anchor the intraperitoneal PTFE mesh. The use of external sutures was gradually eliminated as we noticed that the mesh was quickly, securely and satisfactorily anchored to the abdominal wall when properly tacked.

As a result, the original technique was modified, allowing the placement of large mesh prostheses without the need for external sutures, thereby preventing suture problems and significantly shortening the surgery time.

Our first series comparing mesh suturing versus the new intraperitoneal tack technique using a double crown of tacks for incisional and ventral hernia repair was initially presented to surgeons at the Joint Euro-Asian Congress of Endoscopic Surgery (2). The technique was rapidly implemented by other surgical teams interested in laparoscopic repair for this type of condition.

DIFFERENT RESULTS WITH DIFFERENT VENTRAL HERNIAS

From the standpoint of results, the various types of hernias exhibit display intrinsic differences. A distinction can be made between three different models: primary ventral hernias, incisional hernias and multiple hernia recurrences.

Primary ventral hernias are the simplest and fastest to treat since they rarely include hernia content except (on occasions) omentum or round ligament and, therefore, any problems that occur will be related to the mesh.

Incisional hernias are a significantly more complex challenge which includes the surgical approach; fatty, visceroparietal and viscerovisceral adhesiolysis; releasing of the entire surface of the previous incision and sufficient space to place the mesh; hemostasis of surfaces of dissection; insertion of the mesh and preventive measures to eliminate or minimize seroma. Moreover, various problems that can influence the results may arise, depending on the hernia site. Subcostal, subxiphoid or suprapubic hernias have a poorer prognosis than hernias of the midline, periumbilical region, or lateral or lumbar flanks (Fig. 1 and 2).

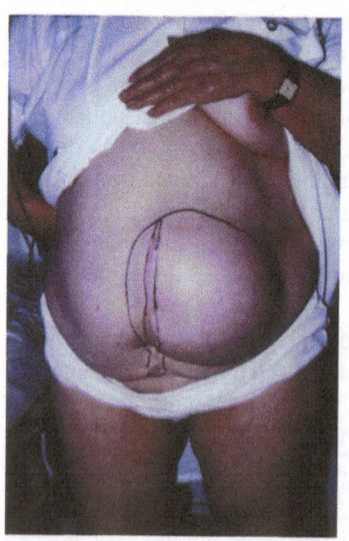

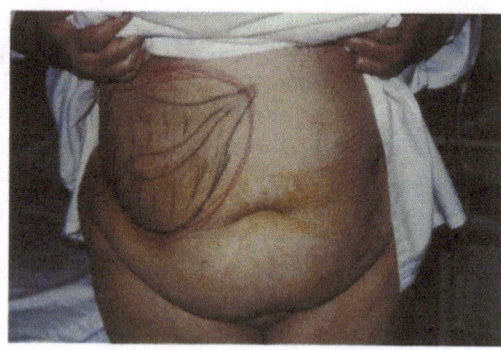

◄ **Fig. 1.** Large incisional hernia in the upper left quadrant.

▲ **Fig. 2.** Right subcostal incisional hernia.

Extensive experience in laparoscopic surgery is necessary for operating on multi-recurrent hernias, particularly if they have been previously repaired with polypropylene mesh. Visceral adhesiolysis can become extremely complex and risky, and there can be catastrophic consequences in the case of missed lesions of the bowel or improper repairs. Ensuring good results is more important than ever and, therefore, the mesh must be sized as generously as possible and anchoring must be done with utmost care.

Another factor to consider in terms of hernia type is the size. Naturally, better results will be obtained with hernias under 5 cm than large incisional hernias with multiple small defects ("Swiss-cheese"), while midline hernias with multiple small defects will have fewer complications than hernias with only one medium-size defect in the same area (Fig. 3). Hernias with narrow necks and large subcutaneous sacs will be easier to cover with mesh, although the respective seroma and complication rates will be much higher.

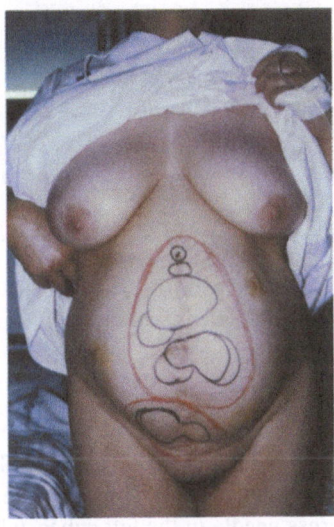

Fig. 3. Multiple midline defects

COMPLICATIONS IN A PERSONAL SERIES OF 200 CASES

All individuals included in this series (operated between January 1994 and November 1999) are part of an observational study in which the patients were operated on by the same surgeon at the same hospital and monitored every three months during the first year and once a year thereafter.

The results obtained with these patients were compiled in a computer database that was controlled and monitored by another evaluator. All patients who were operated in other hospitals or did not meet the follow-up requirements were excluded from the study.

The updated mean follow-up for all patients was 42 months (range: 14-84). All complications were also updated, considering that the longer the follow-up time, the more reliable are the results for long-term complications, one of the cardinal rules of abdominal wall surgery.

The statistical data and the data on hernia classification, defect origin, anatomic site, surfaces to be covered, mesh sizes and surgical technique are mentioned in the literature (3,4,5). Thirty-three patients had a primary ventral hernia and 167 were incisional hernias, of which 65 were multiple recurrences (2-9 times).

Regarding the mesh anchoring technique, external sutures were used in 18 patients and technique of total intraperitoneal fixation with a double crown of tacks in 182 (Fig. 4).

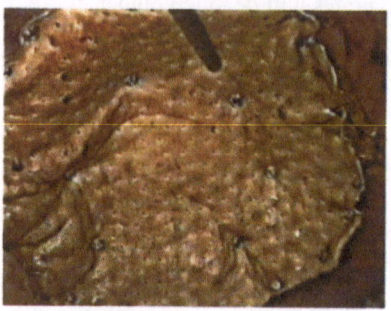

Fig. 4. Mesh positioning which shows double crown (external and internal).

Intraoperative complications

- During the approach. We have not had any complications related to the pneumoperitoneum or placement of the trocars. The pneumoperitoneum is normally created with a Veress needle in the left subcostal space, the safest area to avoid vascular or visceral lesions and for placement of the optical trocar. The two work trocars are placed under direct vision in the left flank. Two cases of wall emphysema due to gas displacement occurred in very thin patients with no subcutaneous cell tissue.

- During adhesiolysis. We had two bowel perforations in two patients with tightly attached fibrotic adhesions between the small intestine and hernia sac; in one case this was due to inadequate traction of the bowel (Fig. 5) and in the other due to progressive tearing of the serosa in severe scar entrapment. The first case was converted to open surgery, being the conversion rate of the series of 0.5%. In the second, intestinal repair by minilaparotomy was performed, with the procedure completed by laparoscopy.
Another four patients had various serosa lesions that were resolved by intraabdominal suturing with no further problems.
We experienced no missed bowel lesions that subsequently required resurgery.
Adhesiolysis is the most common reason for conversion, serious postoperative problems and mortality, particularly when enterotomies are missed during surgery (6). In the case of tightly adhered intestinal bowel, we recommend optimal

exposure by performing blunt dissection, and fine-cutting Metzenbaum scissors, but not laparoscopic traction instruments, cautery or ultrasonic devices. Bowel should be handled from different angles so it can be mobilized from the best side and the procedure should carried out with utmost care and precision (Fig. 6).

The colon may be another source of serious intra-abdominal problems, particularly in medium-high incisions where it can be completely adhered to the abdominal wall; in obese patients, the existence of thick mesocolon can mask the transverse colon and cause missed lesion.

During dissection of left subcostal or subxiphoid hernias, the stomach and liver may be found to be adhered to the wall.

- During mesh placement. We have not had any complications due to mesh anchoring by total intraperitoneal technique. Improperly applied tacks can be easily removed; we have not observed any kind of vascular parietal lesion. It is important to mark the mesh clearly for easy placement with respect to the hernia, then add the initial tacks at the corners for tent-like positioning of the mesh. The entire process should be perfectly controlled with the surgeon's left hand on the abdominal wall. No tack should be applied without first checking from the outside. The tacker should be applied against the surgeon's opposite hand, ensuring complete penetration of the tack in the mesh and abdominal wall (Fig. 7). Surgeon should not leave any loose tacks, in which half the tack does not penetrate or is on top of the mesh without entering the wall, since this leaves the mesh improperly anchored and can produce adhesions to the bowel.

In the first few patients in whom we used external sutures, we observed one severe parietal vascular lesion and another less important lesion that required repair by laparoscopic suturing in both cases.

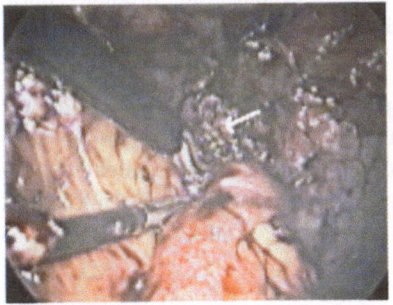
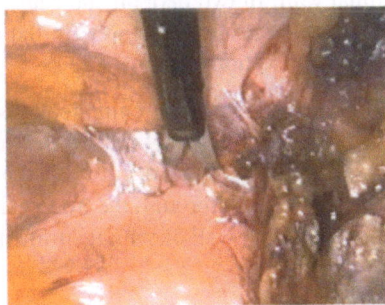

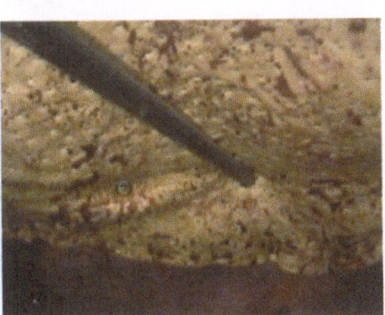

Fig. 5. Enterotomy due to inadequate traction and improper use of the electrocoagulation device.

▲ **Fig. 6.** Use of scissors without any source of energy for dissection near intestinal bowel.

◄ **Fig. 7.** Application of tacks, with external control of the instrument's internal pressure by the surgeon's hand.

Short-term postoperative complications

- Intestinal occlusion. In one of our first patients, in whom the mesh was peripherally secured with the old-style flat staplers, intestinal occlusion occurred on the fourth day post-surgery due to improper anchoring of the mesh to the abdominal wall. The patient had to be reoperated. We did not encounter similar complications with the use of tackers in our series, although incarceration or intestinal occlusion may develop if the tacks are applied with a separation of more than 1.5-2 cm and a second circle has not been applied against the fibrous ring of the hernia sac

- Seroma. Seroma is the most frequently encountered complication, although its importance has decreased with the appearance of Dual-Mesh Plus with holes, a mesh that enhances peritoneal absorption of the exudate. In our series, postoperative seromas developed in 28 patients (14%) and were resolved by fine-needle aspiration and external compression.
We recommend abrasion of parietal dissection surfaces with argon laser terminal for laparoscopy and postoperative external compression on the former hernia sac for 6-7 days. The percentage of seromas currently observed has decreased dramatically with these measures.

- Pain. In 16 cases persistent postoperative pain developed, lasting for the first few weeks. The cases of continued intense pain were observed in patients with external sutures. A sensation of discomfort or "pulling" was reported by several patients with large prostheses or several prostheses that required numerous tacks for placement.

- Abdominal wall hematomas. Four cases presented hematomas of some size in the abdominal wall. In two patients the cause was the vascular lesion produced during placement of the external sutures; in the other two patients, the hematomas were due to trocar insertion.

- Mesh infection. No septic complications related to the mesh or entry ports were observed. Although primary mesh infections have been reported in various series (6,7,8), this is unlikely to occur with the intra-abdominal fixation technique and insertion of the mesh through the trocar, since the mesh does not come into contact with the abdominal wall or with instruments crossing the wall.

General complications. Mortality.

There were no deaths in our series.

Long-term postoperative complications.

- Hernia recurrence. Updated results demonstrated hernia recurrence in eight patients (4%). In four cases recurrence took place during the first three months after the surgery. The patients were reoperated using the same approach and are currently symptom-free. The other four patients presented late recurrences. In two cases the recurrence is small and symptom-free and the patients have declined surgery. The other two patients, who are affected by severe abdominal wall pathology, have presented medium-size recurrences and are pending reoperation. One of the early recurrences was in a patient with sutures (5.5%); the rest occurred in patients with intraabdominal fixation using only tacks (3.8%).

Hernia recurrence is still a major challenge in the field of abdominal wall surgery. We analyzed each of our recurrences and found technical defects in the four early recurrences, placement of a short mesh in two of the late recurrences (Fig. 8) and problems of multiple concomitant associated diseases in the other two.

One of the recurrences was in a primary ventral hernia to which an inadequate mesh had been used; in four cases the hernias were incisional hernias and in the other three, multi-recurrent hernias.

The recurrence rates in the published series are hard to assess because of differences in the procedures used, the type of hernias operated and, particularly in the follow-up time. In our series the recurrence rate increased as the observation period increased. In general, the frequency ranges from 5 to 13% in series with more than 50 cases (7,8,9). Only LeBlanc's study of 100 cases had a mean follow-up time longer than ours (9).

We recommend that surgeons always use large pieces of mesh overlapping at least 5 cm the margin of the hernia defect, that the mesh be secured on the left side first (trocar working site) to prevent improper shifting toward "the easy side", that the tacks penetrate deeply and that the double crown of tacks be properly positioned.

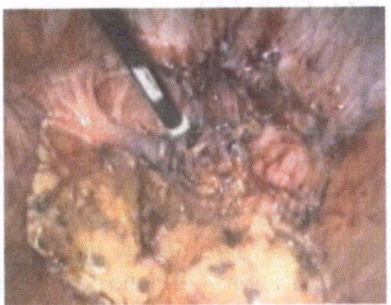

Fig. 8. Late recurrence at 3 years, at the upper margin of a previously implanted mesh (insufficient mesh).

- Implant-related complications. We have not found any problems related to possible conditions of adhesions attached to the mesh, such as chronic abdominal pain or intestinal subocclusion, nor have we observed mesh migration phenomena of any kind, failures of tissue integration or rejection (Fig. 9).

In reoperations for recurrence or other subsequent laparoscopic procedures, we have observed no tight adhesions to the mesh. This is due to rapid PTFE peritonization, which results in the production of peritoneo-peritoneal intraperitoneal adhesions. In vivo biopsies of peritonization tissue from the mesh showed the presence of fibrosis in contact with the implant and peritoneum on the visceral surface (10). In contrast, previously implanted polypropylene prostheses that have penetrated to the abdominal cavity have occasionally shown strong adhesions to the bowel that is difficult and hazardous to dissect. Some laparoscopic intra-abdominal hernioplasty series use Marlex or polypropylene mesh (11-12). However, we do not believe that there is now a well-tested alternative that can replace PTFE (13).

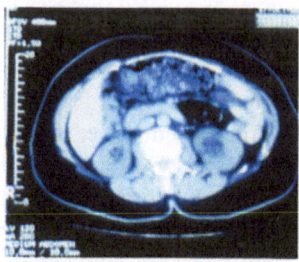

Fig. 9. Follow-up CT study at 3 years, with correct neofor-mation of the abdo-minal linea alba.

RESULTS AND DISCUSSION

Laparoscopic repair of the various types of abdominal wall hernias has developed slowly and found difficulties along the way, in comparison to the rapid growth of laparoscopic surgery in general. Moreover, the interval that has passed since its more generalized use is relatively short for a procedure that needs several years to properly evaluate long-term results.

Nevertheless, the popularity of laparoscopy in recent times is generating a wealth of experience and publications, all indicative of the substantial benefits obtained from these techniques as compared to conventional open surgery (Fig. 10A and 10B). However, a broad multicenter, randomized study comparing the two approaches to abdominal wall repair has still not appeared in the literature. This may be because of the problems arising from fact that there is no suitable "gold standard" in open surgery for comparison and because there are different learning curves and varying degrees of experience in laparoscopic techniques. Along this line, we have performed a random, comparative study of our own as a preliminary step toward discontinuing the use of conventional surgery for this problem (14). In any case, the current evidence appears to indicate that the laparoscopic approach is on the road to becoming a new "gold standard" in abdominal wall surgery.

Another step ahead would be the standardization of laparoscopic procedures, which are basically unified by the most active surgical groups working at present, except in terms of implant placement. External sutures plus tacks or total intra-abdominal fixation with tacks?

Since there is no randomized study comparing any potential differences in the results obtained from the two techniques, we must again recur to the experience of individuals or specific work groups.

Actually the only differences are related to surgery time, potential for mesh infection, postoperative pain assessment and recurrences.

In our experience, surgery time is reduced by about 40-50%. The mean surgery time in our series was 64 minutes (range: 20-180), being about 40% higher in other series (6).

Mesh infection was 0% in our series; other results obtained in series using sutures have been mentioned earlier.

Pain assessment is very difficult to discuss in objective terms. In our series, however, patients with external sutures mentioned pain more frequently than patients without sutures.

The rate of recurrences is very acceptable in our series, which had a mean follow-up of 3 1/2 years. We have mentioned rates reported in the literature that were similar or higher than ours. Nevertheless, the presence of sutures has not been shown to lower the risk of recurrence.

Other parameters such as hospitalization, intraoperative risk and other risks resulting from surgery can be similar and satisfactory in groups with the same level of experience.

New long-term studies will provide more precise data and information that will unquestionably be decisive in the establishment of a definitive common project

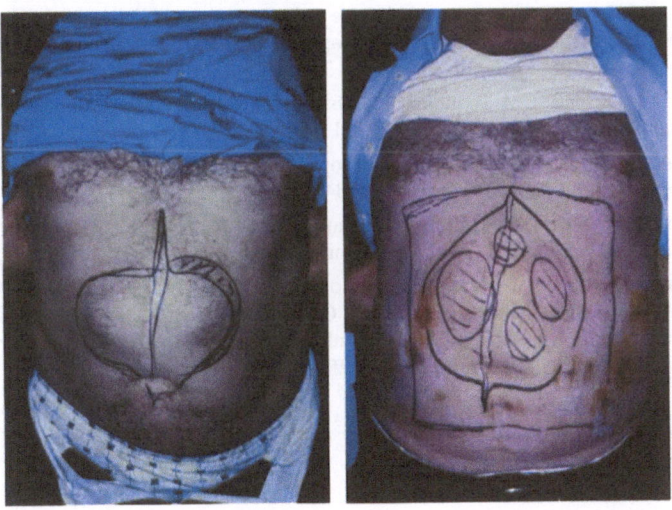

Fig. 10. Large incisional hernia of the midline with multiple wall defects. A: before surgery. B: after surgery.

References

1. LeBlanc KA, Booth WV. Laparoscopic repair of incisional abdominal hernias using expanded polytetrafluoroethylene: preliminary findings. Surg Laparosc Endosc 1993; 3 (1): 39-41.

2. Carbajo Caballero MA, Martín del Olmo JC, Blanco Alvarez JI, Cuesta de la Llave C, Vaquero Puerta C. Laparoscopic treatment of massive periumbilical hernia with expanded PTFE. In: Topuzlu C and Tekant Y, eds. Joint Euro-Asian Congress of Endoscopic Surgery. Bologna: Monduzzi Ed; 1997: 351-354.

3. Carbajo MA, Martin del Olmo JC, Blanco JI, de la Cuesta C, Martín F, Toledano M, Perna C, Vaquero C. Laparoscopic treatment of ventral abdominal wall hernias: preliminary results in 100 patients. J Surg Laparoendosc Surg 2000; 4: 141-145.

4. Carbajo MA, Martín del Olmo JC, Blanco JI, Cuesta de la Llave C, Martín F, Toledano M, Perna C and Vaquero VC. A laparoscopic solution for an old problem: Incisional and abdominal wall hernias. Experience with 200 patients. In: Lomanto D, Kum CK, So JBY and Goh PMY, eds. 7th World Congress of endoscopic surgery. Bologna: Monduzzi Ed; 2000: 437-440.

5. Carbajo Caballero MA, Martín del Olmo JC, Blanco Alvarez JI, Cuesta de la Llave C, Vaquero Puerta C. Volumineuse éventration xipho-pubienne à sacs multiples. La réparation coelioscopique est-elle possible? European J Coelio-Surg 1998; 26: 41-44.

6. Koehler RH, Voeller G. Recurrences in laparoscopic incisional hernia repairs.: A personal series and review of the literature. JSLS 1999; 3: 293-304.

7. Toy FK, Bairley RW, Carey S. Prospective multicenter study of laparoscopic ventral hernioplasty. Preliminary results. Surg Endosc 1997; 12 (7): 955-959.

8. Park A, Gagner H, Pomp A. Laparoscopic repair of large incisional hernias. Surg Lagar Endo 1996; 6: 123-128.

9. LeBlanc KA. Current considerations in laparoscopic incisional and ventral herniorraphy. JSLS 2000; 4: 131-139.

10. Carbajo MA, Martín del Olmo JC, Blanco Alvarez JI, Sastre L, de la Cuesta C, Martín F, Toledano M, Perna C. La prothèse biface de polytetrafluoroethylène expansé destinée aux plasties intrapéritonéales sous coelioscopie est-elle réellement un matériau anti-adhérences?. European J Coelio-Surg 2000; 34: 69-71.

11. Holtzman MD, Purut CM, Reintgen K, Eubanks S, Pappas TN. Laparoscopic ventral and incisional hernioplasty. Surg Endosc 1997; 11: 247-251.

12. Bickel A, Evitan A. A simplified laparoscopic technique for mesh placement in ventral hernia repair. Surg Endosc 1999; 13: 532-534.

13. Carbajo MA, Martín del Olmo JC, Blanco JI. What is the appropiate mesh for laparoscopic intraperitoneal repair of abdominal wall hernia?. Surg Endosc 2000; 14: 408.

14. Carbajo Caballero MA, Martín del Olmo JC, Blanco Alvarez JI, Martín Acebes F, Toledano Trincado M, Cuesta de la Llave C, Vaquero Puerta C, Perna C. Laparoscopic treatment versus open surgery in the solution of major incisional and abdominal wall hernias with mesh. Surg Endosc 1999; 13: 250-252.

CHAPTER 31

Open versus Laparoscopic Ventral Hernia Repair. Prospective Trial

A.Z. Fernandez, E.J. DeMaria

INTRODUCTION

Ventral hernias include both primary abdominal wall defects and incisional hernias. More than 80% of adult ventral hernias are incisional hernias. (1) The incidence of incisional hernias after laparotomy is between 2 and 20%. (2,3,4) Primary repair of ventral hernias has been met with poor results. Recurrence rates vary anywhere from 20% to as high as 52%. (3,5,6,7) In a search to improve recurrence rates, multiple techniques have been developed including the fascia lata technique, the Mayo overlap technique, the Maingot's keel procedure and the Nuttall procedure. (3,5) These repairs were reportedly more successful than simple primary repairs but the rates of recurrence remained unacceptably high.

The use of prosthetic materials for hernia repair began in the 1940's with the introduction of steel mesh. The steel mesh was stiff and impractical. With the advent of plastics in the late 1950's, an alternative to metal mesh was found. In 1963 Usher first reported using knitted polypropylene mesh for hernia repairs. (8) Mesh greatly improved ventral hernia repair results. In a recent multicenter trial, 200 patients were randomly assigned to either a primary suture repair or mesh repair of a ventral hernia. (6) At three years the cumulative recurrence rates for the respective repairs were 43% and 24%. There was a significant difference between the suture and mesh repairs. Other reports have shown recurrence rates below 5% after mesh repairs. (4,9,10,11) The concern with these repairs is that their wound complications, including hematoma, seroma, cellulitis, abscess and skin necrosis, are too high. The rates of complications were between 12% and 44%. (4,9,11,12) This high rate of wound complications was attributed to the extensive dissection required for these procedures, the use of external drains, the mesh, the patient's comorbidities, and the large incision. Furthermore, these procedures were very painful and required long hospital stays. In an effort to improve on these shortcomings, Leblanc first reported a laparoscopic ventral hernia repair in 1993. (13)

RETROSPECTIVE AND PROSPECTIVE SERIES

Since the initial published report of a laparoscopic ventral hernia repair, many retrospective and prospective series have followed (Table I). The largest series to date was reported by Heniford in 2000 (14). They reviewed 415 patients who had undergone a laparoscopic hernia repair. Of the 415 patients, eight (1.9%) had to be converted to an open repair. The remaining 407 patients were comprised of 202 women and 205 men with a mean age of 53.2 years (range 13 to 88 years) and mean body mass index of 32 (range 22 to 60). The mean hernia defect was 100.1cm^2 (range 1 to 480 cm^2). The technique used for the majority of the patients involved using expanded polytetrafluoroethylene (ePTFE) mesh to overlap the defect by 3-4 cm. The mesh was secured into position by means of extracorporeal sutures and intracorporeal spiral staples. The mean operative time was 97 minutes (range 11 to 270 minutes). The patients had an average hospital stay of 1.8 days (range same day to 17 days). The rate of all complications was 13%. The most common complications were prolonged ileus (9), seroma more than 6 weeks (8), and suture site pain more than 8 weeks (8). Twenty-nine of the 53 total complications were wound related (seroma, pain, trocar site cellulitis (5), mesh infection (4), hematoma or bleeding (3), and intraabdominal abscess (1)). All four of the patients with mesh infection required re-operation and mesh removal. Recurrent hernias developed in 14 patients for a rate of 3.4%. This is likely an underestimation in light that the follow-up period was only 23 months. Hesselink has shown that the cumulative primary recurrence after two and five years is 27 and 41 percent, respectively (5). Longer follow-up is needed to be able to truly quantitate the actual recurrence rate for this repair. This report does establish that laparoscopic ventral hernia repair is safe, with morbidity comparable to the best reports of open repairs. One significant benefit is the short hospital stay required. The recurrence rate will require longer follow-up but the initial results are very promising.

Franklin reported another large series in 1998 (15). 176 patients underwent laparoscopic repair of 62 umbilical hernias, 112 ventral, incisional, or recurrent umbilical hernias, and two Spigellian hernias. Their technique involved performing a primary repair if possible followed by reinforcement or placement of intraperitoneal polypropylene mesh. The mesh was secured with staples and "in most circumstances" transfascial sutures. The repaired area was then covered with omentum. 97% of their repairs were completed laparoscopically. Their complication rate was 5.1% with only three trocar site infections and one mesh infection requiring mesh removal. The recurrence rate has also been remarkably low at 1.1% at a mean follow-up of 30 months. One recurrence was in a primary repair of an umbilical hernia and the other in a ventral hernia repair. Isolating the 112 incisional hernia repairs, there was only one recurrence in a mean follow-up period of 2.8 years. Although these results are quite promising, the lack of uniformity of the hernias and the techniques used takes away from their significance.

LeBlanc followed his report of how to do a laparoscopic hernia in 1993 with a review of his first 100 cases in 2000 (16). In this retrospective review, there was a mix of ventral hernias. The majority (90) were incisional, 9 were primary ventral hernias and the last was not reported. Of the 100 hernia defects, 18 were recurrent. The hernias were all repaired laparoscopically with ePTFE. The majority was fixed with staples or tacks alone. Four of the patients had to be converted to open because of either extensive adhesions (3) or an enterotomy (1). The overall outcome was good. 87% of the patients were discharged within 24 hours of the procedure. The mean hospital stay was 1 day. There were a total of fourteen complications, four minor and ten major. Ten of the complications were wound related – seven seromas, one mesh infection requiring removal, one trocar site infection, and one ascitic leak. The mean follow-up was 51 months during which there were nine (9.4%) recurrences. All nine of the recurrences occurred in patients whom only had either staple or tack fixation. Inadequate mesh overlap, large hernia defects (>25 cm^2) and multiple defects were all associated with recurrence.

These studies established laparoscopic ventral hernia repair as a reasonable alternative to the open mesh repair. They had low recurrence and complication rates. The hospital stays were very short. The drawbacks were in the short follow-up periods and varied repair techniques. Furthermore, a comparison to open would further help solidify the laparoscopic repair as an alternative to the open repair.

Table I. Retrospective and prospective series. LOS = length of stay. PTFE = polytetrafluoroethylene patch. NA = not available.

	Study type	Number of patients	Mesh type & fixation	Mean LOS (days)	Complication rate	Recurrence rate
Franklin, 1998(15)	Retrospective review	176	Polypropylene Staples & sutures	NA	5.1%	1.1%
Heniford, 2000(24)	Retrospective review	100	PTFE Staples & sutures	1.6	14%	3%
Reitter, 2000(25)	Prospective series	49 sutures	PTFE Staples & sutures	4.3	NA	7.1%
Heniford, 2000(14)	Retrospective review	407	PTFE 97% Staples & sutures	1.8	13%	3.4%
LeBlanc, 2000(16)	Retrospective review	100	PTFE Staples, tacks, sutures or combination	1	14%	9%

RETROSPECTIVE COMPARISONS

The first to report a comparison study between open and laparoscopic ventral hernia repairs was Holzman in 1997 (17). They retrospectively reviewed two groups undergoing laparoscopic (21 patients) and open (16 patients) ventral hernia repairs. The repairs in each group were all performed by one senior surgeon but varied in technique. Mesh was not used in all the repairs. Furthermore, this study was limited by the fact that it was a retrospective review. The groups were also not well matched. The laparoscopic group was younger and had more patients with obesity, pulmonary insufficiency (defined as either chronic obstructive pulmonary disease (COPD) or chronic cough), steroid use and diabetes mellitus. These factors, age, chronic cough, COPD, steroid use and diabetes, have all been proposed to predispose to hernia recurrence but have not been confirmed (5).

Within the limitations of this review, there were significant results consistent with prior series. The mean length of hospital stay was shorter for the laparoscopic group. The total cost was significantly lower for the laparoscopic group despite greater operating room costs. Furthermore, the overall morbidity was lower in laparoscopic group, 23% versus 31%. In each group, there was only one infection, which resolved with antibiotics in the laparoscopic group but required mesh removal in the open group. After an average follow-up period of 19 months in the open group and 20 months in the laparoscopic group, two recurrences had occurred in each group. Overall, this review showed that it was safe and cost effective to perform laparoscopic ventral hernia repairs. The exact role of laparoscopic ventral hernia repair was yet to be defined.

Park also reported similar results in 1998 (18). They prospectively collected data on 56 consecutive patients having a laparoscopic ventral hernia repair and compared it with 49 patients who had had an open ventral hernia repair in the past. All patients had a prosthetic patch placed for a tension free hernia repair. The groups were not significantly different in age, ASA class, type or size of hernia. The procedures for all repairs were the same though the mesh types varied. The result was a prospective cohort of 56 patients undergoing a laparoscopic ventral hernia repair compared with 49 historical controls.

The results favored the laparoscopic approach. Though the laparoscopic procedure took significantly longer, the postoperative stay was significantly shorter (3.4 versus 6.5 days, p<0.001). The open repair was more morbid resulting in 18 postoperative complications compared to only 10 from the laparoscopic repair. Of the 18 complications for the open repair, eleven were wound related compared with only four wound related complications in the laparoscopic group . The number of recurrences was higher in the open group, 17 versus 6. The disparity in the number of recurrences between the two groups may be related to the difference in mean follow-up. The mean follow-up period in the laparoscopic group was shorter, 24 versus 54 months. The number of recurrences in the laparoscopic group is likely an underestimation because of the shorter follow-up period. The lack of uniformity between the laparoscopic and open procedures makes it difficult to clearly interpret the data Park presented. Though clearly this article showed that the laparoscopic repair is becoming a promising alternative for the ventral hernia repair.

Ramshaw published the last retrospective series in 1999 (19). This study reviewed a large number of patients that underwent hernia repair during the same period of time. During the period November 1995 and December 1998, 253 patients underwent hernia repair either laparoscopically (n=79) or conventionally (n=174). Unlike the laparoscopic repair, mesh was not always used in the open repair. Both groups were large and similar in age, weight, male to female ratio, number of recurrent hernia, and mean number of previous repairs. The groups differed in hernia size. The average hernia area in the laparoscopic group was 73 squared centimeters compared to only 34 in the open group.

The results were not surprising and were comparable to the other two retrospective reviews. The average hospital stay was shorter in the laparoscopic group, 1.7 days versus 2.8 days. The rate of complications was lower, 19% versus 31%. The open group had a higher rate of minor and major infections. The open group had 18 minor wound complications and infections and 6 major complications requiring mesh removal, compared to four and two, respectively, for the laparoscopic group. The recurrence rate was much lower in the laparoscopic group, 2.5% compared to 19.5%. The mean follow-up period was only 21 months for both groups. The large groups added strength to their results, which strongly favored the laparoscopic repair as the preferred approach if technically feasible.

These three retrospective reviews (Table II) provided data establishing laparoscopic ventral hernia repair as a safe and effective procedure. They showed it to be cost effective by reducing the length of the hospital stay, the rate of complications and the rate of recurrence. It was safer than open in that there were fewer complications. This is likely the result of multiple factors including less dissection, smaller incisions and no need for drains. Finally, though the follow-up periods were short, the laparoscopic hernia repair had a reduced rate of recurrence. The studies lacked a prospective comparison of both repairs. One in which both groups of patients were well matched and the procedures performed during the same time period. Standardization of the techniques employed would have reduced bias and strengthened the argument for the laparoscopic approach.

Table II. Retrospective comparison studies. $\S$ = p<0.001. $\ddagger$ = p<0.05.

	Number of patients	Lap Technique	Open Technique	Mean LOS (days)	Complication rate	Recurrence rate
Holzman, 1997(17)	21 Lap 16 Open	Marlex mesh and tacks	Varied	1.6 v. 4.9	23% v. 31%	9.5% v.12.5%
Park, 1998(18)	56 Lap 49 Open	PTFE or polypropylene Sutures & staples	Tension free mesh repair (Polypropylene, PTFE & Polyglactin)	3.4 v. 6.5‡	18% v. 37%‡	10.7% v. 34.7%
Ramshaw 1999(19)	79 Lap 174 Open	PTFE Sutures & tacks	Varied	1.7 v. 2.8	19% v. 31%	2.5% v. 19.5%

PROSPECTIVE SERIES

Two series (Table III) examined the benefits and risks of laparoscopic ventral hernia repair in a prospective comparison. Neither series randomized the patients. Chari examined fourteen consecutive patients undergoing laparoscopic ventral hernia repair and compared them to fourteen matched controls undergoing open repair of a ventral hernia (20). The same surgeon performed all repairs. In the other series we collected data on 39 consecutive patients undergoing either a laparoscopic ventral hernia repair or an open prefascial mesh repair. Both techniques were standardized (4, 21). The results of both series were very different.

The study by Chari was limited by small patient groups and limited follow-up. Both groups were well matched. There was no difference between the groups in length of stay, time to oral intake or operative blood loss. The study showed that the laparoscopic procedure took longer. The authors felt that their results were unexpected. They attributed these to small sample size and poor patient selection. The study did show that laparoscopic ventral hernia repair is as safe as the open repair but requires careful patient selection to optimize its benefits.

We evaluated 39 consecutive patients for ventral hernia repair (22). Of the 39 patients, 21 underwent a laparoscopic repair and 18 an open repair. The groups were similar in age, male to female ratio, previous bariatric surgery, and size of hernia defect. One difference between the groups was the number of recurrent ventral hernias, eleven in the laparoscopic group versus three in the open group. The laparoscopic group had a intraperitoneal PTFE patch placement. The patch was fixed only with tacks. The open group had a primary repair and prefascial polypropylene mesh reinforcement. The outcomes measured were hospital length of stay, total cost, postoperative pain, and complications. At the time of publication, the mean follow-up period was limited.

The findings were significant. 90% of the laparoscopic group was treated as outpatients compared to only 7% of the open group. The mean length of stay was therefore shorter, 0.8 versus 4.4 days. The shorter stay was felt to be influenced by the overall decreased pain and parenteral narcotic usage. The initial hospital costs were also lower for the laparoscopic group as a result of short hospital stays. The rate of complications was not significantly reduced by the laparoscopic approach. Overall there were more wound infections in the open group (six versus two), but two patients in the laparoscopic group required re-operation and mesh removal. Of the patients in the open group, none required re-operation. The rate of seroma was also greater in the laparoscopic group, 43% versus 22%. Despite these complications the cost of the laparoscopic group remained lower. The length of follow-up at the time of the publication was short and limited an accurate measure of recurrence. There had been one recurrence in the laparoscopic group after 18 months and none in the open group. Later additional recurrences within the laparoscopic group were identified and attributed to the use of internal fixation alone. This was improved by the use of both transabdominal sutures and internal fixation. Unfortunately, this increased the operative time and the postoperative pain requiring an extended hospital stay. Still it was cheaper, less painful and just as safe to perform the laparoscopic repair as the open.

Both of these prospective series attempted to further delineate the role of the laparoscopic ventral hernia repair. The weakness of the first report was inadequate sample size. Our follow-up at the time of publication was too short to determine the effectiveness of the procedure. Both prospective reports did not conclusively support laparoscopic ventral hernia repair as the new standard, but supported it as a reliable option in need of further evaluation.

Table III. Prospective series. ‡ = p<0.05. Wound complications were defined as seromas, hematomas, cellulitis, abscess and skin necrosis

	Study type	Number of patients	Lap. technique	Open technique	Mean LOS (days)	Wound complication rate	Recurrence rate
Chari, 2000(20)	Prospective controlled	14 Lap 14 Open	PTFE Screws	Pre-peritoneal mesh repair - polypropylene	5 v. 5.5	NA	NA
DeMaria, 2000(22)	Prospective comparison	21 Lap 18 Open	PTFE Sutures & tacks	Prefascial mesh repair - polypropylene	0.8 v. 4.4‡	19% v. 50%	5% v. 0%
Carbajo, 1999(23)	Prospective randomized	30 Lap 30 Open	PTFE Mixed fixation	Mesh repair – PTFE or polypropylene	2.2 v. 9.1‡	6.7% v. 57%	0% v. 6.7%

PROSPECTIVE RANDOMIZED SERIES

The prospective randomized series is the most clinically significant report produced. It critically looks at one single intervention attempting to find its clinical significance while excluding all other factors that may bias the report's conclusions. Carbajo reported the results of a randomized group of 60 patients that underwent either a laparoscopic or open ventral hernia repair (23). The groups did not differ in age, male to female ratio, primary versus incisional hernia, number of defects or size of the defect. The laparoscopic technique varied only in that the last 12 patients had only intracorporeal fixation of the mesh as opposed to a combination of external and internal fixation. The open technique followed the principles of a tension free closure and tried whenever possible to keep the mesh extraperitoneal. In all cases mesh was used, either PTFE or polypropylene. The laparoscopic technique used only PTFE. The outcomes measured in this report were operative times, length of hospital stay, postoperative complications and recurrence.

The results reported were expected based on the prior studies. First the operative time was shorter for the laparoscopic procedure especially after only internal fixation was used, 87 versus 112 minutes. The postoperative stay was as expected much shorter in the laparoscopic group, 2.23 versus 9.06 days. There were no intraoperative complications in either group, and none of the laparoscopic procedures were converted to open. Postoperative complications were decreased in the laparoscopic group. Wound complications, including seroma, hematoma, cellulitis, abscess, and skin necrosis occurred 14 times in the open group and only once in the laparoscopic group. Each group had one re-operation. The re-operation in the open group was for abscess drainage and mesh removal, and in the laparoscopic group the patient required repeat fixation of the mesh for a postoperative day four hernia recurrence and small bowel obstruction. Long term hernia recurrence occurred twice in the open group, both of which were repaired laparoscopically, and none in the laparoscopic group. The mean follow-up for these groups was 27 months.

The study showed that better results could be obtained with the laparoscopic repair as compared to the open. Though the follow-up was short, recurrence was decreased in the laparoscopic group. The amount of complications was reduced in the laparoscopic group. The operative times and length of hospital stay were also shorter in the laparoscopic group. Overall, the superiority of the laparoscopic procedure was validated, though a larger study with longer follow-up is still needed. The fixation technique itself also still needs to be better defined.

CONCLUSION

The laparoscopic repair of ventral defects is slowly gaining more acceptances as the literature continues to show its advantages over the open repair. By decreasing the incision size, the dissection needed, and the use of drains, the laparoscopic approach has been able to reduce the number of complications and operative time. Furthermore the postoperative pain and hospital stay have also been reduced. The combination of all these factors help to contribute to the decrease in overall cost, despite the expense of the equipment used. The laparoscopic approach is limited, in that all patients are not good candidates, especially those with hostile abdomens or very large hernia defects. Furthermore, the best technique has yet to be developed. The use of intraperitoneal fixation, transabdominal fixation or both has yet to be tested. Intraperitoneal fixation has the advantage of speed and less postoperative pain, but has been felt to be inadequate to prevent recurrences. Transabdominal fixation may cause more pain and take longer to perform, but is associated with less recurrence. The question of which fixation technique to use needs to be answered. Furthermore longer follow-up is still needed to ascertain the true recurrence rate of the laparoscopic approach. Overall, the laparoscopic technique has been proven to be more advantageous than the open repair, but further study is needed to completely delineate its role.

References

1. Larson GM (2000) Ventral hernia repair by the laparoscopic approach. Surg Clin North Am 80: 1329-1340.

2. Mudge M, Hughes LE (1985) Incisional hernia: a 10 year prospective study of incidence and attitudes. Br J Surg 72: 70-71.

3. Santora TA, Roslyn JJ (1993) Incisional hernia. Surg Clin North Am 73: 557-570.

4. Sugerman HJ, Kellum JM, Reines D, DeMaria EJ, Newsome HH, Lowry JW (1996) Greater risk of Incisional hernia with morbidly obese than steroid-dependent patients and low recurrence with prefascial polypropylene mesh. Am J Surg 171: 80-84.

5. Hesselink VJ, Luijendijk RW, de Wilt JHW, Heide R, Jeekel J (1993) An evaluation of risk factors in incisiional hernia recurrence. Surg Gynecol Obstet 176: 228-234.

6. Luijendijk RW, Hop W, van den Tol MP, de Lange D, Braaksma M, Ijzermans J, Boelhouwer RU, de Vries BC, Salu M, Wereldsma J, Bruijninckx C, VJ, Jeekel J (2000) A comparison of suture repair with mesh repair for incisional hernia. NEJM 343: 392-398.

7. Stoppa RE (1989) The treatment of complicated groin and incisional hernias. World J Surg 13: 545-554.

8. Usher FC (1963) Hernia repair with knitted polypropylene mesh. Surg Gynecol Obstet 117: 239-240.

9. Gillion JF, Begin GF, Marecos C, Fourtanier G (1997) Expanded polytetrafluoroethylene patches used in the intraperitoneal or extraperitoneal position for repair of incisional hernias of the anterolateral abdominal wall. Am J Surg 174: 16-19.

10. McLanahan D, King LT, Weems C, Novotney M, Gibson K (1997) Retrorectus prosthetic mesh repair of midline abdominal hernia. Am J Surg 173: 445-449.

11. Temudom T, Siadati M, Sarr MG (1996) Repair of complex giant or recurrent ventral hernias by using tension-free intraparietal prosthetic mesh (Stoppa technique): Lessons learned from our initial experience (fifty patients). Surgery 120: 738-744.

12. White TJ, Santos MC, Thompson JS (1998) Factors affecting wound complications in repair of ventral hernias. Am Surg 64: 276-280.

13. LeBlanc KA, Booth WV (1993) Laparoscopic repair of incisional abdominal hernias using expanded polytetrafluoroethylene: preliminary findings. Surg Laparosc Endosc 3: 39-41.

14. Heniford BT, Park A, Ramshaw BJ, Voeller G (2000) Laparoscopic ventral and incisional hernia repair in 407 patients. J Am Coll Surg 190: 645-650.

15. Franklin ME, Dorman JP, Glass JL, Balli JE, Gonzalez JJ (1998) Laparoscopic ventral and incisional hernia repair. Surg Laparosc Endosc 8: 294-299.

16. LeBlanc KA, Booth WV, Whitaker JM, Bellanger DE (2000) Laparoscopic incisional and ventral herniorrhaphy in 100 patients. Am J Surg 180: 193-197.

17. Holzman MD, Purut CM, Reintgen K, Eubanks S, Pappas TN (1997) Laparoscopic ventral and incisional hernioplasty. Surg Endosc 11: 32-35.

18. Park A, Birch DW, Lovrics P (1998) Laparoscopic and open incisional hernia repair: a comparison study. Surgery 124: 816-822.

19. Ramshaw BJ, Esartia P, Schwab J, Mason EM, Wilson RA, Duncan TD, Miller J, Lucas GW, Promes J (1999) Comparison of laparoscopic and open ventral herniorrhaphy. Am Surg 65: 827-832.

20. Chari R, Chari V, Eisenstat M, Chung R (2000) A case controlled study of laparoscopic incisional hernia repair. Surg Endosc 14: 117-119.

21. Park A, Gagner M, Pomp A (1996) Laparoscopic repair of large incisional hernias. Surg Laparosc Endosc 6: 123-128.

22. DeMaria EJ, Moss JM, Sugerman HJ (2000) Laparoscopic intraperitoneal polytetrafluoroethylene (PTFE) prosthetic patch repair of ventral hernia. Surg Endosc 14: 326-329.

23. Carbajo MA, Martin del Olmo JC, Blanco JI, de la Cuesta C, Toledano M, Martin F, Vaquero C, Inglada L (1999) Laparoscopic treatment vs open surgery in the solution of major Incisional and abdominal wall hernias with mesh. Surg Endosc 13: 250-252.

24. Heniford BT, Ramshaw BJ (2000) Laparoscopic ventral hernia repair. A report of 100 consecutive cases. Surg Endosc 14: 419-423.

25. Reiter DR, Paulsen JK, Debord JR, Estes NC (2000) Five-year experience with the "Four Before" laparoscopic ventral hernia repair. Am Surg 66: 465.

SECTION VII

Laparoscopic Repair on Special Hernias

CHAPTER 32

Laparoscopic Repair of Unusual Hernias: lumbar, spigelian and other special hernias

P. Gentileschi, S. Kini, M. Gagner

Lumbar hernias are rare defects, with approximately 300 cases reported since the first suggestion of their existence (1). Anatomically, the defect involves the extrusion of retroperitoneal fat or viscera through a weakness in the posterior abdominal wall. There are two distinct sites through which lumbar herniation has been described. Petit first, in 1738 (2), described the anatomy of the inferior lumbar triangle: the lateral border of the latissimus dorsi muscle, the posterior margin of the external oblique muscle, and the superior aspect of the iliac crest. The superior lumbar triangle was described by Grynfeltt (3). It is an inverted triangle bound by the internal oblique muscles anteriorly, the erector spinae muscle group medially, and the 12th rib superiorly. Although lumbar hernias may arise in either or both of these anatomic triangles, they are found most frequently on the left side and in the superior triangle (4). Two thirds have been documented in men (5).

Lumbar hernias are divided between congenital and acquired. The acquired hernias are further divided into primary or secondary sets depending on whether there is a causative factor, such as previous surgery, infection or trauma. Fifty-five percent are primary, with 25% being postsurgical or traumatic and the remainder being congenital in origin (6).

The most common symptom is a posterior, protruding bulge found by the patient (Fig.1). It may be associated with lower back pain or, more significantly, with changes in bowel habits. Severe pain and peritoneal signs may occur, usually caused by incarceration or strangulation. Collectively, lumbar hernias have a high risk of complications: a 25% risk of incarceration and a 10% chance of strangulation (5). Of those hernias that occur spontaneously, 24% become incarcerated and 18% will actually be strangulated on presentation (5).

Often, the diagnosis of lumbar hernia can be based solely on physical examination (Fig. 2). The differential diagnosis of a flank bulge with or without pain may include a lipoma, rhabdomyoma, abscess, hematoma, renal tumors or sarcomas. When the diagnosis is uncertain, other modalities may be employed. Computed tomography is commonly used (Fig. 3). It often delineates the defect, as well as any hernia sac contents, which may include bowel, retroperitoneal fat, kidney, omentum, stomach, or appendix, in decreasing order of frequency. Alternatively, ultrasonography can be used, being less costly, quick and effective. However, computed tomography seems to be the diagnostic study of choice, being also able to assist in trocar placement.

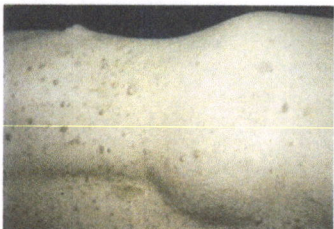
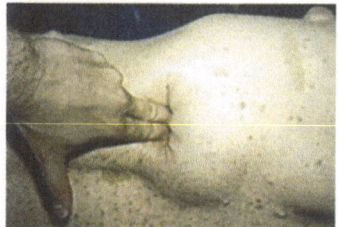

Fig. 1. Upon inspection, lumbar hernias appear as a posterior, protruding bulge.

Fig. 2. The diagnosis of lumbar hernia can be based solely on physical examination.

The natural history of untreated lumbar hernias includes a slow increase in the size of the defect. Given the high risk of complications, and that large defects are more difficult to repair, it is recommended that all lumbar hernias be repaired on presentation as long as no medical contraindications are present.

Over the years, several techniques have been described for the surgical repair of lumbar hernias. Repairing a posterior abdominal wall hernia is difficult, because of the general weakness of the surrounding tissues and the difficulty of sewing onto the bony portions of the hernia boundaries. Furthermore, because few lumbar hernias are described, no one surgeon accumulates enough clinical experience to standardize the surgical technique.

Primary closure has been described, but is often inadequate for repair (7). It may have a role in the management of very small defects, particularly those discovered in infants and in children. In adults and in large defects, this technique is associated with undue tension on the sutured repair and has been abandoned (8). Other methods of closure include rotational flaps and onlay fascial flaps (8, 9). These methods require large planes of dissection with the potential disadvantage of flap ischemia, muscle atrophy, and, eventually, a larger defect than the original. Contemporary reports have strongly advocated abandoning such complicated procedures for an approach using an extensive preperitoneal dissection and placement of a large piece of polypropylene mesh (10). The use of prosthetic mesh to repair lumbar hernias seems reasonable. On the other hand, the technique usually requires a large flank incision, because palpation inadequately defines the hernia defect. For a large lumbar hernia, typically an incision from the 12th rib to the iliac crest is required.

Recently, laparoscopic techniques, which were developed and refined with ventral herniorrhaphies, were applied for the repair of lumbar hernias (11-15). The following is a description of our personal surgical technique for the laparoscopic repair of lumbar hernias. Our experience, together with a review of the literature, is also presented.

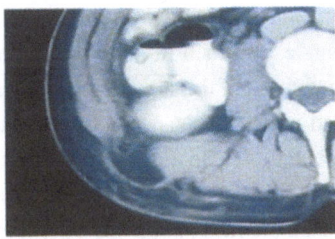

Fig. 3. Computed Tomography often delineates the defect, as well as any hernia sac contents.

SURGICAL TECHNIQUE

Under general anesthesia, the patient is placed in a semilateral position with a 45 degree elevation of the side ipsilateral to the hernia. This position allows the patient to be rolled flat or in a full lateral position to optimize exposure. It also allows the viscera to fall away from the operative field. The surgeon and assistant stand on the opposite side of the hernia (right for a left hernia, left for a right hernia). An incision is made at the umbilicus to insert a 10mm trocar, pneumoperitoneum is established and the laparoscope is introduced. The placement of the remaining trocars is dictated by the location of the defect, its size, and the habitus of the patient. Generally, one port can be placed at the midline infraumbilically and another port in the midline supraumbilically (Fig. 4). Adhesions from previous surgeries are gently dissected and the contents of the hernia are carefully extracted from the sac (Fig. 5,6). Adhesions of these contents to the sac are divided. At this point, the edges of the hernia defect are defined, and the correct size of the hernia is determined (Fig. 7,8).

A polytetrafluoroethylene mesh (Goretex; W.L. Gore and Associates, Flagstaff, Arizona) is used to repair the defect (Fig. 9). The mesh is tailored so that it overlaps the fascial edges of the hernia with at least a 4-cm margin in all directions and introduced in the abdominal cavity (Fig. 9). For superior lumbar hernias, the mesh is secured to the 12th rib by using a polyprolene suture tied around the rib, carefully avoiding the thoracic cavity. For inferior lumbar hernias, the inferior portion of the mesh is sutured onto the iliac crest by passing the suture through the periosteum of the bone (Fig. 10). Alternatively, an orthopaedic 3mm drill bit can be used to create holes in the iliac crest, into which a polyprolene suture can be passed to anchor the mesh. It is important to drill the holes within 1 cm from the edge of the iliac crest; drilling more centrally can damage nerves in this area. At this point, the mesh is secured to the fascia around the hernia defect. A combination of tacking and suturing techniques is used to secure the mesh. A small skin incision (1mm) is made and a suture passer (Karl Storz Endoscopy, Tuttlingen, Germany) loaded with 0 polypropylene suture is passed through the full thickness of the posterolateral abdominal wall and then through the mesh positioned inside (Fig. 11). The end of the suture is released in the abdomen, and the suture passer device is removed. The unloaded suture passer is punctured through the same incision, through the abdominal wall at a slightly different angle, and then through the mesh, grabbing the end of the polypropylene suture. With both ends of the suture outside the abdomen, the suture is tied to itself and the knot is buried in the subcutaneous tissues (Fig. 12). The same suturing technique is used circumferentially to anchor the mesh; a distance of 2-3 cm is left between the sutures. A 5-mm spiral tissue tacker (United States Surgical Corporation, Norwalk, USA) is used to secure the mesh in the gaps between the sutures (Fig. 13, 14). Port fascial incisions are closed using the same suture passer device. Skin incisions are sutured. The small skin incisions are simply reapproximated using Steri-strips.

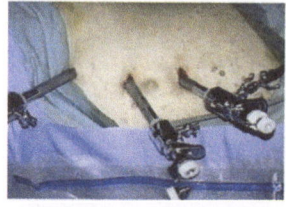

◄ **Fig. 4.** Port positions.

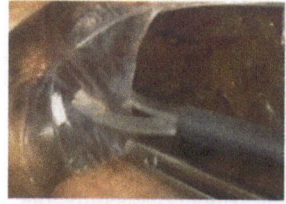
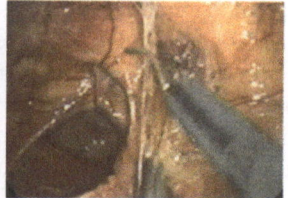

◄ **Figs. 5, 6.** Adhesions from previous surgeries are gently dissected and the contents of the hernia are carefully extracted from the sac.

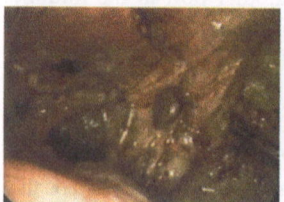
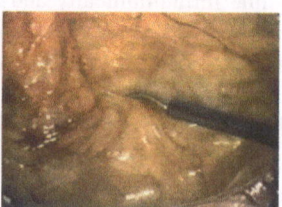

◄ **Figs. 7, 8.** The edges of the hernia defect are defined, and the correct size of the lumbar hernia is determined.

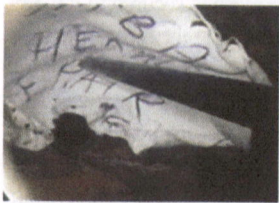

◄ **Fig. 9.** A polytetrafluoro-ethylene mesh (Goretex; W.L. Gore and Associates, Flagstaff, Arizona) is used to repair the defect.

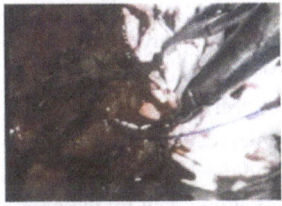

◄ **Fig. 10.** For inferior lumbar hernias, the inferior portion of the mesh is sutured onto the iliac crest by passing the suture through the periosteum of the bone.

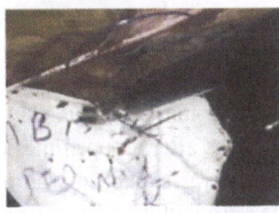

◄ **Fig. 11.** A suture passer (Karl Storz Endoscopy, Tuttlingen, Germany) loaded with 0 poly-propylene suture is passed through the full thickness of the posterolateral abdominal wall and then through the mesh positioned inside.

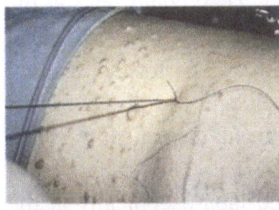

◄ **Fig. 12.** With both ends of the suture outside the abdomen, the suture is tied to itself and the knot is buried in the subcutaneous tissues.

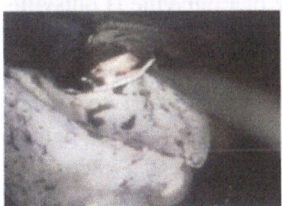
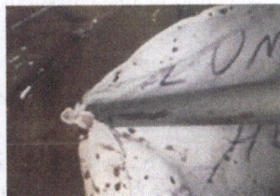

◄ **Figs. 13, 14.** A 5-mm spiral tissue tacker (United States Surgical Corporation, Norwalk, USA) is used to secure the mesh in the gaps between the sutures.

LAPAROSCOPIC APPROACH TO LUMBAR HERNIA

Literature review (Table I)

To date, a total of 10 lumbar hernias have been repaired laparoscopically (11-15). They were 4 case reports and only one series of 7 patients, which included one of the case reports (15) (Table I).

Laparoscopic approach to lumbar hernia was first reported by Burick and Parascandola in 1996 (14). They described a case of acute lumbar hernia as a direct result of blunt trauma. The hernia was repaired by a laparoscopic transabdominal retroperitoneal approach using prolene mesh. In 1997, we reported our first case (13). The patient had a large primary inferior lumbar triangle hernia which was repaired laparoscopically, securing a PTFE mesh to the 12ᵗʰ rib superiorly, iliac crest inferiorly, erector spinae fascia medially, and external oblique fascia laterally. The patient resumed normal activities in less than 2 weeks; 4 months postoperatively, he seemed to have a solid repair. Another case report was published in 1997 by Bickel et al. (12). A morbidly obese woman was found to have an acquired superior triangle lumbar hernia. She was approached laparoscopically. A 3 x 3cm round defect was discovered in proximity to the ureter, between the level of the iliac crest and the 12th rib. A 7 x 11cm piece of prolene mesh was used and fixed to the lumbar abdominal wall by the hernia staples. Postoperative course was uneventful and the patient was discharged on the 3rd postoperative day. During 8 months of follow-up, neither recurrence of hernia nor any related complaints were recorded. Woodward et al. reported in 1999 the only laparoscopic retroperitoneal approach to a recurrent postoperative lumbar hernia (11). The patient presented with a left flank bulge, recurring 3 months after an open mesh repair. After achieving access to the retroperitoneal space, this was expanded with a balloon dissector and a balloon-tipped port was inserted. The retroperitoneal space was insufflated with CO2 and the hernia defect was observed. They could not see the previously placed mesh, quite likely because it was positioned in a more superficial tissue plane. Two more ports were inserted and the repair was performed using a polypropylene mesh. The patient tolerated the procedure well, and was discharged on the 2nd postoperative day. At the 7-month follow-up appointment, the patient was pain free, with no evidence of recurrence.

A retrospective review, of all lumbar hernias repaired laparoscopically at the Cleveland Clinic (Cleveland, OH) and at the University of Louisville (Louisville, KY) over a 16 month-period (August 1996 to November 1997) (15) revealed seven patients. All underwent laparoscopic repair with no conversion to open surgery. Five hernias were acquired defects, and two were congenital. Two patients had previous surgical repairs, which had eventually failed. One to three defects were found per patient. The average size of the hernia defect was 77.8cm^2. We used the surgical technique described before in this chapter. The average size of the PTFE mesh used was 336.4cm^2. The average length of hospital stay was 1.7 days. One patient returned with an abscess over the mesh, which necessitated removal of the graft. Otherwise, there were no complications, and the remaining six patients had no recurrences after follow-up of 1-15 months. The number of hernias per patient, the size of the hernias, the size of the prostheses used, and the total operative time are shown in Table II.

Table I. Laparoscopic repairs of lumbar hernias

Author	Year	No. Patients	Morbidity	Hospital Stay
Burick	1996	1	none	
Gagner	1997	1	none	2 days
Bickel	1997	1	none	3 days
Gagner	1998	7	1 abscess	1.7 days (average)
Woodward	1999	1	none	2 days

Table II. Laparoscopic repair of lumbar hernias

Patient no.	No. of hernias	Hernia size (cm x cm)	Mesh size (cm)	Total OR time (min)
1	2	4 x 3,3 x 3	20 x 36	150
2	1	8 x 11	11 x 15	120
3	3	1.5x1.5(x3)	20 x 16	85
4	1	3 x 10	9 x 18	80
5	1	4.5 x 7.5	10 x 15	130
6	1	15 x 21	20 x 30	325
7	1	3.5 x 5.5	14 x 17	120

DISCUSSION

Laparoscopic techniques to repair incisional, ventral hernias have been developed with promising results (16). We participated to a multicenter prospective study on laparoscopic ventral hernia repair, and the successful outcomes were reported in 1998 (17). Our experience revealed that it is technically feasible, has minimal morbidity and discomfort, and allows a prompt discharge from the hospital and the quick return to normal activities. The same endoscopic methods for the repair of ventral hernias were applied to lumbar hernias.

All literature experiences with laparoscopic lumbar hernia repair are successful, showing short hospital courses and encouraging results (11-15). In the only series reported, of a total of 7 patients, two patients required only oral analgesics; the others required a combination of oral and parenteral analgesics. The largest amount of parenteral narcotic used was 40 mg of morphine sulfate divided in five intramuscolar injections. Four patients were home within 24 hours; two patients stayed in the hospital for 48 hours; one patient stayed for 36 hours. One patient presenting with an abscess above the mesh 2 weeks after surgery, required removal of the graft. He had a prolonged operative time (325 minutes) because of adhesiolysis from a previous open mesh repair. He received intravenous antibiotics for 24 hours. He was obese but had no other risk factors for infection. A definitive repair of the hernia has yet to be performed. In the remaining six patients, no hernias recurred within 1-14 months of follow-up. We had no immediate complications such as bleeding, injuries to the viscera, ureters, or nerves. A thorough knowledge of anatomy aids in the prevention of these complications.

Given the rarity of this disease, many years and a longer follow-up will be needed to determine morbidity, outcomes, and indications of the laparoscopic approach to lumbar hernias. Furthermore, the reported experience is still limited. Nevertheless, some initial conclusions can be made.

Laparoscopic visualization of the hernia affords an excellent view of the hernia contents and the edges of the fascial defect. The laparoscopic view may also help identify unexpected fascial defects, which can be simultaneously repaired with a larger mesh. The size of the hernia can be measured accurately, and the size of the mesh can be tailored as needed. The mesh can be placed inside the defect, allowing intra-abdominal pressure to hold it in position. Patients seem to benefit from a minimally invasive approach with less pain, less analgesic requirements, shortened hospital stay, better cosmetic result, and quick return to normal activities.

Long-term efficacy of laparoscopic repair of lumbar hernias is uncertain until longer follow-up is achieved. However, the repair is straightforward, and easily adapted by surgeons familiar with the laparoscopic ventral hernia repair. We anticipate that the laparoscopic approach will become the best method for repairing lumbar hernias.

SPIGELIAN HERNIA

Spigelian hernias are uncommon hernias of the abdominal wall, representing 0.1-0.2% of all abdominal wall hernias (18). Only 900 cases have been reported to date (18). The area of the aponeurosis that lies between the semilunar line and the lateral edge of the rectus abdominis muscle is called the "Spigelian fascia". The protrusion of a peritoneal sac and/or abdominal organs through a congenital or acquired defect in the Spigelian fascia is referred to as a "Spigelian hernia". The hernia usually enters the transversus and internal oblique muscles covered by the external oblique aponeurosis. The hernia defect is usually oval, with a small diameter, and usually contains omentum, small bowel, or large bowel. Typically, these hernias occur below the level of the umbilicus.

Symptoms are nonspecific, such as pain or a palpable mass in the anterior abdominal wall. Signs of incarceration may be present, with or without intestinal obstruction. The major complication of these hernias is strangulation, occurring in 20% of these patients (18). The preoperative diagnosis is often difficult, and it is missed in approximately 50% of patients (19). This is due to several reasons: symptoms can be vague, vary considerably, or simulate lower quadrant abdominal diseases, and physical examination is often unremarkable. Ultrasonography can be used, especially in obese patients, showing the hernia defect as a discontinuity in the echo line from the aponeurosis (20). Computed tomography is superior to ultrasonography in showing the defect of the abdominal wall, and in identifying the contents of the hernial sac (21).

Spigelian hernias are repaired by a variety of surgical procedures. Open "tension-free" repairs using various types of prostheses are associated with good results and minimal morbidity (19). Laparoscopy approaches 100% accuracy in the diagnosis of hernias (22). It is also very useful to discover unexpected hernias during different procedures (23). Furthermore, laparoscopy can also serve a therapeutic function. Laparoscopic techniques have been applied to various types of herniorrhapies, with excellent results and rapid recovery (16, 17).

The following is a review of the literature on the laparoscopic approach to Spigelian hernia.

LAPAROSCOPIC APPROACH TO SPIGELIAN HERNIA

Literature review (Table III)

To date, a total of 13 patients, with 14 Spigelian hernias, have been approached laparoscopically, using different techniques (22-33)(Table III). The first case was reported in 1992 by Carter (23). A 72-year-old woman was evaluated for a complaint of splitting lower abdominal pain of many years' duration. Physical examination outlined an area of tenderness along the left side of the abdominal wall, and a small umbilical hernia. Diagnostic laparoscopy was eventually performed which revealed a large omental adhesion herniating into a 10 cm defect in the semilunar line. Laparoscopic repair was accomplished by placement of No. 1 Vycril sutures in an interrupted-Figure-eight pattern. Ties were made with an extracorporeal knotting procedure. The umbilical hernia was closed in a similar fashion.

Since then, 13 laparoscopic Spigelian hernia repairs, in 12 patients, have been reported (22,24-33). In 6 patients the diagnosis of Spigelian hernia was obtained only by laparoscopy.

Different surgical techniques have been described, and different prostheses have been used. In 3 patients, laparoscopic Spigelian hernia repair was performed in association with cholecystectomy, in 2 patients, with umbilical hernia repair, in one patient, with bilateral inguinal hernia repair, in one patient, with pelvic lymph node dissection for prostatic carcinoma. No post-operative complication has been reported. Most of the Authors did not report postoperative hospital stay. When reported, it ranged from 24 to 48 hours.

Three main laparoscopic procedures can be identified. Primary closure of the defect, trans-abdominal preperitoneal polypropylene mesh repair, intra-abdominal placement of a PTFE patch (Goretex DualMesh; W.L. Gore and Associates, Flagstaff, Arizona). In one case a composite mesh prosthesis consisting of a sandwich of polyester fiber mesh and polyglactin 910 mesh, sutured together at the operating table was used. Direct preperitoneal repair has not been described for Spigelian hernias.

Although laparoscopic direct suture of Spigelian hernias has been initially reported, we know from open hernia surgery, that this repair is associated in the long-term with a higher rate of recurrence (34). Current evidence shows that abdominal wall hernias must be repaired by mesh hernioplasty, either by open approach or by laparoscopy (35).

Laparoscopic trans-abdominal preperitoneal mesh repair of Spigelian hernias has been described (22-33). The technique is similar to the trans-abdominal preperitoneal approach to inguinal hernias. Basically, the hernia defect is first identified by laparoscopic exploration. Eventual adhesions between intra-abdominal organs, usually bowel loops, and the hernia sac are sectioned. The dissection begins with a peritoneal incision, usually superiorly, medially and laterally to the wall defect. The hernia sac is then reduced out of the fascial defect. The surrounding fascia is exposed, keeping the peritoneal flap distally out of the defect. A polypropylene mesh large enough to overlap 2-3 cm onto the normal fascia is introduced into the abdominal cavity and fixed with a hernia stapler. Finally, the preperitoneal flap is closed with a running suture.

When using a PTFE mesh, after reducing the hernia sac, there is no need of opening the peritoneum because the material does not cause adhesions with intra-abdominal organs. The PTFE patch is placed against the abdominal wall, overlaying the defect with a 3-4 cm margin in all directions. The mesh is anchored either with a tacker device or with the technique described for lumbar hernias. Placement of the mesh posterior to the anterior fascia, adds the benefit of intra-abdominal pressure, holding the mesh in the correct position over a large surface area.

Table III. Laparoscopic approach to spigelian hernia

Author	Year	No.patients	No.hernias	Morbidity	H.stay
Carter	1992	1	1	none	
DeMatteo	1994	1	1	none	
Fisher	1994	1	1	none	
Welter	1994	1	1	none	
Barie	1994	1	1	none	
Sanchis	1995	1	1	none	
Kasirajan	1997	1	1	none	
Amendolara	1998	2	2	none	2 days, 1day
Gedebou	1998	1	2	none	1 day
Teleky	1999	1	1	none	
Appeltans	2000	1	1	none	2 days
Novell	2000	1	1	none	1 day

DISCUSSION

The small number of reported laparoscopic repairs of Spigelian hernias is related to the rarity of these abdominal wall hernias. For this reason, no definite conclusion can be made about the surgical treatment of choice for such hernias. However, the laparoscopic approach seems to offer many advantages for the following reasons.

The preoperative diagnosis of Spigelian hernia is difficult, being missed in approximately 50% of patients (19). In this review, in 6 of the 13 patients (46.1%), the hernia defect was discovered only by laparoscopy. The indications for operation were abdominal pain, abdominal wall tenderness, gallstones and prostatic carcinoma. In a pre-laparoscopy era, these patients would have been approached by a large midline incision, with consequent discomfort and morbidity. All the reports emphasize the difficulty in making a preoperative diagnosis. The nonspecific symptoms and the common intramural location are contributing factors.

Although uncommon, Spigelian hernias are a source of acute and chronic abdominal pain. Strangulation occurs in 20% of such hernias (18). Incarceration is also common (18). Many patients require emergency surgery. Laparoscopic evaluation of abdominal pain can allow diagnosis before eventual laparotomy. With the techniques described here, Spigelian hernias can also be repaired laparoscopically and open exploratory surgery can be avoided.

Spigelian hernias are common in older patients, who may be affected by simultaneous surgical diseases. In 7 of the 13 patients (53.8%), the Spigelian hernia repair was performed in association with other procedures, which, in an open setting, would have required a larger incision, or two different incisions.

In all patients, when reported, laparoscopic repair afforded a short postoperative hospital course, minimal pain and rapid return to normal activities. In older patients, in case of uncertain preoperative diagnosis, or when another abdominal procedure needs simultaneous repair, patients with the suspect of Spigelian hernias may be better approached by laparoscopy. All cases reported in the literature, have shown excellent results.

OTHER UNUSUAL HERNIAS

The only laparoscopic approach to other rare abdominal wall hernias was reported by Lawton in 1998 (36). A large incisional hernia secondary to placement of a subcostal implantable cardioverter defibrillator, was repaired laparoscopically. The patient experienced no complication and prompt resumption of routine activities and work.

Subcostal, suprapubic, or other rare abdominal wall hernias may be approached laparoscopically, using the same technique described for incisional and lumbar hernias.

References

1. Ponka JL. Lumbar hernias. In: Ponka JL, ed. Hernias of the abdominal wall. Philadelphia: WB Saunders; 1980: 465-478.

2. Petit JL. Traité des maladies chirurgicales et des opérations qui leurs conviennent. Paris T.F. Didot 1774 ; 2 : 256-259.

3. Grynfeltt J. Quelques mots sur la hernie lombaire. Montpellier Med 1866 ; 16 : 323.

4. Thorek M. Lumbar hernia. J Int Coll Surg 1950; 14: 367-393.

5. Watson LE. Hernia. 3rd ed. St Louis, Mo: Mosby-Year book Inc; 1948: 443-446.

6. Swartz WT. Lumbar hernias. J Ky Med Assoc 1954; 52: 673-678.

7. Dowd CN. Congenital lumbar hernia at the triangle of Petit. Ann Surg 1907; 45: 245-248.

8. Sutherland RS, Gerow RR. Hernia after dorsal incision into lumbar region: a case report and review of pathogenesis and treatment. J Urol 1995; 153: 382-384.

9. Bolkier M, Moskovitz B, Ginesin Y, et al. An operation for incisional lumbar hernias. Eur Urol 1991; 20: 52-53.

10. Knol JA, and Eckhauser FE. Inguinal anatomy and abdominal wall hernias. In: Greenfield LJ, ed. Surgery: Scientific Principles and Practice. Philadelphia: JB Lippincot; 1993: 1081-1107.

11. Woodward AM, Flint LM, Ferrara JJ. Laparoscopic retroperitoneal repair of recurrent postoperative lumbar hernia. J Laparoendosc Adv Surg Tech A. 1999; 2: 181-6.

12. Bickel A, Haj M, Eitan A. Laparoscopic management of lumbar hernia. Surg Endosc 1997; 11: 1129-30.

13. Heniford BT, Iannitti DA, Gagner M. Laparoscopic inferior and superior lumbar hernia repair. Arch Surg 1997; 132: 1141-4.

14. Burick AJ, Parascandola SA. Laparoscopic repair of a traumatic lumbar hernia: a case report. J Laparoendosc Surg 1996 ; 6 : 259-62.

15. Arca MJ, Heniford BT, Pokorny R, et al. Laparoscopic repair of lumbar hernias. J Am Coll Surg 1998; 2: 147-152.

16. Larson GM. Ventral hernia repair by the laparoscopic approach. Surg Clin North Am 2000; 80: 1329-40.

17. Toy FK, Bailey RW, Carey S, et al. Prospective, multicenter study of laparoscopic ventral hernioplasty. Preliminary results. Surg Endosc 1998; 12: 955-9.

18. Spangen L. Spigelian hernia. World J Surg 1989; 13: 573-580.

19. Eubanks S, Sabiston DC. Hernias. In: DC Sabiston (ed). Sabiston's Textbook of Surgery, 1997. W.B.Saunders, Philadelphia, 1230.

20. Campos SM, Walden T. Images in clinical medicine: Spigelian hernia. New Engl J Med 1997; 336: 1149-1152.

21. Coulier B, Ramboux A, Mailleux P. Strangulated intestinal Spigelian hernia. J Belg Radiol 1997; 80 : 68-70.

22. Kasiragan K, Lopez J, Lopez R. Laparoscopic technique in the management of Spigelian hernia. J Laparoendosc Adv Surg Tech 1997; 7: 385-388.

23. Carter JE, Mizes C. Laparoscopic diagnosis and repair of spigelian hernia: report of a case and technique. Am J Obstet Gynecol 1992; 167: 77-78.

24. DeMatteo RP, Morris JB, Broderick J. Incidental laparoscopic repair of a spigelian hernia. Surgery 1994; 115: 521-2.

25. Fisher BL. Video-assisted spigelian hernia repair. Surg Laparosc Endosc 1994; 4: 238-40.

26. Welter HF. Laparoscopic management of a spigelian hernia. Chirurg 1994; 65: 898-9.

27. Barie PS, Thompson WA, Mack CA. Planned laparoscopic repair of a spigelian hernia using a composite prosthesis. J Laparoendosc Surg 1994; 4: 359-63.

28. Salvador Sanchis JL, Laguna Sastre M, Adel Carceller R, et al. Laparoscopic repair of spigelian hernia. Rev Esp Enferm Dig 1995; 87: 759-60.

29. Amendolara M. Videolaparoscopic treatment of Spigelian hernias. Surg Laparosc Endosc 1998; 8: 136-9.

30. Teleky R, Duda M, Brezina L. Spigelian hernia and cholecystolithiasis treated laparoscopically. Rozhl Chir 1999; 78: 610-2.

31. Appeltans BMG, Zeebregts CJAM, Hoedemaker C. Laparoscopic repair of a Spigelian hernia using an expanded polytetrafluoroethylene (ePTFE) mesh. Surg Endosc 2000; 14:1189.

32. Novell F, Sanchez G, Sentis J, et al. Laparoscopic management of spigelian hernia. Surg Endosc 2000; 14:1189.

33. Gedebou TM, Neubauer W. Laparoscopic repair of bilateral spigelian and inguinal hernias. Surg Endosc 1998; 12: 1424-25.

34. Paul A, Troidl H, Williams JI, et al. Randomized trial of modified Bassini vs Shouldice inguinal hernia repair. The Cologne Hernia Study Group. BR J Surg 1994; 81: 1531-4.

35. Amid PK, Shulman AG, Lichtenstein IL. The Lichtenstein open tension-free mesh repair of inguinal hernias. Surg Today 1995; 25: 619-25.

36. Lawton JS, Embrey RP, DeMaria EJ. Laparoscopic hernia repair of an incisional hernia secondary to placement of an implantable cardioverter defibrillator. Pacing Clin Electrophysiol 1998; 21: 1492-3.

CHAPTER 33

Laparoscopic Repair of post-sternotomy Incisional Hernia of the Subxiphoid Region

H.R. Freund, I. Charuzi

INTRODUCTION

Hernias of the subxiphoid region following median sternotomy incisions are unique for two reasons. Firstly, the abdominal wall hernia is the result of a non-abdominal operation, mainly cardiac surgery. Secondly, the hernia occurs in a difficult location for repair.

Post median sternotomy incisional hernia is an infrequent complication and was reported by Davidson and Bailey (1) in the only large series dealing with this issue, to occur in 4.2% of their patients undergoing cardiothoracic surgery. They report retrospectively on 475 cardiothoracic procedures through median sternotomies in which 20 incisional hernias developed (4.2%) in the subxiphoid linea alba. No single etiological factor was found to be responsible for the formation of the incisional hernia in the epigastrium. The hernias appeared between one month to three years following surgery, 70% within three months.

Predisposing factors as listed by the authors are: male sex, aortic valve replacement, obesity, reoperation, postoperative wound infection and postoperative left ventricular failure.

The Anatomy of the Xipho-Epigastrium Area and its Relation to the Type of Incisional Hernia Repair

The rectus abdominis muscle arises from the pubic bone and is embedded in the cartilages of ribs 5, 6, and 7, the costoxiphoid ligament and the xiphoid process.

The muscle is enclosed by the rectus sheath with its anterior leaf composed of the aponeuroses of the external oblique and the anterior leaf of the internal oblique, while its posterior leaf is composed of the aponeuroses of the transversus abdominis and internal oblique muscles. The anterior and posterior layers of the rectus sheath fuse at the midline to create the linea alba, which, lacking muscular support, is the weakest point in this area.

The entire area of xiphoid process and linea alba in this region are closely enclosed by bony structures creating a rigid frame (Fig. 1) which prevents, under normal circumstances, laxity and mobility of tissues or eventual mobilization and approximation of tissues for repair in the event of a hernia.

Cohen and Starling (2) described three muscular attachments to the xiphoid:

1. The costoxiphoid ligament arising from the 7th rib and inserting on the lateral xiphoid process (Fig. 1).

2. The transverse muscles of the thorax arising from the 6th rib and inserting on the xiphoid process (Fig. 1).

3. The sternal portion of the diaphragm inserting on the xiphoid process.

They also reported a consistent finding of a bifid xiphoid in 14 patients with hernias located in the subxiphoid region following an extended median sternotomy for cardiac procedures. They speculated that the split xiphoid has a major role in the pathogenesis and recurrence of these hernias.

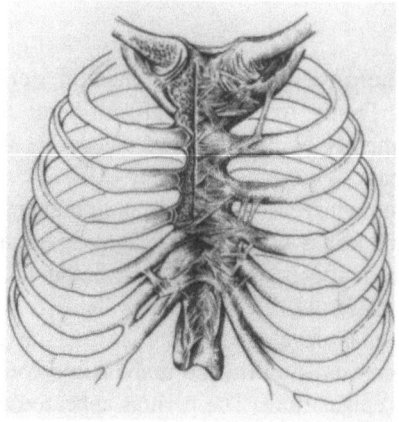

Fig. 1. The skeletal and ligamental anatomy of the sternum, xiphoid and thorax. Note the costoxiphoid and transverse ligaments and their relation to the xiphoid process.

Combining these facts, Cohen and Starling (2) claim that the creation of a bifid xiphoid by midsternotomy enhances displacement by lateral and posterior forces exerted by the three muscular attachments mentioned above, resulting in increased lateral tension and subsequent fascial dehiscence. However, it should be noted that a bifid xiphoid process can also occur as a result of congenital malfusion of both sternal parts. Cohen and Starling were also the first to describe and report on the subxiphoid incisional hernia after median sternotomy and to advocate the use of a mesh repair for these hernias, after experiencing an 80% failure rate with a primary suture repair (2).

Indeed, the unique anatomy of the xiphoid and subxiphoid area, coupled with its rigid bony frame, should discourage any attempt to repair subxiphoid incisional hernias by primary suturing.

In 1987, Davidson and Bailey published their initial experience of three patients with huge subxiphoid hernias repaired by the Wells technique (3). They later reported on a total of seven patients with excellent results of this relatively tedious procedure which involves the creation of rotating flaps of the anterior rectus sheath to cover the hernial defect, reminiscent of the Chevrel and Welti-Eudel procedures.

A simpler and much safer method seems to be the use of a prosthetic mesh. The mesh can either be used in the time - proven open operation or in the more recently introduced laparoscopic technique.

THE OPEN MESH REPAIR

The procedure is accomplished under general anaesthesia. Cephalosporin prophylaxis is routinely used, but if there is a history of a previous repair complicated by wound infection, vancomycin is preferable. The previous scar is often excised and the subcutaneous tissues carefully dissected along the plane between the hernial sac and fatty tissue until the musculofascial borders of the hernia are clearly identified. Superiorly the xiphoid process should be clearly identified and exposed. Two techniques are available. With the underlay method an attempt is made to avoid, if possible, opening the hernial sac. The hernial sac should be dissected and simply reduced. If the sac is large, plication might help to reduce its size and tuck it out of the way. A plane is developed between the posterior rectus sheath and the peritoneum and the mesh laid out in this plane. This dissection should extend far enough so that the sutures anchoring the mesh should be positioned all around in healthy tissues, sufficiently distant from the weakened hernial musculofascial margin.

We prefer the onlay technique (Fig. 2, 3, 4). After the hernia sac is dissected off the skin and subcutis, the sac is opened. Adhesions in the abdomen are released, and the abdominal wall cleared so that the anchoring sutures for the mesh can be safely placed far enough from the hernia margin. The polypropylene mesh is laid flat over the rectus musculofascial edge, covering the entire hernia defect and about 5 cm beyond the hernia edges in all directions. The mesh should be anchored with closely placed #0 Prolene full thickness mattress sutures with 1 to 1.2 cm bites of the musculoaponeurotic tissue of the abdominal wall (Fig. 2, 3, 4). The sutures holding the mesh should be placed 1.0 to 2.0 cm apart and approximately 3 to 5 cm away from the margins of the hernia. The ends of the sutures are left long and held in hemostats until all of them are placed and then tied and cut successively (Fig. 2, 3). The prosthesis should lie flat but a 20% laxity and redundancy should be allowed for future shrinkage of the mesh. The excess mesh is trimmed and perfect hemostasis must be achieved. The wound is irrigated to remove any debris of fat and blood and the subcutaneous tissue snugly approximated. If possible, some of the subcutaneous sutures should also be anchored to the mesh to avoid dead space and eventual collection of a seroma (Fig. 4). Any unhealthy or superfluous skin should be excised and the skin closed. The use of drains should be avoided.

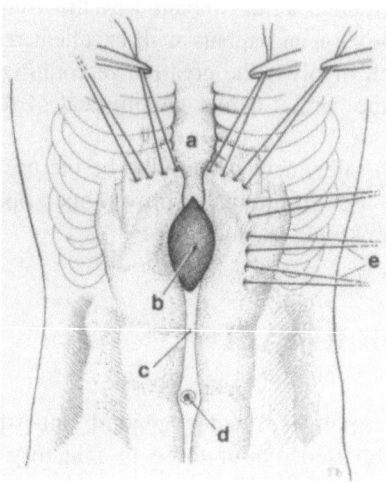

Fig. 2. Placement of interrupted full thickness Prolene sutures in healthy tissue around the hernia defect. Note: bifid xiphoid (a); hernia defect (b); linea alba (c); umbilicus (d); mattress sutures placed and held with hemostats (e).

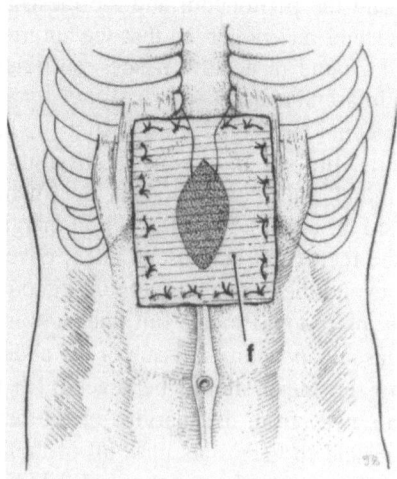

Fig. 3. Large size mesh (f) placed over hernia defect and anchored by previously placed sutures well beyond the hernia edges.

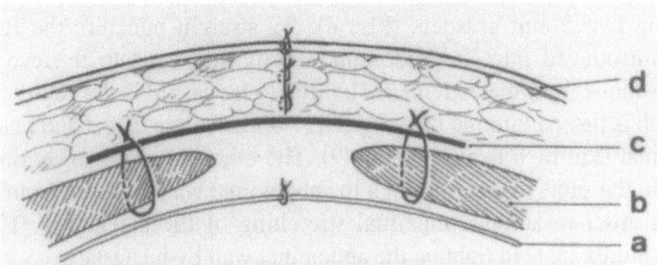

Fig. 4. Schematic view of the abdominal wall with mesh placed and anchored to the musculofascial layer (onlay repair techmique). Note: peritoneum (a); musculofascial layer (b); mesh anchored to musculofascial layer (c); subcutis and skin snugly approximated (d).

The Laparoscopic Repair

Visualized through the laparoscope the subxiphoid incisional hernia is characterized by its rhomboid appearance with the xiphoid split or missing in the upper corner of the defect with the fascia retracted towards the costal margins. The laparoscopic repair of this type of hernia is easier as no previous abdominal surgery occured and usually no intra-abdominal adhesions are present. Other advantages of the laparoscopic repair are easy fixation of the mesh to adjacent structures (fascia and periosteum), sufficient space to spread a large-size mesh, minimal postoperative morbidity, rapid convalescence, and possibly a low recurrence rate.

Operative Technique

The laparoscopic repair is performed with the patient under general anaesthesia in the supine position. Cephalosporin prophylaxis is routinely used. Pneumoperitoneum is established by insufflating the abdomen to 15 mmHg with carbon-dioxide through a Veress needle or through a subumbilical trocar placed by the open technique. Two additional 5 mm trocars are inserted under vision in the mid-abdomen at the left and right anterior axillary line (Fig. 5).

Usually there are no intra-abdominal adhesions permiting immediate placement of the mesh. We routinely use a Gore-Tex DualMesh® prepared to cover the hernia defect with at least 3 cm margins all around. Five long Vicryl 2/0 anchoring sutures are placed on the mesh (Fig. 6). One suture is placed exactly in the centre of the patch. Two sutures are placed in the two caudal corners and two sutures are placed half-way on the lateral borders of the mesh (Fig. 6). Three additional loops are placed on the cranial edge of the patch to assist with grasping, placing and anchoring the patch over the area of sternum and ribcage (Fig. 6).

The patch is then rolled from the cranial and caudal borders towards the centre creating a tight scroll (Fig. 7). The laparoscope and the umbilical trocar are removed and the scrolled patch is introduced into the abdomen directly through the subumbilical opening. Following introduction of the patch into the abdomen the trocar and laparoscope are re-introduced. The patch is unfolded in the abdominal cavity using two 5 mm graspers (Fig. 8). By straight puncture the EndoClose needle is introduced into the abdominal cavity and used to retrieve the long anchoring sutures from the abdomen. The first to be passed is the centre anchoring suture which is passed through the very centre of the hernia defect and held tight on the abdominal skin by a hemostat (Fig. 9). The other four long anchoring sutures are pulled in the same manner through the abdominal wall far away from the patch margins in order to achieve maximal stretching of the patch (Fig. 10). These anchoring sutures are held tight on the abdominal wall by hemostats.

Once the patch is firmly held in place it is fixed to the abdominal wall, sternum and ribcage using endoscopic tackers placed all around the patch, 10 to 12 mm apart and 2 to 3 mm away from the edges of the patch (Figure 10). The anchoring sutures are cut, the abdomen emptied of gas and trocars removed.

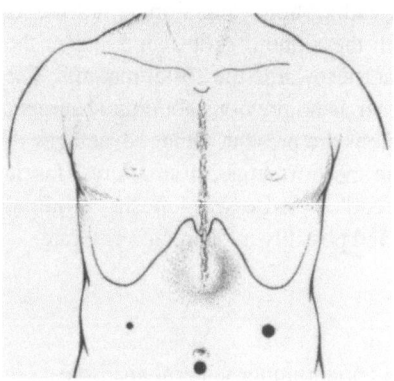

Fig. 5. Location of the hernia and placement of trocars for the laparoscopic repair. A 10-11 mm trocar for the laparoscope is placed under the umbilicus. Two working ports (two 5 mm or one 5 mm and a second 10-11 mm) are placed laterally at the anterior axillary lines.

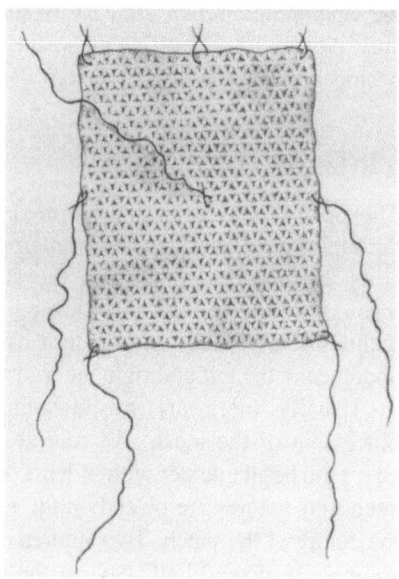

Fig. 6. The Gore-Tex DualMesh is fashioned to cover the hernia defect and at least 3 cm margins all around the defect. Long Vicryl 2/0 anchoring sutures are placed one in the centre and the other four as marked. The three loops are located on the cranial aspect of the patch to facilitate grasping and anchoring.

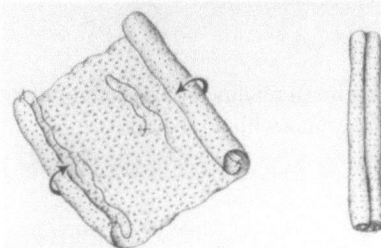

Fig. 7. The patch is rolled from the cranial edge to centre and from the caudal edge to centre to form a tight scroll which is introduced into the abdominal cavity through the subumbilical opening.

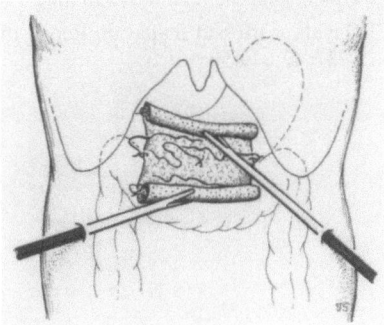

Fig. 8. The patch is unfolded in the abdominal cavity using two 5 mm graspers.

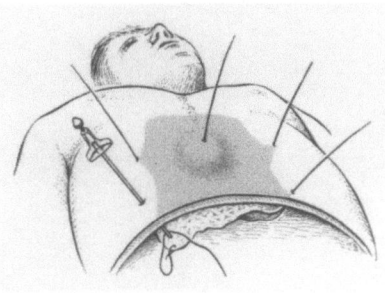

Fig. 9. The EndoClose instrument (needle) is used to retrieve the long anchoring sutures. The centre suture is passed through the centre of the hernia defect while the other four are pulled out far away from the patch margins to achieve maximal stretching of the patch.

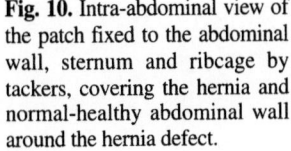

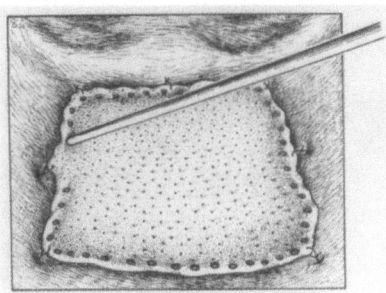

Fig. 10. Intra-abdominal view of the patch fixed to the abdominal wall, sternum and ribcage by tackers, covering the hernia and normal-healthy abdominal wall around the hernia defect.

CONCLUSION

During the past seven years we performed 8 open mesh repairs and 20 laparoscopic repairs of post sternotomy subxiphoid incisional hernias with no recurrence.

References

1. Davidson BR and Bailey JS. Incisional herniae following median sternotomy: their incidence and etiology. Br J Surg 1986; 73:995-6.
2. Cohen MJ and Starling JR. Repair of subxiphoid incisional hernias with Marlex mesh after median sternotomy. Arch Surg 1985; 120:1270-1.
3. Davidson BR and Bailey JS. Repair of incisional hernia after median sternotomy. Thorax 1987; 42:549-50.

CHAPTER 34

Laparoscopic Paraostomal Hernia Repair: indications, technique, and results

D. Berger

Parastomal hernias are defined as fascial defects around enterostomies such as colo- or ileostomies. Also the creation of urological conduits can be complicated by parastomal herniation. Whereas the repair of incisional hernias is recommended whenever such a hernia can be detected and the hernia is growing or hurts the indication for surgical repair of parastomal hernias is much more restrictive (1). Only about 30% of patients with parastomal hernias undergo surgical repair. Today a rapidly growing and symptomatic parastomal hernia should be corrected. Symptoms may be problems with defecation especially in patients which use irrigation for controlled evacuation as well as problems concerning the stoma care. An emergency indication is represented by incarceration. The great number of patients who do not need surgical repair according to todays official opinion is clearly based on the lack of a safe and effective reparation principle. Conventional procedures result in sometimes more than 50% recurrence rate and local infections up to 30% (2-5).

REPARATION PRINCIPLES

Before the laparoscopic era simple fascial closure was propagated in cases with a small hernia. Mostly the parastomal hernia is very big with a small fascial gap. So local repair seemed to be an adequate principle. However the recurrence rate exceeded 50%! The same fact passes for the relocation of the enterostomy (6). The high number of recurrencies after mesh-free repair is today explained by intrinsic defects of wound healing (7). Mesh techniques developed for the repair of incisional hernia were also applied to parastomal hernias and a growing number of publications is now available demonstrating better results by sub- or epifascial placement of nonresorbable meshes (8-10). Recurrence rates of below 10% have been reported. However these studies involve only a small number of patients, the observation period is short and the infection rate sometimes exceeds 10%. Also the procedure is difficult because of the coexistence of incisional and parastomal hernia.

As it is known from the repair of incisional hernia the disadvantages of conventional surgery are the need of creating large flaps of the layers of the abdominal wall followed by hematoma or seroma with further complications such as infection. Furthermore the fascial gap is usually closed resulting in remarkable tension of the abdominal wall. The trauma of the abdominal wall is accompanied by further trauma of the gut because extended adhesiolyis is necessary. As to the case of parastomal hernia the meshes must cut in order to round the stoma loop implying considerable weakness of the mesh itself as well as the possibility of stenosis due to shrinkage of the mesh. So conventional repair represents a stressing operation for the patient with a variety of complications.

In order to overcome some of these problems Sugarbaker described a conventional "IPOM-technique" in 1985, at a time when mesh methods are very rarely used (11). He did not report any infections or recurrencies in 7 patients being observed for 4-7 years.

With the increasing acceptance of laparoscopic repair of incisional hernias using the "IPOM-technique" which is principally based on the low recurrence and infection rate that procedure was also applied to parastomal hernias (12). The obvious advantages of the laparoscopic technique are: (a) no necessity of abdominal wall dissection (b) tension-free closure of the fascial gap by the intraperitoneal-onlay-mesh technique (c) easy coverage of parastomal and incisional hernia with one mesh. The disadvantages may be: (a) expensive procedure (b) time consuming procedure (c) no closure of the primary fascial defect (d) lack of long observation periods.

TECHNIQUE

The principle of the laparoscopic repair relies on the described coverage of the fascial gap with a mesh and the lateralisation of the stoma loop. The latter point ist extremly important and needs further explanation. In almost all cases the fascial gap of parastomal hernias develops medially and cranially to the stoma loop. Lateralisation means that the stoma loop should be covered by the mesh for at least 3-5 cm. So the loop is placed between the mesh and healthy fascia entering the abdominal cavity 3-5 cm laterally from the stoma site.

We usually need 4 trocars, the first one being placed by minilaparotomy as far from the hernia as possible. The complete abdominal wall should be freed of adherent greater omentum or bowel in order to detect any further incisional hernia which is not visible at the preoperative examination. Coagulation is almost never necessary as well as we do not use ultrasound dissection. The content of the parastomal hernia must be completely reduced. So the stoma loop needs to be clearly identified. The fascial gap is left open. We insert a Goretex-Dualmesh of W.L. Gore & Assoc. overlapping the fascial edges for at least 5 cm. When an incisional hernia is present both defects are usually covered by 1 mesh. The corners of the mesh are marked by nonresorbable sutures which are tied through and through leaving the knots in the subcutaneous tissue. In cases with meshes bigger than 20 cm further sutures between the corners are used. Using spiral tacks we finally fix the mesh under slight tension. The trocar sites need to be exactly closed to prevent trocar hernias.

BADEN-BADEN EXPERIENCE

Patients

15 patients, 10 female and 5 males ageing between 34 and 80 years (median age: 70 years) were enrolled in the study. The body mass index varied between 22 and 37 (median: 28). 1-5 previous surgical procedures per patient have been performed. 5 recurrent parastomal hernias after mesh repair were included. 5 ileostomies and 10 colostomies were repaired with 8 concomitant incisional hernias. The median observation time amounted to 6 months and ranged from 3-12 months. The hernia and mesh size ranged between 10 and 240 cm^2, and 84 and 550 cm^2 respectively. The median operating room time was 125 min (85 to 205 min). 1 cholecystectomy and 1 subcutaneous mastectomy were performed simultaneously as well as 1 permanent venous access was implanted.

Results

No conversion was necessary up to now as well as no enterotomy occurred. Even no superficial lesion of the bowel could be detected. All patients needed oral analgesia until discharge. After 4 weeks pain completely disappeared. Only 1 clinically obvious hematoma was seen but there was no need of further treatment. There was no infection in the series. 1 patient was reoperated at day 4 because of an ileus due to inadequate placement of a tack. Only 1 tack was dislocated leading to a small opening between mesh and abdominal wall followed by incarceration of a small bowel loop. 3 parastomal hernias recurred between 2 and 4 months, 2 of them remaining constant without any symptoms.

Pitfalls

The recurrencies which occurred in our series can be simply explained by technical mistakes. In these patients the mesh was to small and the lateralisation of the stoma loop which is essential for effective repair was not adequate. The way from sufficient lateralisation to stenosis seems to be very short but in fact despite a long tunnel between mesh and abdominal wall we did not observe any postoperative stenosis in our later patients. Therefore it should be pointed out once more that the stoma loop must be covered by the mesh for at least 3-5 cm.

A further difficulty is the clear identification of the stoma loop and the differentiation between prolapsed small bowel adherent to the hernia and the stoma loop especially in ileostomies. If a small or large bowel loop is left in the hernia the recurrence is obligate because the prolapsing loop pulls further bowel into the hernia. On the other hand radical preparation may disturb the blood supply of the stoma leading to necrosis or ischemic stenosis. Fortunately we have not observed such a complication. In the case of an enterotomy of the large bowel a mesh should not be implanted. If small bowel is injured and no ileus with suspected bacterial overgrowth is present a mesh repair can safely be performed.

Today only meshes with proven antiadhesive properties on one side should be used as intraperitoneally placed prosthesis. The side to the abdominal wall should induce strong adhesions whereas the side to the bowel must be inert. Up to now only the "Dualmesh" of W.L. Gore & Assoc. fullfills these criteria. Whether doublelayer meshes which are commercially available are really comparable cannot be decided. The intraperitoneal use of polypropylene- or polyestermeshes is strongly forbidden because of massive adhesions and fistula.

The fixation of the mesh is another open question which should be discussed in detail. It is generally recommended that through and through sutures should be used every 3-5 cm. As described in the technique section we use sutures only at the corners and sometimes in between when meshes of more than 20 cm are necessary. The final fixation by spiral tacks is generally used but it should be kept in mind that the tacks must be anchored in the fascia and not only in the peritoneum in order to prevent slippage of the whole mesh. Also the use of a polypropylene layer to the parietal peritoneum would not prevent the slippage of the whole mesh because the ingrowth of tissue into the mesh involves only peritoneum. In most cases the parastomal hernias are located in the lower quadrants. The concomitant incisional hernias therefore extend to the symphysis. For safe and effective fixation of the mesh in the lower abdomen the peritoneal layer should be incised and removed from the fascia and muscle. The symphysis and both Cooper's ligaments must be prepared so that the mesh can be fixed in the bone and the fascia at the lateral edges. Sometimes the removal of epiperitoneal fat between both plicae mediales may be sufficient. However the tacks should never be placed in fatty tissue!

OPEN QUESTIONS

The main open questions concern the long term results and a considerable number of patients. Both aspects are not available today. Furthermore it is not clear whether the fascial defects which are left open may impair the function of the abdominal wall as it is discussed for laparoscopic incisional hernia repair. The fixation with spiral tacks also is a point of debate. During relaparoscopy after hernia repair we find more than filmy adhesions mainly at the tacks. Especially when the tacks do not completely disappear in the mesh these tacks may be the origin of further complications. However as to the case of incisional hernia repair up to now no tack related long- term complication has been described. On the other hand the fixation of the mesh with sutures tied transfascially is clearly associated with more pain during 1-3 months postoperatively. Patients with meshes fixed with tacks only suffer from significantly lower pain. Up to now we do not know whether the suture fixation is really necessary. Concerning the material provided for intraperitoneal use I would like to refer to other chaperts in this book.

SUMMARY

The laparoscopic repair of parastomal hernia is a technically challenging but feasible procedure with some theoretical advantages over the conventional repair. From a clinical point of view it could be shown that the technique is safe and effective. The short term recurrence rate seems to be lowered as well as the postoperative complication rate is dramatically reduced by the laparoscopic technique. Nevertheless we need more patients treated by laparoscopy and strictly followed up in order to support the preliminary but very promising results.

References

1. Martin, L, Foster, G. Parastomal hernia. Ann R Coll Surg (1996) 78: 81-84.

2. Cheung MT, Chia NH, Chiu WY. Surgical treatment of parastomal hernia complicating sigmoid colostomies. Dis Colon Rectum (2001) 44: 266-270.

3. Tekkis PP, Kocher HM, Payne JG. The continuing challenge of parastomal hernia: failure of a novel polypropylene mesh repair. Ann R Coll Surg (1999) 81: 140-141.

4. Byers JM, Steinberg JB, Postier RG. Repair of parastomal hernias using polypropylene mesh. Arch Surg (1992) 127: 1246-1247.

5. Kohler L. Parastomal hernia - technique and results. Zentralbl Chir (1997) 122: 889-892.

6. Rubin MS, Schoetz DJ, Matthews JB. Parastomal hernia. Is stoma relocation superior to fascial repair? Arch Surg (1994) 129: 413-418.

7. Klinge U, Si ZY, Zheng H, Schumpelick V, Bhardwaj RS, Klosterhalfen B. Collagen I/III and matrix metalloproteinases (MMP) 1 and 13 in the fascia of patients with incisional hernias. J Invest Surg (2001) 14: 47-54.

8. De Ruiter P, Bijnen AB. Successful local repair of paracolostomy hernia with a newly developed prosthetic device. Int J Colorectal Dis (1992) 7: 132-134.

9. Tekkis PP, Kocher HM, Payne JG. Parastomal hernia repair: modified thorlakson technique, reinforced by polypropylene mesh. Dis Colon Rectum (1999) 42: 1505-1508.

10. Kasperk R, Klinge U, Schumpelick V. The repair of large parastomal hernias using a midline approach and a prosthetic mesh in the sublay position. Am J Surg (2000) 179: 186-188.

11. Sugarbaker, PH. Peritoneal approach to prosthetic mesh repair of paraostomy hernias. Ann. Surg. (1985) 201: 344-346.

12. Kozlowski PM, Wang PC, Winfield HN. Laparoscopic repair of incisional and parastomal hernias after major genitourinary or abdominal surgery. J Endourol (2001) 15: 175-179.

CHAPTER 35

Special Considerations for Laparoscopic Ventral Hernia Repair of Large and Multirecurrent Incisional Hernias

M.A. Carbajo, F. Martín Acebes, M. Toledano

INTRODUCTION

The surgical treatment of large or multirecurrent incisional hernias has always been a major challenge in abdominal wall repair, regardless of the technique used. The laparoscopic approach is not completely free of difficulties and complex problems, some of which are hard to solve.

Large ventral hernias are generally considered to be those that are more than 10 cm in length. However, this definition may not be sufficiently precise, since the magnitude of defects in the transversal direction, the possibility of additional hernias at some distance and the concomitant multirecurrent nature are not included. In this regard we will deal mainly with the problems associated with the laparoscopic repair of large and multirecurrent incisional hernias, since laparoscopy has already been shown to be possible and beneficial for the patient with massive abdominal wall defects (1).

INDICATIONS AND PATIENTS

General speaking these are complex patients who may have had multiple prior surgeries, which often leave long incisions at several anatomic sites and external sequelae that indicate the intensity of the degree of parallel intra-abdominal adhesions. There may be severe destruction of the abdominal wall (occasionally at different levels) with chronic abdominal pain and omental or visceral incarceration, in which the intra-abdominal "laparoscopic landscape" displays massive visceroparietal and viscerovisceral adhesions that can include not only the small or large intestine, but also the stomach and liver. Many are obese patients over 60 years old with other associated diseases.

Because of these factors we should take special care in preparing these patients, including the following measures, in addition to the general preparation:

- Analysis of medical history of prior surgeries (particularly if incisional hernia repair was previously performed), including technique, mesh used and position.

- When the patient has had polypropylene mesh implantation, one must be aware that serious visceral adhesions may be present.

- Study of respiratory function, with initiation of preoperative respiratory physiotherapy if necessary.

- CT scan and, if possible, MRI studies of the abdominal wall, in order to assess the nature and content of the incisional hernia, the position of firm wall margins, the anatomical involvement, the possibility of multiple sacs and the visceral adhesions (Fig. 1)

- Controlled weight-loss program, if needed. If the patient is morbidly obese, our protocol proposes preliminary bariatric surgery to treat the obesity, followed by repair of the incisional hernia at least 1 1/2 years later.

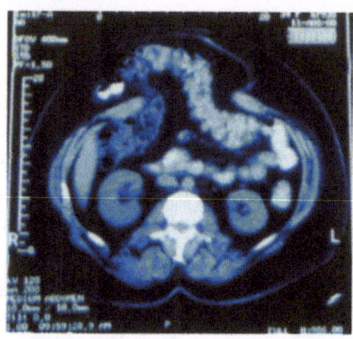

Fig. 1. Preoperative abdominal CT image shows intestinal loops inside a large incisio-nal hernia

In what type of large hernia is laparoscopic repair indicated?

- In general, all those over than 10 cm at any point in any anatomic site or prior any type of surgery, including low gynecological, urological, vascular or cardio-thoracic procedures with intra-abdominal extension.

- Recurrent or multirecurrent incisional hernias, regardless of the number of times operated and the prosthetic materials used previously (Fig. 2A and 2B).

- Incisional hernias with multiple defects that can affect longitudinally from the pubis to the xiphoid (Fig. 3).

- Co-existing ventral hernias at various anatomic sites in the same patient, regardless of number.

- Incisional hernias with other concomitant organic or non-septic condition that would allow simultaneous laparoscopic repair (Fig. 4).

- Incarcerated incisional hernias with any type of abdominal viscera, with or without previous occlusion or subocclusion crises.

- Hernias with early-stage intestinal strangulation and viable bowel, without sepsis, ischemia or necrosis.

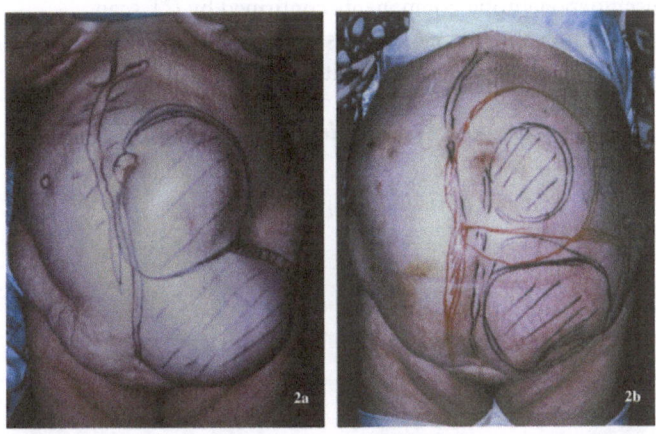

Fig. 2A. Large multirecurrent and multi-cavity incisional hernia. A: Before surgery. **Fig. 2B.** After surgery. Two prostheses were implanted; the first measured 30x20 cm and the second 19x15 cm.

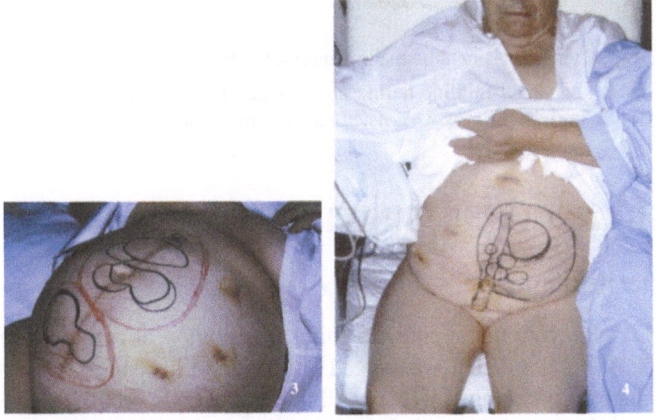

Fig. 3. Xiphopubic multi-cavity incisional hernia.

Fig. 4. Patient with multi-cavity incisional hernia and symptomatic cholelithiasis. Laparoscopic cholecystectomy was also performed during the operation.

For what types of patients is laparoscopic approach contraindicated?

Absolute contraindications include the following:

- Specific anesthesia-related contraindications for all laparoscopic surgery.
- Extremely large incisional hernias where the reintegration of visceras in the abdominal cavity is physically impossible, associated obesity and absence of parietal musculoaponeurotic components confirmed by CT scan.
- Presence of multiple enterocutaneous fistulas or an intra-abdominal septic focus.
- Decompensated liver cirrhosis with ascites.

Relative contraindications can include the following:

- Morbid obesity (Fig. 5)
- Presence of enterocutaneous fistulas (Fig. 6)
- Immunosuppression

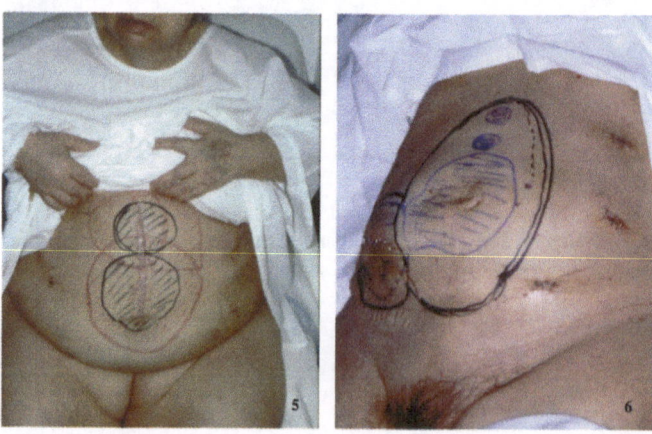

Fig. 5. Double incisional hernia in a morbidly obese patient.

Fig. 6. Incisional midline hernia and isolated entero-cutaneous fistula (colon), in right iliac fossa. Assisted laparoscopic repair

TECHNICAL CONSIDERATIONS

Pneumoperitoneum

The patient is placed in the supine decubitus position, with compressive bandage on both legs. A bladder catheter is placed in infraumbilical surgery and possibly a nasogastric tube in subxiphoid surgery. All parietal defects should be drawn on the skin and all solid areas of the wall should be located.

The pneumoperitoneum is created with a Veress needle in the left subcostal space between the anterior axillary line and the midline (Fig. 7) The right subcostal space is used to create the pneumoperitoneum only when repairing large hernia defects in the left abdomen.

Even in the case of multirecurrent incisional hernias with abdominal cavities
that are completely blocked by adhesions, we have always been able to
successfully create the pneumoperitoneum with a Veress needle in the left
subcostal space. In obese patients, an extra-long veress needle may be required.

A pressure of at least 14 mmHg is needed to produce maximum visceral
release from the abdominal wall and facilitate insertion of the first trocar without
complications. The flow of the inssufation and the presence of the
pneumoperitoneum in the hernia sac provide some indication of the severity of the
adhesions and of the content of the hernia (Fig. 8).

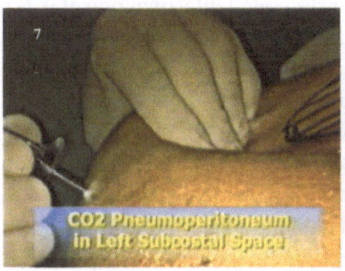 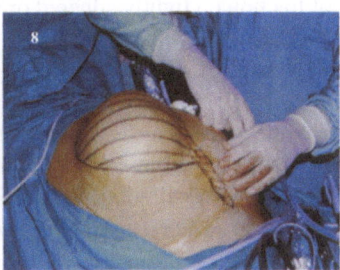

Fig. 7. Introduction of the Veress needle in the left subcostal region, anterior-
medial axillary line.

Fig. 8. View of the abdominal wall defect, perfectly visible when the
pneumoperitoneum is created. The parietal defects should be traced before
the surgery is undertaken.

Parietal and visceral adhesiolysis

A 10-mm trocar (USSC, Norwalk, CT, USA) is introduced at the same site as the
Veress needle (Fig. 9), and a 30-degree scope is used to meticulously examine the
abdominal cavity, severity of the adhesions and visceral involvement, and to
perform an initial assessment of the hernia defects.

Two 5-mm trocars are placed in the left flank, in order to carry out the surgical
procedure (Fig. 10). All hernia conditions at any level of the abdominal midline or the
right flank must be approached in this way. Large hernias of the left flank are repaired
using the same procedure, but from the right side (Fig. 11).

Supplementary trocars in the contralateral hernia abdomen may be necessary if
releasing is required for firmly attached visceral adhesions located below the
working trocars.

Adhesions must be released over the entire incision and it should be extended
at least 8-10 cm peripherally to allow a sufficiently large space for implantation of
the mesh. We recommend the use of ultrasonic harmonic scissors for fatty
adhesiolysis and omental vascularization, while carefully monitoring at all times
the position of neighboring intestinal or colon tissue (Fig. 12). The content of the
hernia sac must be completely released, keeping in mind that small intestine or
colon may be present in the margins of, or adhered to, the hernia sac in large or
recurrent hernias (Fig. 13).

Intestinal adhesiolysis is the underlying cause of the morbidity and mortality described in laparoscopic treatment of incisional hernias. It is also one of the most serious problems to solve, particularly in multirecurrent hernias, where we can find genuine intestinal "entrapment" syndromes, with the serosa layer of the intestine and the scar tissue of the abdominal wall fused in a single plane. The difficulty is even greater when the firmly attached adhesions are inside the hernia sac and are deep, lateralized and in areas with difficult visualization.

Our procedure in these complex situations is based on the following:

- Use of any type of electric or ultrasonic energy near the intestine should be avoided.

- Use of traction on tightly adhered or incarcerated intestinal bowel is forbidden.

- Release adhesions with Metzembaum fine scissors, using blunt dissection (Endo-punt, USSC, Norwalk, CT, USA) to find the area of dissection or to maintain traction on the bowel (Fig. 14). If necessary, section of the peritoneum in order to gradually release the intestine without touching the serosa layer, maintaining the curved side of the scissors against the abdominal wall to control the sectioning without producing a lesion of the intestine (Fig. 15). Some bleeding can occur during the dissection, but is no reason for concern. Hemostasis should not be performed until the adjacent intestine is released.

- Frequent changes of the area of dissection are sometimes required in order to gradually release the less compromised intestinal loops and facilitate access to the most tightly adhered loops.

- One should constantly check the tissue being released and ensure that there is adequate visualization and a clear operative field.

If, despite all these precautions, the serosa layer of an intestinal loop is affected or an enterotomy occurs, immediate repair is the best option. The procedure can then be continued, as in the case of conventional surgery. All intestinal segments affected by the dissection and parietal release must be meticulously examined before the procedure is completed. The most important concern is to prevent missed enterotomies at all costs, since reoperation would be necessary and the mortality rate of the series would be higher (2). If there are any doubts or there are any significantly affected long intestinal segments, a minilaparotomy may be sufficient to examine the released intestinal segments in detail and repaired if necessary (including intestinal resection) and continue with the procedure. An enterotomy does not imply the need for conversion unless the surgeon has little experience and is concerned about the safety of the procedure.

The colon is another viscera frequently found in large and recurrent hernias, particularly in the high supraumbilical incisions. In obese patients with redundant mesocolon the risk may be very high since during the dissection of fatty tissue visualization of the large intestine, particularly the transverse colon, is often more difficult, a fact that favors lesions. This must be kept in mind at all times when releasing medial and high scars. Non-traumatic instruments or blunt dissection should be used until the colon is adequately exposed, and then fine scissors without coagulation to section the parietal adhesions without the risk of lesions. Missed perforation of the colon would have disastrous immediate consequences, and the transmission of electric or ultrasonic energy could cause perforation after patient discharge, requiring readmission in critical condition. All colon lesions, even when they only affect the serosa, must be carefully sutured before continuing with the procedure. If there are any doubts, conversion or a minilaparotomy is advisable.

The stomach can also be adhered to the abdominal wall in the case of very
high incisions, and particularly when gastric surgery or surgery for morbid obesity
has been performed before. Visualization is not a problem in this case, but if the
stomach needs to be mobilized we may encounter major technical difficulties
related to the intense vascularization and possible firm attachment to the liver.

In right or sub-xiphoid subcostal incisional hernias, the liver can be involved in
the hernia process (Fig. 16). Release of the liver is not usually difficult, except for
problems due to bleeding caused by possible rupture of Glisson's capsule, an
easily controlled situation.

Once full adhesiolysis has been performed, the abdominal wall should be carefully
examined and the size of the various hernia defects assessed. All wall surfaces that are
bleeding or show signs of bleeding must be completely cauterized. We recommend
performing this operation with an argon laser terminal for laparoscopy (Fig. 17).
Likewise we also recommend applying argon laser terminal for laparoscopy to the
surface of the hernia sac to minimize the development of postoperative seromas.

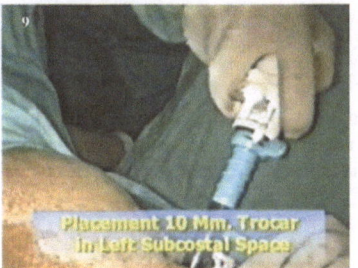
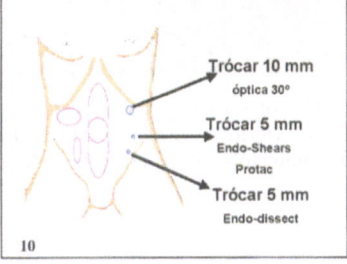

Fig. 9. Introduction of the initial trocar in left subcostal space, the site where
the Veress needle was inserted. **Fig. 10.** Trocar positioning

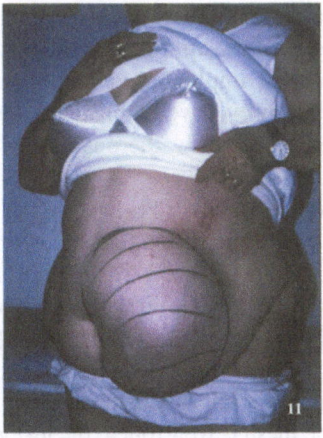

Fig. 11. Example of large incisional
hernia that must be approached from
the patient's right side.

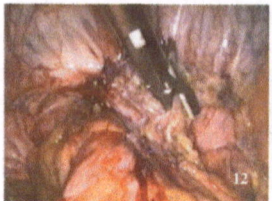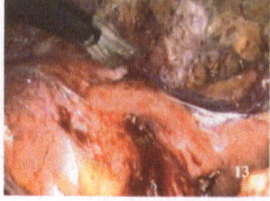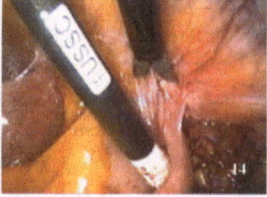

Fig. 12. Use of harmonic scissors. **Fig. 13.** Adhesions firmly attached to the small intestine near the defect margin. **Fig. 14.** Careful traction and use of scissors without any kind of energy during dissection maneuvers. The use of blunt dissection may be very useful.

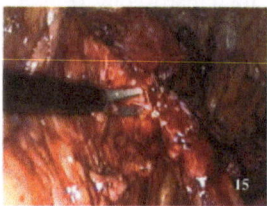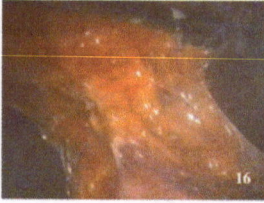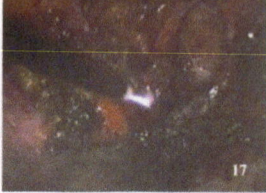

Fig. 15. Use of scissors with the curved side resting on the parietal surface for firmly attached visceroparietal adhesions. **Fig. 16.** Liver and stomach adhesions to the abdominal wall. **Fig. 17.** Application of the argon laser terminal for laparoscopy to dissection surfaces.

Selection and placement of the mesh

Among the various biocompatible materials currently available, PTFE is the most frequently used in intra-abdominal applications. It is the most well-tested in humans (3) and has been proven in experimental studies (4). New composite-type materials have been used in some series, but further studies in larger patient populations and with longer follow-up times are necessary (5) to determine their effectiveness. Intra-abdominal implantation of polypropylene mesh has been performed on occasion (6), however we emphatically advise against it. Although no "ideal" prosthetic material yet exists, there is no obvious alternative at present that improves upon the PTFE (7).

Hence, we recommend the use of PTFE Dual Mesh Plus (WL Gore & Assoc. Inc., Flagstaff, AZ, USA), to repair hernia defects, extending the patch at least 5 cm beyond the margins of the hernia. We are, therefore, using several large prostheses that may cover almost the entire abdominal wall and could be hard to handle intraabdominally if the surgeon does not have sufficient experience.

The mesh will be introduced through one of the trocar. We advise against introduction directly through the wall, as it involves an unnecessary risk of infection of the mesh (2, 8). When the mesh is well-rolled, the inside of the trocar is lubricated and highly resistant laparoscopic traction instruments are used, 2-mm-thick Dual Mesh Plus up to 19 x 15cm in size can be inserted through a 5-11 mm trocar. Larger prostheses up to 20 x 30cm will require a 12 mm trocar. Before rolling, the mesh must be oriented in the final position and marked along its longitudinal and transverse diameters to facilitate intra-abdominal placement (Fig. 18).

The mesh is opened completely by using two curved instruments, prepositioned with respect to the surface being covered and anchored to the wall at the level of the previously marked ends. Each staple point must be controlled from the outside with respect to the hernia defects and the position of the firm components of the wall and placed at a distance of at least 5 cm from the margin or hernia defect (Fig. 19). In order to manage large prostheses, we recommend starting at the longitudinal ends and continuing with the lateral, stapling the entire side of the trocars first in order to ensure that the mesh is properly positioned on the "difficult" flank and does not shift too much toward the opposite side. Once the "tent-like" shape of the mesh has been established, progressive application of tacks (Protack, USSC. Norwalk, CT, USA), is simple. At the inner crown the distance between tacks should not be more than 1.5-2 cm and each tack should penetrate the mesh deeply. This is controlled by external pressure applied by the surgeon's left hand (Fig. 20). A second crown of tacks is applied around the fibrous margin of the hernia defect. The mesh should be taut and firmly anchored on top of the hernia orifices and no tacks should be applied to the mesh when it is connected to the sac near the skin (Fig. 21).

Difficulties are found when extensive xiphopubic surfaces or large lateral defects of the entire wall abdominal must be covered. We currently recommend the use of large prostheses that cover all the defects without the need to place additional mesh. This can be technically more difficult, but it avoids a possible "fracture" line between two or more prostheses. Nevertheless, in very large abdominal cavities and massive lateral hernias, supplementary several prostheses must be used because sufficiently large single pieces are not available (Fig. 22). The same problem arises in case of concomitant hernias in different anatomic positions; more than one mesh patch must be implanted.

In obese patients with large abdominal walls, we recommend decreasing the intra-abdominal pressure at the time the mesh is positioned, as this will make it easier to properly implant the mesh.

Greater difficulty will be found with large hernias in the subcostal or subxiphoid region with a prominent xiphoid appendix, particularly if they are recurrent hernias and several prostheses were used previously. Mesh placement is a challenging task, as it requires applying the tacks over the costal arches, and proper anchoring on prominent xiphoids is practically impossible. To prevent the high risk of recurrence, if the final costal arches allow, we recommend using large prostheses held with external intercostal sutures that help to hold the mesh as stationary as possible and prevent involuntary displacement of the thoracic cavity.

Finally, if adhesiolysis and intestinal adhesiolysis is extensive, a ferric hyaluronate solution (Intergel, Ethicon, Somerville, NJ, USA.) can be instilled to prevent visceral adhesions in the future.

Compressive external bandage over the hernia orifice should be maintained for 5 to 7 days, in order to prevent the appearance of seromas and to promote adhesion of the mesh to the hernia sac.

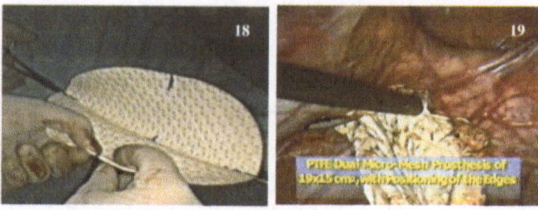

Fig. 18. Preparation of the mesh, after longitudinal and transverse reference marking. **Fig. 19.** Fixation of the first tack. The distance to the defect must be more than 5 cm.

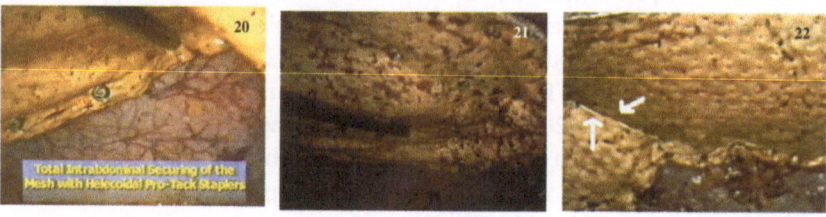

Fig. 20. Fixation is performed with tacks, creating an initial outer crown with an inter-tack distance of no more than 1.5-2 cm. **Fig. 21.** Close-up of the double crown of tacks (outer and inner). **Fig. 22.** In large defects, the use of several several prostheses may be necessary.

RESULTS

In a personal series of 200 patients completed in November 1999 with a current mean follow-up of 3 1/2 years, there were 80 patients with large hernias, among which 65 cases were hernias that had recurred between one and nine times (9). All had incisional hernias and external sutures were added in only one case.

None of these patients required conversion; in one case we performed a minilaparotomy to perform an intestinal resection, completing the procedure by laparoscopy. Three intestinal lesions were sutured intraperitoneally and there were no missed enterotomies.

Minor complications such as seroma were treated on an outpatient basis. No general complication, mesh infection or mortality was observed. The mean postoperative hospitalization of this group of patients was 48 hours.

Five patients in the group presented recurrence, at subcostal or subxiphoid sites in all cases. Two cases were reoperated and are asymptomatic at present; one refused another operation because symptoms were minimal. The other two are pending surgery.

Among the group of patients with recurrent hernias, 26 x 18- or 30 x 24-cm single several prostheses were used in 14 cases, a 26 x 18-cm mesh plus 19 x 15-cm mesh was implanted in 4 patients, 19 x 15-cm twin prostheses were used in 10 cases, and a 19 x 15-cm mesh with additional 15 x 10-cm prostheses were used in all others.

Comments

The indication of laparoscopic repair for small, medium-size or large defects of the abdominal wall is well established nowaday (10).

The benefits of laparoscopic repair for large hernias or recurrent incisional hernias are even more striking if we compare them with the adverse effects of classic surgery (Fig. 23A and 23B). All series with extensive experience have shown this to be true (8, 11-12).

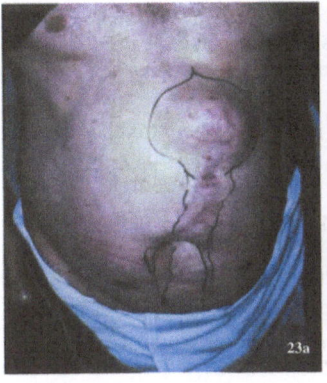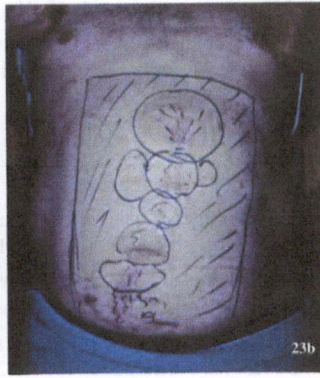

◀ **Fig. 23A.** Multiple midline defects prior to surgery.

◀ **Fig. 23B.** The same case, after surgery.

Nevertheless, laparoscopic repair of this type of large and complex incisional hernia requires an extended learning curve for the technique and specific skills and expertise in laparoscopy. We recommend concrete learning sessions under an expert in the procedure and prior training with simpler cases before attempting the repair of complicated defects in the abdominal wall (Figs. 24A and 24B). We consider the above recommendations on visceral adhesiolysis and mesh implantation to be vitally important, since errors in the former could be very detrimental to the patient and poor technique in the latter could mean hernia recurrence.

We must make ongoing efforts to improve the technique and carry out a well-controlled follow-up of these patients during the next few years to obtain long-term assessment that has not yet been possible, due to the short time during which laparoscopy has been used for this condition.

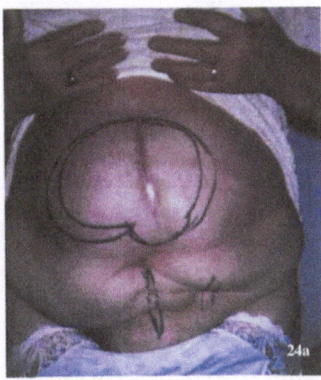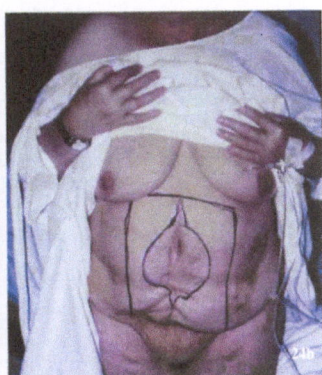

▶ **Fig. 24A.** Large recurrent incisional hernia. A, prior to surgery.

▶ **Fig. 24B.** B after surgery.

References

1. Carbajo Caballero MA, Martín del Olmo JC, Blanco Alvarez JI, Cuesta de la Llave C, Vaquero Puerta C. Volumineuse éventration xipho-pubienne à sacs multiples. La réparation coelioscopique est-elle possible? European J Coelio-Surg 1998; 26: 41-44.

2. Koehler RH, Voeller G. Recurrences in laparoscopic incisional hernia repairs: a personal series and review of the literature. JSLS 1999; 3: 293-304.

3. Carbajo MA, Martín del Olmo JC, Blanco Alvarez JI, Sastre L, de la Cuesta C, Martín F, Toledano M, Perna C. La prothèse biface de polytetrafluoroethylène expansé destinée aux plasties intrapéritonéales sous coelioscopie est-elle réellement un matériau anti-adhérences? European J Coelio-Surg 2000; 34: 69-71.

4. Bellon JM, Contreras LA, Pascual G, Bujan J. Análisis experimental en la respuesta de la fase aguda al implante de diferentes tipos de biomateriales en la pared abdominal. Cir Esp 1999; 4: 286-291.

5. Himpens JM, Leman GM, Deloose KR. Technique of introducing large Composite Mesh while performing laparoscopic incisional hernioplasty. European J of Coelio-Surg 2000; 34: 78-80.

6. Holtzman MD, Purut CM, Reintgen K, Eubanks S, Pappas TN. Laparoscopic ventral and incisional hernioplasty. Surg Endosc 1997; 11: 247-251.

7. Carbajo MA, Martín del Olmo JC, Blanco JI. What is the appropriate mesh for laparoscopic intraperitoneal repair of abdominal wall hernia? Surg Endosc 2000; 14: 408.

8. Toy FK, Bairley RW, Carey S. Prospective multicenter study of laparoscopic ventral hernioplasty. Preliminary results. Surg Endosc 1997; 12 (7): 955-959.

9. Carbajo MA, Martín del Olmo JC, Blanco JI, De la Cuesta C, Martín F, Toledano M, Perna C, Vaquero C. A laparoscopic solution for an old problem: Incisional and abdominal wall hernias. Experience with 200 patients. In 7th World Congress of Endoscopic Surgery. Eds. Monduzzi Ed Bologna, Italy 2000: 437-440.

10. Carbajo Caballero MA, Martín del Olmo JC, Blanco Alvarez JI, Martín Acebes F, Toledano Trincado M, Cuesta de la Llave C, Vaquero Puerta C, Perna C. Laparoscopic treatment versus open surgery in the solution of major incisional and abdominal wall hernias with mesh. Surg Endosc 1999; 13: 250-252.

11. Le Blanc KA. Current considerations in laparoscopic incisional and ventral herniorraphy. JSLS 2000; 4: 131-139.

12. Carbajo MA, Martin del Olmo JC, Blanco JI, de la Cuesta C, Martín F, Toledano M, Perna C, Vaquero C. Laparoscopic treatment of ventral abdominal wall hernias: preliminary results in 100 patients. JSLS 2000, 4: 141-145.

CHAPTER 36

Laparoscopic Incisional Repair in Emergent Situations

J.A. Almeida, M.E. Franklin

Treatment of ventral and incisional hernias has evolved during the past years. The availability of prosthetic material to either reinforce or bridge defects in the abdominal wall has made possible to reduce recurrence rates compared to suture-only techniques. The adoption of the Rives-Stoppa technique as the procedure of choice for incisional hernia repair, as well as the improvement in materials have been of significant help, but the overall results are still somewhat disappointing. The need of extensive dissections to assure a proper exposure of the different layers of the abdominal wall in order to accomplish a good mesh placement also has lead to an increased hospital stay, postoperative complications and return to normal activity.

The wave of minimally invasive techniques has also extended to abdominal wall surgery, including the repair of incisional and ventral hernias. The laparoscopic repair has steadily gained acceptance among the surgical community and there are numerous reports in the literature demonstrating the feasibility of the technique and good short and intermediate term results (1-4). There is yet some reluctance, however, to use this approach in emergent situations, such as incarcerated and/or strangulated hernias. In these instances, a traditional, open approach is preferred, and for the most part, no mesh is used. Rather, a suture-only repair or with an absorbable mesh such as Dexon® or Vicryl® is employed, at the expense of a high recurrence rate, and a delayed, definitive repair is performed after the potential infection has subsided.

The vascular compromise that occurs during incarceration – decreased venous return – or strangulation – frank ischemia, with possible development of necrosis - may cause a contaminated serous effusion within the sac, exposing the prosthesis to an unacceptable risk of infection. In these cases, according to most experienced surgeons, the use of heterologous prostheses becomes prohibitive, owing to the risk of infection, which is greater for nonabsorbable materials. The laparoscopic approach mandates the prosthesis to be placed intraperitoneally, adding an extra risk factor to the whole picture.

One important aspect to consider is that emergency surgery has as its goal the relief of a life-threatening strangulation. The evaluation of the risk of recurrence in the short term is also part of the ethical duty of the surgeon, particularly for aged and fragile patients, but emergency situations rarely permit the rigorous preparation of safe conditions for the use of prostheses.

CHOOSING THE MESH

The ideal prosthesis should be strong and inert, should provide a lattice for incorporating connective tissue while resisting the formation of adhesions, and should be stable in the presence of infection.

Several prosthetic materials are currently available for abdominal wall repair. Non-absorbable meshes have become very popular in incisional hernia repair as they provide good tensile strength over time and are ease to use. However, as there are concerns about their role in infected settings, absorbable meshes represent an alternative to repair incisional or strangulated hernias. They are eventually reabsorbed by the host and that diminishes chances of a foreign body reaction and thus, possibilities of infections are very low. The diminished strength of the repair is responsible, in part, of the high recurrence rate observed in these patients. Clinical experience has demonstrated that an absorbable prosthesis, if not used as a reinforcement to autoplasty, is destined to lose tensile strength within 10 weeks, with recurrences in 100% of cases (5).

Non-absorbable prosthesis

Polypropylene mesh has been the most widely used material in hernia repair since it was first introduced by Usher in 1958. Experimental models of wound infection have shown that more bacteria adhere to polypropylene mesh than to ePTFE (6, 7). Because of these findings, some authors have suggested that this material should not be used in contaminated fields. Others argue that the macroporous structure of polypropylene may allow free egress of contaminated material, thus making it a beneficial prosthetic choice (8). It is interesting to note that the levels of adherent bacteria are similar in models of peritonitis when comparing this prosthesis to ePTFE. On the other hand, Law demonstrated in an experimental study that the wound strength of polypropylene mesh was unaffected by the presence of bacteria when compared to ePTFE repair (9). We have been using in our institution the Surgipro® mesh (USSC, Norwalk, CT) (braided strands of polypropylene compared to monofilament as in Marlex® mesh) in instances of acutely incarcerated incisional hernias with success and few complications.

Expanded polytetrafluoroethylene (ePTFE) meshes have become very popular during the last years. Macroscopically the prosthesis is smooth and pliable, designed to elicit a minimal tissue response. According to several experimental studies ePTFE seems to promote less intraabdominal adhesions and has eventually replaced polypropylene as the material of choice in laparoscopic repairs where the prosthesis is placed intraperitoneally (10-12). As previously mentioned, bacteria seem to be less adherent to the surface of ePTFE when compared to knitted polypropylene in both the presence and absence of antibiotics. Whether these experimental findings are clinically significant is unclear. According to some authors, however, if ePTFE prosthesis becomes infected, the chances of removal are greater that for polypropylene mesh.

Absorbable and Biocompatible prosthesis

Dexon® mesh (polyglycolic acid) was considered the material of choice as it does not require operative removal if infection develops, because it reabsorbs rapidly and inhibits bacterial growth (13). Dexon mesh has been successfully implanted in contaminated abdominal wall in humans (14) but at the expense of a high recurrence rate. Vicryl® mesh (Polyglactin 910) has similar characteristics but with a more rapid absorption rate.

A new prosthetic material has been recently released in the market (Surgisis®, Cook Biotech. Bloomington, IN USA). This prosthesis is made of small intestine submucosa, also referred to as SIS, a bioengineered acellular collagen matrix composed of proteoglycans and several growth factors. Initially developed as a vascular prosthesis (15), further studies showed its ability to serve as a bioscaffold for more specialized tissues including the abdominal wall (16-19). A very attractive feature of SIS is this material promotes neovascularization in the host tissue, rendering it resistant to infection; thus, this very promising prosthesis may represent a valid alternative for those cases in which there is a concern of infection, as occurs in incarcerated/strangulated hernias. Since its release, this mesh constitutes the material of choice for potentially contaminated fields, such as in concurrent surgeries (Altemeier class 2) as well as infected settings and emergent operations (Altemeier class 4). It is currently available in different sizes and as a 4-ply mesh (Surgisis®-ES, Cook Surgical. Bloomigton IN) or, more recently, as a 8-ply mesh (Surgisis® Gold, Cook Surgical. Bloomigton IN), the latter being specifically designed for ventral hernia repair. (Fig. 1) (20).

Fig. 1. Surgisis® Gold Mesh. This material needs rehy-dratation in normal saline during at least 10 min. prior to use.

TECHNIQUE

The technique demands general anesthesia as well as placement of a nasogastric tube and a Foley catheter. It is advisable to perform a bowel cleansing prior to surgery is the clinical situation makes it feasible. The patient must be firmly attached to the table to allow for alterations in position to Trendelenburg, reverse Trendelenburg, or extreme side-to-side "airplaning" to allow bowel displacement and adhesions to be dissected. We prefer to secure the patient to the table with tape at the shoulder level. Sequential compression devices are applied to the legs to prevent venous thrombosis and the video monitors are positioned at the foot of the table, or at a place convenient for viewing by all involved. In a significant number of cases, reduction of hernia contents occurs spontaneously or with gentle maneuvers after institution of general anesthesia and muscle relaxation. This maneuver will help considerably the operative procedure. The authors prefer pneumoperitoneum access with a Veress needle at an alternate site away from the incision scar or hernia, usually in the upper quadrants lateral to the rectus muscle. Rarely an open Hasson technique is chosen but has for the most part abandoned this technique. After insertion of the first trocar, a 0° laparoscope is inserted and the abdomen is thoroughly inspected. If any necrotic bowel is seen, a decision can be made at this point to exteriorize the intestine, resect it and perform the anastomosis extracorporeally or rather, to continue the procedure laparoscopically, according to surgeon's experience and preference. If no necrosis is found, then the adhesions opposite to the initial ports are carefully taken down and additional ports are placed under direct vision. Each of these additional trocars should be considered as a port through which a stapler (or laparoscope) can be placed. Therefore, 10 -12 mm trocars are desirable at all ports, although we have drifted to all 5mm ports except for the ones used to introduce the mesh and staples. Adhesion take-down and reduction of hernia contents are a crucial step of the procedure, and judicious use of electrocautery is strongly advised. We prefer instead to use blunt dissection to minimize the chances of bowel injury. As the planes may be difficult to identify in the acute setting, we have found that the use of irrigation and suction to be of great help (Fig. 2). Bleeding must be meticulously controlled and bowel injury avoided as the anterior abdominal wall is being cleared. All large defects should be closed with sutures, if at all possible, and can be placed either percutaneously or laparoscopically. In our practice this is usually accomplished percutaneously, using the Carter - Thomason® needle point suture passer (Inlet Medical, Inc., Eden Prairie, MN) with placement of #2 Tycron® (Ethicon, Somerville, N.J.) as described previously by us (21).

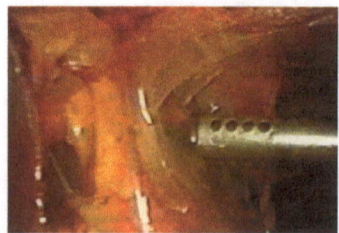

Fig. 2. Use of high-pressure irrigation to facilitate reduction of hernia contents.

Taking into consideration the thickness of the abdominal wall, the chosen mesh is tailored to approximately 10% smaller than the area judged adequate for coverage of the defect, as estimated by laying the mesh out on the skin. As many defects as possible should be covered with each piece of mesh while, at the same time, maintaining minimum margins of 3-5 cm circumferentially around each defect. Although one piece of mesh is ideal, it may not be possible in all instances, especially those abdomens where extensive or multiple, widely spaced defects are present. The mesh must be placed over the defect and held in place with staples and, in most circumstances, transfascial sutures placed (Fig.3). If the peritoneal fluid is not cloudy on initial exam and strangulated bowel immediately has resumption of normal color, a mesh could be placed after a culture of the peritoneal fluid is obtained. The trocar ports should all be carefully and completely closed (again, we prefer the Carter - Thomason® needle point suture passer, Inlet Medical, Inc.) and the abdomen desufflated after covering the repaired area with omentum. The omentum is then spread over and tacked (stapled) in place to serve as a barrier to separate the mesh from the bowel.(Fig. 4) Operative times may vary with severity of adhesions, number of defects, bowel involvement and need for concurrent procedures.

The postoperative course is relatively benign. When excessive bowel manipulation was present due to adhesions or hernia involvement it is preferable to leave the nasogastric tube for 12 to 24 hrs. postoperatively. Hemoglobin, hematocrit, and electrolyte levels are checked the next day. We expect to see occasionally subcutaneous fluid in the hernia sites (serous) and explain this possibility to the patient preoperatively. This occurs at a much lower rate when the fascial defects are closed and "dead space" obliterated. The patient is given a diet when bowel sounds are present, which can vary from immediately to several days postoperative, depending on the amount of dissection, handling of bowel, and bleeding. Patients are allowed to go home when they are afebrile, their wounds are clean, a regular diet is tolerated, and minimal pain is present.

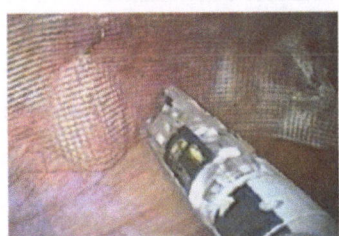 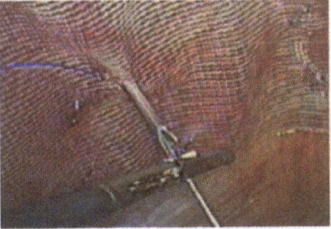

Fig. 3. Fixing the prosthesis with staples(a) and transfascial sutures (b).

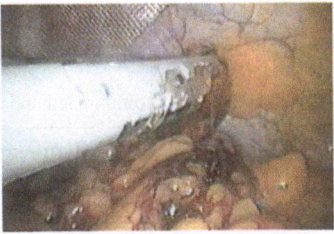

Fig. 4. Tacking the omentum to protect the intraabdominal viscera.

THE TEXAS ENDOSURGERY EXPERIENCE

Two hundred and sixty seven patients have undergone a laparoscopic ventral hernia repair during the past 9 years. The distribution of this series is shown in table I. One hundred and twenty patients showed some degree of complication (incarceration and/or strangulations) and, among these, 39 were operated on an emergent basis (Table II). Operative time and intraoperative complications are listed in table III and table IV. Interestingly, enterotomies only obligated to convert to an open procedure in 2 cases.

Mesh infection occurred in only one patient, requiring its removal at 14 months postoperative. Significant seromas were noted in only two patients but the temptation to aspirate was overcome and the fluid collections finally resolved on their own (average 6 weeks).

Mean follow up is 32 months, with a range of 1-73 months. We have experienced 6 recurrences (2.42%)

Table I. Distribution of patients of our series

	Males	**Females**
No. of patients	119	148
Mean age	58.2 ± 17.67	
Weight	88.47 ± 23.37	
Height	165.3 ± 12.3	

Table II. Types of ventral hernias treated at the Texas Endosurgery Institute. The hernias incarcerated with intestine and strangulated were all treated as emergency cases

Recurrent	91 (34%)	
Complicated	Incarcerated with epiplon	81
	Incarcerated with intestine	23
	Strangulated	16
No complicated	147 (55%)	

Table III. Operative times. Laparoscopic repair of complicated and non-complicated hernias

Incisional	No Complicated	60 min	47-118 min
	Complicated	**120 min**	**70-210 min**
Ventral	No Complicated	40 min	30-60 min
	Complicated	**105 min**	**72-165 min**

Table IV. Intraoperative complications

Event	Number
Conversion	3
Enterotomies	4
Thermal lesions in bowel	0
TOTAL	2.6%

SUMMARY

Although laparoscopic surgery has been gained increase acceptance among surgeons for laparoscopic ventral and incisional hernia repair, there are still few reports on its use in emergent situations. This may be due to the concern of placing a prosthetic material in a potentially infected setting as long as lack of experience. Although technically more demanding, we feel that with experience this type of repair has the potential of becoming more incorporated to the surgeon's armamentarium. The availability of newer prosthetic materials will help in this advance.

References

1. DeMaria EJ, Moss JM, Sugerman HJ. Laparoscopic intraperitoneal polytetrafluoroethylene (PTFE) prosthetic patch repair of ventral hernia. Prospective comparison to open prefascial polypropylene mesh repair. Surg Endosc 2000; 14(4):326-329.

2. Franklin ME, Dorman JP, Glass JL, Balli JE, Gonzalez JJ. Laparoscopic ventral and incisional hernia repair. Surg Laparosc Endosc 1998; 8(4):294-299.

3. Heniford BT, Park A, Ramshaw BJ, Voeller G. Laparoscopic ventral and incisional hernia repair in 407 patients. J Am Coll Surg 2000; 190(6):645-650.

4. LeBlanc KA. Current considerations in laparoscopic incisional and ventral herniorrhaphy. JSLS 2000; 4(2):131-139.

5. Amid PK Silulman AG. Selecting synthetic mesh for the repair of groin hernia. Postgraduate Gen Surg , 150-155. 1992.

6. Brown GL. Comparison of prosthetic materials for abdominal wall reconstruction in the presence of contamination and infection. Ann Surg 1985; 201:705-711.

7. Law NW EH. Adhesion formation and peritoneal healing on prosthetic material. Clin Mater 3, 95-101. 1988.

8. Walker PM LB. Marlex for repair of abdominal wall defects. Can J Surg 1976; 19:211-213.

9. Law NW EH. A comparison of polypropylene mesh and expanded polytetrafluoroethylene patch for the repair of contaminated abdominal wall defects--an experimental study. Surgery 1991; 109(5):652-655.

10. LeBlanc KA, Booth WV. Laparoscopic repair of incisional abdominal hernias using expanded polytetrafluoroethylene: preliminary findings. Surg Laparosc Endosc 1993; 3(1):39-41.

11. Tsimoyiannis EC, Tassis A, Glantzounis G, Jabarin M, Siakas P, Tzourou H. Laparoscopic intraperitoneal onlay mesh repair of incisional hernia. Surg Laparosc Endosc 1998; 8(5):360-362.

12. Voeller GR, Ramshaw B, Park AE, Heniford BT. Incisional hernia. J Am Coll Surg 1999; 189(6):635-637.

13. Edlich RF. Physical and chemical configuration of sutures in the development of surgical infection. Ann Surg 1973; 177:679-688.

14. Dayton MT. Use of an absorbable mesh to repair contaminated abdominal wall defects. Arch Surg 1986; 121:954-960.

15. Egusa S. Experimental study on vascular graft. II. Replacement of inferior vena cava and abdoninal aorta with the autogenous segment of small intestine submucosa. Acta Med Okayama 1968; 22(3):153-165.

16. Chen MK, Badylak SF. Small bowel tissue engineering using small intestinal submucosa as a scaffold. J Surg Res 2001; 99(2):352-358.

17. Xie H, Shaffer BS, Wadia Y, Gregory KW. Use of reconstructed small intestine submucosa for urinary tract replacement. ASAIO J 2000; 46(3):268-272.

18. Dalla VL, Engum S, Kogon B, Jensen E, Davis M, Grosfeld J. Evaluation of small intestine submucosa and acellular dermis as diaphragmatic prostheses. J Pediatr Surg 1999; 34(1):167-171.

19. Clarke KM, Lantz GC, Salisbury SK, Badylak SF, Hiles MC, Voytik SL. Intestine submucosa and polypropylene mesh for abdominal wall repair in dogs. J Surg Res 1996; 60(1):107-114.

20. Almeida JA, Franklin ME. Laparoscopic ventral hernia repair with Surgisis. Personal Communication presented at the ACS 2001 Technical exhibit. Chicago, IL 2001.

21. Rosenthal D, Franklin ME, Jr. Use of percutaneous stitches in laparoscopic mesh hernioplasty. Surg Gynecol Obstet 1993; 176(5):491-492.

Postoperative Aspects
after Laparoscopic Ventral Hernia Repair

CHAPTER 37

Postoperative Management of Patients after Laparoscopic Ventral Hernias Repair

J.A. Guerrero Fernández-Marcote, J.L. Tovar Martínez, E. Segovia Cornejo

INTRODUCTION

In general, laparoscopic surgery is used to treat many pathologies that can benefit from this surgical treatment, in a similar manner and with identical effectiveness as classical surgery procedures but by means of a different approach.

The difference between the two surgical techniques lies precisely in the approach used. Laparoscopic surgery is less aggressive and, therefore, the organic response to the potential internal imbalances resulting from it will be lower.

In the particular issue we are addressing, "Laparoscopic Repair of Ventral Hernia", there is another major difference that contributes to the reduced aggressiveness of the laparoscopic approach. In laparoscopic repair involving, for example, funduplication to treat gastroesophageal reflux disease (GERD), cholecystectomy to treat cholelithiasis or hemicolectomy to treat a colon tumor, the aggressiveness of the procedure and the associated morbidity are reduced. However, the solution to the problem is much the same as in classic laparotomy. In contrast, laparoscopic repair of ventral hernias involves less aggression not only in terms of the approach, but also in the technique used to solve the problem, as there is less tissue disection, no tension and practically no bleeding.

Laparoscopic repair of ventral hernias results in a lower inflammatory response because of this reduced aggression. As a consequence, the postoperative treatment is directed more toward preventing potential complications than toward correcting internal imbalances and their clinical manifestations.

PATHOPHYSIOLOGICAL ASPECTS OF LAPAROSCOPIC SURGERY THAT CONDITION POSTOPERATIVE TREATMENT

Inflammatory response

Surgical trauma induces an endocrine-metabolic response that has traditionally been divided into four stages:

1) **Catabolic or inflammatory phase:** After trauma, the body reacts by releasing several substances known as mediators which trigger the endocrine-metabolic response. This is responsible for all the alterations described as inherent to the immediate postoperative period.

2) **Corticoid withdrawal or phase of crisis:** As an indication of the body's defense mechanism, hormone secretion normalizes and metabolic alterations return to normal once the aggression has begun to subside.

3) **Anabolic phase:** Anabolism dominates in this stage and restoration of tissue integrity begins.

4) **Fat deposit phase:** Definitive recovery stage in which the body returns to normal.

A brief analysis of the first and most essential phase reminds us that surgical aggression involves local and general stimulation of the hypothalamo-hypophyseal-adrenal axis as well as the sympathetic nervous system (1, 2). The humoral mediators (e.g., the cytokines produced at the trauma site) play an important role in triggering this response (3). These mediators are released in proportion to the intensity and duration of the surgical trauma, being this response lower after laparoscopic surgery than open surgery (4,5).

The proteins of the inflammatory phase could be used as an example (6). Cytokines such as interleukin-1 (IL-1), tumor necrosis factor (TNF) and interleukin-6 (IL-6) are the main mediators of the inflammatory phase response. In particular, IL-6 (the most sensitive to trauma) enhances the hepatic production of proteins inherent to this phase such as C-reactive protein. The levels of this protein rise 4 to 12 hours after the surgical procedure and peak at 24 to 72 h. Levels remain high for two weeks (7). After laparoscopic surgery this elevation is much lower, as has been demonstrated in laparoscopic cholelithiasis (8) and repair of inguinal hernias (9, 10). Although there are no serious studies in the literature that corroborate these assertions in the case of ventral hernias, laparoscopic surgery is clearly less traumatic for the body.

These biochemical alterations are the basis for, and the triggering element of, the clinical manifestations seen in the postoperative period, e.g., pain, fever, dehydration, fatigue, etc. Since laparoscopic surgery first appeared in the late 1980s, numerous works have shown that this technique involves less pain for patients during the postoperative period and results in earlier food intake, shorter hospitalization and faster return to normal activities, in comparison with open surgery (11,12,13).

Greater patient satisfaction from the aesthetic point of view and fewer rejections to possible future surgeries are also important points (14,15).

Immune Response-infection

The surgical intervention triggers a series of immune system alterations(16,17) that are partially responsible for postoperative infectious complications. It is now widely recognized that laparoscopic surgery has fewer effects on the immune system than open surgery, since it causes significantly less tissue aggression. Recent studies have analyzed this assertion in depth (18,19), describing the effect produced by laparoscopic surgery on various immune system components, such as T-cells, delayed hypersensitivity, polymorphonuclear neutrophils, and the superoxide anion (5). All these components display considerable alterations after open surgery, a fact that has led to the conclusion that laparoscopic surgery *per se* decreases the incidence of postoperative infectious complications.

Bowel motility

Another important facet of a patient's recovery after surgery is re-establishment of bowel motility, regardless of whether the gastrointestinal tract is directly involved in the operation or not. This aspect of laparoscopic surgery has been well investigated experimentally (20, 21), but not in clinical studies with patients. Hyperactivity of the sympathetic nervous system is generally understood to produce an inhibition of bowel motility. This reflex hyperactivity is triggered by physical events such as laparotomy, intestinal manipulation, blood loss or pain. Laparoscopic surgery obviously minimizes these aggressions, with reduced stimulation of the sympathetic system. As a result, it is not surprising that patients who undergo laparoscopic surgery regain peristalsis earlier than in open surgery and that postoperative ileus symptoms such as nausea or vomiting are much less frequent.

Pain

From the pathophysiological point of view, there are not many reasons for pain following laparoscopic repair of ventral hernias; the incisions are so small that respiratory movement is not hindered and drains are not normally needed. In fact, since there are no major incisions or drains, the role of abdominal wall irritation as a cause of pain is much less important in this type of surgery than in open surgery. This is indirectly evident from respiratory parameters observed 4-6 hours after performing laparoscopic surgery (22, 23). There is one typical pain common to any laparoscopic procedure, the pain due to irritation of the diaphragm. The patient often describes this pain as located in the back, scapula or shoulders because of metameric similarity. The CO_2 used to create and maintain the pneumoperitoneum seems to be highly implicated in the genesis of this pain.

On occasions we may find an inherent aspect of this surgery which although trivial, should not be ignored. This concerns the discomfort produced by the material used to secure the mesh intraperitoneally, usually tacks that attach the mesh to the peritoneum and posterior muscle fasciae. Sometimes, patients describe sporadic pain when pressing with a finger on a specific spot distant from the hernia defect, a symptom they find disconcerting. This must be taken into account during the postoperative period.

Therefore we can say that, although there is some pain after laparoscopic surgery, it is usually not considerable. And this is the reason for earlier recovery from postoperative ileus, greater patient comfort and particularly, more immediate reintegration in the social-family atmosphere.

POSTOPERATIVE TREATMENT

We have devoted the first part of this chapter to presenting the facts that show that laparoscopic surgery, known as "minimally invasive" is also "minimally aggressive" and will cause "minimal physiologic alterations". In conventional surgery, these changes warrant or even require utmost surveillance and careful action during the postoperative period to ensure that the body's systems (renal, respiratory, cardiocirculatory, metabolic, etc.) function perfectly and that the mechanisms characterizing the anabolic phase of the postoperative response activate as soon and as efficiently as possible.

During laparoscopic repair for ventral hernia, the inflammatory phase is almost negligible and, therefore, the related alterations will be minimal. Nevertheless, there are several unquestionable events (e.g., general anesthesia, pneumoperitoneum, introduction of foreign material in the body, small incisions) that require careful monitoring, supervision and action to prevent complications.

As mentioned earlier, these steps are related more to prophylaxis of the possible complication than to specific treatment of an established alteration.

The postoperative care can be divided into:
- Hospital care
- Home care

Hospital care

By definition, laparoscopic surgery involves a very short hospital stay, with patients remaining in the hospital for 24-48 hours or less. During this time, particular attention must be paid to the following points:

Water and electrolyte balance

Since the duration of surgery is relatively short (often shorter than in open surgery), the loss of fluid will be minimal and the anesthesiologist should not find difficulties in maintaining the hemodynamic balance. After the surgery, once the patient is awake, he or she will continue to receive isotonic infusion with an adequate source of glucose and electrolytic balance at a rate of 40 ml/kg of weight per day to preserve hemodynamics and renal perfusion. Naturally this amount may vary, depending on the needs of the patient (e.g., in the case of abundant vomiting, sweating, etc.). Fluid therapy must be maintained until patients can tolerate on their own sufficient fluid intake in terms of quantity and quality to maintain an internal balance.

Nutrition

As in the case of fluids, the organic energy deposits will not decrease since trauma is minimal; therefore, there is no need for extraordinary sources of nutrition. In addition, as has already been mentioned, the alteration of gastrointestinal peristalsis in laparoscopic surgery and specifically in ventral hernia repair is almost imperceptible. In fact, patients can begin to take water and liquid foods on the same day of the operation, provided the intake is moderate and gradual. On the first postoperative day (usually the day of discharge), the patient can begin to eat solid foods. However, carbonated beverages or hard-to-digest foods should be avoided.

Elimination of gases and feces

Rectal elimination of gases usually starts soon due to the early recovery of peristalsis. Nevertheless the elimination of feces is a cause of concern for some patients. In our experience, for example, all patients undergoing this type of surgery are given an antiseptic colon preparation in the form of enema solutions the day before the procedure, either at home or in the hospital. This decreases the risk of infection, in the event that a lesion to the gastrointestinal tract is produced during or after the surgery.

Pain

As mentioned earlier in the pathophysiology section, if there is no intraoperative complication that conditions the normal course of the laparoscopic surgery, pain is generally minimal and can be managed during hospitalization with non-narcotic analgesics as indicated in the protocol and later conditionally at home. Several measures that can be taken to minimize or prevent postoperative pain in laparoscopic surgery in general are applicable to this type of surgery:
- Pain caused by the pneumoperitoneum
- Pain at the trocar incisions
- Pain at the tack anchor sites

The literature contains data indicating that the incidence of back pain due to the pneumoperitoneum is 35-63% (24). In addition to meticulous removal of all gas, some authors recommend irrigation of the diaphragm with bupivacaine at the end of the surgery; the application of 10 ml at 0.5% dissolved in 500 ml of saline solution, 250 ml on each side, significantly reduces the incidence of such pain in the postoperative period (25).

The incisions made to insert the trocars are rarely painful. Nevertheless, infiltration with 5% bupivacaine in the port sites is recommended to further prevent any possible postoperative pain.

Occasional, isolated pain caused by the staples tends to remit spontaneously in a few days with no need for any special measures.

Nausea and vomiting

These are external manifestations of a postoperative ileus. Although we have already mentioned that this is practically non-existent in laparoscopic surgery since peristalsis is recovered immediately, sometimes motility is not recovered as quickly, mainly due to the effect of CO_2 on the intestinal bowel, and this manifests as nausea and vomiting.

Various techniques for controlling nausea and vomiting have been proposed, including intradermal scopolamine, which reduces these symptoms by half. The use of this substance, however, may cause serious side effects such as dry mouth and blurred vision that should be taken into account. Ephedrine (0.5 mcg/kg i.m.) is frequently very effective and has few excessively unpleasant side effects. In any case, ondasentron (an HT3 receptor antagonist), has also been shown to be highly effective in both treatment and prevention. When nausea and vomiting persist, abdominal surgery complication(s) that could be the cause must be ruled out before continuing therapy.

Prophylaxis of deep venous thrombosis

The pneumoperitoneum leads to increased intra-abdominal pressure that hinders venous return from the lower limbs, and this situation can be exacerbated by the inverted Trendelenburg position; thus in laparoscopic surgery measures must be taken to prevent thromboembolic disease. Some authors believe that physical measures are sufficient, including binding the legs, early ambulation, respiratory physiotherapy and mainly pneumatic intermittent sequential compression (ISC) (26). We have always implemented measures to prevent deep venous thrombosis, using several techniques in situations of maximum risk (27, 28). Together with other authors (29) and with the SAGES guidelines (30) we believe that drug-based prophylaxis using low molecular weight heparin at the same doses as in open surgery according to hospital protocols should be used in addition to these physical measures for laparoscopic surgery.

Antibiotic prophylaxis

This is a widespread, accepted practice in the surgical field, particularly in hernia surgery (31,32). In laparoscopic repair of ventral hernias, however, there is no unanimity concerning the issue. Some authors recommend it, arguing that there is a higher risk of microorganism dissemination due to the presence of pressurized CO_2 (33). Others do not feel it is warranted in simple hernias (34). In our opinion, antibiotic prophylaxis is necessary since foreign prosthetic material is being introduced. We use 1 g of a 2nd-generation cephalosporin prior to the anesthesia and 8 hours after the surgery.

Seroma prophylaxis

On occasion a virtual space may remain between the skin covering the incisional hernia and the mesh, which can fill with a serous collection. This is prevented if we take the precaution to apply an opressive bandage for as long as necessary until the tissue becomes integrated with the prosthesis. The use of a surgical girdle is very useful.

Home care

One of the advantages of this type of surgery is that patients can leave the hospital early and go home, where they will be more comfortable. If required the patient can be helped by nearby health care personnel. Nevertheless, we must provide the patient with a series of recommendations to ensure full recovery and rapid detection of any complications:

- Daily inspection of the wound; exposure of the wound to air after daily hygiene is advisable, notifying the health care professionals of any changes.
- Control of temperature.
- Careful control of diet, with moderate intake and no carbonated beverages or gas-producing meals.
- Moderate activity, mainly ambulation.
- Analgesics should be taken only conditionally.
- In exceptional cases of little or no activity, drug prophylaxis for deep vein thrombosis must be continued, at the physician's discretion.
- Postoperative follow-up of the surgery should be carried out in accordance with the protocol established at each center, with an initial follow-up visit at 2-4 weeks after the procedure to detect possible immediate recurrences.

CONCLUSION

Laparoscopic surgery is of undeniable benefit for the patient and its pathophysiological consequences are less aggressive. Nevertheless, it is still a surgical procedure that must be performed as well as possible and followed up carefully to prevent pain and complications for the patient.

References

1. Weissman C. The metabolic response to stress: an overview and update. Anesthesiology 1990; 73: 308-27.

2. Chernow B, Alexander HR, Smallridge RC et al. Hormonal responses to graded surgical stress. Arch Intern Med 1987; 147: 1273-8.

3. Fong Y, Moldawer LL, Shires GT, Lowry SF. The biologic characteristics of citokines and their implication in surgical injury. Surg Gynecol Obstet 1990; 170: 363-78.

4. Karayiannakis AJ, Makri GG, Mantzioka A, et al. Systemic stress response cholecystectomy: a randomized trial. Br J Surg 1997; 84: 467-471.

5. Redmond HP, Watson WG, Houghton T, et al. Immune function in patients undergoing open vs laparoscopic cholecystectomy. Arch Surg 1994; 129: 1240-.1246.

6. Gauldie J, Richards C, Harnish D, et al. Interferon β2/B—cell stimulatory factor type 2 shares identity with monocyte-derived hepatocyte-stimulating factor and regulates the major inflammatory phase protein response in liver cells. Proc Natl Acad Sci 1987; 84:7251-7255.

7. Ohzato H, Yoshizaaki K, Nishimoto N, et al. Interleukin-6 as a new indicator of inflammatory status: detection of serum levels of interleukin-6 and C-reactive protein after surgery. Surgery 1991; 111: 201-209.

8. Vittimberga F, Foley D, Meyers W, et al. Laparoscopic surgery and the systemic immune response. Ann Surg 1998; 227:326-334.

9. Uzunköy A, Coskun A, Akinci F and Kocygit A. Systemic stress responses after laparoscopic or open hernia repair. Eur J Surg 2000; 166: 467-471.

10. Karayiannakis AJ, Makri GG, Mmantziokaa A, et al. Systemic stress response cholecystectomy: a randomized trial. Br J Surg 1997; 84: 467-471.

11. Akhtar K, Kamalky-asl ID, Lamb WR, et al. Metabolic and responses after laparoscopic and open inguinal hernia repair. Ann R Coll Surg Engl 1998; 80: 125-130.

12. Berggren U, Gordh T, Grama D, et al. Laparoscopic versus open cholecystectomy: hospitalization, sick leave, analgesia and trauma responses. Br J Surg 1994; 81: 1362-1365.

13. Ramshaw BJ, Tucker JG, Mason EM, et al. A comparison of transabdominal preperitoneal (TAPP) and total extraperitoneal approach (TEPA) laparoscopic herniorrhaphies. Am Surg 1995; 61: 279-283.

14. Sawyers JL. Current status of conventional (open) cholecystectomy versus laparoscopic cholecystectomy. Ann Surg 1996; 223: 1-3.

15. Barkun JS, Wexler MJ, Hinchey EJ, et al. Laparoscopic versus open inguinal herniorrhaphy: Preliminary results of a randomized controlled trial. Surgery 1995; 118: 703-710.

16. Lennard TWJ, Shenton BK, Borzotta A, et al. The influence of surgical operations on components of the human immune system. Br J Surg 1985; 72: 771-6.

17. Navarro Zorraquino M. Aspectos inmunológicos de la cirugía. Ed. Prensas Universitarias de Zaragoza, 1997.

18. Hackam DJ, Rotstein OD. Host response to laparoscopic surgery: mechanisms and clinical correlates. Can J Surg 1998; 41: 103-11.

19. Sietses C, Beelen RH, Meijer S, Cuesta MA. Immunological consequences of laparoscopic surgery, speculations on the cause and clinical implications. Langenbecks Arch Surg 1990; 384: 250-8.

20. Laparoscopic colectomy shortens postoperative ileus in a canine model. Davies W, Kollmorgen C, Quang M, et al. Surgery 1997; 121: 550-5.

21. Hotokezaka M, Combs M, Mentis E, Schirmer B. Recovery of fasted and fed gastrointestinal motility after open versus laparoscopic cholecystectomy in dogs. Ann Surg 1996; 223: 413-419.

22. Peters JH, Ortega AE, Campbell JAJ, Schwartz DC, Innes JT, Ellison EC. The physiology of laparoscopic surgery I: pulmonary function following laparoscopic surgery. Surg Laparosc. Endosc 1993; 3(5): 350.

23. Putensen-Himmer G, Putensen, Lammer H et al. Comparison of postoperative respiratory function after laparoscopy or open laparotomy for cholecystectomy. Anesthesiology 192; 77: 675-680.

24. Dobbs FF, Kumar V, Alexander JL, Hul MGR. Pain after laparoscopy related to posture and ring versus clip sterilisation. Br J Obstet Gynaecol 1987; 94: 262-266.

25. Cunnife G, Mcanena O, Dar M, et al. A prospective randomized trial of intraoperative bupivacaine irrigation for management of shoulder-tip pain following laparoscopy. Am J Surg 1998; 176: 258-261.

26. Schwenk W, Bohm B, Fugener A, Muller JM. Intermittent pneumatic sequential compression (ISC) of the lower extremities prevents venous stasis during laparoscopic cholesystectomy. A randomized study. Surg Endosc 1998; 12(1): 7-11.

27. Catheline JM, Gaillard JL, Rizk N, et al. Risk factors and prevention of thromboembolic risk in laparoscopy. Ann Chir 1998; 52: 890-5.

28. Vara-Thorbeck R, Guerrero JA. Le dextran et l'hémodilution dans la prévention de la thrombo-embolie postopératoire. Acta Chir Belg 1980; 79:249-255.

29. Vara-Thorbeck R, Rosell J, Mekinassi K, Prados N, Guerrero JA. Prévention de la maladie thrombo-embolique et des complications post-transfusionelle par l'hémodilution normovolémique en chirurgie arthroplastique de la hanche. Rev Chir Orthop. (Paris) 1990; 76: 267-271.

30. SAGES position statements. Global statement on deep venous thrombosis prophylaxis during laparoscopic surgery. Surg Endosc. 1999; 13: 2000.

31. Song F, Glenny A. Antimicrobial prophylaxis in colorectal surgery: a systemic review of randomized controlled trials. Br J Surg 1998; 85: 1232-41.

32. Vara-Thorbeck R, Ruiz M, Rosell J, Tovar JL, Moreno A, Guerrero JA, Morales OI. ¿Quimioprofilaxis en cirugía herniaria?. Cir Esp. 1993; 53: 105-107.

33. Targarona EM, Balagué C, Knook MM, Trías M. Laparoscopic surgery and surgery infection. Br J Surg 2000; 87: 536-544.

34. Schwetlin R, Barlehner E. Is there an indication for general perioperative antibiotic prophylaxxis in laparoscopic plastic hernia repair with implantation of alloplastic tissue?. Zentralbl Chir 1998; 123: 193-5.

CHAPTER 38

Intraoperative and Postoperative Complications of Laparoscopic Ventral Hernia Repair

S. Kini, M. Gagner

INTRODUCTION

Open repair of incisional hernia has been associated with an unacceptably high recurrence rate of up to 50% (1). The use of prosthetic materials has decreased recurrence rates by 10% (1) but not the high wound complication rate. The application of laparoscopic techniques to different fields led to the development of the laparoscopic hernia repair in 1992 (2). Since then laparoscopic ventral hernia technique has gained acceptance while laparoscopic inguinal hernia repair is still preferred by less than 10% of general surgeons. All the comparative studies have shown that the hospital stay is shorter with the laparoscopic technique. (3-8). Whereas operative times vary improvements in technique have shortened them considerably (9).

Various authors have defined complications differently making the interpretation and comparison of multiple studies difficult. It may account for the wide variance in the complication rates between studies. In one study comparison has been further confounded by the fact that patients undergoing open repair were older and with larger fascial defects (3).

Complications can be classified into peroperative complications, perioperative complications (seen in the immediate post operative period) and late complications. Peroperative complications can be further subdivided into those complications (such as trocar injuries) that are peculiar to the laparoscopic approach and those that are also seen in the open approach. Complications after laparoscopic ventral hernia repair have been summarized on (Table I).

Table I. Summary of Complications

Intraoperative complications
Peculiar to lap Surgery
Complications of trocar insertion
Common to hernia repair
Organ Injury
Early postoperative complication
Ileus
Peritonitis
Urinary retention
Hematoma
Seroma
Skin necrosis
Hematoma
DVT
Bleeding
UTI
pneumonia
Pain
Late complications
Bowel obstruction
Infection
Recurrence

Comparative studies

There have been five studies to date that have compared the laparoscopic approach with the open approach. These have been summarized in (Table II). Two of these studies were retrospective (3, 5) and two studies were prospective (7, 8) but the former one compared the open group retrospectively. The study by Carbajo et al is the only randomized styudy comparing the two approaches (6).

There has been only one multicenter study for laparoscopic ventral hernia repair. The initial cohort of 200 patients are being followed (10). They reported five infections, three cases of prolonged ileus, one bowel obstruction, 23 seromas (15 resolved without intervention), and six hernia recurrences. A recent analysis has shown a recurrence rate of 7.6%.

Table II. Comparative studies between Open and Laparoscopic hernia Repair

Author	Year of publication	Type of study	Lap	Open
De Maria EJ et al	2000	Prospective	21	18
Carbajo MA	1999	Randomized	30	30
Ramshaw BJ	1999	Retrospective	79	174
Park A	1998	Prospective laparoscopic compared with retrospective open	56	49
Holzman MD	1997	Retrospective	21	16

Peroperative complications

These have been summarized on (Table III). The most important amongst them is bowel Injury.

Table III. Peroperative complications

Author	Year	Number of patients	Enterotomy	Others
Szymanski J	2000	44	0	0
De Maria EJ	2000	21	0	0
Farrakha M	2000	13	0	0
Heniford BT	1999	407	5	0
Ramshaw BJ	1999	79	2	0
Toy FK	1998	144	2	2
Franklin ME	1998	112	0	0
Park A	1998	56	0	0
Costanza MJ	1998	31	0	0
Tsimoyiannis EC	1998	11	0	0
Holzman MD	1997	21	0	0
Total		**939**	**9 (1%)**	**2 (0.2%)**

Complications of trocar insertion

Careful insertion of trocars is especially important since there are a lot of adhesions in-patient with laparoscopic ventral hernia. Special care should be taken to avoid the inferior epigastric vessels when the lateral ports are placed.

We advocate the open approach to decrease the incidence of injuries associated with trocar insertion. Also, access to the peritoneal surface is gained through an area adjacent to the ventral hernia. Care must be exercise in making the initial skin incision as herniated abdominal contents often lie immediately beneath the skin surface.

Bowel injury

The incidence of bowel injury in all the series combined was found to be 1%. Bowel can be injured at two points of the operation: Firstly, while inserting the trocars (mentioned above) and secondly during adhesiolysis. Adhesiolysis is the most dangerous part of the ventral hernia repair. Any lysis of adhesions is performed with sharp dissection using extreme caution and under direct visualization. We try to avoid the use of any energy at all, but when it is absolutely necessary, we use the harmonic scalpel, for omental adhesions, to decrease the incidence of conducted current causing damage to the bowel. In the laparoscopic approach, the planes of dissection are easier to see on the magnified laparoscopic image because the omentum and viscera are suspended from a stretched abdominal wall.

Bowel injury is dealt with depending on the amount of spillage. Our approach is that if large bowel is entered then we avoid placing a mesh. However, if there is only a small bowel enterotomy with minimal spillage, the laparoscopic ventral hernia repair is completed in the usual fashion with the placement of a mesh. A similar approach was used in one series wherein five patients with known small-bowel enterotomies at the time of operation with minimal spillage. Four had repair of enterotomy and completion of the procedure. In the fifth, there was a conversion to open. None of the five had a recurrence or removal of the mesh (11). Enterotomy missed at initial operation is worse and may lead to peritonitis.

Early postoperative complication

Ventral hernia repair, by the very nature of the operation is associated with certain complications irrespective of the kind of the approach. The early postoperative complications can be divided into general and local complications. General complications with serious consequences include myocardial infarction, thromboembolism and stroke etc. Ones with lesser consequences include ileus, urinary retention and pneumonia. Postoperative pain is much less in the laparoscopic approach and thus respiratory complications are potentially reduced. These include DVT, Genitourinary, Pulmonary/Hypoxia, Cardiac, Stroke Local complications are seen more frequently in the open approach (Table IV).

Table IV. Early postoperative complications

	Laparoscopic n=187	Open n=287
Wound infection	1	2
Cellulitis	0	2
Hematoma	1	11
Seroma	17	37
Infection	4	15
Skin necrosis	0	1
Prolonged ileus	7	11
Bowel obstruction	3	1
Bowel fistula	0	1
DVT	0	3
Genitourinary	2	7
Pulmonary/Hypoxia	2	2
Cardiac	0	2
Stroke	0	1
Total	**39 (20.8%)**	**98 (34.1%)**

Infection

Laparoscopic hernia repair involves no long incision, no wide fascial dissection or flap creation no opening of the hernia sac and no drains. These reasons should theoretically led to a reduced incidence of infection and indeed in most studies this has been found to be so.

Perioperative antibiotics are given in an attempt to minimize infection. Some surgeons have speculated that the risk of mesh infection from cutaneous pathogens is lower in the laparoscopic group due to the distance between the actual incisions and the prosthesis. This has yet to be proven by clinical studies.

Trocar site induration is common and this typically resolves within 6 to 8 weeks. Removal of a mesh is infrequent and in all the series quoted in this chapter only in 3 cases was this required.

Ileus

There is a reduced need for opioid analgesics in laparoscopic hernia repairs when compared with open hernia repair (8). This could theoretically be one of the reasons in the lower incidence of ileus (Table IV).

Seroma

Small, self-limited collections of fluid developing after laparoscopic ventral hernia repair is a common occurrence. For example, in the multicenter study there were seromas in 16% of the patients but two-thirds did not require intervention (10). In fact there does not seem to be any long-term complications from any of the seromas, regardless of whether they are aspirated early or allowed to persist for a maximum of 10 weeks (11). These fluid collections should be expected and are differentiated from infected fluid collections or hernia recurrence by clinical presentation, laboratory data, and lack of ancillary features associated with true hernia such as presence of hernia sac, herniated mesentery, or bowel obstruction (12). Wide differences in incidence probably reflect the differences in definitions.

Late postoperative complications

See (Table V).

Bowel obstruction

There are three causes of bowel obstruction. Firstly, bowel herniation through gaps between the mesh and the abdominal wall can lead to bowel incarceration. This is a technical complication and can be avoided by applying adequate number of tacks between sutures to ensure that there are no gaps for bowel to herniate through. For large incisional hernias, often two staplers are required to fix the edges of the patch adequately (13). It should be remembered that the security of the fixation depends primarily on the sutures (10).

Secondly, adhesions can lead to bowel obstruction. PTFE can minimize adhesions between the mesh and bowel loops. The undersurface of a Dual-Mesh has a pore size of 3μm and thus does not allow any ingrowth of tissue. Unfortunately, like in open surgery, there is little that can be done to prevent adhesions developing between the bowel loops.

Lastly, as with all laparoscopic procedures involving any trocars more than 10mm in diameter, there is a chance of herniation at the trocar site. The incidence of trocar site herniation is low. It was 0.1% in all the series quoted in this chapter. This can be minimized further, by the use of a sturdy fascial closure device such as the one we use from Karl Storz (Tuttlingen, Germany).

Infection

Long-term infection is peculiar to prosthetic grafts. Cases have been reported of infection developing many years after prosthetic mesh implantation. Long term follow of patients who have had their ventral hernia repair laparoscopically will be able to demonstrate if there is a difference in this incidence with the laparoscopic approach.

Pain

Though patients experience less pain after laparoscopic ventral hernia repair than after open repair, there is considerable amount of pain especially on the evening of the operation with a need for narcotics. This is why we do not advocate laparoscopic ventral hernia repair to be done as an outpatient procedure.

Table V. Late complications - Recurrence

Author	Year	Number of patients	Follow-up In months	Recurrence
Szymanski J	2000	44	7	5%
De Maria EJ	2000	21	18	5%
Farrakha M	2000	13	22	7%
Heniford BT	1999	407	23	3.4%
Ramshaw BJ	1999	79	21	2.5%
Toy FK	1998	144	7	4%
Franklin ME	1998	112	34	0.8%
Park A	1998	56	24	10.7%
Costanza MJ	1998	31	18	3%
Tsimoyiannis EC	1998	11	15	0%
Holzman MD	1997	21	18	9.5%
Park A	1996	30	8	3%
Total		**969**	**215**	**0.5%**

Recurrence

In the different series the incidence vary from 0 to 10.7% (average 0.5%). Partly this could be due to a difference in the case mix with certain series having a greater incidence of recurrent hernias (11, 14). Also, the follow-up varied from 7 to 34 months. After adhesiolysis, the laparoscopic view of the ventral hernia is better is than the open view. Hence there is a lower chance of missing small "buttonhole" hernia.

Recurrence after open surgery is less likely if a large mesh is used, but the wide fascial dissection and required flap creation increase complication rates (1, 11). However in the laparoscopic approach, wide dissection is not required. Therefore, large pieces of mesh with 3 to 5 cm of overlap on all sides of the hernia should be used. The large surface area of the mesh allows for substantial growth of tissue for permanent mesh fixation, for anchoring sutures to be placed in solid, healthy musculofascial layers. Additionally, intra-abdominal pressure tends to hold the mesh in place apposed to the posterior fascia over the wider surface area (10). The ratio of mesh to defect size in the multicenter study is 2.5 (mesh size of 281 cm^2 : mean hernia defectr size of 113 cm^2).

Laparoscopic ventral hernia repair being a relatively recent procedure, the long-term recurrence rate is unknown. However since 66-90% of recurrences occur with 2 years after operation (15,16), a follow-up for 2 years will pick up most of the recurrences. The recurrence after laparoscopic hernia repair seems to be lower than the open approach.

One study looked at the site and possible cause of recurrence (7). They concluded that smaller hernias (<50 cm^2) were significantly less likely to recur than large hernias. They also found a trend towards an increased recurrence rate in patients who had undergone a previous repair.

Recurrent hernias

One series, though small, had over 50% recurrent hernias and a low complication rate (14). 10 of these patients had 2 or more hernia repairs. The average number of previous ventral hernia repairs for the series was 2.4 (range 1 to 7) and the average number of previous abdominal procedures was 4 (range 1-10) The average size of these hernias was 130 cm^2. This demonstrates that one can have a low complication rate even for recurrent hernia.

Choice of graft

Selection of the proper prosthetic material is very important. It is a difficult decision for many surgeons. Most desire tissue ingrowth yet wish to avoid adhesions between the mesh and intestines (10).

PTFE incites a low foreign body reaction and a lower rate of adhesion formation and is less easily infected than polypropylene (17). Expanded polytetrafluoroethylene Dual Mesh-Plus (Gore-Tex, WL Gore and Associates, Phoenix, AZ, USA). is probably becoming the most popular mesh material. The Dual mesh has two surfaces. One is very smooth (with micro pores <3 μm in diameter), resulting in minimal tissue attachment. This side is suitable to be placed against the viscera. The other surface has a pore size of 22 μm and this is placed against the abdominal where tissue incorporation is desired. A recent innovation has been the incorporation of silver and chlorhexidene into the e-PTFE in an attempt to further reduce the rate of infection.

Polypropylene mesh is used by some authors (3, 18). However, polypropylene cannot be used directly in contact with viscera as it provokes an intense inflammatory response and he viscera tend to get adherent tot the material. This can lead to bowel fistula and erosion into intraabdominal organs. Polypropylene is difficult to remove should that become necessary. Some authors have tried to interpose omentum between the mesh and the bowel but we do not advocate this.

The other materials that have been used are polyester and polyglactin (as part of a composite graft).

SUMMARY

Complications of laparoscopic ventral hernia repair appear to be lower than open hernia. Although the follow-up period for the laparoscopic repair is only 2 or 3 years the recurrence rate is likely lower than with open repair. However, long-term follow up is required to substantiate this claim. Also, more prospective randomized studies are needed to determine the complication rate and long-term outcome of this procedure.

Initially patient selection of patients who are relatively fit and have small incisional hernias may be helpful to establish confidence and ensure good surgical outcomes.

References

1. Santora TA, Roslyn JJ. Incisional hernia. Surg Clin North Am 1993; 73:557-570.

2. LeBlanc KA, Booth WV. Laparoscopic repair of incisional abdominal hernias using expanded polytetrafluoroethylene: preliminary findings. Surg Laparosc Endosc 1993; 3:39-41.

3. Holzman MD, Purut CM, Reintgen K, Eubanks S, Pappas TN. Laparoscopic ventral and incisional hernioplasty [see comments]. Surg Endosc 1997; 11:32-35.

4. Tsimoyiannis EC, Tassis A, Glantzounis G, Jabarin M, Siakas P, Tzourou H. Laparoscopic intraperitoneal onlay mesh repair of incisional hernia. Surg Laparosc Endosc 1998; 8:360-362.

5. Ramshaw BJ, Esartia P, Schwab J, Mason EM, Wilson RA, Duncan TD, Miller J, Lucas GW, Promes J. Comparison of laparoscopic and open ventral herniorrhaphy. Am Surg 1999; 65:827-831.

6. Carbajo MA, Martin del Olmo JC, Blanco JI, de la CC, Toledano M, Martin F, Vaquero C, Inglada L. Laparoscopic treatment vs open surgery in the solution of major incisional and abdominal wall hernias with mesh [see comments]. Surg Endosc 1999; 13:250-252.

7. Park A, Birch DW, Lovrics P. Laparoscopic and open incisional hernia repair: a comparison study. Surgery 1998; 124:816-821.

8. DeMaria EJ, Moss JM, Sugerman HJ. Laparoscopic intraperitoneal polytetrafluoroethylene (PTFE) prosthetic patch repair of ventral hernia. Prospective comparison to open prefascial polypropylene mesh repair. Surg Endosc 2000; 14:326-329.

9. Chowbey PK, Sharma A, Khullar R, Mann V, Baijal M, Vashistha A. Laparoscopic ventral hernia repair. J Laparoendosc Adv Surg Tech A 2000; 10:79-84.

10. Toy FK, Bailey RW, Carey S, Chappuis CW, Gagner M, Josephs LG, Mangiante EC, Park AE, Pomp A, Smoot RT, Jr., Uddo JF, Jr., Voeller GR. Prospective, multicenter study of laparoscopic ventral hernioplasty. Preliminary results. Surg Endosc 1998; 12:955-959.

11. Heniford BT, Park A, Ramshaw BJ, Voeller G. Laparoscopic ventral and incisional hernia repair in 407 patients. J Am Coll Surg 2000; 190:645-650.

12. Lin BH, Vargish T, Dachman AH. CT findings after laparoscopic repair of ventral hernia. AJR Am J Roentgenol 1999; 172:389-392.

13. Park A, Gagner M, Pomp A. Laparoscopic repair of large incisional hernias. Surg Laparosc Endosc 1996; 6:123-128.

14. Costanza MJ, Heniford BT, Arca MJ, Mayes JT, Gagner M. Laparoscopic repair of recurrent ventral hernias. Am Surg 1998; 64:1121-1125.

15. Hesselink VJ, Luijendijk RW, de Wilt JH, Heide R, Jeekel J. An evaluation of risk factors in incisional hernia recurrence. Surg Gynecol Obstet 1993; 176:228-234.

16. Van der Linden FT, van Vroonhoven TJ. Long-term results after surgical correction of incisional hernia. Neth J Surg 1988; 40:127-129.

17. Law NW. A comparison of polypropylene mesh, expanded polytetrafluoroethylene patch and polyglycolic acid mesh for the repair of experimental abdominal wall defects. Acta Chir Scand 1990; 156:759-762.

18. Szymanski J, Voitk A, Joffe J, Alvarez C, Rosenthal G. Technique and early results of outpatient laparoscopic mesh onlay repair of ventral hernias. Surg Endosc 2000; 14:582-584.

CHAPTER 39

Laparoscopic Incisional Hernioplasty in Day Case Surgery

A. Moreno-Egea, L. Carrasco Gonzalez, J.A. Castillo Bustos, J. Sanz Campillo, J.L. Aguayo Albasini.

INTRODUCTION

Day case surgery (DCS), also known as outpatient surgery, refers to moderately complex procedures performed on patients, with no associated diagnoses involving morbidity without conventional hospital admission. This concept differs from surgery involving short hospitalization or early discharge, i.e., procedures that handle processes requiring major surgery with hospital stays of 1 to 3 days. This chapter discusses the possibilities of including laparoscopic repair of ventral hernias in a DCS program. The creation of DCS units has made it possible to perform surgical procedures traditionally linked to a hospital stay of several days on an outpatient basis. This approach lowers costs and (without it being the main objective) effectively decrease waiting lists since the main reason for surgery delays is a lack of hospital beds (1). Based on its characteristics and frequency, surgical repair of abdominal wall defects is one of the procedures that can be done on an outpatient basis. Although DCS for hernia conditions has been implemented only in recent years, it has historic precedents that were an indication of its future popularity: In the 1940s Shouldice first recommended patient ambulation on the day after surgery. In the 1960s and 70s, Lichtenstein and Rutkow used tension-free techniques with prostheses and recommended normal activity as soon as 24 hours after the operation. This perspective was based on the fact that no relationship had been demonstrated between early activity and hernia recurrence, and that the risk of postoperative thromboembolic and respiratory complications was lower with this approach (2, 3). The use of DCS has become widespread due to the confidence of both patients and surgeons in the method, and to the need to decrease waiting lists and costs associated with each procedure by efficient use of available hospital beds. Over the past decade, many Spanish hospitals that witnessed the proven safety of the procedure for the treatment of inguinal hernias have adopted DCS programs. This led to the implementation of outpatient unit for the treatment of other procedures, such as the repair of midline hernias and incisional hernias (4, 5). The approach was initially limited to simple incisional hernia repair, but was later expanded to include incisional hernia repair with prosthetic mesh, with excellent results (5, 6). The results obtained using laparoscopic inguinal hernia repair on an outpatient basis have led to consideration of the technique for outpatient treatment of incisional hernias. Laparoscopic hernioplasty offers greater patient comfort as it decreases postoperative pain and accelerates the resumption of normal activities. Early return to work would offset the increased cost of the laparoscopic procedure (7, 8). We believe that laparoscopic incisional hernia repair with placement of an intra-abdominal mesh is feasible on an outpatient basis, since it is the large dissections of the ventral sac carried out in the conventional anterior approach and the required drains that limit this possibility.

PATIENT SELECTION CRITERIA FOR LAPAROSCOPIC INCISIONAL HERNIA REPAIR AS DCS

The selection of potential candidates is the most important clinical aspect related to obtaining peak performance from a DCS unit, since it decreases the rate of DCS failure. The criteria may vary as further advances are made in surgical technique (use of well tolerated prostheses, development of laparoscopic technique, etc.) and the anesthesia used (local anesthesia combined with sedation, generally of short duration, spinal analgesia, etc.). There are three sets of criteria or requirements that must be met by all patients with an abdominal wall hernia process who are candidates for DCS.

Patient-related requirements

Preoperative assessment of the patient's associated pathologies is essential, regardless of the surgical procedure the patient will undergo. The ideal candidate for DCS must not have any acute, unstable or insufficiently analyzed medical problems. In addition, the patient must understand the entire procedure he/she will undergo, accept that it be performed on an outpatient basis and be capable of observing all postoperative instructions. The general patient-related requirements are:

- Age under 65 years. Nevertheless, the biological age is more important than the chronological age and, therefore, this limit is not strictly applicable. After a correct analysis of each individual case with the anesthesiologist, patients aged 65-80 can be included.

- Associated diseases: According to the Classification of the American Society of Anesthesiologists (ASA), type I, II and III (compensated) patients can be accepted.

- Morbid obesity (BMI>35), diabetes mellitus, chronic alcoholism, heavy smoking, drug abuse, airway alterations that may complicate intubation, susceptibility to malignant hyperthermia and epilepsy are not absolute exclusion criteria but should be individually evaluated in each case.

- Mentally handicapped patients: Such patients are good candidates, provided they have family members who can act as guardians, since they generally do not tolerate being away from their normal environment well.

Environment-related requirements

- In general the place where the patient will reside for the first 48 hours after surgery should be less than 1 hour from a unit or care center that can assist them properly, if required.
    - A relative should be on hand to drive the patient home after discharge or to handle the admission paperwork in case of complications.
    - Place of residence: must have appropriate conditions in terms of accessibility and hygiene, as well as a telephone within easy reach.

Surgery-related requirements

In principle, all abdominal wall hernias and incisional hernias can be operated on an outpatient basis. After a detailed preanesthesia evaluation, it is assumed that these procedures will involve minimal associated physiological alterations and small blood losses and that there will be no intense postoperative pain or other hard-to-control complications. To achieve this, the following considerations are important:
    - If possible, procedures should be scheduled early in the morning and should not last longer than 90 minutes.
    - Single or multiple defects greater than 12-15 cm when taken as a whole should be avoided, as they would require a large prosthetic mesh (20x25 cm) and numerous tacks to secure it properly.
    - Patients with a significant risk of intra-abdominal adhesions should be excluded (9,10): i.e. those with prior surgery for peritonitis, pelvic surgery or complex infraumbilical surgery, oncological surgery, or surgery with associated radiotherapy. These patients may require greater dissection of the posterior abdominal wall, with increased risk of bleeding and visceral lesions. Patients may sometimes be considered for DCS after dynamic ultrasound imaging or computed tomography study of the abdominal wall.
    - Multi-recurrent or highly lateralized (broad subcostal, lumbar, iliac or atypical) incisional hernias tend to require mobilization of the colon for full visualization of the hernia margins. This involves the use of additional trocars for visceral retraction and a longer surgery time. In these cases at least 24-48 hours of hospitalization is recommended.

PREOPERATIVE ASSESSMENT OF THE LAPAROSCOPIC INCISIONAL HERNIA IN DCS

Once the surgeon has decided that the surgical procedure can be performed on an outpatient basis, he/she must assess whether or not the patient meets the remaining selection criteria. In our hospital the preoperative assessment is performed in both the anesthesia and surgery consulting rooms. This requires two patient visits to the hospital but permits more complete evaluation before the operation and decreases the DCS failure rate.

Surgical preoperative analysis

The analysis is performed on a personalized basis and obliges the surgeon to assume responsibility for assessing the patient's associated pathologies during the preoperative period. A physical examination is the first step involved in any preoperative study of abdominal wall defects (11) and should include the following:

1. Preoperative classification of the incisional hernia: We use Chevrel's SWR classification (12): location, size and previous recurrences of the defect. We also recommend also considering the estimated number of defects.

2. Cutaneous assessment of the abdominal wall: laparoscopic surgery does not include the extirpation of skin and, therefore, if the skin shows prior lesions such as infections, necrosis due to atrophy, extreme weakness in large defects or pathological scars, the patient must be informed and an appropriate open technique proposed.

3. Assessment of the hernia content: examination in various positions (at rest, when making an effort) can provide information on the hernia content, mobility and parietal attachment. When reduction after Valsalva's manoeuvre is painful, adhesions that could hinder complete parietal dissection are usually found at the margin.

4. Ultrasound and CT scan studies: are indicated in obese patients, inconclusive diagnoses, when there are associated pathologies (e.g., cholelithiasis), episodes of incarceration or prior pain, prior surgeries and recurrent incisional hernias. We recommend CT studies in all incisional hernias larger than 5 cm in order to calculate the volume of the defect, assess the cavity, determine the content (different in small intestine, colon or omentum) and evaluate attachment to the wall. In addition, it provides an overview of the entire wall, with important information for laparoscopic repair (muscle retraction, multiple defects, etc.). During the postoperative period, sonographic study is essential for monitoring seromas, hematomas and abscesses.

5. Obtain informed consent for the surgery.

Anesthetic preoperative analysis

The preanesthesia assessment, performed after the surgical assessment, considers the patient as a whole, evaluating his/her social surroundings, the type of surgery chosen and the type of anesthesia. Hence, the role of the anesthesiologist is decisive in the success or failure of the outpatient procedure. The objectives of this assessment are as follows:

1) Record the medical history, perform a complete physical examination and any additional examinations needed to assess the patient's physical condition and determine whether or not a stable functional level exists prior to surgery.

2) Record the clinical anesthesia history to evaluate prior surgical-anesthesia procedures, assess airways and estimate risk (ASA).

3) Plan the need for special perioperative care.

4) Assess the suitability of outpatient laparoscopic repair on a personalized basis.

5) Establish a good physician-patient relationship.

6) Inform the patient of the procedures that will be performed, the attendant risks of such procedures and the expected postoperative progress.

7) Provide appropriate preoperative instructions (fasting time, preoperative medication, etc.).

8) Fill out the clinical documentation and obtain informed consent for the anesthesia.

INDICATIONS, TECHNIQUE AND POSTOPERATIVE INSTRUCTIONS FOR LAPAROSCOPIC INCISIONAL HERNIA AS DCS

Outpatient surgery is feasible for many common surgical procedures that account waiting lists in our hospitals. Hernias can comprise 10-20% of all surgical activity.

Indications

Generally speaking, any patient over 30 with an abdominal wall hernia who understands and accepts the informed consent form can be included in the outpatient surgery program if there is no anesthesia contraindication.

a) Umbilical hernia: we recommend laparoscopic repair in obese patients (BMI<30 kg/m^2) when the hernia is larger than 3 cm, in all patients when it is larger than 5 cm and in all patients (regardless of hernia size) when it is associated with epigastric hernia, diastasis recti or other conditions suitable for laparoscopic surgery during the same procedure (normally cholelithiasis).

b) Epigastric hernia: same criteria as for umbilical hernia.

c) Multiple hernias: regardless of the size, are always treated in our unit by laparoscopy as a general disease.

d) Midline incisional hernias: in principle, all. Periumbilical and supraumbilical hernias are the most accessible for laparoscopic repair without hospitalization.

e) Incisional hernias at other sites: basically all, except those larger than 10 cm or at a highly laterodorsal site, or those in patients with skin lesions or significant skin weakness. In these cases the laparoscopic technique may be difficult or last longer than 60-90 minutes (see recommendations in surgery-related requirements on patient selection).

f) Large incisional hernias: two conditioning factors should be considered: size and the need for drains. Although not absolute contraindications, we recommend conventional surgery for incisional hernias larger than 15 cm. At present if we consider a drain to be useful, admission is still not necessary. We use a closed suction drain of moderate pressure that is easily controlled in outpatients.

g) Spigelian hernias: all; the small size of the margins make them highly suitable for outpatient surgery by the intra-abdominal or preperitoneal approaches (13).

Cases involving emergency surgery, neoplasms, acute infection or risk of sepsis, mental incompetence or failure to obtain informed consent are normally excluded. Based on our experience in introducing laparoscopic hernioplasty as outpatient surgery, we feel the indications can be modified according to the learning curve, known morbidity and re-evaluation of technique efficacy after about 30-50 cases (14, 15).

Anesthetic technique. Protocol

The patients are allowed liquid intake: water, juice or tea up to 4 hours before surgery, as it has been shown that this increases bowel motility and gastric emptying, making the patient calmer and more willing to cooperate without increasing the risk of regurgitation or aspiration. No solid intake is allowed 6-8 hours before the procedure. Premedication is prescribed on an individual basis. In selected patients (obesity, diabetes, reflux, etc.) we use prophylaxis for bronchoaspiration consisting in ranitidine 50 mg iv and metoclopramide 10 mg iv by intravenous infusion (100 ml of saline solution). When the patient arrives to the surgical room, we administer midazolam 0.5-1.5 mg. The laparoscopic technique is performed under general anesthesia and surgical aggression is limited mainly to the intraoperative period. Among the available general anesthesia techniques, we use total intravenous anesthesia (TIVA), since it provides better results, basing the anesthesia on its analgesic component: propofol and remifentanil are used for anesthesia induction and maintenance. Both drugs are administered in continuous infusion, with propofol given by TCI pump (Diprifusor) at a plasma concentration of 2-3Φ/ml for induction and remifentanil given by syringe pump at a rate of 0.5-1 Φ/kg/min. About 2.5 minutes from the start of infusion of both drugs, a dose of 0.15 mg/kg of cisatracurium or 0.6 mg/kg of rocuronium is administered to achieve adequate paralysis for orotracheal intubation. After intubation, we decrease the infusion rates of propofol (1.5-2.5 F/ml) and remifentanil (0.25-0.5 Φ/kg/min), depending on whether or not there are clinical signs of sympathetic activation associated with the surgical stimulation. A combination of propofol and remifentanil can cause hypotension and bradycardia during induction in some patients with decreased cardiovascular function; this can be prevented by preliminary atropinization and decreasing the rate of infusion to slightly prolong induction. Perfusions are discontinued upon skin closure. Prophylaxis with droperidol 0.625 mg and ondansetron 4 mg iv is always administered before the end of the operation for postoperative nausea and vomiting (16-18).

Surgical technique

The surgical procedure has already been discussed in sufficient details in earlier chapters, hence we limit our remarks to key aspects for outpatient surgery:

- All access points must be infiltrated with local anesthesia before placement of the trocars, as this delays and decreases pain.

- A preliminary study of the defects helps for correct placement of the trocars and prevents unnecessary incisions. The use of 5-mm trocars greatly reduces the risk of bleeding and postoperative hernia.

- Adapt the pneumoperitoneum to the needs of the working field. On occasions a pneumoperitoneum of 8-10 mmHg is convenient and prevents other factors related to postoperative pain such as distention or peritoneal reabsorption.

- Adhesiolysis and hemostasia: The use of an ultrasonic scalpel is recommended, as it enhances adhesiolysis with little trauma and helps to control bleeding. The omentum vessels bleed easily; they also retract and make this maneuver tedious if not performed meticulously.

- Prevent unnecessary maneuvers: on occasions, an intestinal or pelvic examination with traumatic laparoscopic instruments can leave areas of bare or injured peritoneum due to microtraumas that can trigger the formation of adhesions, enhance postoperative ileus and increase postoperative discomfort. The defect or sac must not be sutured or approximated.

- The size of the mesh must be overlap about 5 cm the margins of the defect. The overlap should never be less than 3 cm at any point of the defect. The mesh should be introduced with any type of marks at the cardinal points to facilitate positioning, placement and securing. This movement decreases the overall surgery time.

- Fix the mesh adequately: each type of mesh has specific physico-chemical properties that determine its intra-abdominal response. Sufficient suture material (tacks) must be used to secure the mesh during its integration while avoiding excessive stapling, in order to lessen the pain and quantity of intra-abdominal material.

- Controlling closure: removal of the trocars should be closely supervised to prevent inadvertent bleeding, and the pneumoperitoneum should be emptied as much as possible to prevent massive reabsorption of gas through the peritoneum, which can contribute to pain in the shoulders and back (19,20).

Postoperative recommendations

Analgesia

Pain is the most frequent complication following outpatient laparoscopic repair of an incisional hernia. At present, postoperative analgesia is a significant challenge for anesthesiologists and surgeons who participate in day case surgery, since ineffective analgesia will require patient admission or delay discharge, increasing the morbidity and cost of the procedure. Nociception is the neural response to a traumatic or damaging stimulus; its development triggers the cascade of biochemical events leading to pain. Postoperative pain is acute, being primarily linked to nociception. It is caused by the damaging stimulus produced by tissue lesion during surgery and is associated with neuroendocrine stress which is proportional to the intensity of the pain. Based on our understanding of the physiology of pain, greatest efficacy in outpatient treatment of postoperative pain is obtained by targeting all three phases of this process: preoperative, intraoperative and postoperative. (I) The patient's attitude toward surgery and pain should be assessed during the preoperative period. The first step consists of informing the patient of the characteristics of the anesthesia and surgical procedure which he/she will undergo, explaining why the procedure should be performed and administrating anxiolytics the night before the surgery when necessary (normally we use lorazepan 1 mg, because of its pharmacokinetic profile). (II) In the intraoperative period, the main objective is to use a highly effective anesthetic technique, as this influences neuroendocrine response to the surgery and to pain; in this case we use remifentanil 0.25-1 Φ/kg/min because of its pharmacokinetic characteristics and analgesic potency. Prophylactic analgesia *(preemptive-analgesia)* is the use of nerve blocks or the administration of analgesics prior to surgical tissue damage. Preemptive analgesia is used to interrupt the cascade of biochemical events leading to pain. By preventing central nervous system sensitization, the intensity of postoperative pain is decreased. The synergism and enhancement achieved by combining various drugs is the basis for our approach to pain management. Our protocol is as follows: local infiltration with bupivacaine 0.25% at port site; after anesthesia induction we administer pro-paracetamol (2g iv) and ketorolac (60mg iv) or propacetamol (2g iv) and metamizol (2g iv). (III) During the postoperative period, we combine paracetamol (1 g orally) or metamizole (50 mg orally in 2 capsules) every eight hours with a nonsteroidal anti-inflammatory drug (ibuprofen 600 mg/8 h orally) the first 48-72 hours. In patients on corticoids or with a history of gastroduodenal lesion, we administer H_2-blockers (21,22).

Other recommendations

24-hour bed rest; soft diet with plenty of fruits and vegetables to prevent constipation; home ambulation on day 2, with short walks and a check-up visit (nursing visit) on day 3 trocar incisions. The patient should wear a compressive tubular bandage for 2 months (until the wound has acquired 80% of its final resistance) to ease breathing and alleviate pain when coughing or walking. One week after surgery the patient has a follow-up visit in the nursing ward to check the wound and remove stitches. Exercise or lifting weights must be avoided for 10 days. Physical activity is usually not restricted if the patient so desires (the best restriction is the performance of a proper closure technique).

Postoperative control after hospital admission

The implementation of a day case surgery unit requires the design of proper channels for care once the patient has left the hospital unit, in order to allow early detection and treatment of problems and/or complications that could develop during the first few hours at home. A distinction can be made between two different situations: conventional care and emergency care. Both possibilities must be carefully explained to the patient before he/she is allowed to go home.

Conventional care

We recommend two phone calls after the patient has gone home, one the night of the surgery and another the next morning. The questions are asked by a nurse using a questionnaire drawn up for this purpose by the expert surgeon in laparoscopic incisional hernia repair. This contributes to the patient's comfortability and confidence, since potential problems related to the surgery are detected early: trocar bleeding, local hematomas and seromas, wound infection, vomiting and acute abdomen, etc. It also helps to resolve personal questions (e.g., how to handle the drain), increases the patient's satisfaction and well-being in regard to the technique used and helps to lower the readmission rate. The patient is checked at 48 h in the outpatient visiting room.

Emergency care

For situations or problems requiring rapid resolution, a specific phone-line is available so patients can contact the unit directly (in our case, an anesthesiologist is in charge). If actual contact with a surgeon is necessary, the patient is referred to the emergency room at the hospital. Life-threatening complications after laparoscopic repair of incisional hernias are unusual (intra-abdominal bleeding due to parietal or visceral lesion, postoperative ileus due to missed intestinal lesion, etc.). Nevertheless, our emergency room teams have attended training sessions to learn about the outpatient technique and its potential complications. The patient must be fully aware of these risks to prevent any delay in care in the case of doubt.

OUR PERSONAL EXPERIENCE

Forty patients have undergone laparoscopic repair of ventral hernia at our hospital. The technique has already been described and does not differ from the procedure outlined in other chapters (19, 20). The author uses a double-layer mesh consisting of three-dimensional multifiber polyester with a hexagonal structure, thickness of 1.5 mm and pore size above 700 Φm on one side and a hydrophilic, reabsorbable, nonstick collagen membrane on the other (Parietex composite[R], Sofradim, France). This clear film contains a blend of type I oxidated atelocollagen, polyethylene glycol and glycerol, and is intended to protect the viscera from direct contact with the mesh during the process of integration. The double-layer composition promotes full, early integration on the parietal side and prevents adhesion and visceral erosion on the intra-abdominal side. All patients are selected personally. The results are shown in Tables 1 and 2. Moderate obesity (72%) and prior surgery (85%) were frequent. All patients were completed by laparoscopy, with no conversion to open surgery. Intraoperative complications included three cases of bleeding (two due to trocar puncture and one due to lesion of the omentum during reduction of the hernia content), which were successfully controlled during surgery, and one intestinal injury in a case of reoperated incisional hernia that presented a loop closely adhered to the scar (simple suturing was performed). Five patients (12%) developed local granulomas due to organized hematoma. These were controlled by ultrasound examinations and disappeared in about 6 months. Our morbidity can be explained by (a) trocar placement, (b) reduction of hernia content (trocar or omentum bleeding can cause hemorrhage and adhesions that increase the incidence of postoperative ileus and early intestinal occlusion). Late morbidity can be explained by (c) persistence of the peritoneal sac and mesh properties that lead to the creation of a skin-mesh interface where only the sac is located. In the latter case, the persistence of omentum residues and blood in the interface sac can explain the formation of chronic granulomas that took more than 6 months to be reabsorbed.

Table I. General characteristics of the patients undergoing laparoscopic repair of ventral hernia. Classification by location (L), size (T) and previous recurrence (R). The data are expressed as an absolute value (percentage)

	Parietex (n=40)
Mean age (range)	56(36-76)
Sex (men/women)	16/24
Associated diseases:	
Obesity	29
Diabetes mellitus	3
Surgical history	34(85)
Hysterectomy	9
Umbilical hernia	13
Appendectomy	10
Nephrectomy	4
Caesarean section	5
Cholecystectomy	6
Nissen operation	3
Splenectomy	1
SWR classification	
I. Location	
a) Midline	
Supraumbilical	10
Juxta-umbilical	14
Infraumbilical	8
Xiphopubic	2
b) No midline	
Subcostal	0
Transverse	3
Iliac	2
Lumbar	1
II. Size (in cm)	
<5/5-10/10-15/>15	22/10/6/2
III. Recurrences	
R0/R1/R2/R3	32/5/2/1
Number: single/multiple	16/14

Table II. Clinical progress of patients. The data are expressed as absolute values (percentages)

	Parietex (n=40)
Intraoperative morbidity	
Hemorrhage due to trocar	2
Hemorrhage due to dissection	1
Intestinal perforation	1(2.5)
Postoperative morbidity	
Postoperative ileus	1
Intestinal occlusion	0
Hematoma	6(15)
Recurrent seroma	0
Persistent granuloma	5(12.5)
Conversion	0
DCS	28(70)
Recurrence	1(2.5)

Seventy per cent completed the protocol and were discharged without requiring hospitalization. We did not find any other problems (nausea, vomiting, diarrhea, abdominal distension, abdominal colic pain), rejections or infections of the prosthetic mesh, thereby confirming mesh reperitonization with no adhesion problems in the intra-abdominal cavity (19, 23). We did observe one recurrence at one year of follow-up (2.5%) attributable to a deficient technique: the size of the multiple defects was originally miscalculated and two mesh were needed to complete the repair. In our opinion, therefore, several mesh should not be used and the repair should always be performed with a single mesh of sufficient size to cover all existing defects. We believe that the composition and surface (rough, three-dimensional) of the mesh we use promotes complete, early integration in the abdominal wall (24, 25), preventing the need for significant anchoring. This can facilitate early ambulation and the efficient use of the technique as day case surgery. Hence, our experience confirms that the laparoscopic technique for incisional hernia repair can be performed on an outpatient basis with a high rate of success.

References

1. Giner M. Cirugía ambulatoria y de corta estancia. ¿Objetivos asistenciales o económicos? (ed). Cir Esp 1994; 55 (4): 249-50.
2. Lichtenstein IL. Immediate ambulation and return to work following herniorraphy. Industrial medicine and surgery. 1966; 35, 754.
3. Robbins AW, Rutkow IM. The mesh plug hernioplasty and groin hernia surgery. Surg Clin North Am. 1998; 6, 1007.
4. Carrasco L, Flores B, Aguayo JL y Moreno-Egea A. Aportación de la unidad de Cirugía Mayor Ambulatoria en el Servicio de Cirugía General de un hospital de segundo nivel. Cirugía Mayor Ambulatoria 1999; 4 (3):480-83.
5. Flores B, Carrasco L, Moreno-Egea A, Aguayo JL. Tratamiento de los defectos de la pared abdominal en régimen ambulatorio. Cirugía Mayor Ambulatoria 1999; 4 (3): 484-87.

6. Revuelta S. Procedimientos de Cirugía Mayor Ambulatoria en Cirugía General. Criterios de selección, técnicas quirúrgicas y cuidados postoperatorios. In Maestre JM (ed.): Guía para la planificación y desarrollo de un programa de Cirugía Mayor Ambulatoria. Ergón eds. 1997.

7. Payne JH, Grininger LM, Izawa MT et al. Laparoscopic or open inguinal herniorraphy? A prospective randomized trial. Arch Surg. 1994; 129, 979.

8. Heikinnen T, Haunkipura K, Lepala J et al. Total cost of laparoscopic and open Lichtenstein repair. A randomized prospective study. Surg Laparosc Endosc 1997; 7, 1.

9. Moreno Egea A, Aguayo JL, Zambudio G, Parrilla P. Adhesion response to different forms of treating a peritoneal lesion: an experimental study in rats. Dig Surg 1995; 12: 334-337.

10. Moreno Egea A, Aguayo JL, Zambudio G, Ramirez P, Canteras M, Parrilla P. Influence of abdominal incision on the formation of postoperative peritoneal adhesions: an experimental study in rats. Eur J Surg 1996; 162: 181-185.

11. Moreno-Egea A, Girela E, Canteras M, Martinez D, Aguayo JL. Accuracy of clinical diagnosis of inguinal and femoral hernia and its usefulness for indicating laparoscopic surgery. Hernia 2000; 4: 23-28.

12. Chevrel JP, Rath AM. Classification of incisional hernias of the abdominal wall. Hernia 2000; 4: 7-11.

13. Moreno-Egea A, Torralba JA, Aguayo JL. Totally extraperitoneal laparoscopic repair of Spigelian Hernia. Eur J of CoelioSurg 1999, 32: 83-85.

14. Moreno-Egea A, Aguayo JL, Vicente J, Cartagena J, Sanz J. General vs regional anaesthesia in outpatient treatment for inguinal hernia using extraperitoneal laparoscopy. Hernia 2000, 4(3): 135-139.

15. Moreno-Egea A, Canteras M, Aguayo JL Intraoperative and postoperative complications of totally extraperitoneal laparoscopy inguinal hernioplasty. Surgical Laparoscopy Endoscopy and Percutaneous Techniques 2000 (1): 30-33.

16. Song D, Whitten W, White PF. Remifentanil infusion facilitates early recovery for obese outpatients undergoing laparoscopic cholecystectomy. Anesth Analg 2000; 90: 1111-1113.

17. Thwaites AJ, Smith I. Novel anaesthetics and techniques for ambulatory (day case) surgery. Curr Op Anesth 1997; 10: 421-429.

18. Larsen B, Seitz A, Larsen R. Recovery of cognitive function after remifentanil-propofol anesthesia: a comparison with desflurane and sevoflurane anesthesia. Anesth Analg 2000; 90: 168-174.

19. Moreno-Egea A, Lirón R, Girela E and Aguayo JL. Laparoscopic repair of ventral and incisional hernias using a new composite mesh (Parietex[R]): initial experience. Surgical Laparosc Endosc 2001 (in press).

20. Moreno-Egea A, Lirón R, Girela E, Aguayo JL. Laparoscopic repair in multirecurrent incisional hernia. World J of Video-Surg 2000; 4: 22-25.

21. Bayer TL, Coverdale JH, Chiang E, Bangs M. The role of prior pain experience and expectancy in psychologically and physically induced pain. Pain 1998; 74: 327-331.

22. Albrech S, Fechner J, Geisslinger G. Postoperative pain control following remifentanil based anaesthesia for mayor abdominal surgery. Anaesthesia 2000; 55: 315-322.

23. Benchetrit S, Debaert M, Detruit B, Dufilho A, Gaujoux D, Lagrutte J, Lepere M, Martin L, Pavis X, Rico E, Sorrentino J, Therin M (1998). Laparoscopic and open abdominal wall reconstruction using Parietex[R] meshes: clinical results in 2700 hernias. Hernia 2: 57-62

24. Bellón JM, García A, Jurado F, Carrera A y Bujan J. Reparación de defectos de pared abdominal con prótesis composite. Estudio del comportamiento peritoneal. Cir Esp 2000; 67: 432-437.

25. Bellón JM, Contreras L, Pascual G y Bujan J. Neoperitoneal formation after implantation of various biomaterials for the repair of abdominal wall defects in rabbits. Eur J Surg 1999; 165: 145-150.

CHAPTER 40

Management of the Hernia Sac after Laparoscopic Ventral Hernia Repair: is there a place for plastic surgery reconstruction?

A. Iuppa, A. Cuzzocrea

The rapid diffusion of laparoscopic surgery in all ambits of general surgery has also involved, during the past few years, the surgical treatment of the abdominal wall, and particular, the repair of post-operative ventral hernias, which just until a short time ago; seemed to be an exclusive pertinence of open surgery.

This approach, minding the right precautions and indications, is undoubtedly promising for the surgical resolution of laparocele (1, 2, 3, 4). Nevertheless, it has aroused another problem of aesthetic nature: what is to be done of the hernia sac and how can the problem related to an eventual excess of skin and abdominal fat be resolved?

The residual hernia sac, in the case of a laparoscopic treatment of laparocele, is an undesired result, closely related to the treatment mentioned above, and it can be particularly complex to solve this problem.

The advantages of this type of laparoscopic treatment remain confirmed in comparison with the traditional open treatment, firstly because of the minor incidence of infections of the prosthesis (4, 2), and secondly the briefer hospitalisation and the fewer post-operative sequels (1). It is also evident that the consecutive external surgical aggression of the abdominal wall, with its more or less invasive surgical methods, is safe and reliable once the hernia defect is repaired and stable.

In open surgery, in fact, the majority of surgeons are orientated towards a one time operative resolution of the patients' needs. It is on the other hand possible, when and where necessary, to treat in a "sole solution" the parietal defect, the hernia sac and also the abundant fat and skin excess with a lipectomy (16, 10).

Not all surgeons, however, agree to this one time solution treatment (7, 8, 9) as it is subject to major morbidity due to a wide cutaneous dissection with a higher risk of subcutaneous seromas and haematomas that could cause prosthetic infections (6, 9).

The laparoscopic surgery of ventral hernias is not usually associated, on the basis of its own characteristics, with any treatment of aesthetic nature of the hernia sac or excess of subcutaneous skin and fat, and it tends to exclusively repair the parietal defect by the intraperitoneal positioning of a biomaterial. For this reason, one of the most common problems we must face with this particular kind of surgery is the persistency of the hernia sac, which can be only partially removed during surgery.

As a matter of fact, even though there are several similarities with the problem related to secondary seromas in the laparoscopic surgery of inguinal hernias, especially of large direct hernias, the intraoperative treatment of the sac in laparocele shows different technical aspects and characteristics.

In laparocele, for instance, the hernia sac usually consists in a sole involucrum (the peritoneal sac) that at direct contact with the subcutaneous tissue to which it is extremely adherent, makes its detachment complicated and traumatic.

This procedure turns out to be much more simple in the laparoscopic repair of inguinal hernias. This is because right between the peritoneal sac, and subcutaneous tissue is collocated the false sac moulded by the expansion of the transversalis fascia, which is also connected in a more loose manner to the subcutis, in this way enabling an easier traction and fixing it in the abdomen to reduce its volume.

Only in a few cases it is possible, in a simple way, to reduce the volume of the hernia sac of the laparocele, otherwise this occurs with a most traumatic dissection that, by itself, is a cause of seromas.

Even the drainage of the sac with a closed system on the outside, as proposed by some authors (10, 11), leaves us concerned as the drainage itself would expose the prosthesis to external contamination, overlooking one of the main goals of the laparoscopic treatment, and that is to minimize post-operative infections.

Table I. Characteristics of abdominal wall components (1)

SKIN		FAT	MUSCULOFASCIAL
Elasticity		*Extra-abdominal*	*Laxity*
Good*		Minimal*	Mild*
Poor		Moderate	Moderate*
		Severe	Severe
Excess	*No excess*		
Minimal*		*Intra-abdominal*	*Diastasis*
Moderate*		(usually male)	None
Severe			Moderate
Severe			
Striae	*No Striae**		*Hernia*
Minimal*			*Midline*
Moderate*			Epigastric
Severe			Umbilical
			Non Midline
Pattern of Striae			Spigelian
Low*			Inguinal
High*			Other

*Candidate for endoscopic abdominoplasty

In order to standardise the post-operative treatment of patients affected by laparocele that have already undergone laparoscopic operations, we have individualised eight morphological types (Tab. 1-2), each of which requires its own therapeutic iter, keeping in mind the necessities of the patient.

We can standardise two large groups of patients on the basis of the presence of a large or a small residual sac.

In fact, it is the combination of these elements and the conditions of upper tissues that necessitates a secondary reconstructive or aesthetic treatment of the open or endoscopic type.

Generally, in the case of a small hernia sac (Tab. 1), it is the gravity of skin laxity that determines the invasiveness of the treatment, as the excess of skin has to be corrected with extensive panniculectomy.

The diastasis of rectus muscles, which is analysed in detail later, usually requires a minimal invasive treatment (12, 13). Due to cases such as these, the surgeon becomes more familiar with the endoscopical techniques. It is also interesting to note that over the last five years, in particular, endoscopic abdominoplasty techniques in the ambit of reconstructive plastic surgery have become more common.

Table II. Patients with small sac. Selection of candidates for plastic surgery after laparoscopic repair of ventral hernias

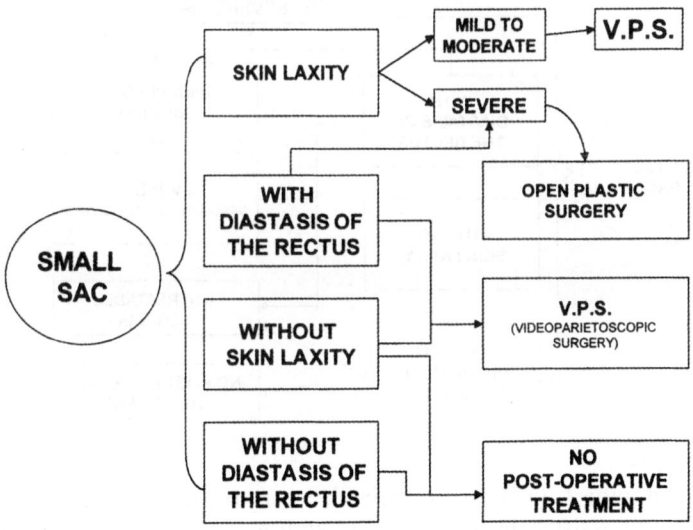

Should the patient have a large hernia sac (Tab. 2), the problem becomes more complex. The sac could be the cause of an open treatment of reduction, especially when we encounter a relapsing fluid collection that could indicate a particular sequela of aesthetic nature or could mimic a recurrent bowel herniation or even an infected post-operative seroma.

In such cases, a CT scan can be useful in order to define the diagnosis and an eventual operation (14) can be planned. The first endoscopic observation of the subcutis tissue was described by Teimourian and Kroll in 1984.

Faria Correra (15) gave the first description of endoscopic abdominoplasty after using a y-shaped longitudinal incision at the umbilicus and another suprapubic transversal incision.

Particular attention is paid in the selection of the patients: postgestional abdominal wall deformity characterized by diastasis recti, lipodystrophies, and widening or protrusion of the umbilicus.

The endoscopic adominoplasty approach, of which the correct indication is tightly correlated with the characteristics of trophicity of the different components of the abdominal wall (Tab. 3), may be extended to patients with abdominal hernias.

As experience with hernias using endoscopy in the subcutaneous space is limited at this time, it is recommended limiting endoscopic hernia repair to small hernias (<6cm in diameter), which are non recurring, midline, and easily reducible (16).

Table III. Patients with a large sac. Selection of candidates for plastic surgery after laparoscopic repair of ventral hernias

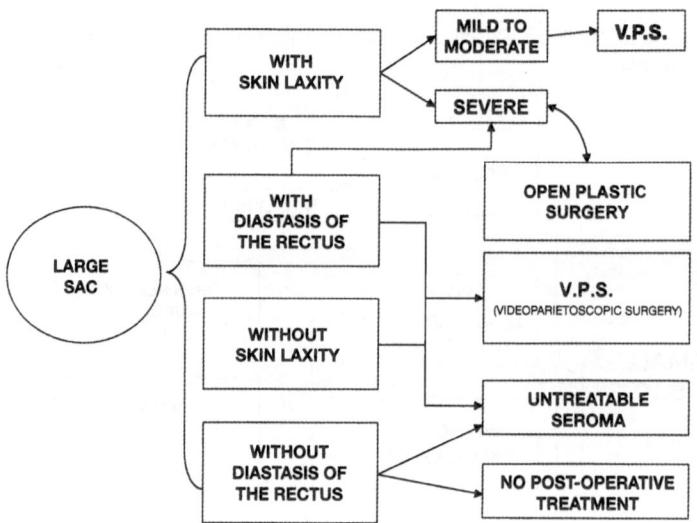

Jackson and others (17) remit their data on rectus abdomimis plication endoscopically assisted in male patients with a gravity of laxity of the mid-abdominal region that ranges from mild to moderate. The surgical manoeuvre consisted in a sole incision at the umbilical site, a dissection on the front side of the anterior fascia of the rectum without insufflation and suture plication under endoscopic guidance. The post-operative results were comparable to those obtained by standard rectus abdominis plication.

Furthermore, in order to increase the potentiality of the technique, an endoscopic abdominal liposuction and, eventually, a minimal suprapubic cutaneous resection may be associated to the procedure (18, 19). More recently, in a review regarding 85 cases, Zukowsky and other colleagues (20) propound an endoscopic intracorporal abdominoplasty. The technique combines traditional abdominal wall liposuction with endoscopic intraperitoneal plication of the rectus fascia by using a series of horizontal mattress sutures. The advantages that have been verified in this procedure include a briefer duration of the surgical treatment, brief hospitalisation (one post-operative day in comparison with an average of three days with the open techniques) and a post-operative morbidity of 15% compared to 24% in the traditional techniques (1, 2, 21). It is however important to keep in mind that the intracorporal approach should be reserved to those rare cases in which the laparocele has been treated without the use of patches as the intraperitoneal plication performed could cause a curling of the prothesis applied as a tissue substitute. Moreover, this approach implies the conversion of an extraperitoneal procedure to an intraperitoneal one.

In general, the presence of umbilical, epigastric or incisional hernias is not a contraindication to the endoscopic approach, unless they are large, complex or associated with extensive scarring that could be improved with an open technique (16, 22).

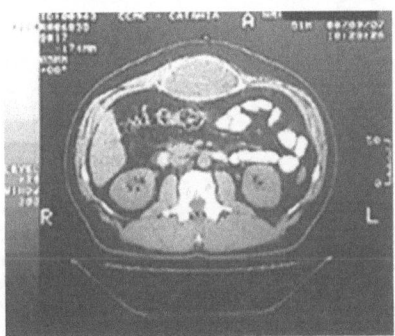

Fig. 1. Position of patient, equipment and operating room team for V.P.S., right-handed surgeon (from Grady B. Core mod.).

An efficient aid for the mini-invasive treatment of the residual sac and the unaesthetisms that have not been resolved during the laparoscopic laparocele is represented by videoparietoscopic surgery (V.P.S.).

This is a new video-surgical approach which creates, in front of the musculo-aponevrotic area, a large space allowing repair of small abdominal wound defects or residual sac, with excellent plastic results.

An important technical aspect of the abdominoplasty via V.P.S. involves the pneumatic dissection of the subcutaneous tissues. After an initial dissociation of the cellular tissue, progressive insufflation with CO_2 produces extensive detachment of the cutaneous plane upward and laterally (23). Using 1mm or 2mm trocars, the aponeurotic plane is progressively freed and the pathological zone is identified and repaired with percutaneous sutures using a Revedin Needle, or according to the preferences of the surgeon, an endoscopic needle-holder.

It is such a methodology that, in the appropriate cases (see table), proves to be useful in the treatment of the residual hernia sac. After the isolation of the sac from the subcutaneous tissue with the aid of CO_2, the sac may be sectioned or plicated by using standard endoscopic sutures and in the meantime avoiding the prothesis, that has been previously applied at a deeper level laparoscopically. During our experience it was necessary to treat the hernia sac using the videoparietoscopic procedure only once, due to an untreatable seroma (Fig. 4) six months after the surgical repair of laparocele. In two cases we performed an endosopic plication in young women due to the diastasis of the rectum 10 and 12 months after the laparoscopic treatment.

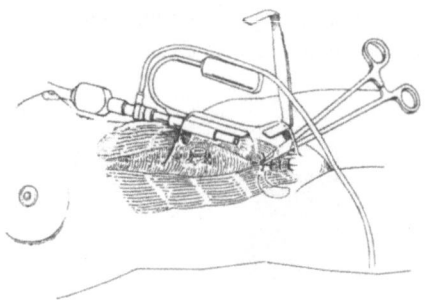

Fig. 2. Beginning plication under direct vision. Endoscope is used as a retractor and as a light source (Core).

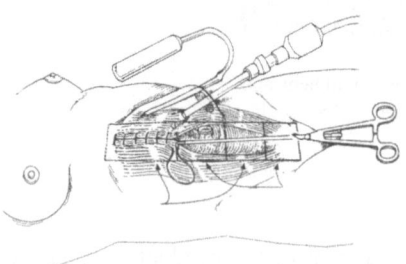

Fig. 3. Plication begins at the xiphoid and carried out under endoscopic control (Core).

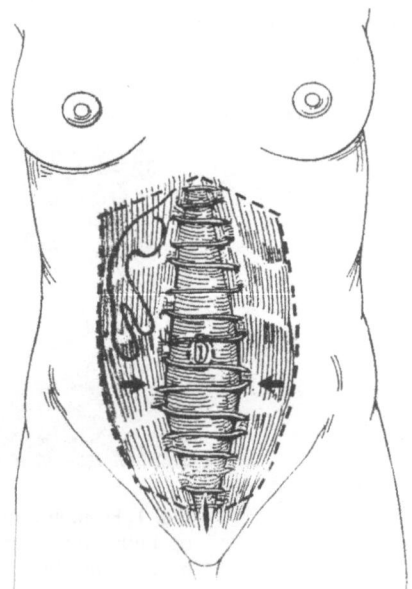

Fig. 4. Tapering plication: if started at the xiphoid process a looped, double-stranded suture should be used to avoid necessity for a knot that can be palpable on this area. At the umbilicus and pubis, knots generally can be inverted to avoid palpation.

However, it must be remembered that the risk of embolization related to the use of CO_2 pressurized in the subcutaneous tissues requires caution in the application of this methodology (15). As described by Core and Ferraro (16, 18), we can access the musculo-aponevrotic area without CO_2 insufflation. This has engendered the new elaboration of the optical instrument, the retractor and the needle-holder alike (24).

Initial undermining is at the interface between the rectus fascia and the subcutaneous tissue and is carried out under direct vision using a headlight for illumination and small retractors to aid with the visualization. This is performed as far as possible with direct vision through each of the two incisions: umbilical and suprapubic.

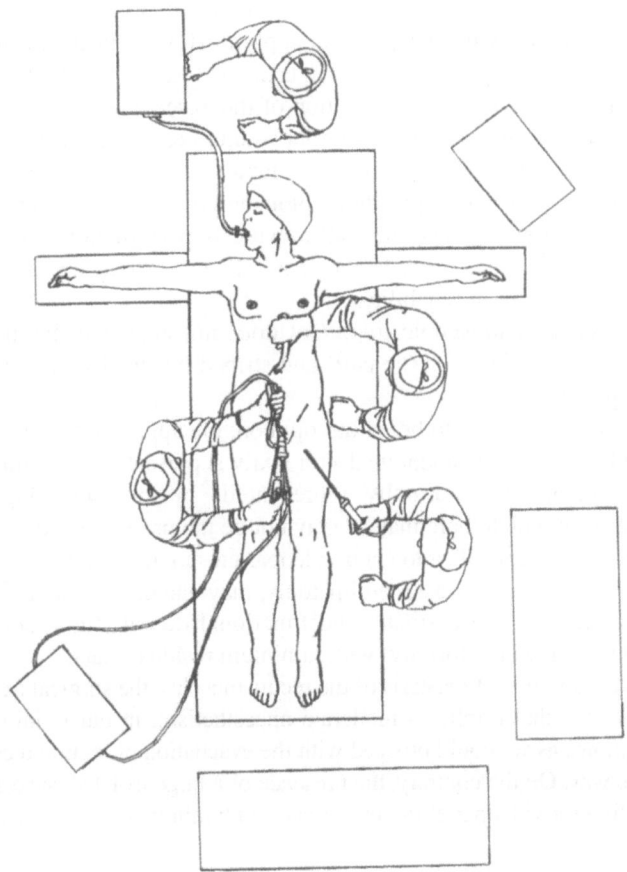

Fig. 5. CT Scan: Fluid collection with mimic recurrent bowel herniation or infected post-operative seromas.

The dissection technique and, above all, the creation of an optical cavity in the context of the subcutaneous tissue can be facilitated by a balloon dissector, that has, among others, the merit of preserving the perforating vessels (18, 25). Proper placement of the balloon is critical or the dissection plane will not be made and endoscopic completion of the procedure may be jeopardized (Fig. 5). After creation of the optical cavity in such a fashion, the laparolift, or a retractor, is introduced to maintain the optical cavity, and division and ligation of vascular perforators are performed under direct vision. Midline attachments at the linea alba and in the area of previous scars require manual dissection.

The videoparietoscopic surgery in the subcutaneous tissue, especially if not aided by gas, is very different compared to endoabdominal laparoscopy and thus must be carried out by a well-trained team (12).

The plastic-reconstructive treatment constitutes thus, in our opinion, an important moment in the general therapeutic approach; the surgeon must pay attention to a few fundamental aspects during planification. To simplify, we consider it useful to divide the patients applying for a plastic reconstructive treatment into two groups: patients with skin laxity and patients without skin laxity.

In the first case, the one time resolution of the exceeding fat, the diastasis of the rectum and the hernia sac (apart from its volume) can be effected, at least six months after the surgical reduction of laparocele and the endoscopical fortification of the wall with a prosthetic biomaterial, through a traditional open procedure. The reinforcement of the wall previously performed internally allows us to attack the hernia sac, already lacking any relation with the abdominal cavity, with a reasonable margin of reliability.

Furthermore, the endoscopic treatment does not appear to be appropriate when in the presence of non-elastic cutis and striped by streaks and scars caused by previous operations.

More complicated seems to be, in our opinion, the approach for those patients in whom a mild to moderate abdominal skin laxity is present, along with an adipic subcutaneous panniculus normally represented. In this subgroup we can distinguish cases in which there may or may not be the presence of diastasis recti. If diastasis exists, a rectus plication and videoparietoscopic resection of the hernia sac, associated with a suction assisted lipetomy, may enable the resolution, during the same treatment, of the aesthetic and functional deficit (for example, post-gestional abdominal wall deformity) with minimum residual scars.

Lastly, in the absence of diastasis of the rectus muscles, the surgical treatment of a small hernia sac, that implies a moderate unaesthetism, in our opinion induces limited indications, as we could proceed with the evacuation of its liquid contents in a conservative way. On the contrary, the presence of a large isolated sac can develop a valid indication for videoparietoscopic surgery with minimal residual scars.

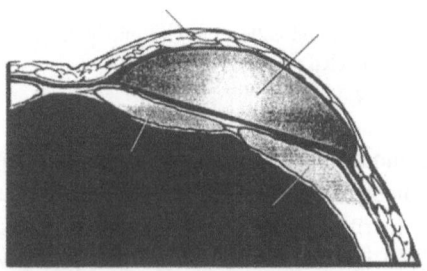

Fig. 6. Coronal section of the optical cavity created by the balloon dissector. Placement of the dissector precisely on the fascia is critical (from Ferraro F. – mod.).

In conclusion, we could assert that the approach towards the hernia sac after laparoscopic ventral hernia repair should be placed within a more ample context of aesthetic and functional defects of the abdominal wall. In this sense, after an accurate selection of the patients on the basis of the following parameters: the extent of cutaneous laxity and, rectus laxity, the quality of the skin, the presence of scars and striae, and the thickness of the adipose layer, the plastic reconstructive treatment finds a precise collocation and, although the techniques for endoscopic abdominoplasty continue to be refined, minimally invasive techniques seem to be safe and efficacious in these well selected patients.

References

1. Carbajo MA, Martin del Olmo JC, Blanco JI, de la Cuesta C, Toledano M, Martin F, Vaquero C, Inglada L. Laparoscopic treatment vs open surgery in the solution of major incisional and abdominal wall hernias with mesh. Surg Endosc 1999 Mar; 13(3): 250-2.

2. Heniford BT, Park A, Ramshaw BJ, Voeller G. Laparoscopic ventral and incisional hernia repair in 407 patients. J Am Coll Surg 2000 Jun; 190 (6): 645-50.

3. Le Blanc KA, and Booth WV. Laparoscopic repair of incisional abdominal hernias using expanded polytetrafluoroethylene: preliminary findings. Surg Laparosc Endosc 1993: 3: 39-41.

4. Toy FK, Bailey RW, Carey S, Chappius CW, Gagner M, Josephs LG, Mangiante EC, Park AE, Pomp A, Smoot RT Jr, Uddo JF Jr, Voeller GR. Prospective, multicenter study of laparoscopic ventral hernioplasty. Preliminary resutls. Surg Endosc 1998 Jul; 12(7): 955-9.

5. Chevrel JP, Flament JB. Rapport présenté au 92e Congrès Français de Chirurgie. Masson, 1990, Paris, Milan, Barcelone, Mexico, 149.

6. Lichtenstein IL. The repair of massive multiple incisional hernias by an intraperitoneal binder technique. Contemp Surg 1982; 20: 29-34.

7. Gareth J. Morris-Stiff, MB, BCh FRCS, and Leslie E. Hughes, DS, FRACS, FRCS. The Outcomes of Nonabsorbable Mesh Placed Within the Abdominal Cavity: Literature Review and Clinical Experience. J. Am. Coll. Surg, Vol. 186, No. 3, March 1998.

8. Louis D, Stoppa R, Henry X, Verhaeghe P. Les éventrations postopératoires. J. Chir (Paris), 122, 523, 1985.

9. Stoppa R. Le risque infectieux dans les réparations prothétiques de la paroi abdominale, p. 134-146.

10. Dufilho A. Les complications des prothèses en tulle de dacron à propos de 414 observations. Thèse Med Paris/Pi, 1981.

11. Francioni G. Surgical complications linked with synthetic prostheses for hernia repair. Communication personelle, 1992.

12. American Society of Plastic and Reconstructive Sugeons: "ASPRS Endoscopic Resource Guide: Arlington Heigts, II 1994, p. 2.

13. Lockwood T. Rectus muscle diastasis in males: primary indication for endoscopically assisted abdominoplasty. Plast Reconstr Surg 1998 May; 101 (6): 1685-3.

14. Lin BH, Vargish T, Dachman AH "CT Findings after Laparoscopic Repair of Ventral Hernia". AJR 1999 Feb., 172 (2): 389-92.

15. Faria-Correa MA. Endoscopic abdominoplasty, mastopexy, and breast reduction. Clin Plast Surg. 1995 Oct; 22(4): 723-45.

16. Core GB, Mizgala CL, Bowen JC, Vasconez LO. Endoscopic abdominoplasty with repair of diastasis recti and abdominal hernia. Clin Plast Surg. 1995 Oct; 22 (4): 707-22.

17. Jackson TL, Jacsor RF, Freeman L. Minimally invasive abdominoplasty: surgical technique development and discussion of three cases. Surg Laparosc Endosc. 1995 Aug; 5 (4): 301-5.

18. Ferraro FJ, Zavitsanos GP, Van Buskirk ER, Rehenke RD et al. Improving the efficiency, ease, and efficacy of endoscopic endoplasty. Plast Reconstr Surg 1997 Mar; 99(3): 895-8.

19. Teimurian B, Kroll SS. Subcutaneous endoscopy in suction lipectomy. Plast Reconstr Surg 1984; 74: 708-11.

20. Zukowsky ML, Ash K, Spencer D, Malanosky M, Moore G. Endoscopic intracorporal abdominoplasty: a review of 85 cases. Plast Reconstr Surg. 1998 Aug; 102 (2): 516-27.

21. Park A, Birch DW, Lovrics P. Laparoscopic and open incisional hernia repair: a comparison study. Surgery 1998 Oct; 124 (4): 816-21; discussion 821-2.

22. Eaves FF 3rd, Nahai F, Bostwick J 3rd. Endoscopic abdominoplasty and endoscopically assisted miniabdominoplasty. Clin Plast Surg. 1996 Oct; 23(4): 599–616.

23. Champult G, Catheline JM, Barrat C. Video-parietoscopic surgery of the abdominal wall. A study of 15 cases. Chirurgie 1998 Nov; 123 (5): 474 – 7.

24. Felmont F. Eaves III, M.D., Foad Nahai, M.D. and John Bostwick III, M.D. "Endoscopic Abdominoplasty and Endoscopically Assisted Mini abdominoplasty". Clin. in Plastic Surgery, Vol. 23 – n° 4, P. 599-616.

25. O'Brien JJ, Glasgow A, Lydon P. Endoscopic balloon-assisted abdominoplasty. Plast Reconstr Surg. 1997 Apr; 99 (5): 1462-3.

CHAPTER 41

Causes and Mechanisms of Recurrence after Laparoscopic Ventral Hernia Repair

B. Bokobza

Treatment of ventral and incisional hernias continues to pose problems in surgical management to repair abdominal wall defects. Many techniques, of greater or lesser complexity, have been proposed by laparotomy (1, 2, 3), each of which has its own proponents, but none of which has received widespread acceptance, due to the high rate of complications and recurrences. Since the first report on the laparoscopic repair of incisional hernias was published in 1992 (4), it has gradually become clear to surgeons, convinced of the usefulness of laparoscopic "tension-free" repair of inguinal hernias, that such procedures could be extended to include repair of abdominal hernias. In this regard, minimum invasive surgery seems to be of obvious interest, insofar as the remaining abdominal wall tissue is left intact as much as possible. The procedure consists in reinforcing the damaged abdominal wall with a resistant intraperitoneal prosthesis, after laparoscopic lysis of adhesions, and which induces a minimum of adhesions. Improvements in prosthetic materials, surgical dissection instruments, and systems for securing the prosthesis, have made this type of surgery relatively standardized (5).

However, laparoscopic repair of abdominal hernias depends greatly on surgical technique, and the quality of results obtained depends on many factors which have been demonstrated over the last few years by the proponents of this technique.

Thus, a study of the causes and mechanisms involved is a basic requirement for the surgeon, who wants to use a surgical technique for which the technical causes of recurrence have been eliminated, and is subject only to the random hazards of surgery.

We will begin with a review of the literature on the surgical repair of such hernias by laparotomy, followed by laparoscopic techniques, showing the evolution of techniques, their results, and the solutions proposed. Then, we will present our own personal series of cases, comparing them to a recent series of cases published, the study of which results enabled us to define the causes and consequences of recurrences after laparoscopic repair of abdominal hernias. We will conclude by presenting our own surgical technique.

SERIES OF CASES TREATED WITH LAPAROTOMY

Usefulness of reinforcement with a prosthetic patch

Two series of cases published in 1985 (6) and 1986 (7), reported the results of repairs by suturing abdominal defects, with recurrence rates of 31 to 46%, the lowest being 44% in cases involving a second repair. Hesselink (8) reported a recurrence rate of 41%, but which depends on the size of the incisional abdominal hernia, with a rate of 25% if the hernial orifice is less than 4 centimetres, and 41% if greater than 4 centimetres.

These poor results obtained with repair by suturing, even after suturing the abdominal aponeuroses using the overlapping technique (9), have led surgeons to use a prosthetic patch to reinforce the abdominal wall, often to replace a damaged abdominal wall in subjects who are often obese (10, 11), and by decreasing tension on the abdominal wall, the cause of postoperative pain and recurrence (12).

Indeed, the recurrence rate appears to decrease considerably by using a prosthetic patch for reinforcement (13). A study in Switzerland in 1995 (14) has confirmed this progression, demonstrating a recurrence rate after simple suturing ranging from 23.2% to 50%, in cases of recurrence. In comparison, use of a non-resorbable prosthetic patch is associated with a recurrence rate of 12.5 to 14.3%. A recent retrospective study (10) reported similar figures, with a recurrence rate of 54% in the case of simple suturing, versus 29% if a prosthetic patch is used.

Which position should the prosthetic patch be placed in?

Intraperitoneal placement of the prosthesis decreases abdominal wall dissection, the cause of bleeding, hematomas, and postoperative infection (15). Other authors (16, 17) have also recommended intraperitoneal placement, which is especially well-suited, without a doubt, to laparoscopic insertion of the prosthesis.

What type of patch?

A study in 1998 (18) comparing polypropylene, ePTFE (expanded polytetra-fluoroethylene), and polyester, showed poor results in terms of complications (4.7 vs 1.4%), fistulas (16 vs 0%), infection (16 vs 6%), and recurrence rates (34 vs 10%), in cases where polyester (Mersilene®) was used. On the contrary, there appears to be no difference with regard to use of mono-filament polypropylene (Marlex®), double-filament (Prolène®), or PTFE (Goretex®) in this series. Otherwise, the use of ePTFE is recommended by Bauer (19, 20), while Arnaud (16) recommends Dacron, and Champetier (21) Mersilene®.

But, intraperitoneal placement of the prosthesis requires use of a material which is little adhesion-inducing to decrease the risk of fistula formation, and the extent of postoperative adhesions in the event of reintervention (22) (Fig. 1, 2). ePTFE meets these requirements, based on results of an experimental study (23) comparing the use of ePTFE and polypropylene in rats.

A consequence of this low adhesion-inducing potential is less optimal encapsulation in adjacent tissue, which can result in an increased recurrence rate (24). This requires placement of a prosthesis which widely overlaps the edges of the incisional hernia, and which is firmly secured to the abdominal wall (25, 26, 27).

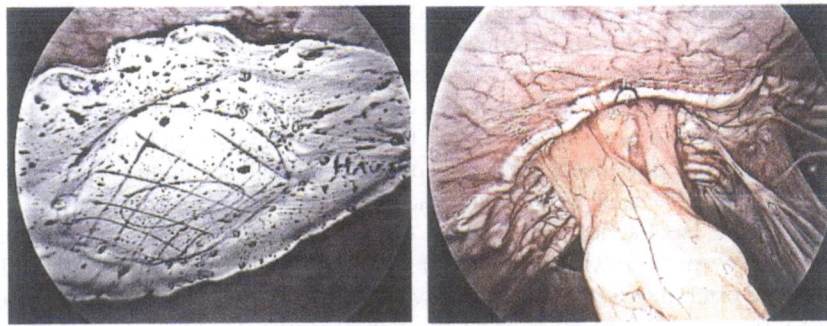

Fig. 1. Little adhesions with ePTFE mesh. **Fig. 2.** Wide adhesions with ePTFE mesh

Conclusion

After reviewing the literature on surgical repair of abdominal hernias by laparotomy, it is clear that recurrences are frequent after simple suturing of the abdominal wall or using the overlapping technique, thus requiring the use of a prosthetic patch to reinforce the abdominal wall defect, especially in obese subjects, and/or in cases of recurrent incisional hernias. Intraperitoneal placement of the prosthesis appears preferable to decrease the rate of complications associated with major dissection of the superficial layers of the abdominal wall, a cause of possible recurrence. A prosthetic patch of ePTFE, which has low adhesion-inducing potential, appears best suited for contact with the small bowel to decrease the risk of fistula formation, another cause of possible recurrence, provided that the prosthesis widely overlaps the edges of the abdominal hernia, and that the prosthesis is firmly secured in place.

SERIES OF CASES TREATED WITH LAPAROSCOPY

The laparoscopic approach has been used since 1991 to treat incisional hernias (28), proving the feasibility of this technique, whose encouraging results have been confirmed by other authors (5, 6, 7, 25, 26).

Several comparative studies have demonstrated the usefulness of the laparoscopic approach compared to conventional techniques using laparotomy.

DeMaria (29) made a prospective comparison of the intraperitoneal ePTFE patch (21 patients) versus the polypropylene preaponeurotic polypropylene patch (18 patients). The results showed the superiority of laparoscopy in terms of postoperative pain, the length and cost of hospital stay, in spite of two serious complications (colocutaneous fistula, infection of the patch), and one recurrence.

Ramshaw (30) performed a retrospective comparison of 174 laparotomies and 79 laparoscopies, and observed favourable results for the laparoscopic approach in terms of the duration of surgery (58 vs 82 minutes), hospital stay (1.7 vs 2.8 days), serious complications (16.5 vs 21.8%), and recurrence rates (2.5 vs 20.7%).

Park (31) compared 56 laparoscopic repairs to a previous series of 49 repairs with laparotomy. The duration of surgery was longer, but the length of hospital stay and complication rates were lower.

The results of these studies are dissimilar, and the only prospective study conducted had a sample size which was too small. However, these results appear at least as good as those obtained with the open abdominal approach. DeMaria (29) insists on the need for an excellent surgical technique to prevent complications associated with learning the technique.

A recent, large series (26) reported on 407 patients who were operated on between November 1993 and December 1999, with the placement of an ePTFE prosthetic patch in 97% of cases. The average size of the abdominal hernia was large (100 cm²), and the mean duration of surgery was 97 minutes. The authors found 14 recurrences, i.e. 3.4%, with a mean follow-up of 23 months. In 6 cases, these recurrences were associated with defective fixation of the prosthesis by the authors, i.e. a recurrence rate which could have been only 1.97% if percutaneous sutures had been used in combination with surgical staples. But the authors did not specify whether fixation was inadequate or if the patch was improperly positioned, perhaps its position was eccentric in relation to the edges of the abdominal hernia. This interpretation confirms the need to define the causes of recurrence associated with the technique, in order to offer the safest possible procedure.

Conclusion

The laparoscopic approach appears both feasible and desirable, with results equivalent to those obtained by laparotomy, and with the additional advantages of endoscopy in terms of postoperative pain, length of hospital stay, and duration of occupational sick leave. The ePTFE prosthetic patch is the preferred material, but although its low adhesion-inducing potential is an advantage with regard to the small bowel in the intraperitoneal position, this can be a disadvantage with regard to the quality of adherence to the abdominal wall. Fixation of the prosthesis should be performed with rigour in order to decrease the number of recurrences associated with the loosening of the prosthesis.

Thus, we will report our own personal series of cases (25), in an effort to identify the causes and mechanisms of recurrences and to propose a desirable surgical technique.

PERSONAL SERIES OF CASES

Patients

Between December 1993 and May 1999, 135 patients (88 women and 47 men) mean age 55 years (range: 24-92 years), were candidates for laparoscopic repair of a ventral hernia (VH).

The mean weight of patients was 81.4 kg (range: 46-135 kg), and 74 patients (54.8 %) were obese. The mean length of the longest diameter of the LRVH was 8.3cm (range 1.5-34.5 cm).

103 patients had a painful VH, and 32 patients had gastrointestinal disorders which could be related to the VH.

127 procedures (94%) were performed by elective hospitalization and 8 (6%) were performed as cases of complicated VH.

81 VH were located along the midline, 37 were juxta-umbilical, 6 were subcostal, and 11 were in a peripheral location.

Technique

The 135 procedures were carried out by three surgeons, each of whom operated on 86 (BB), 40 (JFR) and 9 (CL) patients, respectively.

Surgery was performed under general anesthesia with oro-tracheal intubation, and a nasogastric tube was systematically placed, while a urinary catheter was installed in selected patients.

The surgeon and his assistant placed themselves alongside the patient, to the right or left, depending on the incision and site of the VH. In the case of a subcostal VH, the surgeon took position between the patient's legs.

Patients were installed in two types of position: right lateral recumbent position at a 45° angle with use of 0° optical system (40 patients), or supine with use of a 30° optical system (95 patients). In both cases, the patient's arms were positioned alongside of the body. A video screen was placed at the foot or the head of the patient, depending on the site of the VH.

Pneumoperitoneum was induced using a Veress needle in a scar-free area (generally, the left lower quadrant) in 37 patients (27.4%). As a precautionary measure, open laparoscopy along the left anterior axillary line was performed in 98 patients (72.6%), either conventionally, or by using the Visiport system in 77 patients (BB), for introduction of the first 10 mm trocar.

Two other 5 mm trocars were placed along this same line in the left lower quadrant and the left iliac fossa. In case of a very large VH, three other trocars were symmetrically placed on the opposite side in order to continue the dissection, insert the prosthesis and secure it to the side opposite the surgeon. Lysis of adhesions of the anterior abdominal wall, the VH sac left in place and its contents were performed using monopolar scissors (95 patients), or with a Harmonic Scalpel Ultracision® in 40 patients.

After marking off the skin to determine the desirable size of prosthesis using a rigid ruler, a 1 mm thick ePTFE (Dualmeshl) rectangular-shaped patch was marked, using a sterile felt-tip pen on its smooth aspect for contact with the internal organs, with an " X " indicating the centre of the patch, and the middle of each side also was identified (upper, lower, right, left).

The patch was inserted rolled-up lengthwise, either via the 10mm trocar for the optical system, or, if a large patch was needed, via the 10mm trocar, or a transcutaneous approach after temporary removal of the optic system and widening of the orifice digitally for manual insertion.

The prosthesis was spread over the internal organs and then was turned over so as to position its smooth aspect against the internal organs. Then, the prosthesis was secured to the anterior abdominal wall in intraperitoneal position, using the Endohernia® system at the start of our experience with this series, and later using

5mm Tacker4 or Protack® type helical surgical staples. Generally, two or three cartridges of staples were used to secure the peripheral part of the prosthesis and to apply two additional rows of circular stapling (Fig. 4). A single operator (CL) used prefixation transcutaneous sutures to centre the prosthesis.

When we first began to use our procedure, the prosthesis overlapped the edges of the VH by only 3 cm, while currently a minimum of 5cm seems necessary.

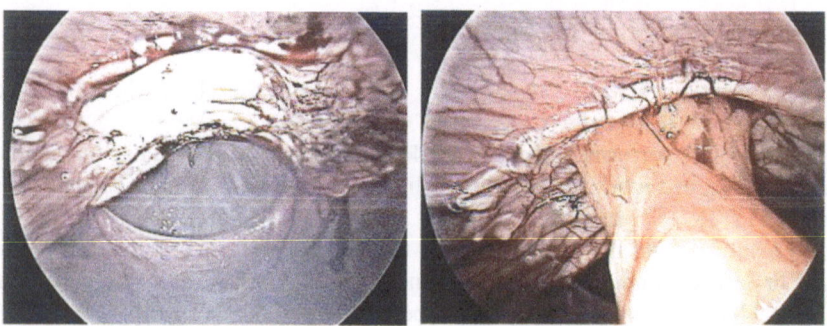

Fig. 3. Recurrence because of a too small a mesh. **Fig. 4.** Mesh fixed to the abdominal wall.

Results

In 130 patients (96.3%), repair of the VH was performed with the laparoscopic approach, with a mean duration of surgery of 58 min. (range: 15-240 min) and a mean hospital stay of 4.5 days (range 1-17 days).

7 perioperative complications (5.2 %) occurred, 5 of which necessitated conversion to open surgery (3.7 %):
- 3 intestinal perforations during the lysis of adhesions phase of the operation,
- 1 dissection was impossible due to the presence of major adhesions, and 1 case of dysfunctioning of the stapling system.

2 other complications were treated with laparoscopy:
- 1 injury to the bladder treated by suturing,
- 1 hemostatic treatment of the inferior epigastric artery.

The mean duration of surgery in the group of 5 patients converted to open-surgery was 110 minutes and the mean length of hospital stay was 13 days (range: 6-25 days).

Postoperative complications:

Mortality was 1.5%: 2 patients died postoperatively, one from a pulmonary embolism, the other from a myocardial infarction despite the fact that they had previously undergone CABG (coronary artery bypass grafting).

Morbidity involved 27 patients (20%):
- 4 abdominal wall suppurations which required removal of the prosthesis 1 to 12 months after the initial procedure; 3 of these cases of sepsis occurred after CPP and 1 in the aftermath of a procedure converted to laparotomy,
- 1 postoperative incisional hernia after conversion to laparotomy,

- 11 haematomas (5 whose outcome was spontaneously favourable, 3 of which were evacuated by needle-puncture, and 3 which were surgically evacuated),
- 1 postoperative hernia through a trocar incision,
- 6 with abdominal wall pain opposite the area of stapling (Tacker® or Protack®) 1 of which required partial removal of the patch in month 4 in another medical centre.

4 general complications:

- 1 digestive hemorrhage,
- 1 pneumonopathy,
- 2 cases of respiratory decompensation.

Currently, the mean follow-up of patients is 18.2 months (range: 0-66 months).

Eleven recurrences were reported (8.3%):

- 2 in the early postoperative period: 1 case of unfastening of the Endohernia® staples, the other as a result of the use of an inadequate patch size (Fig. 3),
- 9 late-onset recurrences: 6 cases of unfastening of the Endohernia® staples and 3 of an inadequate patch size.

No recurrence occurred in patients in whom the prosthesis overlapped the edges of the VH by 5 cm and in patients in whom the prosthesis had been fixated by helical staples (Figure 4). Statistical analysis (chi^2 test) demonstrated a significant difference in the group of patients with a VH whose size was greater than or equal to 7 cm, in terms of duration of surgery (74 mins versus 46 min), hospital stay (5.5 days versus 4 days), rate of conversion (6.3% versus 1.4%), or frequency of postoperative complications (34.4% versus 11.3%). No significant difference was found in the group of obese patients.

Comparison of references

	Patients	Defect (cm^2)	Patch (cm^2)	DOS (min)	Sick-leave days	Complication removal	Recurrences	Follow-up months
Kyzer Surg endosc 13, 1999, 928-31 (32)	53	117	180	89	3.3	1 (1.8 %)	1 (1.8 %)	17
Chowbey J Lap Endosc 10, 2000, 79-84 (33)	148	---	---	70	1.8	---	2 (1.35 %)	---
Heniford Surg Endosc 14, 2000, 419-23 (26)	100	87	287	88	1.6	2 (2 %)	3 (3 %)	23
Bokobza SCL 2001 (34)	147	74	302	62	5	4 (2.7 %)	13 (8.8 %) 4 (2.7 %)	8

CAUSES AND SOLUTIONS

Insertion of trocars

Positioning of trocars was not found to be a cause of recurrence, but it is a cause of technical failure since, if the trocar is placed too close to the edges of the ventral hernia, surgery cannot be performed, and in any event, it is impossible to widely overlap the herniated organs when installing the prosthesis.

Thus, the optic system trocar should be placed as laterally as possible, either to the left or the right. Open laparoscopy is difficult laterally because of muscle thickness, and thus the usefulness of an optical system equipped with a knife such as the Visiport®, which allows the operator to cut through the abdominal wall layers under visual control, preventing injury to a loop of the bowel.

Size and fixation of the prosthesis

The results of our series show that recurrences are related to an insufficient patch size in relation to the size of the hernia, and poor quality fixation of the prosthesis, with both factors combined increasing the risk of failure even more.

Thus, the prosthetic patch should overlap the edges of the hernia by at least 5 cm.

The prosthesis should be firmly secured with helical staples, the only type which can deeply penetrate a 1mm - thick patch and muscle, with percutaneous sutures in addition, if necessary.

Positioning of the prosthesis

Another mechanism which can cause a recurrence, despite the use of an adequate size patch, is the improper positioning of the prosthesis, eccentric in relation to the edges of the ventral hernia, and which subsequently becomes detached.

There is a high risk in the case of large hernias if the operator proceeds only on one side of the patient, since during positioning of the patch there is a tendency to widely cover the opposite edge, and then have too little material to use on the operator's side.

Thus, in cases of large ventral hernias, it is necessary to use controlateral trocars to fixate the patch opposite the operator, starting by anchoring the patch above and below along the midline. Locating the limits of the patch by using a sterile felt - tip pen aids in positioning, and, in addition, helps in locating the intestinal aspect. Another option is percutaneous fixation, as specified by Voeller (26), but the risk of infection is not negligible.

Tension on the prosthesis

However, apart from recurrences, improper patch fixation can result in organ protrusion during exertion, which can be termed "a functional recurrence".

Thus, proper tension is essential to prevent such protrusion, which will be obtained by pushing on the patch during its fixation, which is facilitated by its elasticity. Decreasing the pneumoperitoneum is also a solution, but at the end of the procedure the patch should be horizontal in relation to the operating table, with the hernia sac protruding above. Therefore, it is necessary to securely anchor the patch in place to avoid leaving a superficial pocket, in which a possible source of infection can occur.

Conclusion

Prevention of recurrence with laparoscopic repair of a ventral hernia using a ePTFE patch requires that the trocars used be placed very laterally, with placement of a prosthetic patch more than 5 centimetres over the edges of the hernia, proper positioning of the patch, firm fixation under tension, and securing it to the abdominal wall to prevent possible suppuration.

Future improvement will consist of development of a patch material which encapsulates well into the abdominal wall, but is little adhesion-forming with bowel loops, is not opaque to facilitate its fixation, is resistant to avoid tearing, with an internal structure which facilitates its installation. A sandwich of ePTFE, a mesh-like framework, and an abdominal wall aspect made of polypropylene may be a solution (35), but the answer rests with manufacturers of prosthetic materials and their ability to understand the requirements of surgery, beyond any conflict of interest.

References

1. Chevrel JP, Flament JB. Les éventrations de la paroi abdominale. *Rapport présenté au 92ᵉ Congrès Français de Chirurgie Monographies de l'AFC*. Paris, Masson, 1990.

2. Paul A, Korenkov M, Peeters S, Kohler L. Unacceptable results of the mayo procedure for repair of abdominal incisional hernia *Eur. J Surg*. 1998, 164, 361-367.

3. Rives J, Pire JC, Flament JB, Convers G. Traitement des éventrations *Encycl. Med. Chir.* Paris, Techniques chirurgicales, 40165 - 40207.

4. Leblanc KA, Booth WV. Laparoscopic repair of incisional abdominal hernias using expanded polytetraflucroethylene : preliminary findings *Surg. Laparosc. Endosc.* 1992, 3, 1, 39 - 41.

5. Franklin ME, Dorman JP, Glass JL, Balli JE. Laparoscopic ventral and incisional hernia repair *Surg. Laparosc. Endosc.* 1998, 8, 4, 294 - 299.

6. Langer S, Christiansen J. Long-term results after incisional hernia repair *Acta Chir Scand* 1985, 151(3), 217-9.

7. George CD, Ellis H. The results of incisional hernia repair: a twelve year review *Ann R Coll Surg Engl* 1986, 68(4), 185-7.

8. Hesselink VJ, Luijendijk RW, De Wilt JH, Heide R, Jeekel J. An evaluation of risk factors in incisional hernia recurrence *Surg Gynecol Obstet* 1993, 176(3), 228-34.

9. Luijendijk RW, Lemmen MH, Hop WC, Wereldsma JC. Incisional hernia recurrence following "vest-over-pants" or vertical Mayo repair of primary hernias of the midline *World J Surg* 1997, 21(1), 62-5, discussion 66.

10. Anthony T, Bergen PC, Kim LT, Henderson M, Fhaey T, Rege RV, Turnage RH. Factors affecting recurrence following incisional herniorrhaphy *World J Surg* 2000, 24(1), 95-100, discussion 101.

11. Horhant P, Le Du J, Chaperon J, Lavenac G, Mambrini A. Treatment of postoperative abdominal eventrations with a resorbable prosthesis. Apropos of 160 cases *J Chir (Paris)* 1996, 133(7), 311-6.

12. Santora TA, Roslyn JJ. Incisional hernia *Surg Clin North Am* 1993, 73(3), 557-70.

13. Shaikh NA, Shaikh NM. Comparative study of repair of incisional hernia *JPMA J Pak Med Assoc* 1994 , 44(2), 38-9.

14. Kung C, Herzog U, Schuppisser JP, Ackermann C, Tondelli P. Abdominal cicatricial hernia--results of various surgical techniques *Swiss Surg* 1995, (6), 274-8.

15. Bonnamy C, Samama G, Brefort JL, Le Roux Y, Langlois G. Long-term results of the treatment of eventrations by intraperitoneal non-absorbable prosthesis (149 patients) *Ann Chir* 1999, 53(7), 571-6.

16. Arnaud JP, Tuech JJ, Pessaux P, Hadchity Y. Surgical treatment of postoperative incisional hernias by intraperitoneal insertion of dacron mesh and an aponeurotic graft: a report on 250 cases*Arch Surg* 1999, 134(11), 1260-2.

17. Oussoultzoglou E, Baulieux J, De La Roche E, Peyregne V, Adham M, Berthoux N, Ducerf C. Long-term results of 186 patients with large incisional abdominal wall hernia treated by intraperitoneal mesh *Ann Chir* 1999, 53(1), 33-40.

18. Leber GE, Garb JL, Alexander AI, Reed WP. Long-term complications associated with prosthetic repair of incisional hernias *Arch Surg* 1998, 133(4), 378-82.

19. Bauer JJ, Salky BA, Gelernt IM, Kreel 1. Repair of large abdominal wall defects with expanded polytetrafluoroethylene (ePTFE) *Ann. Surg.* 1987,206, 765-769.

20. Bauer JJ, Harris MT, Kreel I, Gelernt I. Twelve-year experience with expanded polytetrafluoroethylene in the repair of abdominal wall defects *Mt Sinai J Med* 1999, 66(1), 20-5.

21. Champetier J, Leoublon C, Chaland P, Alnaasan I, Bouchard F, Granger P. The repair of recurrent postoperative incisional hernias. Objectives and therapeutic indications (68 cases) *J Chir (Paris)* 1990, 127(4), 191-8.

22. Carbajo MA, Martin Del Olmo JC, Blanco J. What is the appropriate mesh for laparoscopic intraperitoneal repair of abdominal wall hernia ¿ *Surg Endosc* 2000, 14, 408.

23. Simmermacher RK, Schakenraad JM, Bleichrodt RP. Reherniation after repair of the abdominal wall with expanded polytetrafluoroethylene *J Am Coll Surg* 1994, 178(6), 613-6

24. Ambrosiani N, Harb J, Gavelli A, Huguet C. Failure of the treatment of eventrations and hernias with the PTFE plate (111 cases) *Ann Chir* 1994, 48(10), 917-20.

25. Renier JF, Bokobza B, Leturgie C, Merveille M, Selman M, Sfihi A. Cure des éventrations sous laparoscopie par plaque intrapéritonéale d'ePTFE. Technique et résultats : A propos de 135 cas *J. Coeliochir.* 1999, 32, 35 - 39.

26. Heniford BT, Park A, Ramshaw BJ, Voeller G. Laparoscopic ventral and incisional hernia repair in 407 patients. *J Am Coll Surg* 2000, 190(6), 645-50.

27. Heniford BT, Ramshaw BJ. Laparoscopic ventral hernia repair: a report of 100 consecutive cases *Surg Endosc* 2000, 14(5), 419-23.

28. Brown RB. Laparoscopic hernia repair: a rural perspective *Surg Laparosc Endosc* 1994, 4(2), 106-9.

29. Demaria EJ, Moss JM, Sugerman HJ. Laparoscopic intraperitoneal polytetra-fluoroethylene (PTFE) prosthetic patch repair of ventral hernia. Prospective comparison to open prefascial polypropylene mesh repair *Surg Endosc* 2000, 14(4), 326-9.

30. Ramshaw BJ, Esartia P, Schwab J, Mason EM, Wilson RA, Duncan TD, Miller J, Lucas GW, Promes J. Comparison of laparoscopic and open ventral herniorrhaphy *Am Surg* 1999, 65(9), 827-31, discussion 831-2.

31. Park A, Birch DW, Lovrics P. Laparoscopic and open incisional hernia repair: a comparison study *Surgery* 1998, 124(4), 816-21, discussion 821-2.

32. Kyzer S, Alis M, Aloni Y, Charuzi I. Laparoscopic repair of postoperation ventral hernia. Early postoperation results *Surg Endosc* 1999, 13(9), 928-31.

33. Chowbey PK, Sharma A, Khullar R, Mann V, Baijal M, Vashistha A. Laparoscopic ventral hernia repair *J Laparoendosc Adv Surg Tec h A* 2000, 10(2), 79-84.

34. Bokobza B, Renier JF, Leturgie C, Selman M, Sfihi A. Cure laparoscopique des éventrations : A propos de 147 cas, *Congrès Société Française de Chirurgie Laparoscopique* Paris, 01/18/2000.

35. Farrakha M. Laparoscopic treatment of ventral hernia. A bilayer repair *Surg endosc* 2000, 14, 1156-1158.

CHAPTER 42

Laparoscopic Management Of Recurrences after Laparoscopic Ventral Hernia Repair

S. Kyzer, I. Charuzi

Recurrence rate following laparoscopic repair of incisional or ventral hernia varies in the published literature between 1.1% and 10.7% (1-8). In part of the publications, the median follow-up is not mentioned or is very short. In the others (1,4,7,8), a median follow-up period that varies between 23 and 30 months is mentioned. Also in these series, the recurrence risk varies between 1.1% and 10.7% (4). In the study of Park et al., the median follow-up period was 24 months, and the recurrences occurred only up to 12 months post operatively. For these reasons, it is still not clear whether an increased follow-up period will increase the recurrence rate significantly. Park et al. in evaluation of their recurrent cases were able to demonstrate that some factors can contribute significantly to the recurrence. Those factors are as follows: lateral defect, use of polypropylene mesh, occurrence of perioperative complications and presence of larger hernia (> 50 cm²). A nonsignificant trend toward an increased recurrence rate in patients who had undergone a previous non-laparoscopic repair was demonstrated.

Our experience demonstrates that hernia recurrence occurs due to inexact or insufficient coverage of the edges of the hernia with mesh. In most cases, this occurs due to the use of a too small mesh or to deficient fixation of the mesh to the surrounding fascia. Another reason for "recurrence", although it is not a real recurrence, is an unrecognized additional incisional defect(s) which were not covered with mesh. For the above mentioned reasons, it is very important to cover the abdominal wall defect at least 3 cm beyond its edges. In addition if possible, the whole previous incision must be covered with mesh.

In order to prevent infection of the previously used mesh by its exposure to the skin, we think that the repair of recurrent hernia after laparoscopic repair must be also performed, if possible, laparoscopically. We had performed laparoscopic repair of recurrent ventral and incisional hernia in few cases. One of these cases was even admitted with clinical signs of incarceration. Our literature survey of the literature revealed that most authors did not mention the way they managed their recurrences. However, some of the authors stated that they repaired all (3,6) or part (4) of the recurrent cases laparoscopically. During repair of recurrent ventral or incisional hernia, care must be taken to prevent any bowel injury during introduction of the first trocar. In addition, puncturing of the previously introduced mesh by the introduced mesh by the trocars must be prevented. An impression about the exact location of the mesh can be made by performance of a plain abdominal film and identification of the tackers or staples used for fixation of the mesh edges or by performance of CT examination. After loosening of the mesh from the edge of the hernia, tacks or staples remain adherent to the mesh. For this reason, the location of the recurrent hernia can be identified on plain abdominal x-ray because tacks or staples are present inside the usual contour of the mesh (Fig. 1).

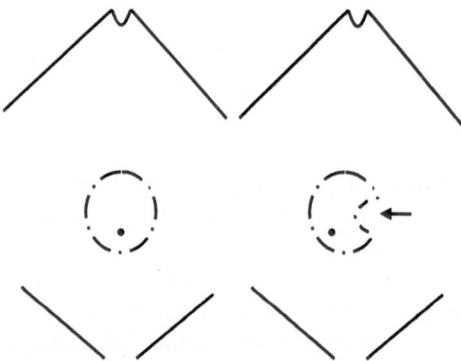

Fig. 1. Schematic illustration demonstrating how recurrent hernia appears on plain abdominal x-ray: left - no recurrent hernia; right - recurrent hernia.

After release of the hernia content, the defect must be covered by mesh (Gore-Tex® or composite mesh) in the usual manner. Because the space of the hernia sac between the mesh and the skin is filled with fibrous tissue, fixation of new laid mesh to the previously laid mesh is possible.

In our experience, we have not encountered recurrence after reoperation for recurrent hernia.

ACKNOWLEDGMENT

We thank Ms. Judy Brandt for her English editing, word processing and contributions.

References

1. Franklin ME, Dorman JP, Glass JL, Balli JE, Gonzalez JJ. Laparoscopic ventral and incisional hernia repair. Surgical Laparoscopy and Endoscopy 1998;8:294-299.

2. Kyzer S, Alis M, Aloni Y, Charuzi I. Laparoscopic repair of postoperation ventral hernia. Early postoperation results. Surg Endosc 1999;13:928-931.

3. Holtzman MD, Puput CM, Reintgen K, Eubanks S, Pappas TN. Laparoscopic ventral and incisional hernioplasty. Surg Endos 1991;11:32-35.

4. Park A, Birch DW, Lovrics P, Hamilton LK. Laparoscopic and open incisional hernia repair: A comparison study. Surgery 1998;124:816-822.

5. Park A, Gagner M, Pomp A. Laparoscopic repair of large incisional hernias. Surgical Laparoscopy and Endoscopy 1996;6:123-128.

6. Szymanski J, Voitk A, Joffe J, Alvarez C, Rosenthal G. Technique and early results of outpatient laparoscopic mesh onlay repair of ventral hernia. Surg Endosc 2000;14: 582-584.

7. Heniford BT, Park A, Ramshaw BJ, Voeller G. Laparoscopic ventral incisional hernia repair in 407 patients. J Am Coll Surg 2000;190:645-650.

8. Reitter DR, Paulsen JK, Debord JR, Estes NC. Five-year experience with the "four-before" laparoscopic ventral hernia repair. Am Surg 2000;66:465-469.

CHAPTER 43

Cost-Effectiveness of Laparoscopic Ventral Hernia Repair

J.D. Tutosaus, S. Morales-Conde, F. López Bernal,
S. Morales-Méndez

INTRODUCTION

In the early 1990s, few literature references to the organization and management of laparoscopic surgery could be found. The tide is turning, however, and now in the year 2001, literature addressing these issues is increasingly available. Nevertheless, the most demonstrative studies, e.g., clinical trials, are still lacking, and, according to the monographic issue of the National Coordinating Centre for Health Technology Assessment (no. 100, June 2001), only fifty per cent of the available studies admit generalization.

By the begining of the 20th century, the classic specialties in medicine had been well established and in some countries such as the U.S., physicians were trained through a residency program. Even so, it was only many years later (in 1984, to be precise) before the first residents trained in health care management came out of these residency programs in the U.S. Now, at the beginning of the 21st century, health management is still a not a formally accepted medical specialty in most of the world. It is not surprising that one area in this field, management related to laparoscopy, a technique first used in 1987, is only now starting to build up a retrievable body of information in the literature.

When discussing the issue of costs and their relationship to effectiveness, we must first look at the actual meaning of effectiveness: This concept represents the extent to which the objectives are achieved. As applied to the specific field under discussion, effectiveness would be something resembling the impact attained by surgeries in daily practice (1). *Efficiency is the term used when effectiveness is related to cost, i.e., when the objectives achieved are assigned an economic value*[1]. This is the concept that will be discussed in this chapter. The issue is not the price, because the concept includes the cost plus the profit, with the latter varying considerably. Therefore, our aim is not to perform a cost-benefit study(2) as this would be another, albeit similar, approach.

We will look at the objectives attained with laparoscopic surgery applied to incisional hernias and analyze the cost of these operations. We will also look at the clinical objectives and their cost in traditional open surgery.

In order for this study to be decisive in terms of comparison of the relative efficiency of one technique over another, the study should be formulated as a clinical trial. However, laparoscopy is a new surgical approach that is still in the developmental stage and there is not sufficient available knowledge on the impact of the procedure. Moreover, to perform a clinical trial only half the hernia repairs would be by laparoscopic access because of the required random distribution into two groups (conventional vs. laparoscopic surgery). Hence, a significant amount of time would be needed to define the current status of the objectives and cost of traditional surgery and to determine whether the objectives of laparoscopic surgery have been reached and how much they cost, i.e. if they are effective.

Despite being the most comprehensive approach to an investigation, clinical trials have two key disadvantages (3): they are costly and they require lengthy development. In time comparative clinical trials will be undertaken. However, we must first present and analyze the currently available knowledge. Some studies have been started in a few surgery services. However, it is extremely important to understand what occurs in an environment such as the one where the authors work (a large 1800-bed teaching hospital with pre- and post-graduate students) and to avoid automatically extrapolating the results from other centers, with all the errors this can produce.

MATERIALS AND METHOD

A total of 78 patients operated between June 1998 and September 2000 were analyzed. The patients were divided into three groups as homogeneous as possible in terms of the series of characteristics being studied: All patients had similar characteristics regarding their pathology (size of hernia defect, etc.) and similar demographic characteristics (weight, height, sex, etc.), and all were operated on by the same team (four surgeons), in the shortest possible period of time (last three years). Although the patients were not chosen randomly, an attempt was made to selectively create homogeneous groups. Naturally we could not be excessively strict in the inclusion criteria, as few patients would be eligible, more surgeons from the department would be needed (leading to greater variability) and/or the recruitment period would be longer. This latter factor would have introduced variations in other characteristics, such as increasing surgical experience with time, changes in the teams and in the conditions of the setting, and a delay in data collection.

The distribution by sex was 51 women (65%) and 27 men (34%). Mean age was 55.9 years (standard deviation, or SD=12.3). Mean weight was 79.3 kg (SD=15.6). Mean height was 161.2 cm (SD=8.2), with a body mass index (BMI) of 30.7 (SD=7.0). The anesthesia risk was ASA 2.75 (SD=0.63).

The *first group* contained 19 patients who were treated by conventional open surgery using polypropylene mesh (PPL).

Table I. Characteristics of the groups

	OPEN	OPEN	LAPAROSCOPIC	S. E.
	19 PPL	14 ePTFE	44 ePTFE	
AGE	57.2	56.2	54.9	NS
SEX	F 13 M 6	F 9 M 6	F 28 M 16	NS
WEIGHT	83.2	84.4	73.9	S
HEIGHT	154.6	161.7	162.4	NS
BMI	32.8	32.7	28.2	S
ASA	3	2.4	2.8	NS
SURGERY TIME	130	119	80	S
PERISTALSIS	55	40	24	S
FLUID INTAKE	54	64	24	S
HOSPITALIZATION	10.3	14.6	2.5	S

Table II. Immediate complications in the groups

	OPEN 19 PPL	OPEN 14 ePTFE	LAPAROSCOPIC 44 ePTFE
INFECTION	1	0	0
HEMATOMA	1	1	0
SEROMA	0	2	1
PERFORATION	1	0	1
DYSPNEA	0	2	0
AGITATION	0	1	0
ILEUS	0	0	1

Table III. Short- and medium-term complications in the groups

PPL, open	1 month	6 months	12 months
TENSION	0	0	1
PAIN	0	0	4
SEROMA	0	0	0
RECURRENCE	0	1	2
ePTFE, open	1 month	6 months	12 months
TENSION	0	1	0
PAIN	0	0	1
SEROMA	6	6	2
RECURRENCE	0	0	0
ePTFE, lapar.	1 month	6 months	12 months
TENSION	0	0	0
PAIN	0	0	0
SEROMA	1	1	1
RECURRENCE	0	1	1

Table IV. Costs according to group (euros)

Group	Hospitalization	Prosthesis	Suture	Materials	Total
1. PPL, open	4.790	105	22	--	4.917
2. PTFE, open	7.196	723	22	--	7.941
3. PTFE, lapar.	1.082	1.140	356	739	3.317

Table V. Statistical differences in group costs

Group	Hospitalization	Prosthesis	Suture	Materials	Total
G1/G2	NS	S	NS	NS	NS
G1/G3	S	S	S	S	S
G2/G3	S	NS	S	S	S

S = Significant, i.e., with p< 0.05
NS = Not significant, i.e., with p>0.05

Table VI. Statistical differences in characteristics of the groups

	Open/Open G1/G2	Open 1/Lapar. G1/G3	Open 2/Lapar. G2/G3
AGE	NS	NS	NS
SEX	NS	NS	NS
WEIGHT	NS	S	S
HEIGHT	NS	NS	NS
BMI	NS	S	S
ASA	NS	NS	NS
SURGERY TIME	NS	S	S
PERISTALSIS	NS	S	S
FLUID INTAKE	NS	S	S
HOSPITALIZATION	NS	S	S

S = Significant, i.e., with p< 0.05
NS = Not significant, i.e., with p>0.05

The *second group* consisted of 14 patients also operated by conventional open surgery, but using expanded polytetrafluoroethylene mesh (ePTFE).

These two groups comprise the macrogroup of 34 patients operated by conventional open surgery.

The *third group* was composed of 44 patients operated by laparoscopic surgery using an ePTFE Dual Mesh prosthesis. The first ten patients treated by laparoscopic technique were considered to be a learning group and, therefore, were not included although the surgeons had extensive general laparoscopic experience.

The **method** used was a crossover descriptive analysis of the results using simple statistical variables such as the mean and standard deviation and a purely descriptive comparison of the groups, with no attempt to present decisive results for the reasons mentioned in the introduction.

The *statistical analysis* was performed using the SPSS statistical program (3). The analysis was based on non-parametric tests, due to the distribution of the variables and the fact that two of the groups had fewer than 30 individuals. The overall significance of a variable with respect to the group was analyzed using the Kruskal-Wallis test.

In order to compare the two groups (with the exceptions mentioned), the Mann-Whitney U-test was used, understanding the significance level (SL) to be significant (S) if the differences had a probability (p) of error under five per cent ($p < 0.05$).

RESULTS

The epidemiological and surgical **characteristics** of each patient group are shown in Table I.

Since surgical **effectiveness** is defined as obtaining the expected results, i.e., *resolution* of the condition and few or no *complications*, these data should be mentioned: All the pathologies in all the groups were initially resolved, although there were three recurrences in the first open surgery group (Group 1) and one in the laparoscopic surgery group (Group 3). The complications for each group are listed in Tables II (immediate) and III (short and medium-term).

The **cost** of hospitalization and the surgical procedures (itemized as hospital stay, prosthesic implant cost, suture cost, and cost of disposable and total surgical material) is shown in Table IV.

Statistical comparisons among the variables for the groups are shown in Tables V and VI.

DISCUSSION

In terms of the **analysis of the study variables**, we should briefly comment on the *number of patients* mentioned in similar studies published in prestigious journals with strict selection committees screening the studies they accept. Park

(5) described 30 cases, Costanza (6) 31, Kyzer (7) 53 and Sanders (8) 20. In studies comparing open surgery with laparoscopic surgery, Holzman (9) presented 21 cases, Carbajo (10) 30 and Park (11) 56. The present study had a total of 78 cases (44 laparoscopic and 34 laparotomic) and, therefore, it falls within the scope of other publications on this subject. However this does not mean that either this study or the others mentioned meet the requirements defining minimal sample size to draw comparisons from the epidemiological point of view.

In terms of *distribution by sex*, the present study had 30% more women (65%) than men (35%). Carbajo's study (10) had 23.3% more; whereas Toy's study (12) showed the opposite, namely 9.6% more men, along the lines of Park's study (13) which had 4.2% more men. Such large differences could be important and should be compared with those existing in the patients' parent population and with the epidemiological mean for gender in the postoperative hernia condition. In Spain, the percentage of men to women (14) for hernias as a whole is 75:25%, although this figure includes inguinal hernias; if limited only to incisional hernias, the percentage is 71% men versus 29% women (15). The percentage shows the opposite trend to that existing in hernia patients in general, being in any case extremely different from the natural mean of the human population, with differences of about 2% more women. The reasons for this are unknown. It should be determined whether this could be related to a higher demand for health services by women in the hospital area of Hospitales Virgen del Rocío, although a selection bias cannot be ruled out.

The distribution by *age* in the present study resulted in a mean of 54.9 years, similar to that reported in the previously cited publications (14) (55 years).

The *weight (and BMI)* ranged from a mean of 73.9 kg (BMI=28) in Group 3 (laparoscopic surgery) to 84.4 kg (BMI=33) in Group 2 (open surgery). The difference between these groups was significant. This is probably due to a bias in patient selection, since one might be more restrictive (consciously or unconsciously) when indicating laparoscopic surgery in very obese patients since the technique is still being introduced.

In this study, the *size of the defect being repaired* was 114.2 cm^2. In the different studies consulted, defect size varied considerably being 8.6 cm^2 in the Coleman study (13) to 139.4 cm^2 in Carbajo's study (10), with a mean of about 110 cm^2 (Toy (12) 98.3 cm^2, Holzman (9) 99 cm^2, Park (5, 11) 105.4-104 cm^2, Costanza (5) 130 cm^2, etc.).

The *surgery time* ranged from 80 minutes for laparoscopic surgery (Group 3) to 130 minutes for Group 1 (open), with these differences being significant. In the medical literature, surgery time ranges from 52 minutes, as reported by Coleman (16) to 210 minutes, as reported by Sanders (8). The duration varies considerably due to differences in the technique (staples or sutures), surgeon characteristics, surgical team and position on the learning curve.

The **surgical results (effectiveness)** were initially positive in 100% of cases for all the types of techniques, although the incidence of complications (different for each approach and prosthetic material) and recurrences must be subtracted from this favorable percentage (in terms of achieving short-term surgical resolution of the hernia). Longer term results (5 years or more) should be analyzed, particularly in terms of recurrences.

Complications are perhaps the hardest aspect to observe and quantify. In an ideal, objective study, the complications should be quantified "blindly", i.e. by an investigator-evaluator who is not a member of the work team and is not aware (to the extent possible) of the technique used (e.g., type of prosthesis). Naturally, this should be done after defining and validating what is understood by complications since differences between tension and painful discomfort or degrees of pain are highly subjective and because Table VII (prepared individually) should be validated extensively. In the light of these qualifying comments, the complications in Tables II and III can be examined.

Table VII. Effectiveness in the groups

	%	G1 PPL Open	G2 PTFE Open	G3 . PTFE Lapar
COMPLICATION-FREE CURE	100	x 8 = 800	x 3 = 300	x 38 = 3800
TENSION	95	x 1 = 95	x 1 = 95	0
PAIN	90	x 4 = 360	x 1 = 90	0
SEROMA	90	0	x 6 = 540	x 1 = 90
HEMATOMA	90	x 1 = 90	x 1 = 90	0
PROLONGED ILEUS	85	0	0	x 1 = 85
INFECTION	80	x 1 = 80	0	0
EMBOLISM	70	0	x 2 = 140	0
PERFORATION	70	x 1 = 70	0	x 1 = 70
RECURRENCE	0	x 3 = 0	0	x 3 = 0
MEAN		1495:19=78.7	1255:14=89.6	4054:44=92.1

Hospitalization is shown in Table I. Hospitalization was 2.5 days in the laparoscopic surgery group, 10.3 days in open surgery Group 3 with PPL and 14.6 days in open surgery Group 2 with ePTFE. In all published studies, this is the gold standard on which all health care cost-cutting measures are based. However, not all the authors of this chapter agree with this. Some believe that this basis should be corrected and the cause of patient hospitalization should be estimated from strictly clinical criteria, i.e., when discharge is not possible for clinical reasons rather than other considerations. The hospital discharge process is highly subjective, as it looks at patient progress during the hospital stay: Before laparoscopy came into use, major surgery patients were never discharged until the sutures had been removed. Once experience with laparoscopic surgery had been gained, major surgery patients operated by conventional laparotomy began to be discharged much earlier. Several studies have been published (in all pathologies and specialties, surgical and non-surgical (17, 18) showing the variability of the hospital stay. Thus one should not attribute more hospitalization savings than are actually attained with use of the laparoscopic approach. Considerable work must be done to ensure the adoption of discharge criteria that are strictly clinical (rather than cultural, traditional or legalist) and true objectivity in the use of such criteria based on the actual status of the patient instead of the surgical technique used. Perhaps objective signs such as the recovery of peristalsis (rather than subjective symptoms such as pain, which can be pharmacologically and psychologically modified) should be the guide for establishing discharge criteria.

This links with the philosophy of many of the authors of this book and of those who support laparoscopic surgery (including hospital directors-managers (19) in that laparoscopic surgery will be increasingly widespread because patients (acting more and more as clients) will demand it, rather than because of its lower cost.

Based on our analysis of the characteristics of the three patient groups, we can comment on the **effectiveness obtained** (Table VII). Effectiveness was considered to be 100% if the condition was resolved with no complications or recurrences and 0% if the outcome was recurrence (i.e., the surgery was totally ineffective). Based on the type of complication, varying percentages were established that could be deducted from total effectiveness. Thus, a feeling of tension at the wound site decreased effectiveness by 5%; pain, seroma and hematoma decreased it by 10%, prolonged ileus by 15%, infection by 20%, and embolism and perforation by 30%. By making the respective calculations, the mean effectiveness of each group was 78.7% in open surgery with PPL, 89.6% in open surgery with ePTFE and 92.1% in the laparoscopic surgery group; the overall effectiveness for all open surgery was 83.3%.

The average **cost** in euros (€) per patient in each group is shown in Table IV. This showed great variation depending on the group, since there were important, significant differences in the cost of the prostheses and hospitalization. The average cost was 4,917 € ($4,305 at an exchange rate of US $0.8757 per euro) in Group 1 (less expensive prosthesis, intermediate mean stay), 7,941 € ($6,954) in Group 2 (longest mean stay, prosthesis of medium-high cost) and 3,317 € ($2,905) in the laparoscopic surgery group (shortest stay, more expensive prosthesis and surgical material). Other surgical costs were not considered (e.g., staff costs). Nevertheless, this would have favored the laparoscopic surgery group because of the lower surgical theater time required, with all that this implies in terms of staff costs or alternative cost for other uses. The cost of depreciation of the inventory apparatus used in laparoscopic surgery (insufflator, video camera, monitors, etc.), was not taken into account since they are already depreciated for other normal uses (gall bladder surgery). Disposable instruments were, however, included in the calculation (if reusable material had been utilized, there would only have been depreciation costs). Cost differences between the groups were statistically significant, although we maintain the qualifying factors regarding our results mentioned earlier.

In order to calculate the quotient mentioned in the chapter title, namely, the *"cost-effectiveness ratio"* (CER), we used the average cost of each group multiplied by 100 (maximum effectiveness) in the numerator and the actual relative percentage obtained for effectiveness in the denominator.

As a result, in the open surgery *Group 1 with PPL prosthesis*, the CER was

$$\frac{Cost}{Effectiveness} = \frac{4,917 \text{ € x } 100\%}{78.7\%} = 6,248 \text{ "efficient" euros}$$

We have called the resulting quotient, or "cost-effectiveness ratio", "actual" euros since efficiency is defined as the ratio of effectiveness to its cost, as stated in the introduction.

In open surgery *Group 2 with ePTFE prosthesis*, the CER was

$$\frac{Cost}{Effectiveness} = \frac{7,941 \text{ € x } 100\%}{89.6\%} = 8,863 \text{ "efficient" euros}$$

The overall CER for the *open surgery macrogroup* (19 PPL and ePTFE) was

$$\frac{Cost}{Effectiveness} = \frac{6,200 \text{ € x } 100\%}{83.3\%} = 7,443 \text{ "efficient" euros}$$

when cost and efficacy are considered as averages.

In the laparoscopic surgery *group with ePTFE-DM prosthesis (Group 3)*, the average cost per procedure was 3,317 euros, hence the cost-effectiveness ratio or "efficiency" was

$$\frac{Cost}{Effectiveness} = \frac{3,317 \text{ € x } 100\%}{92.1\%} = 3,607 \text{ "efficient" euros}$$

Some authors such as Traverso (17) estimate the *"value"* of the procedures as the quotient between health *process quality* and cost. In our study, process quality would be equivalent to effectiveness, as we have just mentioned. Hence, the maximum quality would be successful surgical outcome (hernia resolution) with no complications, defined as 100%. In contrast, a recurrence would be the poorest outcome (without mentioning death or more important sequelae), assigned a value of 0%. Table VII would be used to define deductions for quality in the same percentages. Hence, the result would be:

$$\text{"Value" of open surgery} = \frac{Quality = 93.1\% \text{ x } 100}{Costs = 6,200 \text{ €}} = 1.34 \text{ (efficiency)}$$

$$\text{"Value" of laparoscopic surgery} = \frac{Quality = 93.1\% \text{ x } 100}{Costs = 3,317 \text{ €}} = 2.81 \text{ (efficiency)}$$

We have called 1.34 and 2.81 the *"efficiency points"*, although we could also use another designation; the idea is to have a system to be able to numerically quantify the cost-effectiveness relationship ("efficiency"), as we have explained. As can be seen, the efficiency value for laparoscopic surgery is more than twice that of conventional surgery.

Before completing our general analysis of the matter of cost and effectiveness, we should comment on the highly regarded opinions of Harvard professor Peter F. Drucker. Perhaps the most influential thinker in management issues, Prof. Drucker stated in 1989 that as of the year 2000, companies who wished to be excellent would have to function as a hospital (21). Drucker's theories include an old concept that is specifically related to the subject at hand. He formulated his postulate of innovation, considering that "the core of economic theory must be moved from cost, where it has always been, toward risk. This would, in turn, lead to a reevaluation of the nature, role and function of profit" (22). Traditionally, the issue of profit was a cornerstone in conventional economics, with a lack of information considered to be the most important risk and, therefore, a risk that must be minimized (23).

Drucker was an advanced thinker in terms of innovation. Managers, directors and supervisors must have an ongoing capacity for influencing and driving change. Laparoscopic surgery is a change that represents an innovation in surgery. We cannot forget that innovations are motivations. For a hospital service to function, its members must be motivated; and management must involve all members of the service; One surgeon, Dr. Gil Goñi published the following in Cirugía Española (24): "...we will implement modern management techniques to measure and quantify our medical care because otherwise 'others' will do it for us, and you can be assured that 'they' will not do it as well as we would because 'they' do not understand surgery." Someone who is not a surgeon or even a physician would have to be rather audacious to get involved in evaluating patient prognoses and results.

As mentioned earlier, laparoscopy will become the standard because the clients demand it. This is a key, crucial concept. Patients will continue demanding it because the outcome is more comfortable and offers fewer complications than conventional surgery. We must move toward a management formula in marketing terms. However, politicians do not have sufficient technical capacity and the technical staff do not have the necessary power. Only by asking will we know how patients prefer to be operated.

Since 1969 the theory that marketing was the exclusive territory of business has changed, thanks to Kotler's theories (25). Marketing is more a concept of exchange than a market transaction, and can be applied to health services. Hospital structures must be adapted to the requirements of their clients, as these are the parties sustaining such structures with taxes, fees and invoices paid to national insurance programs and public and private hospitals. The best possible care must be provided at the lowest possible cost, and the range of services that can be offered to the population must be defined and made known publicly. They should be defined in terms of additional quality, patient comfort, personalized treatment and the participation of the patient and his or her family in the healing process.

Patients are seeking less trauma, less aggression, smaller scars, fewer complications, and faster return to normal life; and they want this if possible (and it is) in the company of their family, even in the surgical theater. Laparoscopic surgery can provide them with all these benefits. Surgeons must use this last advantage, which, until now, has not been not disseminated. Moreover, one should remember that operations are now being broadcast on commercial television. This is happening because a major public sector has demanded it; people want to know what happens to their body in the surgical theater. Is there a better occasion to show them? Within only a short time, this will become part of the quality objectives of a laparoscopic surgery department, i.e., its quality level (namely, value) of efficiency or, as mentioned in the title, cost-effectiveness.

References

1. Muir Gray JA. Atención sanitaria basada en la evidencia. Ed. Churchill Livingstone, Madrid, 1979, p. 126.

2. Cabasés JM. Análisis costo-beneficio. Ed. EASP, Granada, 1994; p. 7.

3. Burgos R, Chicharro JA, Bobenrieth MA. Metodología de investigación y escritura científica en clínica. Ed. Escuela Andaluza de Salud Pública, Granada 1994, p 98-110.

4. SPSS Real Stats. Real Easy. v 8.0. Ed. SPSS Inc. New Jersey, 1997.

5. Park A, Gagner M, Pomp A. Laparoscopic repair of large incisional hernias. Surg Laparosc Endosc 1996; 6: 123-128.

6. Costanza MJ, Heniford BT, Arca MJ. Laparoscopic repair of recurrent ventral hernias. Am Surg 1998; 64(12): 1121-1127.

7. Kyzer S, Alis M, Aloni Y. Laparoscopic repair of postoperation ventral hernia. Surg Endosc 1999; 13: 928-931.

8. Sanders L, Flint L. Initial experience with laparoscopic repair of incisional hernias. Am J Surg 1999; 177: 227-231.

9. Holzman MD, Purut CM, Reintgen K, Pappas TN. Laparoscopic ventral and incisional hernioplasty. Surg Endosc 1997; 11: 32-35.

10. Carbajo MA, Martín del Olmo JC, Blanco JI. Laparoscopic treatement vs open surgery in the solution of major incisional and abdominal wall hernias with mesh. Surg Endosc 1999; 13: 250-252.

11. Park A, Birch DW, Lovrics P. Laparoscopic and open incisional hernia repair: a comparison study. Surgery 1999; 124: 816-822.

12. Toy FK, Bailey RW, Carey CW. Prospective multicenter study of laparoscopic ventral hernioplasty; preliminary results. Surg Endosc 1998; 12: 955-959.

13. Park A, Gagner M, Pomp A. Laparoscopic repair of large incisional hernias. Surg Laparosc Endosc 1996; 6: 123-128.

14. Hidalgo M, Figueroa JM, Córdova H. Hernia de la pared abdominal. Estudio multicéntrico, en Porrero JL. Cirugía de la Pared abdominal. Ed. Masson, Barcelona 1997.

15. Pailler JL, Le Coadou A. Tratamiento quirúrgico de las eventraciones abdominales: principios y técnicas, en Porrero JL. Cirugía de la Pared abdominal. Ed. Masson, Barcelona 1997.

16. Coleman MG, Kua KB. Laparoscopic repair of ventral incisional hernias, en Abstracts del 7° Congreso Mundial de Cirugía Endoscópica. Ed. Lomanto, Kum So. Singapur 2000.

17. Rodríguez E, Martínez R, Gili M, Tutosaus JD, Castillo J: Ingresos de causa neumológica en hospitales de Andalucía: 1993-1994. Arch Bronconeumol 1997; 33: 185-189.

18. Oterino D, Peiró S, Portella E, Marchan C, Aymerich S. Utilización innecesaria de la hospitalización: Importancia de la gestión a nivel de servicio. Rev Calidad Asistencial 1994; 9 (1): 8-16.

19. Tutosaus JD, Díaz-O J, Gómez-B I, Morales-M S. La opinión de los gerentes de hospitales sobre las nuevas tecnologías: la cirugía laparoscópica. Gestión Hospitalaria 1999; 10: 53-57.

20. Traverso LW. Tecnología y cirugía. Clínicas Quirúrgicas de Norteamérica, McGraw Hill ed., 1996, p 129-138.

21. Drucker PF. What Business Can Learn from Nonprofits. Harvard Business Review, 1989: 4.

22. Drucker PF. The Age of Discontinuity: Guidelines to Our Changing Society, Ed. Harper & Row, New York, 1969, p. 132.

23. Stein G. El arte de gobernar según Peter Drucker. Ed. Gestión 2000, Barcelona, 1969, p. 63.

24. Gil-G A. Editorial. La formación en gestión: Una necesidad para los cirujanos de hoy. Cir Esp 1992; 51 (6): 399-400.

25. Kotler P, Clarke RN. Market segmentation and targeting. Chap. 9, in: Marketing for health care organizations. Ed. Prentice Hall, New Jersey 1990. P 231-255.

_____

Valuation of other Uses of Meshes placed intraperitoneally in other Abdominal Cavity Defects

_____

CHAPTER 44

Laparoscopic Repair for Inguinal Hernias : is there a place for IPOM technique? Indications, technique and results

J.A. Almeida, M.E. Franklin

INTRODUCTION

The description by Edoardo Bassini in 1890 of his herniorrhaphy marked the beginning of a new era in the treatment of inguinal hernia. Widely accepted in the western world, the results were not, however, as effective as the ones reported by him. This fact was due in part by an inaccurate description of Bassini's original "triple layer repair", particularly in the United States and thus, division of the *transversalis fascia* was not emphasized. Recurrence rates of up to 10% in some American series lead to seek different approaches to this common pathology. In 1959 Francis Usher described the use of polypropylene mesh for non-tension repair of inguinal hernia (1), later popularized by Irving Lichtenstein in California (2). Shouldice in Canada rediscovered the Bassini's repair and championed the short-stay repair, and Ira Rutkow in New Jersey described the "plug and patch" repair. All of these techniques represent anterior approaches.

The history and rationale of the preperitoneal repair of groin hernias has been described in detail by Mikkelsen et. al., Musgrove et. al., Nyhus et. al., and Read (3-8). The absence in the preperitoneal area of adequate fascial or aponeurotic structures that could be approximated to bridge the hernia defect led to the abandonment of this particular technique. Stoppa in Amiens, and Rives in Reims revived interest in the preperitoneal area to repair the hernia defect by placing a large sheath of mesh in this area. This technique has gained wide acceptance in France for the treatment of many inguinal hernias. In the United States its use had been generally limited to recurrent groin hernias (3).

Placing a prosthetic veil in the preperitoneal area for repair of a recurrent hernia alleviates the need to re-enter previously divided planes and dissect the cicatrized cord. This avoids the ever-present incidence of ischemic testicular and nerve injuries occurring after such dissections. The mesh placed preperitoneally, if large enough, will not only cover the area of recurrence but will also cover other potential groin herniation sites including the femoral canal. The preperitoneal placement of mesh for "first time" and recurrent hernias has been well described in numerous publications.

With the development of laparoscopic surgery and continuous refinements in techniques occurring in that field (9), the authors tried to establish whether the principles of preperitoneal placement of synthetic mesh could be used expeditiously and safely laparoscopically.

When we began studying a procedure for laparoscopic mesh placement in humans in early 1990, attempts at placing the large portion of mesh (12cm x 15cm) preperitoneally required a large amount of dissection. The post operative scrotal discomfort experienced by some patients when using this technique lead us to try the much simpler intraperitoneal placement of the mesh. Arbitrarily we decided not to operate on patients under 18 years of age, or patients having large inguino-scrotal hernias. Later we have dropped the latter exclusion.

INDICATIONS

Table I. Current Indications for IPOM Technique

• Recurrent inguinal hernias
• Inguinal hernias after a previous laparoscopic repair
• Repair of inguinal hernias in patients with previous infraumbilical surgeries (violation of the preperitoneal space)
   – Appendectomies
   – C-section

Table II. IPOM technique. The Texas Endosurgery Institute experience

Location	Hernia Type	No of patients	% cases
Right IH	Direct	27	39.05%
	Indirect	143	
	Pantaloon	4	
	Femoral	8	
Left IH	Direct	15	31.75%
	Indirect	127	
	Pantaloon	2	
	Femoral	4	
Bilateral IH		116	38.44%
TOTAL		**466**	**100%**

At the beginning of our experience, all patients with inguinal, femoral or obturator hernias underwent this procedure. During the last years the authors have chosen the TEP (totally extraperitoneal) laparoscopic approach as the procedure of choice for inguinal hernia repair. This technique is described and discussed elsewhere in the book. However, the IPOM technique still has nowadays its indications (Table I).

One of the most attractive indications is the repair of inguinal hernias which have undergone a previous laparoscopic repair. This situation is becoming more commonly encountered, as we are starting to observe the recurrences from laparoscopic repairs. In these cases, the preperitoneal space has been already violated (TAPP or TEP techniques) making the dissection of this plane somewhat difficult. Similarly, when dealing with recurrences after open repairs, this approach avoids re-enter scar tissue present at the anterior abdominal wall. The onlay placement of prosthesis is a straightforward procedure and the newly designed, two-sided prosthesis have reduced the risk of intraabdominal adhesion formation significantly. An anterior, open approach represents a valid alternative as well.

The contraindications are the usual for laparoscopic procedures. Patients, who can not undergo general anesthesia, have intractable bleeding dyscrasias, or severe cardiopulmonary conditions are not candidates for IPOM. There is some concern on the usage of prosthesis under the age of 18, as the body is still growing and the fate of mesh in younger patients is unclear. Schumpelick et al have recently reported about the potential carcinogetic effects of mesh, although most of the clinical and experimental data proves the contrary.

Although obesity and multiple prior abdominal operations were considered as contraindications for laparoscopic surgery, the increasing experience and advances in instrumentation have both made possible to include this subgroup of patients as candidates. However, they have to be assessed in an individual basis.

TECHNIQUE

With the patient under general anesthesia, a catheter is placed in the bladder and a nasogastric tube is placed in the stomach, both are removed at the end of the procedure. The surgeon places himself on the contralateral side of the hernia (Fig. 1). Pneumoperitoneum is established by Veress technique on an alternate site, lateral to the umbilicus and on the opposite side of the hernia, particularly if the patient has prior abdominal surgeries. After inflating the peritoneal cavity, a 5 mm trocar is inserted followed by a 0° laparoscope. The abdominal cavity is surveyed and two additional trocars, a 12 mm trocar at the umbilicus and a 5 mm trocar lateral to the umbilicus at the the same level of the first trocar, are inserted under direct vision. For bilateral repairs the same configuration applies.

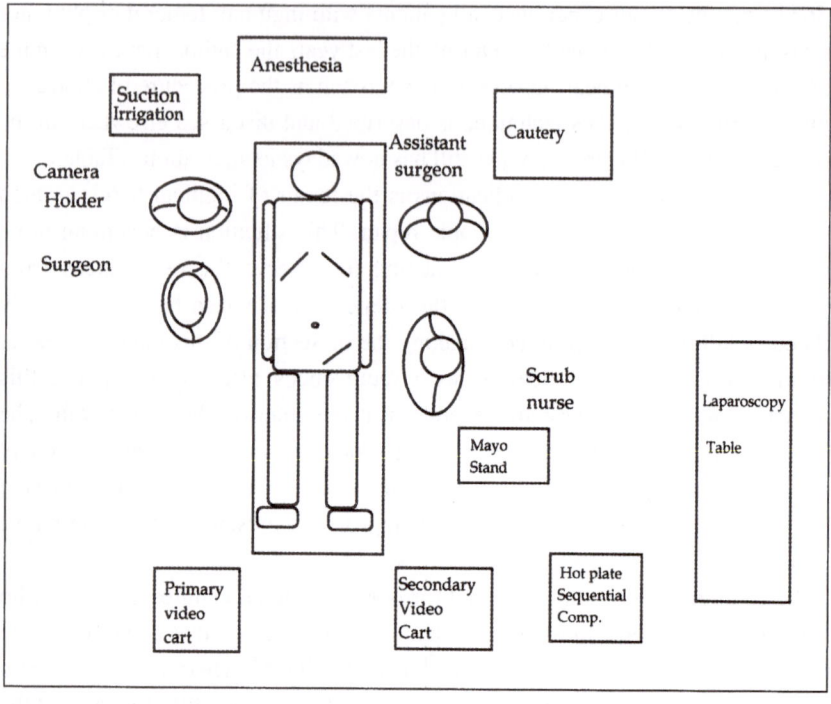

Fig. 1. Operating Room Setup

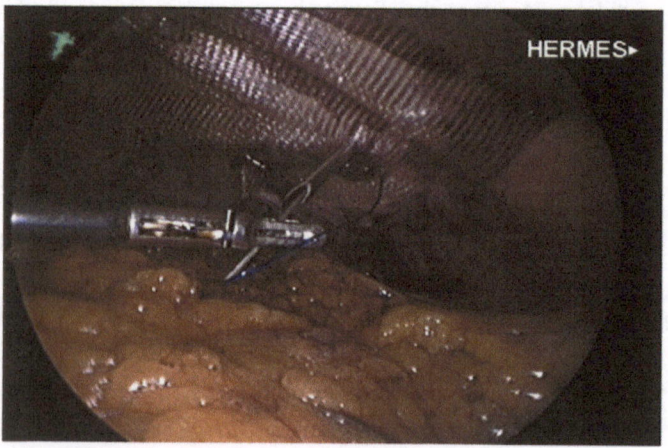

Fig. 2. Insertion of transabdominal sutures with the aid of a spinal needle
to fix the mesh

After inspecting the peritoneal cavity, the hernia site and the contralateral inguinal area are carefully evaluated. For proper orientation the surgeon should recognize the median, medial, and lateral umbilical ligaments. Just below the posterior parietal peritoneum the external iliac vein and artery, the gonadal vessels, and in males the vas deferens should be identified (Fig. 3). The hidden course of the genito-femoral nerve and the approximate course of the lateral femoro-cutaneous nerve should be recalled and mapped and care taken to avoid cross or rough dissection in this area. The exact location of the ureter bilaterally should also be noted.

We now routinely remove direct and indirect hernia sacs, since in our experience leaving the sac may perpetuate a bulge in the groin, a bulge that patients and inexperienced surgeons interpret as an operative failure despite repeated assurances that no bowel can enter the sac or space. Division of the sac also gives access to the preperitoneal area, where a "lipoma" of the cord if present can be excised. When operating for left sided hernias we often find it necessary to divide the embryonic adhesions that the sigmoid colon contracts with the parietal peritoneum next to the hernia defect. We excise the sac using laparoscopic scissors connected to an electro-surgical unit.

First the sac is progressively inverted into the peritoneal cavity using gentle traction. Once the inversion is completed, the sac is incised starting 1 or 2 cm from its base at the 12 o'clock position and proceeding clockwise to about the 4 o'clock position. The incision is then restarted at the "top" and carried in a counter clockwise fashion until approximately the 8 o'clock position. The inversion of an indirect inguinal hernia sac drags within it the fatty areolar tissue in which the gonadal vessels and the vas may be embedded. This tissue must be bluntly and carefully swept away from the sac anteriorly. Once fully separated from the elements of the cord, the sac can now be safely circumferentially excised and removed through a 10/12mm port.

Small or capillary vessel bleeding during this phase of the operation is easily controlled by pinpoint electro-coagulation. Large inguino-scrotal sacs and sacs in multiple recurrent hernias are ringed at the neck (incising the peritoneum circumferentially) and are left in place as bleeding and extensive edema may ensue if these sacs are aggressively pursued.

Once the sac is removed, a piece of mesh is prepared. The size of the mesh should be such that it covers the hernia defect and extends 3 cm beyond its rim at a minimum. We have found that a 12 x 15cm. portion of mesh covers most defects adequately. The folded mesh is introduced into the abdominal cavity; if the mesh is folded rather than rolled, once opened it will not have a tendency to curl and will be much easier to manipulate and hold in place. Once the mesh is unfolded, it is placed over the defect and held there with grasping forceps.

The superior border of the mesh in its mid portion is then tightly held against the anterior abdominal wall. Transfascial sutures are now inserted as previously described.[8] A Keith needle attached to a 00 strand of Prolene® is pushed through the abdominal wall and through the mesh (Fig. 2). The spot where the incision is to be made and where the needle is to pierce the abdominal wall, can be established by gently depressing the abdominal wall and visualizing the indentation laparoscopically. Through the same incision a 13 gauge needle is then placed through the abdominal wall and the mesh, parallel to the Keith needle.

Once the Keith needle is passed through the abdomen and mesh, it is grasped, turned around and pushed back through the lumen of the 13 gauge needle exiting through the small skin incision. A clamp is applied to the Prolene® suture at skin level holding the mesh tightly against the abdominal wall. The same procedure is repeated at both upper corners of the mesh.

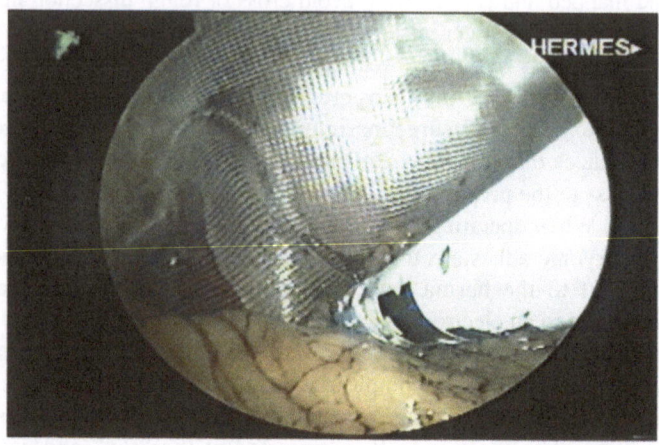

Fig. 3. Omental fixation with staples to cover the polypropylene mesh

Once placed, these three sutures hold the mesh securely in place, spreading it evenly and allowing for the rest of the mesh to be precisely and easily stapled in place. The staples are placed first on vertical sides of the mesh approximately 1 - 1.5 cm apart, then along its lower edge. Care should be taken to place the staples vertically along the inferior edge of the mesh to minimize the chances of entrapping the femoral branch of the genitofemoral nerve or the lateral-femoral cutaneous nerve. Along the lower margin of the mesh, staples should be placed lightly and further apart (2 cm) to avoid damage to the iliac vessels and the vas deferens. A few staples are also used to fix the superior and central portion of the mesh to the anterior abdominal wall. Medially, an every effort should be made to secure the mesh to Cooper's Ligament. The anteriorly placed inferior epigastric vessels immediately beneath the peritoneum should be avoided in the stapling process. Staples should not be used near the inferior and infero-lateral aspect of the internal ring for fear of injuring the structures passing through it.

Omentum is interposed between the mesh and bowel, and fixed to the abdominal wall by several lightly placed staples (Fig. 3).

The area is irrigated with saline solution and inspected for hemostasis. The subcutaneous fat below the skin incisions through which the Prolene® strands were placed is spread with a fine tip hemostat, allowing the sutures to be tied over the external oblique aponeurosis. Firm anchoring of the mesh by transabdominal stitches and staples in Cooper's Ligament prevents, in our opinion, displacement of the mesh when the abdomen is deflated and when the patient assumes the erect position. We firmly believe that it is early migration of the mesh away from its intended position that causes recurrences; therefore, we do not rely solely on staples, grasping only mesh and peritoneum, to hold the mesh in place.

To repair a contra-lateral hernia, the same procedure is carried out on the opposite side. The two pieces of mesh should overlap in the midline to diminish the chances of recurrence.

As the trocars are sequentially removed, the video camera examines the trocar sites to ensure that no bleeding is present. Finally the umbilical insertion site is observed by slowly withdrawing together the camera and its cannula. To prevent potential herniation, all 10 mm trocar sites are closed by repairing the underlying fascia or aponeurosis with 0 Vicryl® or Polysorb® sutures with the aid of a Carter-Thomason suture passer. The skin edges are approximated using Monocryl® and adhesive tape. The patients are generally discharged the evening of surgery or the following morning

RESULTS

Our experience with laparoscopic mesh hernioplasty consists of 520 hernia repairs performed on 466 patients from January 1990 through May 2001 (Table I).

Our follow-up extends for up to 84 months with a median of 68 months. There were 109 females and 357 males. We have had to date 5 (0.96%) recurrences after a unilateral laparoscopic mesh hernioplasty. One was performed on a non-previously operated hernia and at re-operation, the obvious technical mistake that caused the recurrence was the use of an inadequate size patch applied only partially over the hernia defect. The second case was that of a 67 year old male with three recurrent right inguinal herniae prior to a laparoscopic repair (Bassini, McVay, Lichstenstein). The postoperative complications in our series are listed in Table III.

In summary, IPOM laparoscopic inguinal repair still posses advantages similar to other minimally invasive procedures. Although it has been widely replaced by other laparoscopic procedures, we feel that it has to be included in any laparoscopic surgeon's armamentarium.

Table III. Main postoperative complications

Complication	No. of patients
Neuropraxia Genitofemoral 3 Femorocutaneous 9	12 (2.5%)
Seroma	15 (3.2%)
Testicular Pain	3 (0.6%)
Infection	0
Trocar herniation	0
Abdominal wall hematoma	4 (0.8%)
TOTAL	**33 (7%)**

References

1. Usher F. The repair of incisional and inguinal hernias. Surg Gynecol Obstet 1970; 131(3):525-530.

2. Lichstenstein IL, Shulman AG, Amid PK. The tension free hernioplasty. Am J Surg 1989; 157:188-193.

3. Mozingo D, Walters M, Otchy D, Rosenthal D. Properitoneal synthetic mesh repair of recurrent inguinal hernias. Surg Gyn Obst 1992; 174:33-35.

4. Musgrove J, McCready F. The Henry approach to femoral hernia. Surgery 1949; 26: 601-611.

5. Nyhus L, Condon R, Harkins H. Preperitoneal hernia repair for all types of hernia of the groin. Am J Surg 1960; 100:234-244.

6. Read R. Preperitoneal exposure of inguinal herniations. Am J Surg 1968; 116:653-658.

7. Rignault D. Properitoneal prosthetic inguinal hernioplasty through a Pfannenstiel approach. Surg Gyn Obst 2001; 163:465-468.

8. Rosenthal D, Watlers M. Properitoneal synthetic placement for recurrent hernias of the groin. Surg Gyn Obst 1986; 163:285-286.

9. Nguyen N, Camps J, Fitzgibbons R. Laparoscopic Intraperitoneal Onlay Mesh Inguinal Hernia Repair. Seminars Lap Surg 1994; 1(2):24-32.

CHAPTER 45

Paraesophageal Hernias: indications and methods for closure of the crura

M. Martín-Gómez, A. Cano, S. Morales-Conde

Hernias that develop in the esophageal hiatus have traditionally been classified into three well-defined types as proposed by Akerlund in 1926: Type I, or sliding hernia (also known as partial thoracic stomach), characterized by sliding of the cardia toward the mediastinum due to a short esophagus, whether congenital or acquired, Type II hernia (also known as paraesophageal) in which the gastric fundus slides toward the mediastinum but the cardia retains its normal position (Fig. 1), and Type III hernia (known as gastroesophageal, or mixed) in which the stomach slides toward the mediastinum, rotates 180° around its longitudinal axis (taking the cardia and the pylorus as fixed points) and assumes an intrathoracic position.

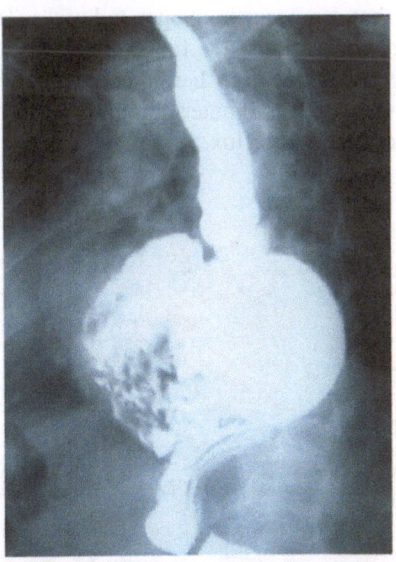

Fig. 1. Type II paraesophageal hernia, in which the gastric fundus slides toward the mediastinum but the cardia retains its normal position.

The incidence of paraesophageal hernias varies from 3.5 to 33%, depending on the series, with this type of hernia appearing more often in the second half of life. They may be primary or secondary to surgery performed in the area of the esophageal hiatus and particularly after antireflux surgery, irrespective of whether conventional surgery or laparoscopy was performed. In the latter case, the development of paraesophageal hernia or migration of the wrap to the thoracic cavity can occur in 7 to 18.8%, depending on the published series. When these patients are reoperated, many cases show that the crura, have been sectioned by the sutures placed in previous surgery. This has been attributed to the movements of the diaphragm on a sutured area in tension.

From the clinical standpoint, unlike sliding hernias, paraesophageal hernias tend to produce symptoms, predominantly dysphagia and postpandrial fullness. In 23% of cases, upper gastrointestinal bleeding may develop due to ulceration of the herniated stomach, with respiratory symptoms secondary to aspiration or compression dyspnea also being frequent. In cases with associated gastroesophageal reflux, pyrosis and regurgitation can also present. Nevertheless, the greatest risk associated with paraesophageal hernias is the high rate of extremely serious complications that is estimated at 20% (1) and that can range from massive bleeding to strangulation of the herniated stomach within the mediastinum, causing fatal mediastinitis.

INDICATIONS FOR SURGICAL TREATMENT

Paraesophageal hernias must always be repaired surgically, due to the high rate of serious complications that can occur in unoperated cases. Traditionally it has been considered that surgery must pursue the following objectives, some of them still subject to controversy: a) reduction of hernia content, b) resection of the sac, c) suture of the diaphragmatic crura, d) anterior pexis, and e) fundoplication in cases associated with gastroesophageal reflux.

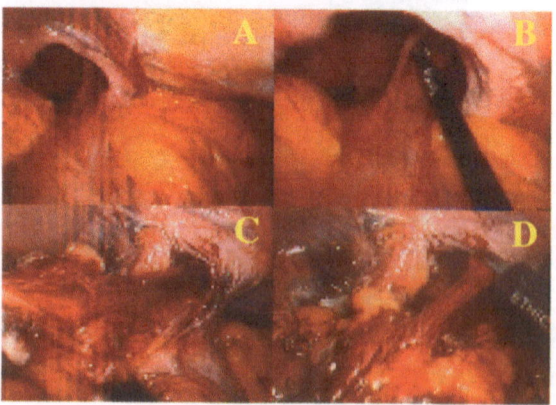

Fig. 2. A and B show the defect of the hernia with the sac, which is being resected in C and D.

Based on Cuhshieri's description in 1989 of laparoscopic fundoplication for the repair of hiatal hernias and gastroesophageal reflux disease, this minimally invasive approach was also implemented in the case of paraesophageal hernias, with a considerable number of cases already reported in the literature.

Sac content reduction is relatively easy by laparoscopy since there are generally no major adhesions to the sac and, therefore, stomach reduction is performed by simple traction. In cases where there are adhesions to the sac, the adhesions must be sectioned so that the stomach can be displaced to the abdominal cavity without difficulty.

A more controversial issue is sac resection (Fig. 2). Not all authors are in agreement as to whether complete or partial resection should be performed or whether the sac should be left in situ (2-6). Some feel that retention of the sac could lead to the development of a fluid collection within, and the appearance of complications, particularly infection (7). In contrast, sac resection facilitates exposure of the esophagus and especially the diaphragmatic crura, despite the fact that this procedure is difficult and not free of possible complications such as intraoperative hemorrhage or late postoperative hemorrhage and pleural rupture with the development of pneumothorax (4).

Another controversial question concerns whether or not the esophageal hiatus should be closed with simple suture or mesh. The rates for hernia recurrence or fundoplication migration to the thoracic cavity as well as the appearance of paraesophageal hernias in operated fundoplication patients are similar for open (8, 9) and laparoscopic surgery (10-13) and are cited at 5.7% by Stein (12), 11% by Williamson and Cadiere (8,10), 16.7% by Frantzides (14) and 18.8% by Carlson (15). Basso (16) published a series in which a 360° fundoplication was performed in 65 gastroesophageal reflux or hiatal hernia patients from November 1992 to August 1995. Fundoplication migration to the thorax was observed in nine cases (13.8%), with six of these patients being reoperated by laparoscopy. An analysis of the video tapes of the initial surgical procedure and the findings of the subsequent operation led to the conclusion that in the recurrent cases, the crura had been sutured with tension, since the reoperation showed disruption of the muscle fibers of the right crus, probably due to suture tension during the inspiratory movements of the diaphragm. Afterwards tension-free hiatoplasty was performed using a 3 x 4cm polypropylene mesh secured to the diaphragm by means of tacks. This technique was performed in 67 GERD patients from August 1995 to February 1998, with no mesh-related recurrences or complications during the mean follow-up period of 22.5 months.

In order to prevent or lower this rate of hernia recurrence, various authors (14, 15, 17, 18) have proposed closure of the crura with support or reinforcement from prosthetic materials. The use of prosthetic materials is decisive in terms of lowering hernia recurrence, as evident in several published articles. Hawasli (17) reported 27 cases that were operated for paraesophageal hernia using hiatoplasty with mesh in all cases, with no hernia recurrence in the follow-up period of 56 months. Carlson (15) conducted a study comparing 31 patients divided into two groups, one including 16 patients in which mesh was not used during crus closure, and another including 15 patients in which hiatoplasty with PTFE mesh was used. In the follow-up period, a hernia recurrence rate of 18.8% was observed in the group operated without mesh versus 0% in those repaired with mesh. In a similar study Frantzide (14) compared a group of 17 patients treated without mesh versus another group of 18 patients in which hiatal repair with PTFE mesh had been used, obtaining 16.7% of recurrences in the first group versus 0% in the second.

Based on the published data, therefore, we can conclude that mesh-reinforced cruroplasty should be used in all patients who undergo antireflux surgery in which there is a large hiatal hernia, with a ring equal to or greater than 8 cm (14), in all paraesophageal hernias and in all cases in which the sutures used to close the crura demonstrate residual tension.

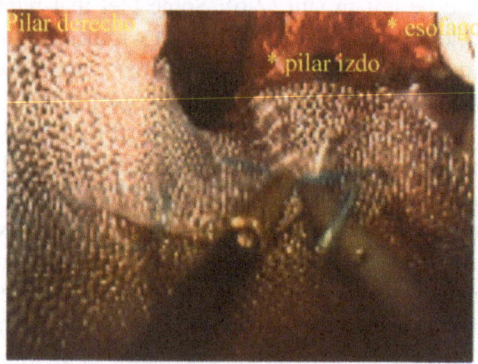

Fig. 3. Tension-free hiatoplasty with polipropilene mesh suture to the crura with non-absorbable sutures.

In terms of the type of mesh to be used, several authors (16, 20, 22) use polypropylene mesh with good results (Fig. 3). This type of mesh has the advantage of rapid tissue integration, allowing the patient early mobilization. The tendency to create adhesions when in contact with the posterior side of the esophagus and the gastric fundus would favor the fixation of these organs to the mesh, thereby preventing hernia recurrence due to migration of the wrap (21). Nevertheless, polypropylene is known to erode the lumen of viscera (23), leading to intestinal fistulas and even migration of the mesh to the visceral lumen although no published case of mesh migration or fistulization to the esophagus or stomach in cruroplasty for laparoscopic repair of hiatal hernia has been reported to our knowledge. To prevent these possible complications, authors such as Carlson (15) and Frantzides (14) advocate the use of expanded polytetrafluoroethylene mesh (ePTFE). These prosthetic materials have an advantage over polypropylene, in that they do not attach to the esophagus or stomach walls since the adhesive capacity of the side in contact with the viscera is low. Nevertheless, they should not be used in patients who are hypersensitive to chlorhexidine or silver, and have the drawback of being much more costly than polypropylene.

CRURA CLOSURE METHODS

The hiatal orifice can be closed in a number of ways, e.g., simple suture with individual stitches, suture supported on prosthetic material, crus suture with placement of a mesh (either polypropylene or PTFE) or simple placement of the mesh without bringing the crura together, which is known as tension-free hiatoplasty, a term derived from tension-free hernioplasty of inguinal hernias.

Simple suture

The V of the crura can be closed by means of simple suturing with a nonabsorbable material, consisting of suturing with individual stitches that bring together the right and left crura. This suture may be entirely done retroesophageally (Fig. 4). This approach is known as posterior cruroplasty or hiatoplasty and it requires good dissection and exposure of the crura to be performed. In this case, the hernia sac must be resectioned and retroesophagically dissected, identifying the posterior nervus vagus, until the "V" of the crura is exposed. Identifying and preserving if possible the hepatic branch of the vagus is essential. In these patients this dissection may be very difficult and significant bleeding may occur due to lesion of an aberrant hepatic artery, which can occur in 7-10% of patients.

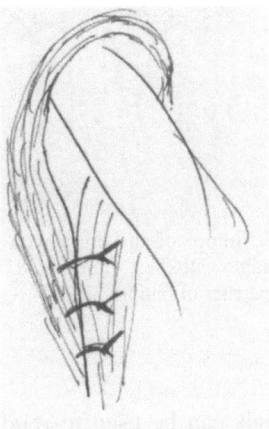

Fig. 4. Posterior cruroplasty

In anterior cruroplasty the esophageal hiatus is sutured with individual stitches of a nonabsorbable material in front of the esophagus, a tactic that may be easier in the laparoscopic approach. In both cases, either intracorporal or extracorporal tying of the sutures can be used. Nevertheless, when these sutures are made on extremely separate crura, tension may be result and tearing can occur with the respiratory movement of the diaphragm.

Mesh-reinforced suture

In order to prevent tension at the suture line or tearing of the crus muscle by the sutures with subsequent recurrence due to migration of the wrap, the use of small rectangles of mesh may be useful to support the suture thread as shown in Fig. 5.

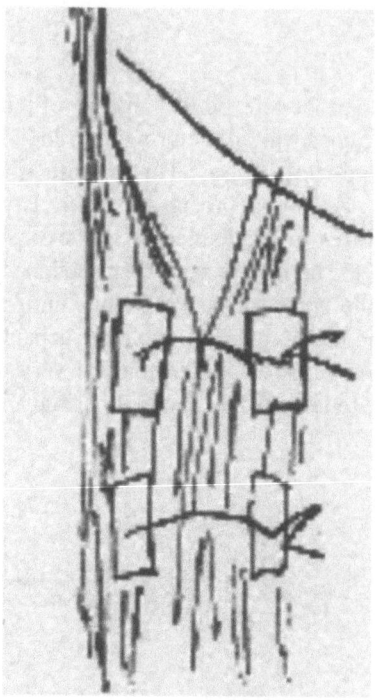

Fig. 5. Suture of the crura with non-absorbable stitches, reinforced with small patches of polipropilene.

Larger prosthetic materials can be used to reinforce the crus closure with simple sutures or as tension-free hiatoplasty, allowing some distance between the crura and closing the defect by placing a mesh that is sutured to both crura (Fig. 6 and 7).

These sutures can be done with individual stitches of nonabsorbable material with intracorporal or extracorporal tying as preferred, or by the use of tacks (Fig. 8 and 9), which enormously facilitate the procedure.

In patients with proven gastroesophageal reflux by 24-hour pH-metry, a floppy Nissen fundoplication is indicated as an antireflux procedure, although we perform the fundoplication in all cases.

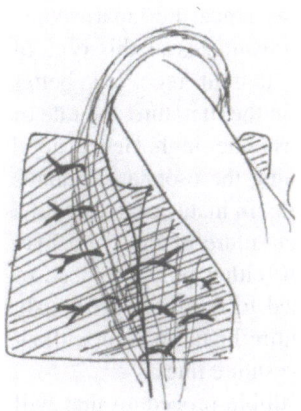

Fig. 6. Tension-free hiatoplasty with mesh sutured to the crura.

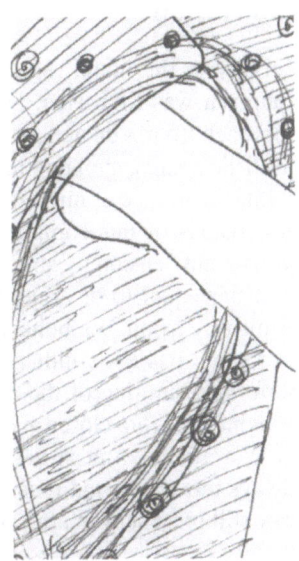

Fig. 7. Tension-free hiatoplasty with mesh fixed to the crura with tacks.

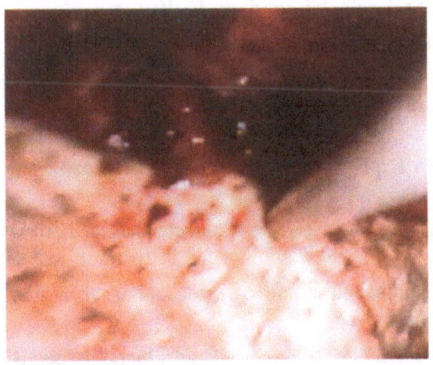

Fig. 8. Tension-free hiatoplasty with PTFE-e mesh fixed to the crura with tacks.

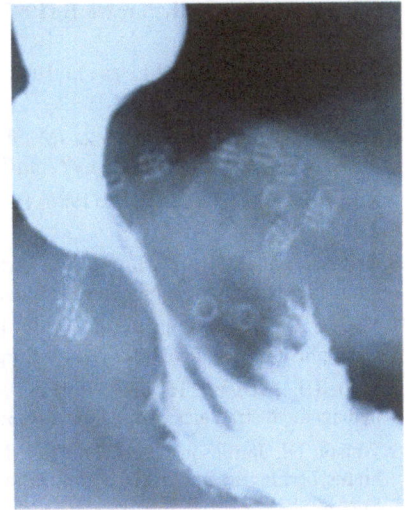

Fig. 9. Postoperative control of a tension-free hiatoplasty using a PTFE-e mesh fixed to the crura with tacks, as shown in figure 7.

Conclusion

Surgery in the hiatal region has increased considerably since the laparoscopic approach was first used. Despite the unquestionable advantages of this type of approach (e.g., decreased postoperative pain, rapid patient recovery, better aesthetic results, etc.) and in view of the data published in the literature, the rate of hernia recurrence or migration of the wrap to the thorax is rather high. Hence, good prophylaxis of this complication would consist of closing the esophageal hiatus without any tension by simple suturing whenever possible. In hiatus orifices with a diameter equal to or greater than 8 cm in which direct suture of the crura may result in tension, we believe that placement of a mesh (either polypropylene or preferably PTFE) is indicated, with the mesh positioned to reinforce previously performed suturing of the crura or securing it to the entire hiatal margin without bringing the crura closer in order to prevent tension at the suture line.

Nevertheless, mesh-based hiatoplasty is not an infallible procedure that will always prevent hernia recurrence. As occurred in one of our patients, recurrence may still present even after placement of a mesh.

References

1. Walther B, DeMeester TR, Lafontaine E et al. (1984) Effect of paraesophageal hernia on sphincter function and its implication on surgical therapy. Am. J. Surg. 147:111.

2. Fisher BL, Little AG (1995) Paraesophageal hiatal hernia. In Cameron JL (ed) Current Surgical therapy, 50th ed. Mosby-Year Book, St. Louis, Missouri, pp 36-40.

3. Kuster CG, Gilroy S (1993) Laparoscopic technique for repair of paraesophageal hiatal hernias. J Laparoendosc Surg 3: 278-281.

4. Perdikis G, Hinder RA et al. (1997) Laparoscopic paraesophageal hernia repair. Arch Surg 132:586590.

5. Rosati R, Bona S, Fumagalli U et al. (1996) Laparoscopic treatment of paraesophageal and large mixed hiatal hernias. Surg Endosc 10:429-431.

6. Wilekes CL, Edoga JK, Frezza E (1997) Laparoscopic repair of paraesophageal hernia. Ann Surg 225:31-38.

7. Oddsdottir M, Franco AL, et al. (1995) Laparoscopic repair of paraesophageal hernia. Surg Endosc 9:164-168.

8. Williamson WA, Ellis FH, Streitz JM, Shahian DS (1993) Paraesophageal hiatal hernia: is an antireflux procedure necessary? Ann Thorac Surg 56:447-452.

9. Ellis FH, Crozer RE, Shea JA (1986) Paraesophaegeal hiatus hernia. Arch Surg 121: 416-420.

10. Cadiere GB, Bruyns J, Himpens J, Vertruyen M (1996) Intrathoracic migration of the wrap after laparoscopic Nissen fundoplication. Surg Endoc 10:187 (S43).

11. Munro W, Brancatisano R, Adams IP, Falk GL (1996) Complications of laparoscopic fundoplication: the first 100 patients. Surg Laparosc Endosc 6: 421-423.

12. Stein HJ, Feussner H, Siewert JR (1996) Failure of antireflux surgery: causes and management strategies. Am J Surg 171:36-40.

13. Watson DI, Jamieson GG, Devitt PG, Mitchell PC, Game PA (1995) Paraesophaegeal hiatus hernia: an important complication of laparoscopic Nissen fundoplication. Br. J. Surg.82: 521-523.

14. Frantzides CT, Richards CG, Carlson MA (1999) Laparoscopic repair of large hiatal hernia with polytetrafluoroethylene. Surg Endosc 13 (9): 906-908.

15. Carlson MA, Richards CG, Frantzides CT (1999) Laparoscopic prosthetic reinforcement of hiatal herniorrhaphy. Dig Surg 16(5): 407-410.

16. Basso N, De Leo A, Genco A, Rosato P, et al. (2000) 360 degrees laparoscopic fundoplication with tension-free hiatoplasty in the treatment of symptomatic gastroesophageal reflux disease. Surg Endosc 14(2):164.169.

17. Hawasli A, Zonca S (1998) Laparoscopic repair of paraesophageal hiatal hernia. Am Surg 64 (8):703-10.

18. Gautert WA, Patti MG et al. (1998) Laparoscopic repair of paraesophageal hiatal hernias. J Am Coll Surg 186(4):428-32.

19. Frantzides CT, Carlson MA (1997) Prosthetic reinforcement of posterior cruroplasty during laparoscopic hiatal herniorrhaphy Surg Endosc 11:769-71.

20. Barlehennetz E, Heukrodt B (1998) Laparoscopic repair of large hiatal hernias with polypropylene mesh Zentralbl Chir 123(11):1303-5.

21. Edelman DS (1995) Laparoscopic paraesophageal hernia repair with mesh. Surg Laparosc Endosc 5:32-37.

22. Pitcher DE, Curet MU, et al. (1995) Successful laparoscopic repair of paraesophageal hernia Arch Surg 130:590-96.

23. Kaufman Z, Engelberg M, Zager M (1981) Fecal fistula: a late complication of Marlex mesh repair. Dis Colon Rectum 24:543-44.

CHAPTER 46

Paraesophageal Hernia: technique and method of fixation a mesh by laparoscopy

S. Morales-Conde, J.F. Ponce, S. Morales-Méndez

INTRODUCTION

Hiatal hernias have been traditionally associated with gastroesophageal reflux disease (GERD). Nevertheless, there are cases of reflux in which this anatomic alteration is not present and conversely, cases of hiatal hernia in which there are no associated symptoms of reflux. A clear distinction should be made between the two types of hiatal hernias in terms of anatomic characteristics, associated symptoms, management and surgical treatment.

Sliding hernias, which account for 90 to 95% of all hiatal hernias, are characterized by a migrating of the gastroesophageal junction toward the mediastinum (1). In paraesophageal hernias, the gastroesophageal junction is located in its normal position, with part of the stomach displaced cephalad and parallel to the esophagus. Cases of paraesophageal hernias with the gastroesophageal junction positioned in the mediastinum are considered "mixed" hernias.

As a result of these anatomic differences, the clinical presentation of these conditions can also show several differences. Patients presenting sliding hiatal hernias often exhibit reflux symptoms resulting from the anatomic alterations that are intrinsic to this type of hernia (2). Although paraesophageal hiatal hernias can also be accompanied by reflux, they are typically associated with another set of symptoms, derived mainly from herniation of the stomach itself, a site where erosions, ulcers and bleeding can develop. Paraesophageal hernias can also be accompanied with episodes of incarceration with retrosternal pain and dysphagia. When the herniated content is sufficiently large, it can exert pressure on the left lung, resulting in respiratory symptoms, and gastric volvulus may even occur.

Paraesophageal hernia symptoms require surgery for resolution in all cases. Hence, these patients must be handled differently from those with sliding hiatal hernias, in whom simple management of the symptoms (reflux) with medical treatment can often provide excellent results.

However, surgical repair of paraesophageal hiatal hernias or mixed hernias should be discussed separately since the management is quite different from the approach used to resolve a reflux condition or reflux associated with a sliding hiatal hernia. Surgical treatment of paraesophageal hernias constitutes a challenge for the laparoscopic approach to the abdominal cavity because of the technical difficulties involved in achieving resolution. Moreover, there are many points of controversy concerning the determining factors of surgery that influence recurrence of the hernia.

Controversies associated with laparoscopic surgical repair of paraesophageal hiatal hernias

The morbidity associated with surgical resolution of paraesophageal hiatal hernias by laparotomy or thoracotomy (3) caused a decrease in the surgical indications for this condition. However, the potential danger of developing major complications in patients who are not operated and in those managed with conservative treatment is so high, with rates of 33% (4, 5) and 45% (6) depending on the series, that attitudes toward this condition have changed, particularly since the appearance of laparoscopic surgery. Laparoscopic repair of paraesophageal hernia is associated with lower morbidity than open repair (7, 8) and results in earlier patient recovery, shorter hospitalization and faster return to normal activities. In addition, with the laparoscopic approach the anatomical structures are highly visible, allowing higher dissection of the esophagus in the mediastinum than is possible in open surgery, that is, a correct dissection of the area.

However, laparoscopic repair for this condition is relatively difficult compared to conventional antireflux surgery to treat gastroesophageal reflux disease, regardless of whether the disease is associated or not with sliding hiatal hernia. Morbidity is higher and surgical time is more lengthy (9, 10), in addition to the fact that most cases are real challenges for the surgeon. Nevertheless, there are fewer general complications arising from surgical treatment than conservative, non-surgical management of this condition (11). In our series of 353 procedures for esophageal hiatus, we had two gastric perforations (0.56%). One of them required conversion and the other was resolved by laparoscopy. Both cases were included in the 61 operated paraesophageal or mixed hernias. Our series had three conversions (0.84%), in patients with paraesophageal and mixed hernias, which in addition to the patient with gastric perforation, included two patients who developed major subcutaneous emphysema.

In addition to the technical difficulties associated with laparoscopic repair of this type of hernia, one of the main problems related to this technique is the high recurrence rate and resulting reappearance of symptoms, as high as 100% of cases in some series (12). Due to this high recurrence rate, various technical details have been proposed to avoid reappearance of the hernia, and these have been a source of controversy among authors. The debate focuses on the need to remove the sac or not, on the performance or not of fundoplication as an attachment method, gastropexy to the diaphragm or to the anterior wall of the stomach, and the discussion over the actual need for and safety involved in the use of mesh at this level to perform tension-free repair.

There now seems to be some consensus on the question of whether or not to remove the sac. For years there has been a great deal of controversy surrounding the possible need to excise the sac entirely or partially, or simply to leave it in situ (13-17), since sac removal can be associated with pleural lesions with subsequent tension pneumothorax (15). It appears to be clear, however, that removal of the sac technically aids hernia repair by facilitating mobilization of the esophagus. In addition, fluid collections in the sac have been reported in patients in whom the sac was not removed (18), with some authors making a direct correlation between hernia recurrence and maintenance of the sac (19).

One of the points of discussion centers on the need to perform a systematic fundoplication-type antireflux mechanism in all patients operated for paraesophageal hernia. There are various opinions in this regard, with some working groups only recommending the creation of fundoplication in patients presenting reflux symptoms (10). However, the need to create a systematic 360° fundoplication (20) is based on the following arguments: on the one hand, dissection of the esophageal hiatus involves destroying the anatomy of the area, thereby leading in many cases to reflux symptoms in the postoperative period (5, 8). On the other hand, depending on the series between 33% (10) and 52% (21) of patients operated for paraesophageal hernia present reflux-related symptoms, making it necessary to create an antireflux mechanism. Lastly, we should take into account that the gastric wrap is used as an anchoring mechanism to prevent hernia recurrence since it facilitates fixation of the gastroesophageal junction in the subdiaphragmatic position. Based on these arguments, we are in favor of performing a 360° fundoplication in our patients. Moreover, in our experience creation of the fundoplication is not associated with the development of dysphagia or other post-funduplication symptoms, since the elongation of stomach ligaments due to fundus migration in the hernia sac means that tension-free repair is possible. Some authors (22) take the middle ground in this discussion by recommending anterior hemifunduplication as an antireflux method and as a key component for attaching the gastroesophageal junction at the abdominal level. We used this technique in 7 patients in our series (11.5%) because of technical difficulties; these were early patients from our initial experience, in whom we did not perform sac removal.

The performance or not of a gastropexy is also debated, with some authors preferring routine fixation of the stomach to the anterior wall of the stomach to prevent further gastric rotation (20). As other authors (23), we consider that simple attachment of the stomach to the diaphragm is sufficient to prevent recurrence. Attachment to the anterior wall of the stomach is not a key factor in preventing recurrence and may be associated with complications in the case that the patient must be operated by midline laparotomy.

Another factor involved in paraesophageal hernia recurrence is the existence of a short esophagus. One of the advantages of laparoscopic repair regarding this factor is the visibility of the area, which allows correct mediastinal dissection of the esophagus. It has been shown that the actual number of patients with a short esophagus is less than might be initially believed on the basis of preoperative images. However, if the esophagus is actually short, it may be possible to perform a Collis gastric wrap using the laparoscopic approach (24) while repairing the paraesophageal hernia.

Indications for the use of mesh in esophageal hiatus

Several mechanisms have been described as the cause of failure of the antireflux mechanism when patients are treated by laparoscopy for gastroesophageal reflux disease, regardless of whether or not this is associated with sliding hernias. Among these mechanisms, the most important is migration of the fundoplication to the thoracic cavity (13, 25-30) followed by disruption of the fundoplication. Among the mechanisms to account for fundoplication migration, the following have been described (25, 30, 31): premature mobilization of the patient, resumption of normal activities and diet before adequate scar tissue is formed, excessive dissection of the esophagus in the mediastinum, accidental lesions in the left pleura with the instrumentation causing creation of a pneumothorax under tension, and disruption of crura fibers due to tension between the crura during the inspiratory movements of the diaphragm. Hence, in reflux patients with a sliding hernia in which the basic problem is the reflux condition and not the hernia, fundoplication migration due to tearing of the crura fibers resulting from tension has been reported as one of the most important problems relating to surgical failure. This becomes even more relevant when discussing closure of the crura during paraesophageal hernia repair and has led to the concept of performing the closure with prosthetic materials to prevent tension and therefore recurrence of the hernia. Some authors have already proposed the systematic use of mesh prostheses to reinforce the hiatus in patients operated for a reflux condition (regardless of whether or not it is associated with a sliding hernia) as a key component to preventing tension when closing the crura and preventing fundoplication migration (31). These authors argue that the fibrosis created by a small piece of polypropylene mesh in the hiatus ensures that there is no tension, thereby preventing migration of the wrap.

The use of mesh in the esophageal hiatus is especially indicated in paraesophageal hernias in which simple closure often involves tension with the resulting danger of recurrence. A series of large paraesophageal hiatal hernias repaired by laparoscopy has been described in which crura closure without mesh led to a recurrence rate of 100%, which subsequently dropped to 0% when the hiatus was closed with the use of mesh (12). This has led some authors to recommend the systematic use of mesh in the esophageal hiatus as a basic component to prevent recurrence (10). One randomized prospective study (32) has demonstrated that the use of PTFE mesh prostheses to close the hiatus in patients presenting hiatal hernias larger than 8 cm is associated with a statistically significant decrease in the rate of recurrence. It should be taken into account that there are no reports of complications related to the use of mesh in the hiatus (31, 32). However, some working groups have advised that mesh should not be implanted at this site because of the potential danger resulting from its use and they only recommend the use of these prostheses in cases where it is strictly necessary (20).

Currently our indications for mesh use in the hiatus are recurrent paraesophageal hernias and patients with a hiatal defect larger than 8 cm. We also believe that mesh placement is indicated in closures with excessive tension at the sutures or where the crura are not in good condition, having a small number of fibers that will tear readily.

Another point of discussion centers on the type of mesh that should be used. Some authors prefer polypropylene mesh (31) for the esophageal hiatus on the basis that the prosthesis only comes into contact with the posterior gastric wall and that the left lobe of the liver serves as a protection from possible adhesions with other intra-abdominal viscera. In addition, they defend this type of mesh because of its macroporous structure, which results in rapid incorporation and allows the patient to move freely soon after the procedure (14). Another reported advantage that supports the use of this type of mesh in the hiatus is that clear visualization of the posterior structures facilitates the anchoring of the mesh to the crura with staples (31). Moreover, polypropylene mesh is much less expensive than PTFE mesh. However, a number of experimental studies, including those carried out in our experimental surgical theater by our working group (33), contraindicate the use of polypropylene mesh at the intraperitoneal level due to the quantity of adhesions they cause and the possibility of intestinal fistulas. Hence, we prefer the use of the ePTFE mesh to avoid a possible fistula from the polypropylene mesh to the stomach or esophagus.

Management of the mesh in the esophageal hiatus

The approach to the abdominal cavity for paraesophageal hiatal hernia repair in which a mesh is to be placed is initially done in the same way as in patients undergoing fundoplication for gastroesophageal reflux disease. We typically create the pneumoperitoneum by using a Veress needle inserted in the left hypochondrium. Once the pneumoperitoneum has been established, the approach to the cavity is performed with five trocars, two of 10 mm and three of 5 mm, placed as follows: a 10-mm trocar is placed in the midline at the midpoint of the line between the umbilicus and xiphoid appendix for introduction of the scope. This approach will vary depending on the patient's physical characteristics and a more cephalad location is necessary in many cases. Once the initial trocar is in place, the remaining trocars can be introduced under direct vision. A 10-mm trocar is placed about 5-10 cm to the right of the midleline trocar. This will be used by the surgeon to handle the instrument with the right hand, to insert the ultrasonic scalpel and to introduce the suture holder system, which is also used to insert the mesh inside the cavity. A 5-mm trocar is introduced at the same distance (but on the left side) and used by the surgeon to hold the instrument with the left hand. The two remaining trocars are placed on both sides but lower than the previous trocars; one of these trocars is used to tense the stomach and the other to introduce the liver retractor. The resulting trocar arrangement creates an inverted arch (Fig. 1).

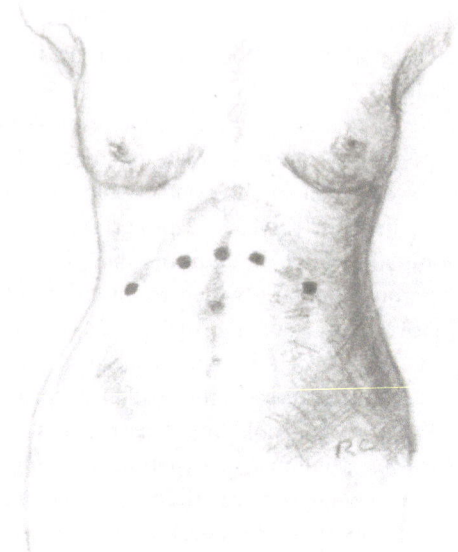

Fig. 1. Trocar position used to repair a paraesophageal hernia.

Once the scope is introduced, the hernia sac content must be reduced by tensing the stomach with one clamp to prevent the hernia content from returning to its original position and to expose the esophageal hiatus properly (Fig. 2).

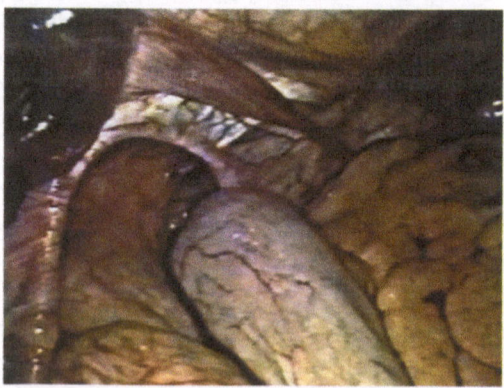

Fig. 2. Hernia defect of a paraesophageal hernia.

The hernia sac must then be dissected, starting in some cases with the left crus and taking utmost care to avoid opening the pleura (Fig. 3a and 3b). Once the sac is reduced, the various structures of the area (esophagus, vagus nerves and both diaphragmatic crura) must be correctly identified (Fig. 4).

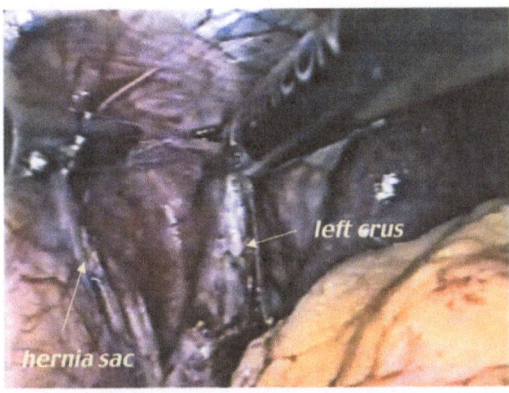

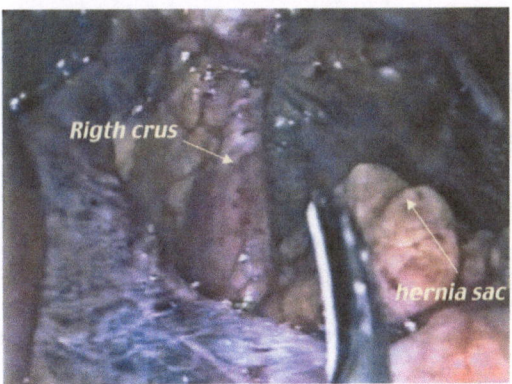

Figs. 3a and 3b. Reduction of the sac of the hernia starting in the left crus (3a), identifying later the rigth crus (3b).

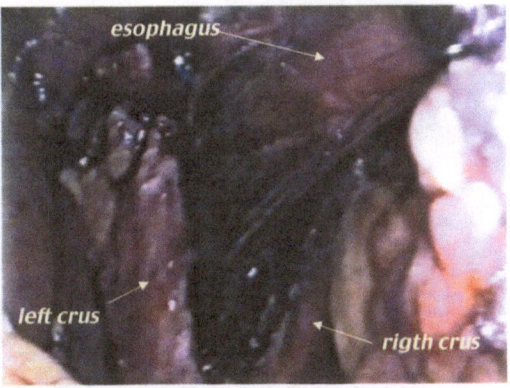

Fig. 4. Identification of the different structures of the area: esophagus and both diaphragmatic crura.

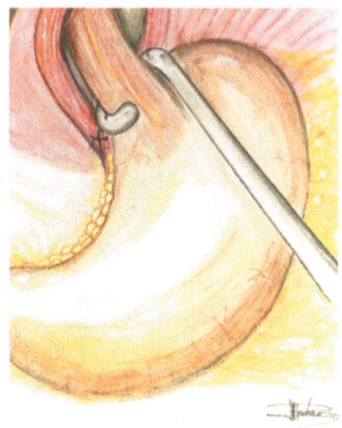

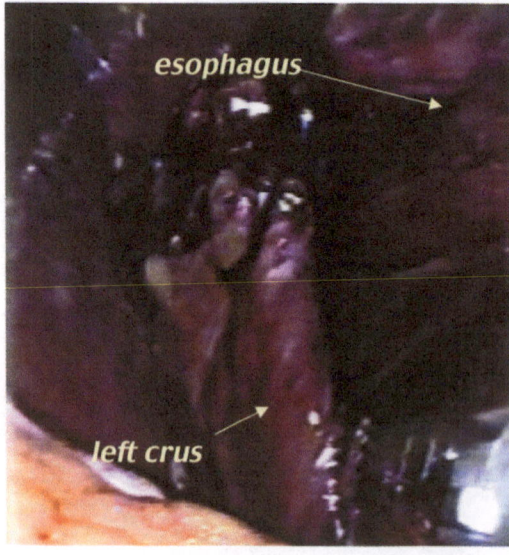

Figs. 5a, 5b and 5c.
Stitch at the junction of both crura.

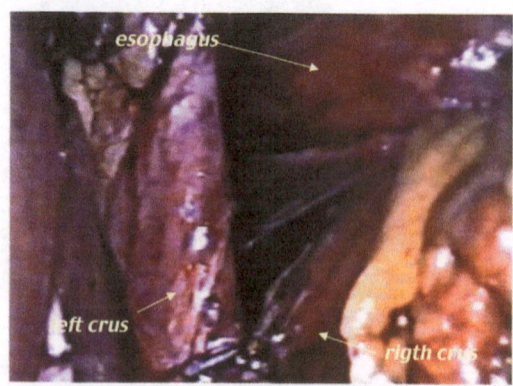

As mentioned earlier, a mesh is placed in patients with a hiatus larger than 8 cm and in patients operated on for recurrence of hiatal hernias. Comprehensive dissection of both crura to their "V" intersection is first performed. At this level a stitch with nonabsorbable material must be place at their junction to create a solid area for initial anchorage of the mesh, and to obtain a place to attach the mesh with the tacks without the risk of lesion to the aorta (Fig. 5a, 5b and 5c).

In all our cases, we used a 10 x 15cm ePTFE mesh known as "Dual-mesh plus with holes" (W.L. Gore & Associates, Flagstaff, AZ, USA) that has an oval shape, with the side of the mesh in contact with the viscera toward the abdominal cavity. We prepare the mesh for placement in the hiatus by shaping it into a "U", creating a central orifice for the esophagus with a diameter of about 5 cm in the upper half of the mesh and leaving two upper tabs that will be crossed over to hold the entire esophagus. Once the mesh is prepared, it is rolled as a cigarette and introduced in the abdominal cavity through one of the 10-mm trocars, then subsequently unrolled inside the cavity using two forceps.

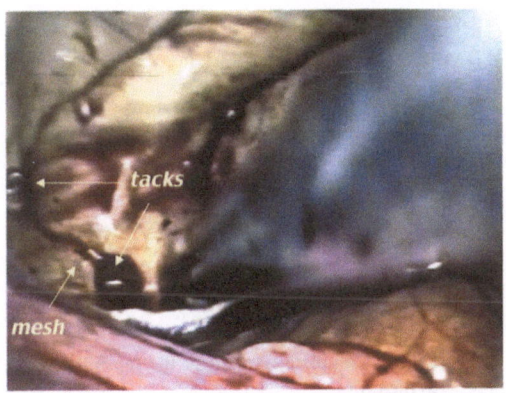

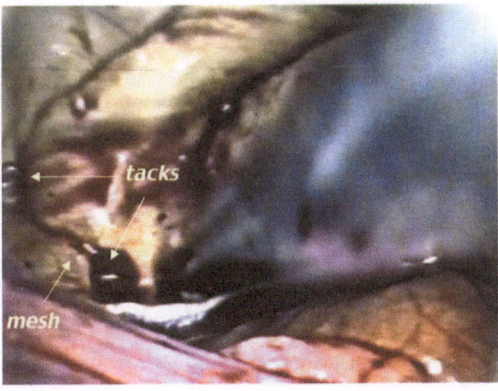

Figs. 6a and 6b. Attachment of the mesh to the lower midpoint to the area where the stitch was placed.

To place the mesh, we pass one of the tabs behind the esophagus, marking the lower midpoint and attaching it to the crura V in the area of the stitch, using a tacker (Fig. 6a and 6b). We then attach the mesh completely to both crura at both sides of the esophagus. The upper tabs are crossed in front of the esophagus and anchored one against the other with several tacks (Fig. 7). The esophagus is subsequently checked to ensure that it is not confined and that the mesh does not compress it excessively, thereby ensuring proper esophageal mobility while swallowing.

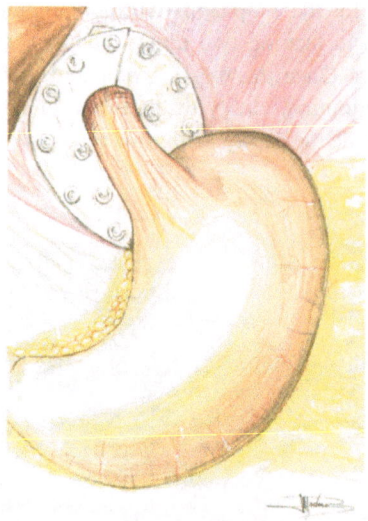

Fig. 7. Complete fixation of the mesh to the crura

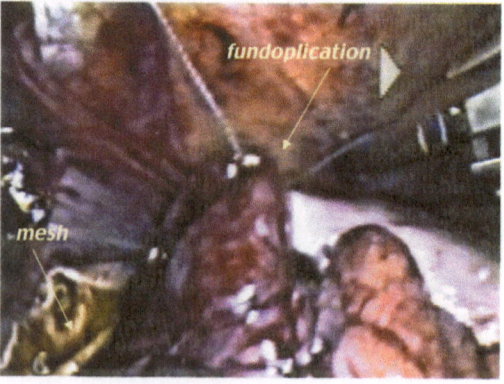

Fig. 8. Creation of a short and floppy 360° fundoplication.

Subsequently a loose, short 360° fundoplication is created (Fig. 8). Sectioning the short vessels was not required in any case in our series, since the presence of a paraesophageal hernia results in stomach displacement producing elongation and allowing a tension-free fundoplication to be created.

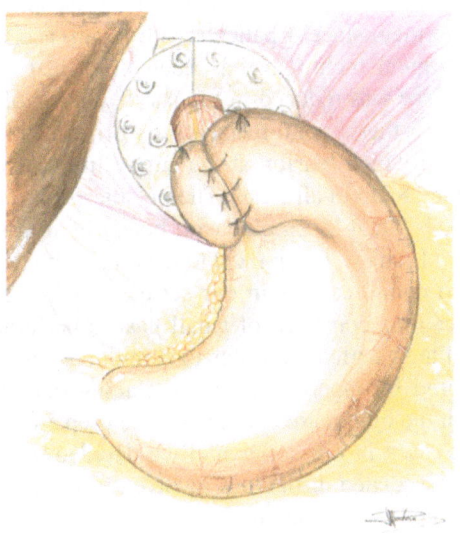

Fig. 9. Stiches from the fundoplication to the mesh to prevent recurrences.

Once the fundoplication is created, the mesh is attached to ensure that the gastroesophageal junction is anchored at the subdiaphragmatic level in order to prevent recurrence of the hernia (Fig. 9). The fundoplication is attached to the mesh with 4 or 6 nonabsorbable sutures using the endostitch. A suture (of key importance) from the postewer part of the fundoplication to the mesh is then placed. This is the area where we experienced recurrence in one patient due to insufficient attachment of the mesh at this level. As also described by other authors (34), our aim is to avoid adherence of the mesh to the posterior wall of the gastric wrap rather than the posterior wall of the esophagus which will function as a gastropexy, after fixing it to the mesh, anchoring the stomach in its normal anatomical position and preventing migration. The fundoplication is then attached to the mesh on both sides with one or two sutures (one higher and one lower) that reinforce the posterior fixation of the mesh. On occasion we have enclosed the fundoplication, the crus and the mesh in these lateral sutures, to ensure mesh attachment to the crura. Lastly, we add one suture of the fundoplication to both tabs of the mesh where they cross at the anterior level. As a result, we are able to ensure correct attachment of the fundoplication to the mesh in a manner similar to gastropexy, preventing migration and hernia recurrence.

OUR EXPERIENCE

Three hundred and fifty-three patients were operated on by our gastroesophageal reflux working group using the laparoscopic approach. We retrospectively evaluated the outcome of 61 consecutive patients with type II (22 patients) or III (39 patients) paraesophageal hernias treated laparoscopically, in which 65 operations were performed, since 4 patients with recurrence were reoperated by laparoscopy. The surgical technique has been described earlier, taking into account only that the sac was reduced in the last few cases of our series and -as we have mentioned- prosthesis reinforcement was performed in recurrent hernias and primary hernias in which tension at the suture line was observed, with the defect being larger than 8 cm in all cases. The prosthesis placed in the hiatus was a 10 x 15 ePTFE mesh (Dual-Mesh plus with holes) in all cases. The mesh was prepared by creating a U shape, being fixed to the crura with tacks.

We had only two complications in our series, which accounts for 3.1% of cases; these complications consisted of small gastric perforations that resulted from manipulation of the gastric fundus due to continuous traction of the stomach. One case was repaired by laparoscopy after placing one suture to close the perforation. Although the other case could have been repaired laparoscopically, it was one of the first cases in our series and we decided to open for the repair because of potential associated difficulties involved in laparoscopic resolution of the giant hernia presented by this patient.

Four patients of the 65 cases were converted to open surgery (6.1%): one of them was the above case of gastric perforation in an obese patient with a giant mixed hiatal hernia. The reason for conversion was related more to the difficulties in dissection than to the perforation itself; two of them were due to massive emphysema after a large mediastinal dissection of the esophagus once the dissection of the hernia sac was completed; and the other case was a recurrence presented by a patient with a prosthesis from a previous surgery, in which laparoscopic repair was not possible because of the intense fibrosis created between the mesh and the gastric fundus of the fundoplication.

Simple closure of the crura was performed in 55 cases, with a prosthesis placed in 9 cases: 6 primary and 3 recurrent paraesophageal hernias. A 360° funduplication was associated in all cases, with division of short gastric vessels not necessary in any case. However, paraesophageal hernias present more difficulties for the performance of an antireflux procedure when the sac is not excised, as occurred in our initial experience. Of our initial 61 paraesophageal and mixed hernias, the posterior hiatus could not be dissected in 7 since the posterior part of the sac did not allow us to perform the dissection. As a result, an anterior fundoplication (Dor procedure) was performed.

Mention should also be made of the fact that there were no complications during the postoperative period and no mesh-related complications occurred. Patients did not show any symptoms other than light dysphagia in a few cases, and other post-fundoplication symptoms or reflux were not present.

The recurrence rate of the series was 6.1% (4 of 65 cases). Simple closure was performed in 3 of these 4 patients all of them among the initial cases of our series in which the sac was not excised. One of these patients had a paraesophageal hernia larger than 8 cm in which mesh was not placed due to our lack of experience, and in which the sutures were left under tension. The other recurrence corresponded to one patient in which a cruroplasty with mesh was performed, with subsequent herniation observed due to a failure in posterior fixation of the fundoplication to the mesh.

Table I. Methods used to close the diaphragmatic crura in our series

PARAESOPHAGEAL AND MIXED HIATAL HERNIAS	64 (61 patients)	
Simple closure	55	86.1%
Closure with mesh	9	13.9%

Table II. Complications during laparoscopic repair of paraesophageal and mixed hernias

COMPLICATIONS		
Intraoperative complications	2	3.1%
Conversion	4	6.1%
Gastric perforation	1	1.5%
Massive emphysema	2	3.1%
Fundus-mesh fibrosis	1	1.5 %

CONCLUSIONS

The sac must be excised to avoid recurrences during laparoscopic repair of paraesophageal hernias. Reinforcement of the crura with mesh is a good method to decrease the recurrence rate in large and recurrent hernias. There are no complications related to the use of protheses or to the tack-based fixation method, with a key factor being proper fixation of the fundus to the mesh to prevent recurrences.

References

1. Fleshler B. Esophagitis and hiatal hernia. In: Farmer RG, Achkar E, Fleshler B. Clinical gastroenterology. Raven Press, New York. 1983 (169-83).
2. Morales-Conde, S. Tratamiento por vía laparoscópica de la enfermedad por reflujo gastroesofágico. McGraw-Hill, Madrid. 1998.
3. Paul MG, DeRosa RP, Petrucci PE, Palmer ML, Danovitch SH. Laparoscopic tension-free repair of large paraesophageal hernias. Surg Endosc 1997; 11:303-307.
4. Oddsdottir M, Franco AL, Laycock WS, Waring JP, Hunter JG. Laparoscopic repair of paraesophageal hernia. Surg Endosc 1995; 9:164-168.
5. Perdikis G, Hinder RA, Filipi CJ, Walenz T, McBride PJ, Stephen SL, Katada N, Klingler PJ. Laparoscopic paraesophageal hernia repair. Arch Surg 1997; 132:586-590.
6. Treacy PJ, Jamieson GG. An approach to the management of paraesophageal hernias, Aust N Z J Surg 1987; 57:813-817.

7. Huntington TR. Short-term outcome of laparoscopic paraesophageal hernia repair. Surg Endosc 1997; 11:894-898.

8. Willekes CL, Edoga JK, Frezza E. Laparoscopic repair of paraesophageal hernia. Ann Surg 1997; 225:31-38.

9. Wu JS, Dunnegan DL, Soper NJ. The influence of surgical technique on clinical outcome of laparoscopic Nissen fundoplication. Surg Endosc 1996; 10:1164-1170.

10. Hawasli A, Zonca S. Laparoscopic repair of paraesophageal hiatal hernia. Am Surg 1998; 64:703-710.

11. Trus TL, Bax T, Richardson WS, Branum GD, Mauren SJ, Swanstrom LL, Hunter JG. Complications of laparoscopic paraesophageal hernia repair. J Gastrointest Surg 1997; 1(3):221-228.

12. Basso N, Rosato P, De Leo A, Genco A, Rea S, Neri T. "Tension-free" hiatoplasty, gastrophrenic anchorage, and 360 degrees fundoplication in the laparoscopic treatment of parasophageal hernia. Surg Laparosc Endosc Percutan Tech 1999; 9(4):257-262.

13. Dallamagne B, Weerts JM, Jehaes C, Marchiewicz S. Causes of failures of laparoscopic antireflux operations. Surg Endosc 1996; 10:305-310.

14. Holzman MD, Purut CM, Reintgen K, Eubanks S, Pappas TN. Laparoscopic ventral and incisional hernioplasty. Surg Endosc 1997; 11:32-35.

15. Peters JH, DeMeester TR. Indications, benefits and outcome of laparoscopic Nissen fundoplication. Dig Dis 1996; 14:169-179.

16. Snow LL, Weinstein LS, Hannon JK. Laparoscopic reconstruction of gastroesophageal anatomy for the treatment of reflux disease. Surg Endosc 1995; 9:774-780.

17. Watson DI, Baigrie RJ, Jamieson GG. A learning curve for laparoscopic fundoplication: definable, avoidable or a waste of time? Ann Surg 1996; 224:198-364.

18. Kuster GGR, Innocenti FA. Laparoscopic anatomy of the region of the esophageal hiatus. Surg Endosc 1997; 11:883-893.

19. Van der Peet DL, Klinkenberg-Knol EC, Alonso Poza A, Sietses C, Cuesta MA. Laparoscopic treatment of large paraesophageal hernias: both excision of the sac and gastropexy are imperative for adequate surgical treatment. Surg Endosc 2000; 14(11):1015-1018.

20. Wu JS, Dunnegan DL, Soper NJ. Clinical and radiological assessment of laparoscopic paraesophageal hernia repair. Surg Endosc 1999; 13;497-502.

21. Gantert WA, Patti MG, Arcerito M, Feo C, Stewart L, DePinto M, Bhoyrul S, Rangel S, Tyrrell D, Fujino D, Mulvihill SJ, Way LW. Laparoscopic repair of paraesophageal hiatal hernias. J Am Coll Surg 1998; 186(4):428-432.

22. Athanasakis H, Tzortzinis A, Tsiaoussis J, Vassilakis JS, Xynos E. Laparoscopic repair of paraesophageal hernia. Endoscopy 2000; 33(7):590-594.

23. Kuster GG, Gilroy S. Laparoscopic technique for repair of paraesophageal hernias. J Laparoendosc Surg 1993; 3(4):331-338.

24. Swanstrom LL, Marcus DR, Galloway GO. Laparoscopic Collis gastroplasty is the treatment of choice for the shortened esophagus. Am J Surg 1996; 172:477-481.

25. Cadiere GB, Bruyns J, Himpens J, Vertruyen M. Intrathoracic migration of the wrap after laparoscopic Nissen fundoplication. Surg Endosc 1996; 187:43.

26. Johanson B, Glise H, Hallerbäck B. Thoracic herniation and intrathoracic gastric perforation after laparoscopic fundoplication. Surg Endosc 1995; 9:917-918.

27. Munro W, Brancatisano R, Adams IP, Falk GL. Complications of laparoscopic fundoplication: the first 100 patients. Surg Laparosc Endosc 1996; 6:421.423.

28. Rieger NA, Jamieson GG, Britten-Jones R. Reoperation after failed antireflux surgery. Br J Surg 1994; 81:1159-1161.

29. Stein HJ, Feussner H, Siewert JR. Failure of antireflux surgery: causes and management strategies. Am J Surg 1996; 171:36-40.

30. Watson DI, Jamieson GG, Devitt PG, Mitchell PC, Game PA. Paraesophageal hiatus hernia: an important complication of laparoscopic Nissen fundoplication. Br J Surg 1995; 82:521-523.

31. Basso N, De Leo A, Genco A, Rosato P, Rea S, Spaziani E, Primavera A. 360° fundoplication with tension-free hiatoplasty in the treatment of symptomatic gastroesophageal reflux disease. Surg Endosc 2000; 14:164-169.

32. Carlson MA, Richards CG, Frantzides CT. Laparoscopic prosthesic reinforcement of hiatal herniorraphy. Dig Surg 1999; 16(5):407-410.

33. Ponce JF, Barriga R, Martín I, Morales-Conde S, Morales S. Prosthetic materials in incisional hernia. Experimental study. Cir Esp 1998; 63(3):189-194.

34. Edelman DS. Laparoscopic paraesophageal hernia repair with mesh. Surg Laparosc Endosc 1995; 5:32-37.

CHAPTER 47

Laparoscopic Diaphragmatic Hernia Repair

D.S. Thoman, T. Hui, E.H. Phillips

INTRODUCTION

Extensive experience has been gained with the laparoscopic approach to the diaphragm in recent years. However, this experience is almost exclusively with the various types of hiatal hernia repair. Traumatic and congenital diaphragmatic defects are much less common, and each present unique obstacles to a minimally invasive approach. However, with the proper training, equipment and circumstance most of the unusual diaphragmatic hernias are amenable to laparoscopic repair. Furthermore, patients can expect the same well-known benefits of minimal access surgery, with a recurrence rate similar to the open approach.

ANATOMY AND EMBRYOLOGY

The diaphragm is a dome-shaped, musculotendinous structure separating the thoracic and abdominal cavities. Its embryology is complex and not yet fully understood. The diaphragm is formed by the septum transversum, pleuroperitoneal membranes, dorsal mesentery of the esophagus and body wall muscles (1). During its caudal migration the septum transversum passes the third, fourth and fifth segments of the neck where it is joined by what will become the phrenic nerve (1).

The right phrenic nerve enters directly lateral to the caval opening into the central tendon. The left phrenic enters directly lateral to the left border of the heart and in front of the central tendon into the muscular part of the diaphragm. The intradiaphragmatic branching of the phrenic nerves must be considered when incising or suturing the diaphragm. Fortunately, this branching is fairly constant and is demonstrated in Figure 1 (2). Safe areas for extending a phrenotomy are shown here.

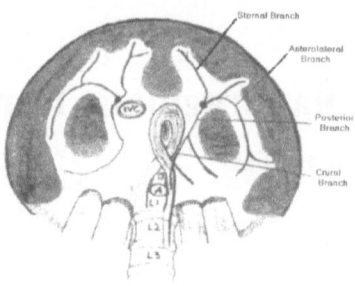

Fig. 1. Major branches of the phrenic nerve as seen from below. Areas where phrenotomy may be performed with relative safety are shaded. (Modified from Nyhus L, Baker R, Fischer J (eds). Mastery of Surgery. Boston: Little, Brown and Co. Reproduced with permission).

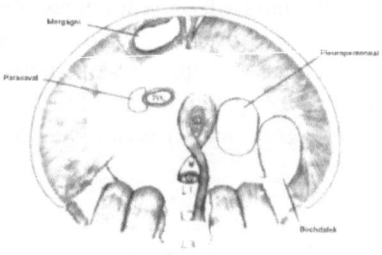

Fig. 2. Typical locations for congenital diaphragmatic hernias as seen from below. (Modified from Nyhus L, Baker R, Fischer J (eds). Mastery of Surgery. Boston: Little, Brown and Co. Reproduced with permission).

The pericardiophrenic, musculophrenic and superior phrenic arteries are smaller vessels supplying the cranial side of the diaphragm. Small direct branches from the aorta also supply the dorsal diaphragm. Most of the blood flow comes from the inferior phrenic arteries, which arise from the aorta or celiac axis just below the median arcuate ligament (1). The venous drainage can be variable but tends to follow the arteries.

The diaphragm contains well-defined openings for the esophagus, vena cava and aorta, as well as, several areas of potential herniation. The foramen of Bochdalek posterolaterally and the foramen of Morgagni and Larrey on either side of the xiphoid process are two common areas of congenital herniation. Rarely congenital hernias, which are difficult to explain embryologically, occur in the pleuroperitoneal, peritoneopericardial and paracaval areas (1). These areas are demonstrated in Figure 2.

The crura arise from the anterior longitudinal ligament, intervertebral discs, and the anterior surface of L1 to L4 on the right and L1 to L2 or L3 on the left.(2) In 90 % of cadavers the crura were found to be tendinous posteriorly and medially, from their vertebral origins to the level of T10 (3). When suturing the crura the tendinous portion, as well as, the endoabdominal fascia must be incorporated in the closure for adequate strength.

The diaphragm is the chief respiratory muscle in the body, with both inspiratory and expiratory functions. On fluoroscopy, diaphragmatic excursion is 3-6cm in 75% of patients, less than 3cm in 23%, and over 6cm in 2% (4). In addition to having a slightly greater excursion, the left hemidiaphragm also moves more rapidly (4).

CONGENITAL DIAPHRAGMATIC HERNIAS

Congenital hernias of the diaphragm can be classified into four different types – eventration of the diaphragm, posterolateral hernia of Bochdalek, parasternal hernia of Morgagni-Larrey and peritoneopericardial hernia (1). However, the term congenital diaphragmatic hernia usually refers to the most common posterolateral type of hernia, first described by Bochdalek in 1848. Development of a Bochdalek type hernia occurs at 8 – 10 weeks of gestation from failure of closure of the posterolateral aspect of the pleuroperitoneal canal (2). This anomaly is invariably associated with pulmonary hypoplasia and pulmonary hypertension with persistent fetal circulation leading to respiratory failure in the neonatal period. Repair of the diaphragmatic defect is usually performed in the postnatal period after improvement in pulmonary function and reversal of pulmonary hypertension. Laparoscopic diaphragmatic repair is generally not feasible in these infants because of the risk of pneumoperitoneum. However, approximately 5% of patients with Bochdalek hernias have small defects which are detected after the neonatal period (2). In addition to two cases of thoracoscopic repair, three attempts at laparoscopic repair appear in the English language literature (5, 6). Al-Emadi reported laparoscopic repair of a Bochdalek hernia on a 38 year-old women presenting with acute epigastric pain (5). Two defects were found in the left hemidiaphragm and were closed with e-PTFE mesh. Van der Zee described a primary laparoscopic repair in a 6 month old boy (6). Mar Fan et al. attempted laparoscopic repair of an incarcerated Bochdalek hernia in a 32-year-old women, but converted to laparotomy when an enterotomy was suspected (7).

Table I. English language case reports of laparoscopic repair of Morgagni-Larrey hernias

Author	Age (yrs)	Defect size (cm)	Sac removed	Mesh	Complication
Kuster (1992) [9]	67	-	No	no	no
Rau (1994) [12]	42	6	Yes	yes	no
Newmann (1995) [13]	57	-	Yes	yes	no
	22	-	Yes	no	no
	70	10x15	Yes	no	no
Smith (1995) [14]	60	2x3, 5	No	no	no
Fernandez-Cebrian (1996) [15]	53	10x15	Yes	no	no
Huntington (1996) [16]	32	4x9	No	yes	no
Orita (1997) [17]	78	2x4	No	yes	no
Vanclooster (1997) [18]	42	10x4	No	yes	no
Contini (1998) [19]	85	7x4	No	no	Enterotomy
Nguyen (1998) [20]	38	5x6	Yes	yes	no
Bortul (1998) [21]	61	6x10	No	yes	Post-op A-fib
Del Castillo (1998) [22]	50	12x15	No	yes	no
Ramachandran (1999) [10]	58	8x5	No	yes	no
Lima (2000) [23]	3	10x5	No	no	no

Unlike the Bochdalek hernia, the Morgagni-Larrey hernia is usually not symptomatic in the neonatal period and may present in adulthood with visceral incarceration. The defect occurs between attachments of the diaphragm to the xiphoid process and the seventh costal cartilage. This retro-xiphoid space is termed Larrey's gap on the left and Morgagni's gap on the right, and is normally filled with the superior epigastric vessels and fat. In asymptomatic patients the defect is often discovered on a routine chest radiograph or CT scan performed for other reasons. Symptomatic patients may present with signs of visceral incarceration and are diagnosed with a CT scan, MRI or contrast study. Surgical repair is usually indicated even in asymptomatic patients because of the risk of incarceration (8). Repair can be achieved via a transabdominal or transthoracic approach. With advances in minimally invasive surgery, laparoscopic repair of these hernias has been performed. Kuster carried out the first laparoscopic repair of a Morgagni hernia in 1992 (9). A total of 16 cases of laparoscopically repaired Morgagni hernias have been reported in the literature and are detailed in Table I.

Morgagni hernias often have a sac that may be quite adherent to the pleura and pericardium making sac excision difficult. In two-thirds of the reported cases, the hernia contents were reduced and the defect repaired without excision of the sac. Whether or not this influences long-term recurrence or cyst formation is uncertain due to the limited experience and lack of objective long-term follow-up.

In the case report by Ramachandran, repair of the hernia without excision of the sac led to almost complete disappearance of the sac on CT scan one month after repair (10). A second area of controversy is the method of defect closure. Small defects can generally be sutured laparoscopically. However, defects larger than 20-30 cm^2 should probably be closed with mesh to avoid tension. A 2-5% fistula rate has been reported when using polypropylene mesh in ventral hernia closure, whereas fistulization has not occurred with PTFE (11). Therefore, PTFE or a composite prosthetic with PTFE and polypropylene is preferred.

TRAUMATIC DIAPHRAGMATIC HERNIAS

Penetrating trauma accounts for more than 90% of diaphragmatic injuries in the U.S.. The diaphragm is lacerated in 10%-15% of penetrating thoracic injuries and 0.8% to 1.6% of patients with blunt trauma (24). Unrecognized diaphragmatic rupture may occur in as many as 66% of patients with polytrauma (4). Spontaneous closure of a rupture does not occur, however omental interposition may temporarily seal a tear (4). Therefore, the identification of a diaphragmatic defect is an indication for repair. Ruptures tend to occur at the central tendon or at the boundary between the tendinous and muscular part of the diaphragm. In blunt trauma, the rupture occurs on the left 65-85% of the time, the right 15-35%, and bilateral 1-12% (3, 4). Reasons for the disparity are protection of the right side by the liver, underdiagnosis on the right, and weakness of the left hemidiaphragm at points of embryonic fusion of the pleuroperitoneal canals.

Although acutely herniated viscera may closely mimic a tension pneumothorax, diaphragmatic injury alone rarely causes hemodynamic compromise. Symptoms of acute injury include dyspnea, orthopnea, and chest or scapular pain. Blunt trauma is often associated with significant concomitant injury and, in fact, one-third of these patients present with hypotension and hypoxia (4). Blunt diaphragmatic injuries are associated with a 40% incidence of pelvic fractures, a 25% incidence of both hepatic and splenic injuries and a 5% incidence of thoracic aortic tears (24). Demetriades reported a 75% incidence of associated intra-abdominal injury with penetrating injury to the diaphragm (25).

Several diagnostic modalities may be used to identify a diaphragm injury including chest radiography (with or without contrast studies), ultrasound, CT scan, and MRI. Laparoscopy and thoracoscopy have also been used successfully. Thoracoscopy does not require insufflation and has a sensitivity and specificity approaching 100% (26). Unfortunately, only one hemidiaphragm can be inspected at a time, and there is no way to evaluate accompanying abdominal injury. It may be best suited for right-sided penetrating injuries less than 3 cm (26) .

The role of laparoscopy in the evaluation of the acutely injured patient is still evolving. The disadvantages include the need for general anesthesia, the risks of access, gas embolism, and tension pneumothorax. However, several reports in the literature confirm the safety and efficacy of laparoscopy for both diagnosis and repair of acute injuries (27-29). Good candidates would be hemodynamically stable, without obvious evidence of serious intra-abdominal injury (protruding viscera, peritoneal signs, blood in the gastrointestinal tract) and have had minimal prior abdominal surgery. Zantut reported the results of 510 diagnostic laparoscopies for penetrating injury at three trauma centers (29). Peritoneal penetration was not found in 277 (54%) patients who were spared laparotomy. Twenty-six patients had a therapeutic procedure performed laparoscopically, including 16 diaphragm repairs. Fabian performed diagnostic laparoscopy on 182 patients with both penetrating and blunt trauma and found 11 (6%) diaphragm injuries (28).

Most reports of laparoscopic diaphragm repair have been in the acute setting. The typical scenario involves a penetrating injury for which laparoscopy was used as a diagnostic tool. Trauma surgeons, with variable laparoscopic experience, often perform the procedure. Primary repair is the rule and can be performed with staples, running or interrupted sutures. Defects larger than $25cm^2$ will usually require prosthetic repair or repositioning of the diaphragm (30). In either case, the associated injuries with that level of trauma would preclude a laparoscopic approach.

For acute injury, the supine position is used most commonly to allow for a thorough abdominal exploration. Cougard reported improved visualization and easier reduction of herniated organs with the lateral position in seven patients with acute diaphragm injury (31). However, abdominal exploration was not performed, and this position should be reserved for patients several days out from injury not requiring a proper diagnostic procedure. Pneumatic compression stockings are used for thromboembolism prophylaxis, if the patient's condition permits. A wide surgical prep from the neck to the knees is performed. The chest must always be included in the surgical field in case urgent anterolateral thoracotomy or tube thoracostomy is required.

A 30-45∞ angled laparoscope is essential for adequate visualization. At least two other working ports will be needed for suturing, one of which should be at least 10 mm to allow introduction of a large curved needle. Alternatively, 5 mm ports may be used with canoe-shaped needles. Additional 5 mm working ports should be placed without hesitation to allow for retraction of the various abdominal organs. Ports should be placed at least 5 cm or, more optimally, 10 cm away from each other to minimize "sword-fighting." Figure 3 demonstrates typical port placement for an acute left-sided defect.

There is no data favoring interrupted over running, permanent over absorbable suture or two layer over single layer closure. Our preference is to use a braided permanent suture in either running or interrupted fashion depending on the size and location of the defect. Polyglactin probably absorbs too quickly. Silk, polypropylene and polydioxanone are easily damaged by handling with the laparoscopic instruments.

Pneumothorax is an obvious and recognized complication of laparoscopic diaphragm repair. Symptoms when present are usually minimal and can be improved by lowering the insufflation pressure and adding PEEP. Zantut et al. had four (0.8%) cases of tension pneumothorax in 510 laparoscopies (29). Tension pneumothorax occurred in one of 24 laparoscopically diagnosed diaphragm injuries by Fabian (28). Ivatury experienced one tension pneumothorax in 17 patients with diaphragmatic defects found on diagnostic laparoscopy (27). All of these patients were diagnosed immediately and responded to tube thoracostomy decompression without sequelae. However, this demonstrates the need for both vigilance and a ready course of action. Pneumothorax has not been reported in the laparoscopic repair of chronic diaphragmatic hernias, possibly secondary to the presence of intrathoracic adhesions.

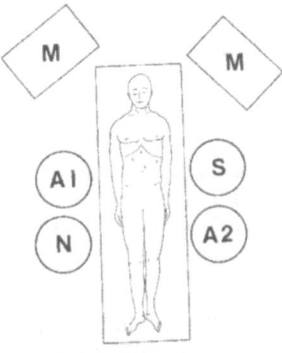

Fig. 3. Patient positioning and typical port placement for abdominal exploration and repair of acute left diaphragmatic hernia. The second assistant is optional.

Concern has also been raised over the potential for gas embolism in patients with acute trauma who may have liver or vascular injuries. Clinically apparent gas embolization is rare, occurring in only 15 of 115,253 gynecologic laparoscopies (32). Patients undergoing repair of acute diaphragmatic injuries may be at increased risk due to a low central venous pressure and the need for reverse Trendelenberg positioning. However, gas embolization has yet to be reported in laparoscopy for trauma. In Fabian's study there were 27 liver injuries and three major vascular injuries without evidence of embolization (28).

CHRONIC DIAPHRAGMATIC HERNIAS

Unlike acute injuries where minimal dissection is required, chronic defects will often have intense fibrosis between the hernia sac, pleura, and abdominal viscera. Dissection planes are often difficult to discern and the chance of injury to the herniated abdominal organs, lung and mediastinum is much greater (33). Consequently at the time of this writing, there are only 11 reports in the English language literature of successful repair. Tables II and III detail these reports.

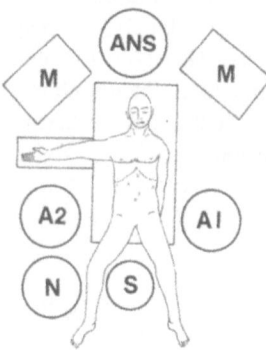

Fig. 4. Patient positioning and typical port placement for repair of chronic diaphragmatic hernia.

When repairing chronic hernias, positioning and port placement will depend on the location and size of the defect. A modified lithotomy position with the surgeon between the legs is usually best for most defects (Figure 4). An optical port is placed four finger-breaths below the costal margin and several centimeters off midline, depending on hernia location, being careful to avoid the superior epigastric vessels. The true lateral position has also been reported to give adequate exposure (31). As with congenital hernias, PTFE should be used to close larger defects in a tension free manner. Although data on complications and recurrence is limited, preliminary results are very favorable.

Table II. English language case reports of laparoscopic repair of chronic diaphragmatic hernias

Author	Location/Size	Time from Injury	Operative time (min)	Type of repair
Pross (2000) [34]	Left/ 10 cm	2 yrs.	145	Polydiaxone patch, pledgets
Meyer (2000) [35]	Right/ -	10 yrs.	125	Nonabsorbable 0 mattress sutures
Torresini (2000) [36]	Left/ 7 cm	6 mos.	45	Mersilene mesh, endo-clips
Matz (2000) [37]	Left/ 5 cm	2-6 mos.	40	Primary repair
	Right/ 10 cm	2-6 mos.	60	PTFE patch
	Left/ 4 cm	2-6 mos.	90	Primary repair
Shah (2000) [33]	Left/ 6 cm	23 mos.	160	PTFE patch
Slim (1998) [38]	Left/ 12 cm	13 mos.	-	Polypropylene patch
Domene (1998) [39]	Left/ 12 cm	12 mos.	-	Primary repair
Rasiah (1995) [40]	Left/ 5 cm	5 wks.	90	Primary repair
Campos (1991) [41]	Left/ 7.5 cm	21 yrs.	-	PTFE patch

Table III. English language case reports of laparoscopic repair of chronic diaphragmatic hernias

Author	Perioperative complications	Length of Stay (days)	Follow-up
Pross (2000) [34]	None	7	2 mos.
Meyer (2000) [35]	None	6	42 mos.
Torresini (2000) [36]	None	-	-
Matz (2000) [37]	Trocar site hernia	3	18 mos.
	None	5	18 mos.
	None	7	18 mos.
Shah (2000)33	None	2	6 mos.
Slim (1998)38	None	7	3 mos.
Domene (1998)39	None	5	-
Rasiah (1995)40	None	2	18 mos.
Campos (1991)41	None	1	1 wk.

References

1. Schumpelick V, Steinau G, Schluper I, Prescher A (2000) Surgical embryology and anatomy of the diaphragm with surgical applications. Surg Clin North Am 80:213-39.

2. Skandalakis LJ CG, Skandalakis JE (1997) Surgical anatomy of the diaphragm. In Nyhus LM, Baker RJ, Fischer JE (eds) Mastery of Surgery. Little Brown and Co., Boston, pp 649 - 670.

3. Gray SW RJJ, Skandalakis JE (1979) Surgical anatomy of the gastroesophageal junction. Am Surg 45:575.

4. Wilson RF, Bender JS (1996) Diaphragmatic Injuries. In Wilson RW, Walt AJ (eds) Management of Trauma. William and Wilkins, Philadelphia, pp 432-448.

5. Al-Emadi M, Helmy I, Nada M, Al-Jaber H (1999) Laparoscopic repair of Bochdalek hernia in an adult. Surg Laparosc Endosc 9(6): 423-425.

6. Van der Zee DC, Bax NM (1995) Laparoscopic repair of congenital diaphragmatic hernia in a 6-month-old child. Surg Endosc 9: 1001-1003.

7. Mar Fan MJ, Coulson ML, Siu SK (1999) Adult incarcerated right-sided Bochdalek hernia. Aust NZ J Surg 69: 239-241.

8. Wong NA, Dayan CM, Virjee J, Heaton KW (1995) Acute respiratory distress secondary to Morgagni diaphragmatic herniation in an adult. Postgrad Med J 71: 39-41.

9. Kuster GG, Kline LE, Garzo G (1992) Diaphragmatic hernia through the foramen of Morgagni: laparoscopic repair case report. J Laparoendosc Surg 2:93-100.

10. Ramachandran CS, Arora V (1999) Laparoscopic transabdominal repair of hernia of Morgagni-Larrey. Surg Laparosc Endosc Perc Tech 9:358-61.

11. Heniford BT, Park A, Ramshaw BJ, Voeller G (2000) Laparoscopic ventral and incisional hernia repair in 407 patients. JACS 190(6) 645-650.

12. Rau HG, Schardey HM, Lange V (1994) Laparoscopic repair of a Morgagni hernia. Surg Endosc 8:1439-42.

13. Newman L, Eubanks S, Bridges WM, Lucas G (1995) Laparoscopic diagnosis and treatment of Morgagni hernia. Surg Laparosc Endosc 5:27-31.

14. Smith J, Ghani A (1995) Morgagni hernia: incidental repair during laparoscopic cholecystectomy. J Laparoendosc Surg 5:123-5.

15. Fernandez-Cebrian JM, De Oteyza JP (1996) Laparoscopic repair of hernia of foramen of Morgagni: a new case report. J Laparoendosc Surg 6:61-4.

16. Huntington TR (1996) Laparoscopic transabdominal preperitoneal repair of a hernia of Morgagni. J Laparoendosc Surg 6:131-3.

17. Orita M, Okino M, Yamashita K, Morita N, Esato K (1997) Laparoscopic repair of a diaphragmatic hernia through the foramen of morgagni. Surg Endosc 11:668-70.

18. Vanclooster P, Lefevre A, Nijs S, de Gheldere C (1997) Laparoscopic repair of a Morgagni hernia. Acta Chir Belg 97:84-5.

19. Contini S, Dalla Valle R, Bonati L, Zinicola R (1999) Laparoscopic repair of a Morgagni hernia: report of a case and review of the literature. J Laparoendosc Adv Surg Tech A 9:93-9.

20. Nguyen T, Eubanks P, Nguyen D, Klein S (1998) The laparoscopic approach for repair of Morgagni hernias. JSLS 2:85-88.

21. Bortul M, Calligaris L, Gheller P (1998) Laparoscopic repair of a Morgagni-Larrey hernia. J Laparoendosc Adv Surg Tech A 8:309-13.

22. Del Castillo D, Sanchez J, Hernandez M, Sanchez A, Domenech J, Jara J (1998) Morgagni's hernia resolved by laparoscopic surgery. J Laparosc Adv Surg Tech 8(2) 105-108.

23. Lima M, Domini M, Libri M, Morabito A, Tani G, Domini R (2000) Laparoscopic repair of Morgagni-Larrey hernia in a child. J Ped Surg 35(8) 1266-1268.

24. Asencio JA, Demetriades D, Rodriguez A (2000) Injury to the diaphragm. In Mattox KL, Feliciano DV, Moore EE (eds) Trauma. McGraw-Hill, New York, pp. 603-632.

25. Demetriades D, Kakoyiannis K, Parekh D (1988) Penetrating injuries to the diaphragm. Br J Surg 75: 824.

26. Koehler RH, Smith S (1994) Thoracoscopic repair of missed diaphragmatic injury in penetrating trauma: case report. J Trauma 36(3): 424-427.

27. Ivatury RR, Simon RJ, Stahl WM (1993) Acritical evaluation of laparoscopy in penetrating abdominal trauma. J Trauma 34(6) 822-828.

28. Fabian TC, Croce MA, Stewart RM, Pritchard FE, Minard G, Kudsk KA (1993) A prospective analysis of diagnostic laparoscopy in trauma. Ann Surg 217(5) 557-565.

29. Zantut LF, Ivatury RR, Smith RS, et al. (1997) Diagnostic and therapeutic laparoscopy for penetrating abdominal trauma: A multicenter experience. J Trauma 42(5) 825-829.

30. Lucas CE, Ledgerwood AM (1998) Diaphragmatic injury. In Cameron JL (ed.) Current Surgical Therapy. Mosby, St. Louis pp.944-947.

31. Cougard P, Goudet P, Arnal E, Ferrand F (2000) Treatment of diaphragmatic ruptures by laparoscopic approach in the lateral position. Ann Chirug 125(3) 238-241.

32. Sternberg DM, Petrick AT, Gharagozloo F, Hannallah MS (1997) Tension pneumothorax precluding laparoscopic repair of diaphragmatic hernia. Surg Laparosc Endosc 7(5) 429-431.

33. Shah S, Matthews BD, Sing RF, Heniford BT (2000) Laparoscopic repair of a chronic diaphragmatic hernia. Surg Laparosc Endosc Percutan Tech 10:182-6.

34. Pross M, Manger T, Mirow L, Wolff S, Lippert H (2000) Laparoscopic management of a late-diagnosed major diaphragmatic rupture. J Laparoendosc Adv Surg Tech A 10:111-4.

35. Meyer G, Huttl P, Hatz RA, Schildberg FW (2000) Laparoscopic repair of traumatic diaphragmatic hernias. Surg Endosc 14:1010-1014.

36. Torresini G, Sozio L, Crisci R, Amicucci G (2000) Laparoscopic repair of diaphragmatic iatrogenic hernia. Endoscopy 32:S2.

37. Matz A, Alis M, Charuzi I, Kyzer S (2000) The role of laparoscopy in the diagnosis and treatment of missed diaphragmatic rupture. Surg Endosc 14:537-9.

38. Slim K, Bousquet J, Chipponi J (1998) Laparoscopic repair of missed blunt diaphragmatic rupture using a prosthesis. Surg Endosc 12:1358-60.

39. Domene CE, Volpe P, Santo MA, Onari P, Szachnowicz S, Pinotti HW (1998) Laparoscopic treatment of traumatic diaphragmatic hernia. J Laparoendosc Adv Surg Tech A 8:225-9.

40. Rasiah KK, Crowe PJ (1995) Laparoscopic repair of a traumatic diaphragmatic hernia. J Laparoendosc Surg 5:405-7.

41. Campos LI, Sipes EK (1991) Laparoscopic repair of diaphragmatic hernia. J Laparoendosc Surg 1:369-73.

Future Considerations
of Laparoscopic Ventral Hernia Repair

CHAPTER 48

Training for Laparoscopic Ventral Hernia Repair and Credentialing

S. Morales-Conde, E. Prendes, V. Fernández, S. Morales-Méndez

INTRODUCTION

With the development and widespread use of laparoscopic cholecystectomy the first laparoscopic technique recognized and accepted worldwide, laparoscopic approach is being applied to more and more pathologic conditions requiring surgical treatment. Because of this fact laparoscopic surgery, enhanced in part by technological breakthroughs, is in a process of continuous improvement and renovation.

At the beginning laparoscopic surgery was the subject of numerous adverse reports due to the complications described. These problems, attributed to the surgeons' null or limited experience in this field and in diagnostic laparoscopy, were excused in part by the so-called "learning curve". For this reason, from the earliest days of laparoscopic surgery, an attempt has been made to establish minimum requirements or guidelines to accredit surgeons for the performance of this type of procedure. This concern has resulted in a number of articles over the years, including those published by surgical associations, such as the Society of American Gastrointestinal Endoscopic Surgeons (SAGES) in 1990 (1,2), that have presented a series of requirements that must be met by all surgeons performing these minimally invasive procedures. Several published surveys have also addressed the issue. One example is a survey conducted by Asbun and Reddick in 1992 (3), which gathered opinions on aptitude and training in laparoscopic surgery from 149 surgeons and concluded that a course covering theory and practice in animals should be a requirement for accreditation. The survey also mentioned the need to establish a minimal number of procedures that a surgeon should perform as an assistant and as a surgeon supervised by an expert before performing a procedure alone.

As part of the effort to establish the requisites for laparoscopic surgery training, in 1993 the European Association of Endoscopic Surgeons (EAES)

proposed a series of requirements considered essential for a surgeon to perform minimally invasive procedures (4).

Based on the foregoing, as well as on ongoing advances and changes in the field, proper, progressive training addressed to the following individuals is necessary:

- Surgeons without experience in laparoscopic techniques, so they can perform these procedures safely and skillfully;

- Surgeons now performing the technique, for their further advancement; and

- Staff members at a standard laparoscopic surgery center, so they can establish the guidelines to be followed in their setting and to evaluate the feasibility of certain procedures.

Ethically we must offer our patients the most beneficial healthcare, and in certain procedures the laparoscopic approach is the best. Nevertheless, we are also morally obliged to offer what we know how to do best and, therefore, must clearly establish the basis for proper training. In this way our patients will benefit from the technological advances that facilitate the development of these minimally invasive techniques.

TRAINING, TEACHING AND ACCREDITATION IN LAPAROSCOPIC SURGERY

Laparoscopic surgery requires ongoing, continuous training which, in our opinion and on the basis of experience gained over the years and compared with other learning centers, can be structured into three main divisions:

- An introductory level for surgeons who will be performing this approach for the first time.

- An advanced level, for surgeons with knowledge on laparoscopic surgery who want to develop more complex techniques in an advanced setting, including laparoscopic repair of ventral hernias.

- Continuous training for experts on these techniques.

Introduction in laparoscopic surgery

This level is directed toward surgeons who want to use this approach for the first time, and toward medical residents, who has not been systematically included in laparoscopy training programs until recently, primarily because the surgical staff of the diffent surgical departments of most hospitals often lacked both basic and advanced training in laparoscopic techniques. The situation is improving as increasing numbers of laparoscopic procedures are performed in hospitals, with no small number actually done by residents (5).

In regard to the subject at hand, candidates who wish to perform laparoscopic procedures must take a theoretical-practical course lasting 3 to 7 days to obtain basic training, with further experience gained by performing the technique in actual clinical practice. At the beginning trainees will always work under the supervision of surgeons with experience in this type of procedure, until they obtain a level of skill, safety, confidence and assurance comparable to that of procedures performed using conventional surgical techniques.

The courses should be taught and supervised by surgeons experienced in laparoscopy and endorsed by an official organisation (university, national endoscopic association or hospital with prestige in terms of laparoscopic surgery). We propose a course organized into three modules (6-8):

- *Module I*: A module primarily centered on theory and consisting of sessions that discuss both theoretical and practical aspects including historical background data, a description of laparoscopic techniques, a description of the instrumentation, anesthesia-related topics, pathophysiology of the pneumoperitoneum, potential complications of the procedures and resolution thereof, etc.

- *Module II*: A module in which the participants use simulators under direct vision and/or a monitor to acquire the necessary skills to perform the differents techniques in experimental animals (9).

- *Module III*: A module consisting of surgery performed on experimental animals, covering both simple and advanced techniques, and simulating actual situations requiring a correct resolution. This section is aimed at acquiring a variety of skills not attainable with inanimate models, including mobilization of anatomical structures, hemostasis, intra-abdominal anastomosis, etc.

These introductory laparoscopic surgery courses are not valid in themselves (10-12) and must be accompanied by an integral training plan that includes close cooperation with surgeons experienced in this type of approach.

In this context medical resident training has several unique characteristics. Since residents receive basic training for all types of surgery, a close contact with laparoscopic surgery is delayed to virtually the final years of training. But, in the first few years, however, residents have gradual contact with the laparoscopic approach, particularly as it relates to instrumentation, technological components, training in the insertion of needles and trocars, and pneumoperitoneum techniques. Over the years this enhanced training effort has favored a significant increase in the number of laparoscopic procedures performed in daily surgical practice in many hospitals. The progressive approach toward training is aimed at ensuring optimal conditions upon completion of the residency, allowing these surgeons to perform basic laparoscopic procedures without the need to participate in additional intensive courses (13).

Training in advanced laparoscopic surgery

Addressed to surgeons well-grounded in laparoscopic surgery using non-advanced techniques (cholecystectomy, appendectomy, explorative laparoscopy, etc.). To achieve training in advanced laparoscopic procedures, three phases that attempt to meet the same objectives reached in the introductory stage must be completed, namely:

- Become familiar with the technique.
- Participate actively in the technique.
- Perform the technique: first in experimental animals, then in clinical practice, initially assisted by expert surgeons and once sufficient experience has been gained, on their own.

We consider the repair of abdominal parietal defects an advanced laparoscopic procedure, as it is usually performed on patients who have undergone previous laparotomy and present intestinal adhesions. These factors require complex management of the bowel, with potentially adverse consequences if the maneuvers are not performed by an expert.

In our setting, which serves as a reference for training surgeons in laparoscopic repair of incisional hernias and other conditions, we discuss the points accepted as basic for advanced laparoscopic training in the morning and evening sessions over a single day. These sessions contain three modules with the following content:

- *Module I*: Presentation of clinical cases and performance of live surgery with the surgeons in the operating theatre.

- *Module II*: Theoretical-practical session analyzing indications, surgical techniques and the results of our group and comparing them with the observations made during the two surgeries performed in the morning.

- *Module III*: Practice of the surgical technique in experimental animals.

As in the introductory courses, we strive to ensure that the course session described is not an isolated aspect of the training. Therefore, we recommend that participating surgeons have prior theoretical and practical knowledge of the technique being discussed and that, after the courses, they contact surgeons with expertise in the technique to complete their integrated training. To monitor their first procedures, we sometimes go to the hospitals of the participating surgeons a few days after completion of the course to perform laparoscopic surgery in which they act as our assistants, followed by surgery in which we assist them.

Continuous training in laparoscopic surgery

In order to keep abreast of advances in laparoscopic surgery, we must attempt to stay up-to-date in terms of the results obtained from new procedures being developed and from new technological breakthroughs being implemented, with the aim of facilitating our work and using these new procedures.

There are currently two methods to this end, an analytical approach that consists in reading related journals and on attending courses in which various aspects related to this surgical approach are debated. Live surgery plays a key role in these courses, as it allows surgeons to acquire resources that will aid them in performing the surgery successfully.

ACCREDITATION

As has been emphasized throughout the chapter, an essential point of laparoscopic training is accreditation of the experts who impart the training and of the course content. But, in a final analysis the surgeon is the person most capable of assessing (his)their capacity to perform a particular laparoscopic technique.

It is evident that scientific societies and universities (or the national committee for medicinal specialties, in the case of residents) are the ones that should accredit the groups in charge of training, and on the basis of some established guidelines, accredit laparoscopic training itself.

Along these lines certain scientific societies such as the Society of American Gastrointestinal Endoscopic Surgeons (SAGES), the Asociación Mexicana de Cirugía Laparoscópica (AMCL), the European Association of Endoscopic Surgeons (EAES), etc. (4,14) have published minimum requirements for credentialing a surgeon to perform laparoscopic procedures. In Spain, during the meeting of the Laparoscopic Surgery Session of the National Association of Surgeons, the first steps were taken toward establishing accreditation criteria for the various courses designed to bring surgeons up to date in this type of approach.

COURSES ON LAPAROSCOPIC VENTRAL HERNIA REPAIR

As mentioned earlier, we believe that courses on laparoscopic repair of ventral hernias fit the context of the description we have made of training courses in advanced laparoscopic surgery. These courses should contain a part consisting of live surgery, several discussions on the subject and surgery in experimental animals to perform the technique. Our first objective is to avoid crowding in the courses in order to ensure direct communication between the instructors and surgeons and maximize the benefit of the interchange. For this reason, we believe there should be no more than four surgeons per course, as this is a manageable number for attending the surgical rooms and permits adequate communication during surgery. The organization of the experimental operating theatre allows us to work with two pigs simultaneously. Two surgeons per animal is considered to be the maximum, since two incisional hernias will be created in each pig, and each hernia will be repaired by one of the surgeons participating in the course. Because the number of participants is limited, we feel that the surgeons attending must be specifically interested in the abdominal wall and in advanced laparoscopic techniques, and that they should have experience in both aspects to maximize their benefit from such an intensive monographic course.

Live surgery

We start by presenting two clinical cases that will be operated on, discussing the indications and the surgical strategy we devise to perform the technique in these patients. We then enter the operating room where the two surgeries will be performed. Direct observation of the surgery inside the operating theatre is highly useful, as it allows the surgeons to take in all the small details we have gained through experience and that help us to execute the technique successfully. While performing any laparoscopic procedure, we believe that the interaction among the surgeon, nursing staff and anesthesiologists is fundamental and that it contributes significantly to the management of this type of patient in the operating room. The details can be lost during simple retransmissions of the procedure. We try to create an environment of continuous interaction among the surgical team and the attending surgeons at all times, in order to achieve maximum rapport and to convey as much information as possible.

Theoretical-practical sessions

Once the surgery is completed, we discuss the latest findings from the related literature and our accumulated experience. At this point we also attempt to explain why we perform our current surgical method, the *double-crown* technique. This is done in theoretical-practical sessions that maintain the climate of close communication and interaction created in the operating room. Our sessions are divided into four main sections: analysis of how to manage the prostheses and suture materials used to attach them based on our experimental studies; description of our surgical technique and why we perform it that way; analysis of the results obtained by using the *double crown* technique for abdominal wall repair; and lastly, analysis of current problems with the technique, such as cost-benefit and future lines of research we have underway based on the doubts that still arise when analyzing ventral hernia repair with this approach.

Surgery in experimental animals

After a comprehensive analysis of the surgical technique during the morning, we feel that it is essential for the participating surgeons to personally carry out ventral hernia repair in experimental animals so that they can put into practice all the fine points of the procedure that have been covered. By performing the technique in experimental animals, each individual participant can see the true value of the multiple small details regarding method observed in the operating room. Additionally certain maneuvers they may not have picked up during the morning surgical session can be directly demonstrated.

Nevertheless, performance of these procedures in experimental animals has somewhat different connotations from those of training courses we organize for other conditions, e.g., cholecystectomy, achalasia, gastroesophageal reflux, etc., since the animals used do not present incisional hernias and the hernia must be created prior to the start of the course.

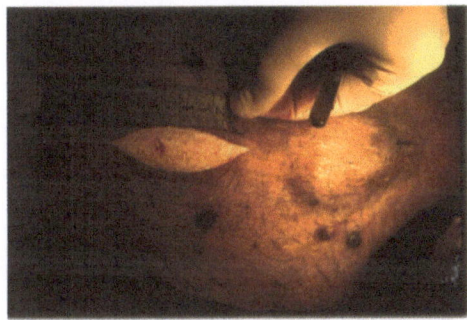

Fig. 1. 8-cm infraumbilical incision in the skin of a pig to create an incisional hernia, performed two weeks before the training course on laparoscopic repair of ventral hernias.

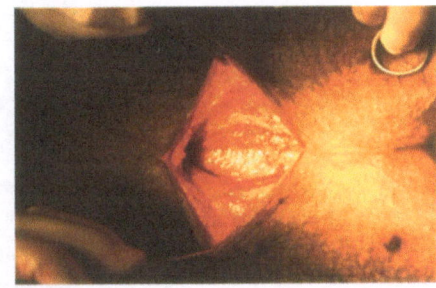

Fig. 2. Opening of subcutaneous cellular tissue and fascia to the peritoneum, leaving the latter untouched.

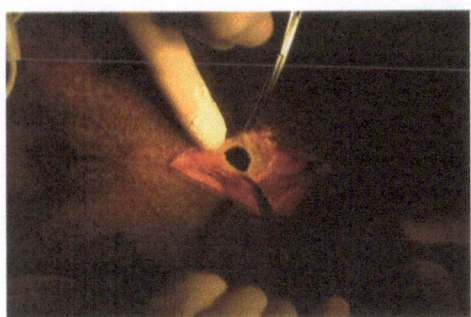

Fig. 3. Creation of an orifice in the peritoneum to introduce the finger with talcum powder, which acts as an irritant for the formation of adhesions.

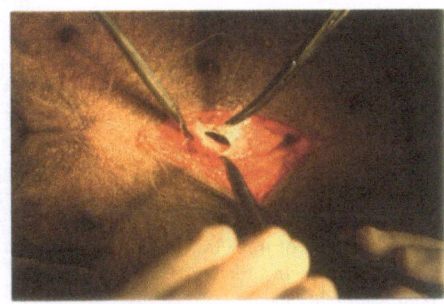

Fig. 4. Closure of the opening made in the peritoneum.

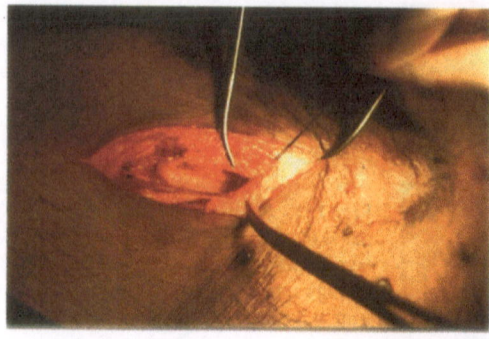

Fig. 5. Sutures at both ends of the fascia to prevent the hernia from lengthening during the postoperative period and to maintain the previously established size.

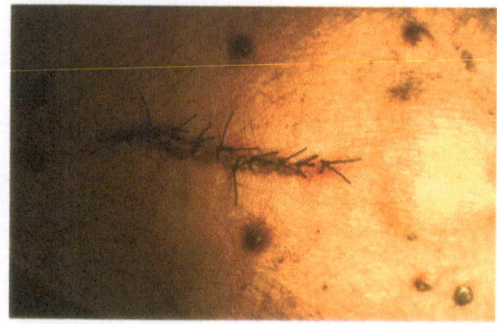

Fig. 6. Final condition after direct closure of the skin with interrupted silk stitches without closing the fascia and subcutaneous tissue.

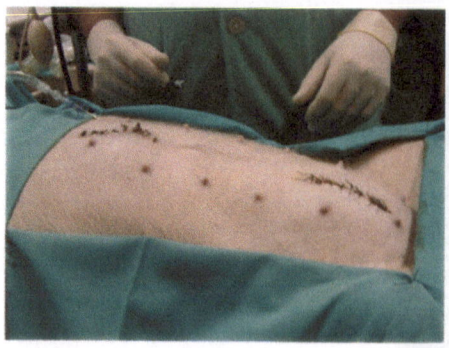

Fig. 7. Creation of the pneumo-peritoneum with the Veress needle by an attending surgeon during one of the courses, observing during insufflation how the two hernias created two weeks before have become distended.

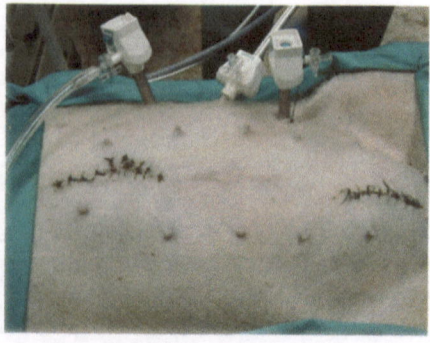

Fig. 8. Placement of three trocars in line in the left abdomen, in order to begin repair of both ventral hernias.

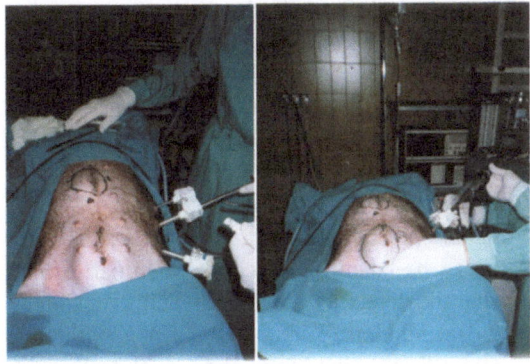

Figs. 9 and 10. After marking the limits of the defect to be covered with the mesh, start of repair of the incisional hernia in the upper abdomen (Fig. 9), followed by repair of the lower defect by the second surgeon (Fig. 10).

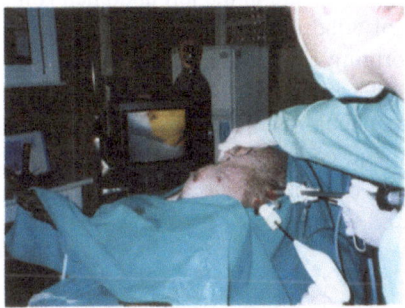

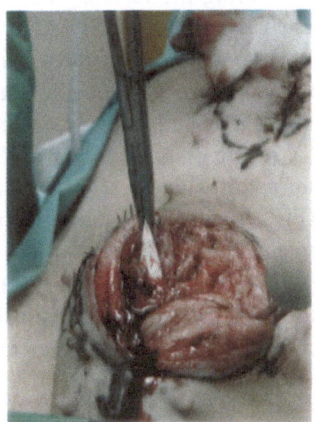

Fig. 11. Once the mesh has been introduced, one of the surgeons attaches the mesh with tacks, exerting pressure from the outside to ensure that it is properly attached.

Fig. 12. After the mesh has been placed by laparoscopy, an incision must be made in the dome of the hernia sac to check that the mesh has been positioned and attached correctly. In this way the potential shortcomings of the procedure can be analyzed while confirming that the repair is properly done.

In this case, two weeks before the course, we create two incisional hernias in both experimental animals needed: one in the upper abdomen and another in the lower abdomen. To create the incisional hernias, we select two pigs weighing at least 20 kilograms and make an incision in the upper and lower compartments of the abdomen (Fig. 1), opening the skin, the subcutaneous cellular tissue and the fascia until reaching the peritoneum which is left untouched (Fig. 2). Then we perform a very small incision in the peritoneum in order to access the abdominal cavity and introduce an irritant substance consisting of two small portions of talcum podwer (Fig. 3). This will produce adhesions in the postoperative period and provide a more realistic situation. Once the peritoneum is closed (Fig. 4), we place two stitches at each end of the fascia to prevent the hernia from lengthening (Fig. 5), then we close the skin directly with interrupted silk stitches, leaving the fascia and subcutaneous tissue open (Fig. 6).

As a result, two weeks after the surgery the animals will present two incisional hernias (one superior and another inferior) with all the characteristics of a real case, including the sac, defect limits and presence of intra-abdominal adhesions. Lastly, the only consideration that must be taken into account when performing the surgery to create the hernias is that the defect produced in the upper abdomen should be made through an incision in the skin of about 10 cm of length. The lower incision should be smaller (about 8 cm) since intra-abdominal pressure in the pig is greater at this level and larger incisions will result in larger defects.

During the teaching course, two groups with two surgeons each are formed. Each group will work with an experimental animal having two incisional hernias so that each surgeon can repair one of them by following the same steps we use in humans: creation of the pneumoperitoneum with Veress needle in the left hypochondrium (Fig. 7), in-line placement of the trocars in the left abdomen (Fig. 8), repair of both hernia defects by means of adhesiolysis and placement of an intraperitoneal mesh fixed with tacks performing the Double Crown technique (Fig. 9, 10 and 11). Once the mesh has been placed by laparoscopy, an incision is made in the dome of both hernia sacs to check that the mesh is correctly positioned and attached, in order to analyze and correct any errors made during the procedure and to check the repair so that the participant can become more confident in their laparoscopic skills (Fig. 12).

CONCLUSION

The basic objectives of laparoscopic surgery training in the repair of ventral hernias or any other condition must be directed toward adequately instructing the surgeons interested in this technique and minimizing or eliminating the morbidity associated with the learning curve. In summary, teaching efforts in this type of approach were not well established until only a few years ago and the various working groups were self-taught, hence the constant mention of a learning curve in all studies reporting any type of laparoscopic procedure. In fact, the relatively large number of biliary tract lesions associated with laparoscopic surgery in the early 1990s (15) and the development of tumoral lesions in the trocar sites can be considered nothing more than the result of this learning curve. In experienced groups these complications have been decreasing to levels equal to or less than those occurring after open surgery, leading us to believe that experienced surgeons have a moral obligation to teach others. Moreover, surgeons in training are likewise obliged to learn in an adequate manner, in order to minimize and finally obtain one of the objectives that should prevail at present: eliminate this learning curve. This is the underlying rationale leading to one of the conclusions of our analysis, namely the need to establish the components required for training and acquiring knowledge about the repair of ventral hernias and treatment of other conditions by means of the laparoscopic approach, as has been presented in this section.

References

1. Society of Surgery of the Alimentary Tract. Resolution concerning privileges to perform laparoscopic cholecistectomy. SSAT. San Antonio, 1990.

2. Statements on emerging surgical technologies and evaluation of credentials. Hult ACS 1994; 6:40-41.

3. Asbun, H.J., Reddick, E.J.: Credentialing in laparoscopic surgery: A survey of physicians. J. Lap. Surg. 1992; 2:27-32.

4. Requirements for basic and advanced courses in endoscopic surgery should fulfill to become recommendation of EAES and training and assessment of competence. Executive Office of the European Association for Endoscopic Surgery. April 1993.

5. Parsa, C.J., Ogan, C.H. Jr., Barkan, H. Changing patterns of resident operative experience from 1990 to 1997. Arch. Surg. 2000. 135(5):570(3).

6. Cushieri, A., Berci, G.: Biliary surgery by Laparoscopy. In: Training for Laparoscopic Surgery. Ed. Arnette. Paris. 1991:1-9.

7. Dent, T.L. Training credentialing and granting of clinical privileges for laparoscopic general surgery. Am. J. Surg. 1991; 161:399-403.

8. Hunter, J.C., Sackler, J.M.: Training for minimally invasive surgery. In: Minimally Invasive Surgery. McGraw-Hill. New York. 1993:5-6.

9. Champion, J.K., Hunter, J., Trus, T., Laycock, W. Teaching basic video skills as an aid in laparoscopic suturing. Surg. Endosc. 1996; 10:23-25.

10. Zucker, K.A., Bailey, R.W., Graham, S.M., Scovil, W., Ibembo, A.L. Training for laparoscopic surgery. World J. Surg. 1993; 17(1):3-7.

11. Ibembo, A.L., Zucker, K.A.: Training for laparoscopic surgery and credentialing. In: Zucker K.A.: Surgical laparoscopy. Quality Medical Publishing, Inc. St. Louis, Missouri. 1991; Chapter 17: 343-350.

12. Entrenamiento de la cirugía biliar laparoscópica. En: Cuschieri, A., Berci, G., Cirugía biliar laparoscópica. Blackwell Scientific Publications. Oxford 1994. Capitulo 1:1-13.

13. Friedman, R.I., Pace, B.W.: Resident education in laparoscopic cholecistectomy. Surg. Endosc. 1996; 10:26-28.

14. Society of American Gastrointestinal Endoscopic Surgeons. Guidelines for granting of privileges for laparoscopic (Peritoneoscopic) general surgery. Los Angeles, California: Society of American Endoscopic Surgeons. 1992. SAGES publication # 0014-10/92.

15. Horvath KD. Strategies for the prevention of laparoscopic common bile duct injuries. Surg Endosc 1993. 7(5):439-44.

CHAPTER 49

The Future of Laparoscopic Ventral Hernia Repair

C. Gracia, S. Morales-Conde

FUTURE OF LAPAROSCOPY

INTRODUCTION

Minimally invasive surgical (MIS) techniques have been evolving over the past decade. The ability to remotely access various body parts through tiny incisions has revolutionized the practice of surgery. Laparoscopic surgery has been recognized as beneficial in the performance of a growing number of surgical procedures. The development of superior optics, video imaging equipment, and design of instrumentation to work remotely, have enabled numerous advances which have centered predominantly around gastrointestinal, gynecologic, urologic, general thoracic procedures, and more recently coronary bypass surgery. Progress continues on three fronts. One is where MIS technique and technologies continue to be applied to an increasing number of additional procedures and specialties. The other front is in the technology itself. This involves advances in video systems, lights, optics, and instrumentation. Most of this technological advancement is now centering on the miniaturization of instrumentation. The final front is in the operating room environment itself and its direct impact on the surgical team's ability to adopt the increasing numbers of complex minimally invasive procedures.

FUTURE OF CORE TECHNOLOGY

There are many procedures, e.g., hernia repairs (inguinal and ventral repairs) and colectomy, where debate continues over the advantages and wisdom of conversion to MIS. Laparoscopic ventral hernia repairs have now gained momentum with consistently good results in terms of morbidity and recurrence rates. Large incisions have been replaced with five and ten millimeter trocar sites. In light of this, what could possibly be the wisdom or role of miniaturization into the realm of two and three millimeter trocars and instrumentation? (Fig. 1).

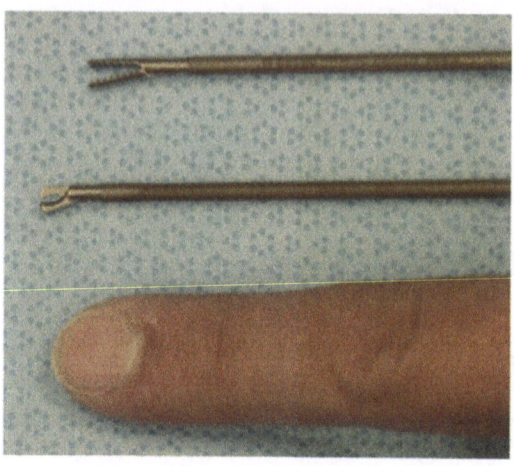

Fig. 1. Close-up view of the 3 mm instruments.

There has been confusion regarding miniaturization over the last several years. Sub-two millimeter fiber optic scopes were introduced several years ago. They were more of a technical curiosity with very limited view and depth of field. There was interest in their role for diagnostic laparoscopy in either an emergency room, bedside ICU, or outpatient office setting. However, it has been the newer wave of instrumentation in the last couple of years that has demonstrated the increased applicability of a smaller size. Diagnostic applications have seemed to be the most popular thus far. Until now, attempts to do more with miniaturization have led to surgeon frustration. As a result, the question is raised of whether or not the added difficulties to the surgeon justify any additional returns to patients over the current crop of laparoscopic techniques with five and ten millimeter tools.

At this point, it becomes very necessary to begin to understand the instrumentation in more detail. The original crop of instrumentation was in the 2mm range. The term "needlescopic surgery" was coined mostly due to the very small size of the scopes, instruments and trocars that frankly resemble more a large-bore needle than a laparoscopic instrument. Differences in instrument behavior have become very obvious. The smaller the tool, the greater the tendency for the instrument to "bayonet" when manipulated. This results in oscillation of the instrument making it difficult to steer to the target and grasp it. Once tissue is targeted, the instrument is obviously not as strong and is more susceptible to bending. The narrower diameter of the tools also give the grasping end limited options for tips and has a smaller "foot print". The latter makes it more difficult to grasp tissue for dissection. The finer tips may also possibly lead to easier perforation or damage of the target tissue or organ. Also, suction capability and the option to insert sponges, etc, in case of bleeding is very limited. More diligence is required to avoid these types of difficulties with more patience required on the part of the operating surgeon

Many have abandoned 2 mm tools for the following reasons: 1/ they are too flexible and subsequently too fragile for routine use, 2/ their footprints were to small and the tips too sharp as a function of their small size, 3/ it was very difficult to either suture or tie knots as they bent easily and would rip suture, 4/ the "bayonet effect" proved quite frustrating, and 5/ most importantly, one is limited to 2 mm scopes due to the size of the trocars. This latter problem proved major, as they were too fragile to use and gave limited images and illumination.

In general, 3-mm instrumentation has proven superior for operative procedures. Several features were responsible, including the short learning curve involved in changing to 3-mm tools. One can suture with 3 mm tools and tie secure knots, even to approximate the diaphragmatic hiatus. Strands of suture can easily be introduced through the 3-mm trocar to ligate structures. This is not possible through 2-mm trocars. The performance of 3-mm instruments is much like that of 5-mm tools, yet without the additional tissue trauma associated with the larger trocar. The familiar 5-mm trocar is actually a minimum of 5.6 mm in outer diameter. The use of 3 mm tools now begins to approach more of a 50 % reduction in size of the instrumentation. As experience grows with mini-laparoscopy, a general gravitation towards 3-mm instrumentation develops.

Excellent imaging is very important to the performance of laparoscopic procedures. Looking into the peritoneal cavity at large can strain the best of current light sources and video systems. The 3-mm rod-lens system is superior in optical performance when compared to 2-mm scopes. Evolving camera technology includes a zoom feature that allows the mini-scope image to be expanded to nearly that seen with a 10-mm scope. New digital camera technologies will continue to enhance imagery will decreasing light requirements. High quality light sources enable excellent images. The 3-mm scopes also prove to be more durable with routine handling in the operating room than the 2-mm fiber optic scopes.

There are specific considerations with laparoscopic ventral hernia repair that influence whether any miniaturizations are reasonable. A mesh needs to be introduced and various mechanical fixation devices may also need to be inserted. Various strategies can be implemented in order to take advantage of the smaller trocar sizes. A "single port" of 10-12 mm can be utilized to deliver the larger materials as necessary. Around this port can be utilized 3 mm trocars through which to work with 3 mm instruments. Ventral hernias and abdominal wall defects occur in a wide variety of locations. The umbilicus may or may not be available nor well suited for visualization of the operative field. An advantage of a decreasing scope size is that a smaller high quality scope can utilize multiple alternative viewing sites. It would not be necessary to have multiple large trocars in place to be able to move the scope about for a different view.

Is it worth it to our patient's outcomes to deal with the additional time, cost, and potential nuisance factor that all of this may introduce? One look at a patient with 3-mm trocar sites would immediately dispel the belief that there is no difference in patients between 3 mm and 5 mm trocars (Fig. 2). Whatever additional time is spent working with "mini" tools can be recovered by the lack of a need to close any trocar site. These are simply infiltrated with local anesthetic at the completion of the case, and steri-stripped closed. These are removed 4-5 days later and rarely is a mark >2-3 mm noticeable.

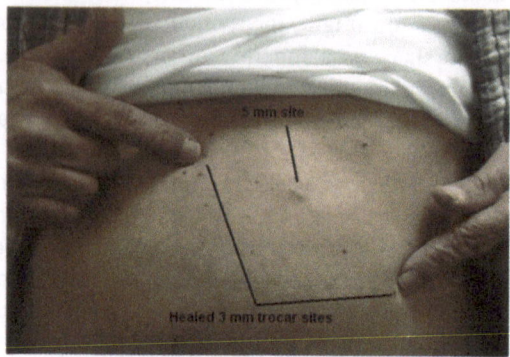

Fig. 2. Comparison between healed trocar sites of 3 mm and 5 mm at 2 weeks from surgery. The 3 mm trocar sites are indistinguishable from other small skin moles. The 5 mm trocar site has a clear scar. Although it may not appear to be significant when looking at the trocars directly, there may be in some cases another 50% reduction in overall surface traumatized by the 3mm trocars when compared to 5 mm trocars.

FUTURE CHALLENGES

There has been incredible advancement in scopes, video systems and instrumentation which has enabled a major revolution to take place in how surgery is performed. The advantages of minimally invasive surgery to our patients has been extensively studied and measured for the last several years since the first laparoscopic cholecystectomy was performed. These advantages have stimulated a tremendous investment in the development of new surgical technology. In turn, this has enabled more specialties in surgery to be able to apply these technologies to their respective fields. This cycle has been further fueled by patient demand, as they are better informed regarding the technologies and outcomes enabling minimally invasive surgery. The result is that there is an unprecedented revolution in surgery. Minimally invasive surgery is here to stay and continues to grow.

Technology has changed the way that surgeons work. Numerous technological advancements have made possible numerous treatments and procedures previously unimagined. However, for the surgeon quality of care is usually seen in terms of technical excellence. Miraculous outcomes or treatments have been generally considered the result of advanced individual skill and ability. Surgical training, in order to develop the necessary skill, experience, and judgment, takes years. In order to not deny patients the advantages of new developments, how does one incorporate all of the new knowledge and obtain the new skills necessary.

Considering how much technology has changed the way that surgeons work, the operating room has changed little, (Fig. 3). Despite all the technology developed, much of it has been introduced to the operating room on large bulky carts that operating room personnel had to roll about. The logistical problems encountered with this are significant. This has in turn help create an atmosphere which has not been supportive of introducing more technology or adopting the procedures that required it.

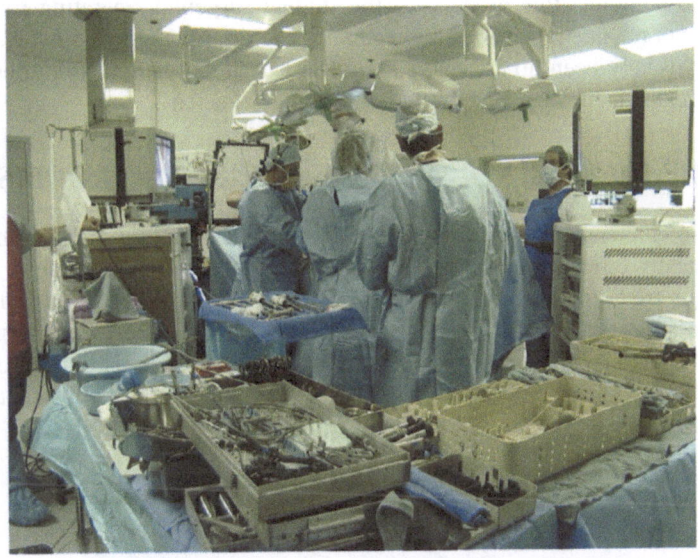

Fig. 3. Photo of modern day operating room cluttered as result of increasing technology. In this case, laparoscopy is being combined with minimally invasive spine surgery for anterior fusion. Basic laparoscopic equipment, extensive orthopedic equipment, and C-arm fluoroscopy all must come into an operating room never designed or planned for this sort of application.

The new technology has created a new way of doing surgery in most circumstances. This means that the surgeon now not only must obtain knowledge regarding the new technologies, but more importantly, the skill set to be successful with the new procedures. Surgical training is known to take years to develop an informed and technically competent surgeon. The challenge has become how to continue this long term educational process outside of the established training programs.

The short term one to two day training course has not proven successful in empowering surgeons the skills or experience to return to their own operating rooms and begin to perform the new procedures. Because of this ineffectiveness and the high cost associated with this type of program, these courses have been dwindling. The financial considerations are significant when one includes the time away from practice, the expenses of modern day air travel, and the cost of running a training facility with animals, personnel, and equipment. Attempts to support surgeons after these short term training programs has also been prohibitively expensive. Consider the costs of taking experts out of their practice and transporting them to the student surgeon's hospital to mentor or preceptor their first few cases. It usually requires more than the one or two proctored cases to become competent in a new procedure. How does one provide for long term support until the student surgeon has acquired the necessary skill and judgment. Other logistical problems exist with this model, in that: 1/ there are not enough experts to complete this process, 2/ the student surgeon's operating room has typically not obtained the necessary technology to do the surgery correctly, and 3/ there has usually been no consideration towards training the remaining members of the surgical team, such as surgical nurses and technicians.

FUTURE OF TECHNOLOGIES IN OPERATING ROOMS

The major challenges include organizing the modern operating room so that it is ergonomically efficient, upgradeable, and enables surgical team training. These three items are critical for the future of minimally invasive surgery. Only as these areas are addressed will there then be an increasing number of surgeons and surgical teams capable of performing more complex tasks. This increases the overall penetration of procedures such as laparoscopic ventral hernia repair into the hands of more surgeons to benefit more patients.

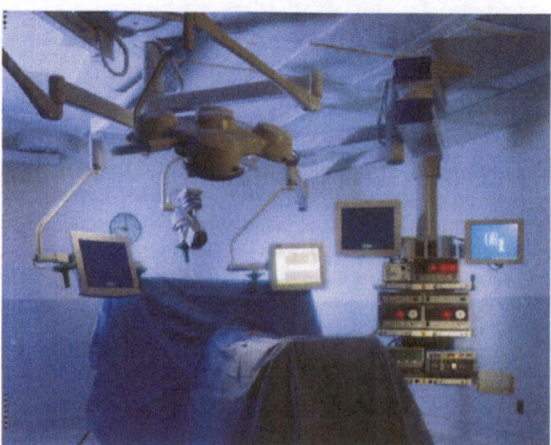

Fig. 4. Photo of a modern day operating designed for minimally invasive surgery. Pre-planned boom configuration lifts and organizes necessary equipment off of the floor. In addition, flat panel technology has been incorporated simplifying boom layout and cost. Touch screen control panels for computer control of surgical equipment and environmental controls have been integrated into boom arrangements.

The first real improvement in operating rooms has included the introduction of booms to simply lift bulky equipment utilized in modern laparoscopic surgery off of the floor. This has led to major improvements in the ergonomics of the operating room (Fig. 4). The environment has also been more critically analyzed to see what would empower surgical teams to be more comfortable and more efficient. In this analysis, it became obvious that control of the operating room technology and environment was also important. Control systems that allow the surgeon to access them real-time from within the sterile field have proven instrumental to improving efficiency while decreasing stress.

The costs of acquiring technology are always a concern. As attention is directed toward this effort, some of the costs of making this type of ergonomic improvement has been offset. An example is the increased daily productivity of an operating room due to the decreased turnover times between surgeries from enhanced ergonomics. The development of this technology itself can help contain costs. Another example is that of video monitors. The current modern ergonomic solution to the video monitor is to suspend it on booms. Realistically the booms are heavy and require expensive conduits and structural reinforcements. As flat panel technology improves, the weight of the monitor will subsequently decrease significantly as will the cost of suspending it. Wireless technologies are also developing which may eliminate the need for expensive conduits.

By organizing operating rooms more efficiently, this has paved the way to begin to introduce other types of technology, not typically associated with the performance of surgery. The most important example of this is modern videoconferencing equipment. This technology has been used routinely for many years in the business world. The cost of the equipment has dropped significantly rather than remain prohibitively expensive. This availability has led to the increased use of videoconferencing equipment at a significant pace. Videoconferencing in the operating room is growing significantly. Surgeons now have the intraoperative ability to obtain face-to-face consultation with colleagues and or mentors. Similarly, the colleagues and mentors have simultaneous access to see what the surgeon is trying to communicate. The opportunity for surgeons to obtain intraoperative consultation regarding a host of issues is revolutionary. Conversely, mentors would be able to monitor a surgeon's progress and be immediately available when a surgeon is having difficulty or requires assistance at that moment.

It may seem that the introduction of more technology might make things more difficult as the surgeon and team have more to learn and keep track of. This would be true if it were not for the introduction of the computer into the operating room. The presence of the computer into the operating room will catapult us into a new era. Computer systems are constantly increasing in power while decreasing in cost. Hardware components can be added or replaced to readily upgrade without significant cost. The software is also readily upgraded, improved, or trouble-shooted. All of this can be accomplished over the internet as needed. The resultant risk of obsolescence of a system is low while the capacity for expanding functionality and usefulness extremely high.

The computer has the capability to take the controls of any operating room equipment, as well as any environmental controls, and integrate it into a simple to use interface. Several control interfaces, such as voice control or touch screens with integration of macro commands, are available (Figure 5 A and B). A major advantage of computer access and control by the surgeon during surgery, is that computers communicate with other computers. The operating room's computer can communicate with the hospital computer system where critical patient data such as laboratory data, radiological images, pathology reports, medical history, pharmacy information, etc., would be instantly available to the surgeon in the operating room when needed.

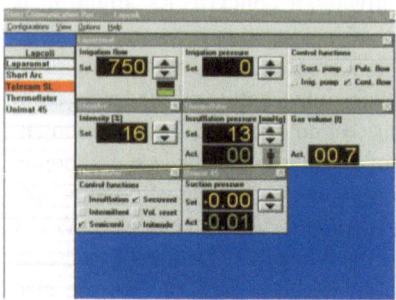
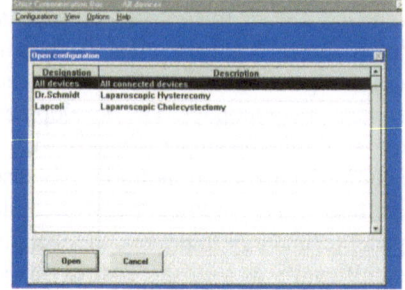

Fig. 5 A. Photo of the touch screen control panel showing snapshots of all surgical devices activated to specific "pre-set" settings. These are activated based on procedure and individual surgeon's preference.

Fig. 5 B. Individual surgeon "pre-sets" are stored in a folder of configuration preferences. Multiple preferences can be saved for each of the different procedures that a surgeon may do. Every surgeon using the operating room can store their individual preferences for each of the surgical devices and environmental parameters.

Intraoperative videoconferencing can be controlled by the surgeon through the computer. The modern day infrastructure for broadband internet communication continues to expand daily. As videoconferencing is integrated into the computer, it will provide this capability by internet which will dramatically further minimize the cost of this type of communication. The involvement of computers for this communication provides the foundation for using wireless technology. Images from an operating room will be transmitted wirelessly to handheld device.

A fascinating future potential may be realized by computers through robots. Current surgical robotic technology is basically a computer placed between the handle of surgical instrument and the end or effector. We are beginning to see some advantages of surgical robots in minimally invasive surgery as a performance enhancing technology. The power of the computer to communicate with other computers may enable us to control robots in distant operating rooms. The advantages of this scenario for teaching complex procedures may be significant.

Computers have provided unparallel integration and control of numerous aspects of our lives. This is accomplished for the most part from behind the scenes. Control systems and functionality are continually improving and easily upgraded. No one would question the advantages and improvements attributable to the computer in the modern day business world or in our everyday lives. It is time for the computer to do the same in the operating room.

FUTURE OF LAPAROSCOPIC VENTRAL HERNIA

INTRODUCTION

Despite the enormous advantages associated with laparoscopic repair of ventral hernias, there are still some questions that need to be answer, an issue that clinical and experimental research, analysis of existing results and cumulative experience will have to solve. The major contributions of laparoscopic surgery in cholecystectomy and other procedures such as fundoplication, splenectomy and suprarenalectomy are evident. Even so, the progressive implementation of laparoscopy has been relatively slow until its establishment as the technique of choice at many hospitals. It is still in the developmental stage in many places and is not yet accepted as an alternative to traditional surgery in others, despite the results in world literature that demonstrate the advantages of laparoscopy over the conventional approach. In addition, there is clear evidence that the same therapeutic measures are performed as with open surgery when treating these pathologies. Hence, the conceptual acceptance of laparoscopy as a technique of choice is not a problem, except for the need for correct training.

However, laparoscopic repair of ventral hernias is different. Performance of the technique does not mean simply taking the same steps as with open surgery, as in the pathologies mentioned. Some principles that are basic for many surgeons must change from the very start in relation to repair of ventral hernias: we do not perform anatomic repair, such as approximation of the anterior rectus muscles in midline repairs, we do not resect the sac, and we place a mesh (i.e., a foreign material) in contact with the bowel. For these reasons, the future acceptance of laparoscopic treatment for ventral hernias requires showing the scientific community that breaking with the conventional basic principles of ventral hernia repair can be associated with good functional results for the patient, an acceptable recurrence rate and no complications related to the prosthetic materials.

The advantages of laparoscopy in ventral hernia repair are evident, and the series published to date show that abdominal wall functionality is retained and that wound-and mesh-related complications are decreased. Moreover, there are no reported complications from intraperitoneal placement of prosthetic materials in contact with the bowel. This results in greater patient comfort and faster recovery, accompanied by a significantly lower recurrence rate than after open surgery.

ESTABLISHING THE INDICATIONS

Nevertheless, there are doubts and problems associated with this type of repair. The development of this technique has been carried out in practically a self-taught manner by the different surgical teams. We feel that now is the moment to reconsider, to analyze what has been done up to now and to establish which patients will actually benefit from this surgical technique, i.e., to clearly establish the indications. Based on our experience, we have sufficient evidence to state that the ideal cases for laparoscopic repair are patients with hernias more than 3-4 centimeters and less than 8-10 centimeters in diameter, with a small-to-medium size sac at least 4 cm from the costal plane, the xiphoids or the pubis, and preferably supraumbilical. These cases include small to medium-size hernias in which wall functionality is maintained regardless of any approximation of the muscles, there are no major problems associated with possible seromas forming in the sac (since they will be minimal), and no difficulty in adequately covering the hernia defect and ensuring proper attachment of the prosthesis. In these cases, obese patients will benefit the most.

The indications for this approach to ventral hernia repair must be more clearly defined in the future: 1) it must be determined whether the repair of large hernias (particularly those greater than 15 centimeters), in which wall functionality is affected, can be properly treated with this approach; 2) it should be established whether laparoscopic repair of hernias with a prominent sac is advisable, because of implications from the cosmetic standpoint and from the standpoint of handling possible seromas forming in such large spaces; and 3) correct technical management must be defined as it relates to proper mesh attachment in hernias near bone structures, as occurs in suprapubic, subcostal or subxiphoid hernias.

IMPROVEMENTS IN THE SURGICAL TECHNIQUE AND MATERIAL

The surgical technique should also be analyzed, although the most widely accepted trend is toward intraperitoneal mesh placement. The use of external sutures or exclusive placement of tacks, as in the *"double crown"* technique, is a point of controversy that should be resolved. Long-term results will indicate whether or not placement of transmural suture points is necessary, since short- and medium-term results already show the advantages of using only tacks. Recurrence rates are similar and the problems related to sutures (e.g., postoperative pain, longer surgery time, etc.) are obviated. We believe that the ideal fixation method has still not been developed. Problems associated with tack placement can also occur and have been reported in both clinical and experimental studies, particularly in terms of potential adhesions created by the tacks. The future solution may lie in covering the ends of the sutures with some kind of material that would avoid the development of adhesions, or in creating new attachment systems.

The concept of minimization will also affect ventral hernia repair, as mentioned earlier, and will have repercussions on patient comfort during the postoperative period and improved cosmetic results. We begin by assuming that mesh placement will be required and, therefore, a 10-mm or 12-mm initial trocar must be inserted. The size of the other trocars can be reduced to 3-mm, depending on the needs of the attachment system.

SEARCH FOR THE IDEAL PROSTHETIC MATERIAL

There are actually several very good prosthetic materials that can be placed inside the abdominal cavity in contact with the bowel. These are quite safe and problems related to intraperitoneal placement are not anticipated; however, the ideal material has yet to be found. Both e-PTFE mesh (particularly the corduroy dual-mesh plus variant) and composite materials have excellent properties for use in laparoscopic procedures and implantation inside the cavity, though the ideal material still does not exist. In the future, basic research --regarding the development of new materials-- and technical research --based on improving existing materials-- should offer prostheses that are even easier to be managed laparoscopically and even safer for intraperitoneal use.

General speaking, the existing mesh materials have a series of drawbacks: 1) Adhesions have been reported at the margins of the mesh, making it necessary to ensure perfect mesh extension to fully integrate the edges to the abdominal wall. Materials that are specially treated at this level should be developed in the future; 2) There are disadvantages of the management of the mesh itself inside the cavity, particularly the pure e-PTFE mesh which does not have like the polypropylene memory. This material is more difficult to manage, making it necessary to develop systems for "automatic extension" of the mesh inside the cavity to facilitate its management; 3) In composite materials, there is some fear that disappearance of the absorbable coating (in composite materials with polypropylene and absorbable substances) or deterioration of the fine layer of e-PTFE due to its management (in prostheses combining this material with polypropylene) could mean that the material will come into contact with the bowel, with the resulting associated dangers of fistula formation, occlusion, etc. The decrease in adhesions associated with using e-PTFE as a prosthetic material does not mean that they will not appear. Hence, it is necessary to improve the material, develop other, new materials or use temporary covering substances in order to prevent adhesions during the mesh integration period. We are now conducting studies along this line in our experimental operating room.

OBJECTIVE OF TRAINING IN THE FUTURE: ELIMINATE THE LEARNING CURVE

Our first task is to present the results and learn from our years of developing this technique so that the learning curve existing in all series disappears entirely in those surgical teams just starting to use the laparoscopic approach. We have learned a great deal from our experience: we know how to perform proper adhesiolysis, how to manage the mesh and suture materials, and how to perform mesh placement. We have gradually added a number of small technical tricks and details to promote the development of the technique and avoid the difficulties we found at the beginning. Like other surgical teams, we have reached the point where we should make our initial faults known to prevent them from being repeated. We must establish training courses and teach what we know, in order to eliminate the learning curve. At present there are enough experienced teams around the world to train and advise the groups that want to start performing laparoscopic repair of ventral hernias using all the technological advances that are available.